# Pharmacologic Analysis of Drug-Receptor Interaction

*Second Edition*

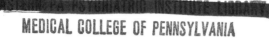
# Pharmacologic Analysis of Drug-Receptor Interaction

*Second Edition*

**Terry Kenakin, PH.D.**

*Department of Cellular Biochemistry*
*Glaxo Research Institute*
*Glaxo, Inc.*
*Research Triangle Park, North Carolina*

Raven 🦢 New York

ress, Ltd., 1185 Avenue of the Americas, New York, New York 10036

© 1993 by Raven Press, Ltd. All rights reserved. This book is protected
by copyright. No part of it may be reproduced, stored in a retrieval system, or
transmitted, in any form or by any means, electronic, mechanical,
photocopying or recording, or otherwise, without the prior written permission
of the publisher.

Made in the United States of America

**Library of Congress Cataloging-in-Publication Data**

Kenakin, Terrence P.
    Pharmacologic analysis of drug-receptor interaction / Terry
Kenakin. — 2nd ed.
        p.   cm.
    Includes bibliographical references and index.
    ISBN 0-7817-0065-5
    1. Drug receptors.   I.  Title.
    [DNLM:   1.  Receptors, Drug.   2.  Drug Interactions.
3. Pharmacology.   QV 38 K33p 1993]
RM301.41.K45   1993
615'.7—dc20                                              93-20235
                                                             CIP

The material contained in this volume was submitted as previously
unpublished material, except in the instances in which credit has been given to
the source from which some of the illustrative material was derived.
    Great care has been taken to maintain the accuracy of the information
contained in the volume. However, neither Raven Press nor the author can
be held responsible for errors or for any consequences arising from the use of
the information contained herein.

9 8 7 6 5 4 3 2 1

*To my wife Debbie*
*for what went before*
*and for what is to come*

# Contents

# Preface to First Edition

The receptor can be considered a crossroads where a vast array of hormones, autacoids, neurotransmitters, drugs, and other foreign substances meet the cell and transmit their messages to another vast array of stimulus-response mechanisms. In this sense, the study of drug-receptor interactions touches all aspects of pharmacology, and a great many aspects of biochemistry and physiology. Thus, by necessity, the discipline of drug-receptor kinetics enters the lives of scientists concerned with a variety of biological mechanisms, forcing them to go into the realm of kinetic processes in diffusion-restricted systems observed in an indirect manner.

This volume considers the pharmacologic analysis of the interactions of drugs and drug receptors as a problem of classification, the ultimate aim of which is to define the properties of drugs on biological systems. In the process, this same exercise is capable of classifying physiological processes as well. Unlike many treatises on drug-receptor pharmacology, little emphasis is placed on the structure of the receptor, the definition of its nature being subordinate to its function as a looking glass into the properties of drugs and physiological mechanisms.

For the pharmacologist, the techniques for study of drug-receptor interaction are major tools in the quest for new drugs of therapeutic benefit. Definition of the properties of drugs is an essential part of this process, and from this standpoint, every newly discovered selective drug *begins* the pharmacologist's primary task of classification. Thus, the discovery of the drug becomes both the endpoint (delivery of a therapeutic entity for the benefit of humans) and the starting point (defining what makes it a benefit to humans) for pharmacologic research. It will be axiomatic that this latter process is essential to the former.

TERRY KENAKIN

# Preface

The first edition of this book concentrated primarily on the classification of drugs and drug receptors in functional systems. Over the intervening years the face of pharmacology has changed immensely, and now the systems available to study drugs and drug responses can be customized and, in some cases, even created. The state of the art of pharmacology as a discipline owes much to this new technology. Perhaps because we sometimes fail to fathom the complexities of chemical perturbation of cellular function, drug selectivity can be a mystery, and one interim way to classify selective drugs is to pass the mysterious property on to the cellular recognition site, i.e., the receptor. This edition discusses the procedures available to determine whether selectivity is a function of the receptor or a result of the collective properties in the drug, receptor, and tissue host.

At present, cells can be made to express drug-receptor proteins at will, with the apparent promise of systems in which drug activity can be quantified without complication. The true import of the findings in such systems remains to be seen and may, in fact, depend on the verisimilitude of the surrogate systems to those operative in humans. The verdict on how well the new technology will ease the process of drug design for therapeutic benefit in humans lies in the accuracy of the quantification of drug effect. This edition also concerns the criteria by which drug selectivity can be ascribed to receptor selectivity and the robustness of the resulting classifications in the therapeutic arena. It has relevance to pharmacologists, physiologists, and cell biologists interested in the strengths and limitations of drugs as chemical scalpels used to dissect biological systems.

TERRY KENAKIN

# Acknowledgments

I wish to thank Sir James Black, for guidance in critical analyses, and Paul Morgan and Mike Lutz, for invaluable assistance in theoretical modeling and calculation. The second edition of this book was made possible by the support of the Glaxo Research Institute to whom I am grateful.

# 1

# Drug-Receptor Theory

*That combining group of the protoplasmic molecule to which the introduced group is anchored will hereafter be termed receptor.*

—PAUL EHRLICH, 1909

## DEFINITION OF THE "KEY"

When a medicinal chemist synthesizes a compound that does something extraordinary to a physiological system, this compound enters an elite class of chemicals and becomes classified as a drug. Let us suppose that this drug has one and only one property in its interactions with all physiological systems and thus possesses the property of specificity. Under these circumstances it can be used to perturb a variety of physiological and biological systems, and by observing the way these systems accommodate the perturbations, we can gain physiological knowledge. In short, the drug becomes a "key." It will be one premise of this book that the obvious value of such keys can lead to tacit assumptions of specificity and that the challenge of these assumptions is a critical function of pharmacologists.

Experience demonstrates that drugs more often are selective rather than specific, in that a specific activity is incontrovertibly linked to a concentration range (therapeutic window). Therefore, a drug is useful therapeutically if the dosage is kept within the range in which only the desired property is expressed. If this range is exceeded, other properties of the drug may complicate the therapy; as stated by Walter Straub (1874–1944), "there is only a quantitative difference between a drug and a poison." A drug discovered to possess one property, when subjected to scrutiny, often is found to have another. For instance, cocaine is known mainly as a central nervous system stimulant and local anesthetic, but it also is a potent inhibitor of the uptake of catecholamines by nerves. Hydrocortisone is a well-known anti-inflammatory drug, but it also blocks the ability of muscle to take up and degrade catecholamines. *It is the major thesis of this book that pharmacologists should be concerned primarily with the discovery of and quantification of*

*1*

*the properties of drugs, not the physiological systems with which they inter-
act*—in essence, the definition of the key. This is not a new idea. It was
proposed more than a century ago by the German pharmacologist Rudolf
Buchheim (1820–1879) in his statement that "we pharmacologists must ac-
quire a knowledge of the tools which we use" (4). Not only pharmacologists
should be concerned with the classification of drugs, but also every biological
scientist who uses drugs to delineate physiological mechanisms.

There are at least three reasons that pharmacology should be concerned
with the definition of the key. First, if specificity is erroneously assumed for
a given drug, then all subsequent classifications utilizing this drug are in
danger of being irrelevant. Considering the numbers of drugs, receptors,
tissues, and species, this could lead to an enormous amount of contradictory
data. For example, suppose a new drug is classified as being a stimulant of
a particular cellular mechanism on the basis of limited data and then is shown
to produce a stimulant response in an organ previously thought, on the basis
of other data, not to possess that particular mechanism. An interesting di-
lemma presents itself: Does one reclassify the drug or reclassify the organ?
If an error is made at this point, a second dissimilitude occurs, because all
subsequent classifications using either the misclassified drug or organ will be
incorrect as well.

The third reason for questioning specificity is the possible therapeutic
benefit of the process. Let us assume that a drug has been discovered that
produces a specific action *in vivo* and that current classifications of the
known receptors cannot explain the specificity attained. One point of view
assumes that the drug is a key that has unlocked another secret of physiology;
it has led to the discovery of a new receptor. Considering the limited numbers
of hormones, autacoids, and neurotransmitters that cells have to deal with,
a parsimonious view of membrane receptors would discourage such specula-
tion unless it is inescapable. In the process of defining possible receptor
heterogeneity, exploration of other possible properties of the drug that could
be responsible for the selectivity would be warranted. Thus, an alternative
point of view would seek to explain the selective effect of the drug in terms
of a more commonly encountered phenomenon, namely, multiple drug properties. In this setting, the selectivity would result from the drug acting on
two or more biological mechanisms that interact in the host (whether this be
cell, tissue, or whole body) in a complex manner. The definition of such
selectivity theoretically could suggest new and better ways to attain selectivity, because delineation of the various processes would suggest to the synthetic organic chemist new structures for future molecular design. If a drug
is selective because it interacts with a newly discovered cellular process, the
chemist has a limited data base on which to design analogues of the drug,
namely, those structures synthesized en route to the drug. If, on the other
hand, the selectivity of the drug is found to result from interaction of the
drug with two already known cellular processes, then all other chemical

structures known to interact with these cellular processes become relevant to the drug design process.

## DRUG NOMENCLATURE

The label attached to a drug often determines how it is used, and some guidelines to drug nomenclature should be noted before discussion of the properties of drugs. Some ambiguities involved in the utilization of drugs as tools arise from their sometimes protean nature, a property that often can be controlled by limiting the concentration, because it becomes evident when selectivity windows are exceeded. In general, a drug is known for and used for its most prominent property, although it may have other properties. This necessitates a procrustean approach to the attainment of pharmacologic specificity. Like the giant Procrustes in Greek mythology, who made his hapless victims lie on a bed and either stretched or truncated them until they fit the bed,[1] pharmacologists often find themselves truncating the concentration ranges of their drugs in order to achieve some measure of specificity. For example, yohimbine can be thought of as a competitive antagonist of $\alpha_2$-adrenoceptors, $\alpha_1$-adrenoceptors, serotonin receptors, and acetylcholinesterase, as well as a local anesthetic (Fig. 1.1A). An even more extreme case of multiple personality is exhibited by amitriptyline, which boasts no fewer than six prominent properties (Fig. 1.1B). However, by using yohimbine within a concentration range of 6 to 60 nM and amitriptyline between 8 and 60 nM, selective $\alpha_2$-adrenoceptor blockade and histamine H-1 receptor blockade, respectively, can be achieved. Thus, a window of selectivity is obtained by judicious restriction of concentration. An example of how the nature of a drug can change when these windows are exceeded is provided by clonidine, which at concentrations below 30 nM selectively depresses electrically stimulated twitch contraction of the rat anococcygeus muscle (Fig. 1.2). When 30 nM clonidine is added to the organ bath, the selectivity window for this property is exceeded, and postsynaptic stimulation, resulting in a powerful tissue contraction, is observed. In general, the concentration of a drug at which a particular activity is observed is critical to characterization of the event, and selective labels must always be qualified by quantitative limits.

Perhaps nowhere is the protean nature of drugs better revealed than in the variations seen in drug stimulant activities. By definition, a drug that produces stimulation is labeled an agonist, whereas that which blocks the effects of an agonist is an antagonist. The tissue producing the response determines the observed maximal response, and the powerful drugs that produce the same maximal responses in any given tissue are termed full agonists, i.e., they produce the maximal tissue response. Those drugs that produce a re-

---

[1] Good for Procrustes, until Theseus did the same to him.

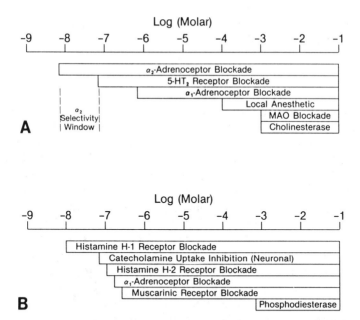

**FIG. 1.1.** The necessity for a procrustean approach to specificity. **A:** Yohimbine concentration ranges (on a logarithmic molar scale) necessary for activity for a series of autonomic receptors and functions. **B:** Similar data for amitriptyline.

sponse that is less than the tissue maximum are termed partial agonists. Thus, a hazardous nomenclature results that is based on biological tissues with all their variances. Clearly, a sensitive tissue may show a drug to be a full agonist, whereas in a less sensitive tissue the same drug may be a partial agonist. Conceivably, in a rather insensitive tissue, the drug can produce no

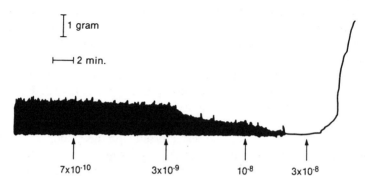

**FIG. 1.2.** Effects of clonidine on electrically stimulated isometric twitch in rat anococcygeus muscle. Concentrations between 0.7 and 10 nM depress twitch by $\alpha_2$-adrenoceptor-mediated inhibition of neurotransmission. At a concentration of 30 nM, clonidine produces a sustained contraction by $\alpha_1$-adrenoceptor activation. (From ref. 19.)

response at all and be an antagonist. For example, prenalterol can be shown to be nearly a full agonist in thyroxine-treated guinea pig right atria, a weak partial agonist in cat papillary muscle, and a pure competitive antagonist in canine coronary artery (Fig. 1.3). Tissues are amplifiers of the effects of drugs and can vary dramatically in their threshold and maximal limits of amplification. To discuss this point further requires definition of the two fundamental properties of drugs: affinity and intrinsic efficacy. The affinity of a drug is the tenacity with which it binds to its biological receptor on the cell membrane. Clark (5), in his classic treatment of drug-receptor theory, discussed affinity as the ability of drugs to be "fixed" to cells. In statistical terms, the affinity is the probability of a drug molecule binding to a free drug receptor at any given instant. The intrinsic efficacy of a drug is that inherent property that imparts the biological signal to the drug receptor (and thus to the cell) to result in a biological response. Intrinsic efficacy is a property of the drug, not the tissue, and is a very important parameter in the classification of drugs and drug receptors (*vide infra*). Thus, the affinity gets the drug to the receptor, and the intrinsic efficacy determines what it does when it gets there. The pharmacologist observes what the tissue does with the signal; it can greatly amplify it to yield a response, or it may deem the signal too weak to bother about and not give a response.

The production of a biological response by a drug can be thought of as the addition of a weight to one side of a lever balance. The weight is the intrinsic efficacy of the drug, an inviolate property. As the weight is added to the lever, the opposite end is displaced in proportion to the weight (Fig. 1.4). Where, along the lever, we view this process determines what displacement we observe. If we equate the magnitude of displacement with maximal response, the different vantage points along the lever represent different tissues. Thus, referring to Fig. 1.4, tissue I would demonstrate very little response for the drug, tissue II would show the drug to be a partial agonist, and tissue III a full agonist. Considering the multitude of tissues and variations in intrinsic efficacies of drugs, it can be seen that the designations full agonist,

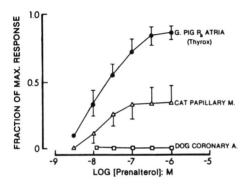

FIG. 1.3. Concentration-response curves in isolated tissues for prenalterol. Ordinate: Responses as fractions of maximal responses to the full agonist isoproterenol. Abscissa: Logarithms of molar concentrations of prenalterol. Responses of right atria from thyroxine-pretreated guinea pigs [($\bullet$)$N = 4$], cat left atria ($N = 6$), and canine coronary [($\bullet$)$N = 4$]. Bars represent SEM. (Adapted from refs. 16 and 17.)

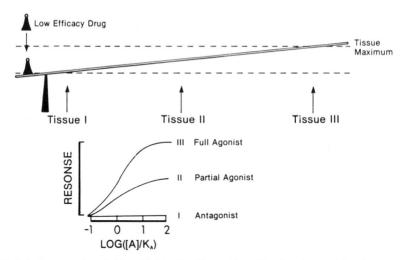

**FIG. 1.4.** An operational view of intrinsic efficacy. **Top:** The drug is considered a mass with a given weight corresponding to its intrinsic efficacy. The tissue response is considered to be displacement of the lever as a result of placement of the weight to the left of the fulcrum. The downward displacement can be thought of as the stimulus, with the upward displacement the amplified maximal response. Where along the lever this process is viewed determines the amplification factor; these vantage points correspond to different tissues. **Bottom:** The predicted dose-response curves to the drug in tissues I, II, and III, these corresponding to the labeled vantage points.

partial agonist, and antagonist may sometimes be ambiguous. In practice, most drugs have intrinsic efficacies that either greatly exceed tissue limits (thus uniformly are full agonists) or are well below tissue thresholds (antagonists). Therefore, ambiguities arise only with drugs of intermediate intrinsic efficacies (partial agonists).

In summary, it would seem to be prudent to interpret drug labels in terms of the nature of the drug activity and extent of selectivity (or claimed specificity) with some latitude, keeping in mind the dependence of these factors on the nature of the test system and the concentration of the drug.

## DRUG RECEPTORS

The definition of a drug as any chemical that perturbs a biological system suggests a broad category of substances. Thus, drugs can produce effects by virtue of their acidic or basic properties (antacids, protamine), surfactant properties (amphotericin), ability to denature proteins (astringents), osmotic properties (laxatives, diuretics), and physicochemical interactions with membrane lipids (general and local anesthetics). However, a vast array of hormones, autacoids, toxins, neurotransmitters, and drugs can transfer information to cells by interaction with specific membrane proteins given the general name receptors. The concept of specific sites residing on cell membranes with cognitive and transitive properties for drugs emerged at the turn of the century as a result of studies by Ehrlich (1854–1915), through his experiments with tissue stains, snake venoms, and bacterial toxins, and Langley (1852–1926), who studied the effects of pilocarpine and atropine on salivary secretion.

There are certain extraordinary properties of drug actions that invite, if not compel, the postulate of a specific receptor on a cell membrane capable of binding drugs and serving also as a transducer for biological stimuli. First, many drug responses are obtained at very low concentrations. Calculations from studies of atropine binding to guinea pig ileum suggest that only 0.02% of the cell surface is composed of specific receptors for acetylcholine. Thus, if a muscle cell were compared to a sphere the size of the earth, an area the size of Iceland would contain the complete acetylcholine-receptor population. Clark (1885–1941) calculated that the area on a frog heart cell covered by a concentration of acetylcholine sufficient to reduce heart rate by 50% would be 0.001%, or an area the size of the Caribbean island of Jamaica if the heart cell were the size of the heart. Such extraordinary potencies suggest specific receptors linked to amplification processes. Second, responses to drugs can be very selectively blocked by other drugs of specific chemical structures. For example, the antihistaminic drug mepyramine blocks isolated tissue responses to histamine at concentrations of 0.4 nM, whereas concentrations 30,000 times higher (12 μM) are required to block the effects of acetylcholine. Third, the selectivities of drugs as stimulants and antagonists are extremely dependent on chemical structures, and very small changes in the structures of drugs can lead to profound changes in pharmacologic activities. Thus, extension of the methylene side chain of alkyltrimethylammonium salts by one methylene bridge (*n*-propyl to *n*-butyl) changes the potency for stimulation of guinea pig ileum by a factor of 145 (Fig. 1.5A). Addition of a single chlorine atom to pheniramine produces a 10-fold enhancement of potency for antihistaminic activity (Fig. 1.5B). The dependence of activity on structure impressed Clark, who wrote that "the most interesting feature of drug action is the extraordinary specificity of action of drugs and the manner in which slight changes in chemical constitution alter their action." These data, and much recent biochemical data, have led to important operational concepts concerning the receptor, a protein usually embedded in the plasma membrane that serves to recognize drugs and transmit their information to the cell.

In general the membrane-bound receptors currently known can be divided by structural, biochemical, and functional data into families (see Fig. 1.6). One such family consists of G protein–linked receptors, which contain seven membrane-spanning regions (as deduced from hydropathicity data) joining extracellular and intracellular loops of amino acids. These receptors transmit information to the cell by binding to membrane-bound coupling proteins that,

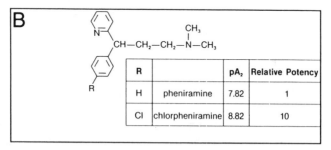

| A | | Relative Potency |
|---|---|---|
| n-propyl TMA | CH₃—CH₂—CH₂—N⊕—CH₃ (CH₃, CH₃) | 1 |
| n-butyl TMA | CH₃—CH₂—CH₂—CH₂—N⊕—CH₃ (CH₃, CH₃) | 145 |

| B | R | | pA₂ | Relative Potency |
|---|---|---|---|---|
| | H | pheniramine | 7.82 | 1 |
| | Cl | chlorpheniramine | 8.82 | 10 |

**FIG. 1.5.** Dependence of drug potency on chemical structure. **A:** Addition of one methylene bridge to *n*-propyltrimethylammonium (to form *n*-butyltrimethylammonium) increases the potency by a factor of 145. Shown are the concentrations producing 50% maximal response in guinea pig ileum. (Data from ref. 25.) **B:** Addition of a single chlorine atom on the pararing position of pheniramine increases antihistaminic potency by a factor of 10. Shown are the $pA_2$ values minus logarithms of the molar concentrations of antagonist producing a twofold shift to the right in a concentration-response curve to histamine in guinea pig ileum. (Data from ref. 23.)

when activated by agonist-receptor complexes, initiate biochemical cellular processes. These coupling proteins utilize guanine nucleotides and thus are called G proteins. Many receptors for neurotransmitters (i.e., α-adrenoceptors and β-adrenoceptors for catecholamines) and hormones are G protein–linked receptors. Another class of receptor are multisubunit proteins that contain ion channels and thus transmit ions from the extracellular space into the cytosol. For example, nicotinic receptors for acetylcholine allow passage of more than $10^6$ sodium ions per second into the cell when activated by cholinergic agonists. Another family of receptor contains enzymatic activity. Insulin, endothelial growth factor, and platelet-derived growth factor are among the substances that utilize receptors linked to tyrosine kinase activity. Yet another group of receptors have membrane-bound guanylate-cyclase enzymatic activity (i.e., atrial natriuretic factor).

The common properties of all of these receptors are the two that are essential for receptors, namely, that of *recognition* of extracellular substances and *transduction* of information of those substances to the intracellular machinery.

There is a substantial branch of pharmacology dedicated to studying the structures and functions of these most important proteins with techniques employing affinity labels, biochemical binding, and reconstitution biochemistry. These studies undoubtedly will furnish valuable data for an understanding of pharmacologic effects and further design of drugs. This monograph will consider drug receptors strictly operationally. In this sense, receptors will be considered somewhat like "black boxes," yielding quantal (but uniform) units of stimuli to biological apparatus in response to drugs that can be quantified. However, it will be seen from subsequent discussion that complete ignorance of the nature of these black boxes is obstructive to the classification of drugs, and consideration of drug binding sites and transducer function, which necessitates discussion of the nature of receptors, sometimes is required.

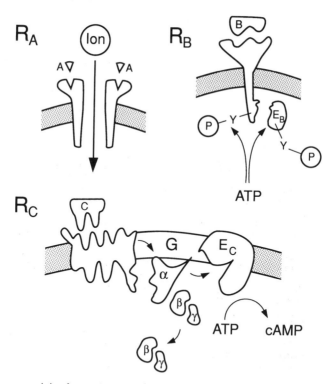

**FIG. 1.6.** Three models of receptor types in cell membranes. $R_A$ is an ion channel modulating ion flux. $R_B$ is a ligand-related transmembrane enzyme. For example, this figure depicts tyrosine kinase activity in which the receptor becomes autophosphorylated in the process of phosphorylating a target substrate. $R_C$ is a receptor that interacts with membrane-bound transducer protein. Depicted is the interaction with an oligomeric G protein leading to the dissociation of the G protein into $\alpha$ and $\beta\gamma$ subunits. The $\alpha$ subunit goes on to regulate the enzyme adenylate cyclase. (From ref. 13.)

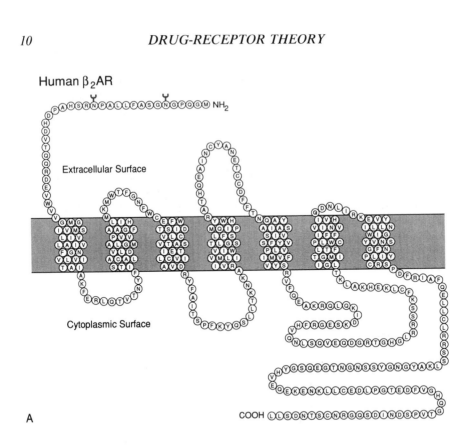

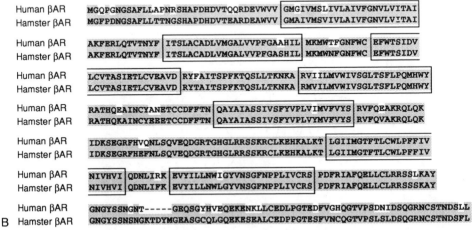

**FIG. 1.7.** Homology of β-adrenoceptors from human and hamster tissue. **A:** Structure of the human β2-adrenoceptor (β2AR) as determined by hydropathicity experiments. Amino acids (*open circles*) show correspondence to those found in hamster β2-adrenoceptors; *filled circles* represent differences in amino acids between the two receptors. (From ref. 7.) **B:** Amino acid sequences of the human and hamster β2-adrenoceptors (βAR). *Shaded areas* show homology and *boxed areas* the transmembrane-spanning regions of the receptors. (Data from ref. 7.)

Considering drug receptors as operational black boxes raises a fundamental question for pharmacologic analysis of drugs as it can be applied to the design of human therapeutic agents, namely, are the black boxes studied by experimental pharmacologists the same black boxes that clinicians deal with in the treatment of disease?

In this regard, pharmacologists appear to have been fortunate in the apparent uniformity of drug properties across animal species and in humans. Figure 1.7A shows the amino acid sequence and tertiary conformation in the membrane of a human $\beta_2$-adrenoceptor. The amino acids shown in open circles denote identity with those in the $\beta_2$-adrenoceptor from the hamster. This 88% sequence homology is shown more clearly in Fig. 1.7B. The differences appear to be of minor consequence to the pharmacologic profile of these two receptors.

The correspondence between some drug receptors in a wide variety of animals and humans, as measured by interactions with selective drugs, can be documented (Table 1.1). In fact, this correspondence forms the basis of experimental pharmacology as it is applied to the drug discovery process.

**TABLE 1.1.** *Equilibrium dissociation constants for drug-receptor complexes in animals and humans* in vitro

| | β-Blockers[a] | | | |
|---|---|---|---|---|
| | Atria | | Bronchi | |
| Drug | Guinea pig | Human | Guinea pig | Human |
|---|---|---|---|---|
| Propranolol | 8.5 | 8.36 | 8.25 | 8.56 |
| Pindolol | 8.67 | 8.8 | 8.83 | 8.64 |
| RO 3-4787 | 8.39 | 8.3 | 7.95 | 8.36 |
| Practolol | 6.5 | 6.44 | 4.87 | 4.65 |
| Atenolol | 7.21 | 6.95 | 5.57 | 5.33 |
| Acebutolol | 6.54 | 6.76 | 5.13 | 5.06 |
| Metoprolol | 7.43 | 7.44 | 6.06 | 6.35 |
| H87/07 | 6.66 | 6.45 | 4.98 | 5.01 |
| Tolamolol | 8.37 | 7.91 | 7.16 | 7.02 |

| | β- and α-Blockers | | |
|---|---|---|---|
| Location | Propranolol | Phentolamine | Bupranolol |
|---|---|---|---|
| Human | | | |
| Left atrium | 8.36[b] | | |
| Bronchus | 8.4 | | |
| Papillary muscle | | | 8.96 |
| Metacarpal artery | | 7.8 | |

*(Continued)*

**TABLE 1.1.** *Continued.*

β- and α-Blockers

| Location | Propranolol | Phentolamine | Bupranolol |
|---|---|---|---|
| Guinea pig | | | |
|   Left atrium | 8.5 | | |
|   Right atrium | 8.35 | | |
|   Trachea | 8.25 | 7.9 | |
|   Vas deferens | 8.9 | | |
|   Esophagus | 8.3 | | |
|   Ileum | 8.7 | | |
|   Aorta | | 8.0 | |
| Rat | | | |
|   Left atrium | | | 8.9 |
|   Aorta | | 8.0 | |
|   Jugular vein | 8.7 | | |
|   Vas deferens | | 8.2 | |
|   Uterus | 8.5 | | |
| Cat | | | |
|   Papillary muscle | 8.7 | | 9.0 |
|   Right atrium | 8.5 | | |
|   Aorta | | 8.0 | |
|   Nictitating muscle | | 7.5 | |
|   Uterus | 8.8 | | |
|   Ventricle | | | 9.1 |
| Rabbit | | | |
|   Aorta | 8.9 | 8.0 | |
|   Stomach | | 8.0 | |
|   Left atrium | 8.4 | | |
|   Duodenum | | 8.1 | |
|   Ileum | 8.7 | | |
| Mouse | | | |
|   Uterus | 8.4 | | |
|   Vas deferens | | 8.3 | |
|   Spleen | | 8.2 | |
| Pig | | | |
|   Coronary artery | 8.4 | | |
| Cow | | | |
|   Trachea | 8.2 | | |

[a] From ref. 12.
[b] Data as $-\log K_{equilibrium}$.

Clearly, a dogmatic belief in the homogeneity of the receptors used to classify drugs can be obstructive to the classification process. However, the fact that new receptor subtypes are discovered only after the discovery of new selective drugs raises the specter of circular reasoning; this will be dealt with more fully in Chapter 11. The general approach to be taken here is that before a new receptor can be convincingly defined, evidence must be presented to *disprove* the null hypothesis that the receptor in question is a sample of a homogeneous population.

It is hoped that it will be apparent that the strictly operational view of receptors used in drug-receptor theory is satisfactory for the pharmacologic purpose of quantifying the elemental properties of drugs, namely, the ability to bind to cells and initiate or block a response. The simple kinetic models that describe these processes on a molecular level provide the basis for what is generally referred to as drug-receptor theory.

## DRUG-RECEPTOR THEORIES

Numerous mathematical, thermodynamic, and biochemical models have been put forth to describe the interactions of drugs with drug receptors. The preeminent theory from the point of view of attempting to describe drug-receptor interaction has been *occupation theory*, in which a response is thought to emanate from a receptor only when it is occupied by an appropriate drug molecule. This model was the first proposed and its historical development traces the essential elements of drug-receptor interactions. A model of drug-receptor interaction that has gained eminence over the past few years is the *operational model*. This model has theoretical and practical advantages over standard occupation theory and describes agonism as a series of hyperbolic functions. The techniques used to quantify drug activity in pharmacologic terms in this book are described both in terms of occupation theory and the operational model.

Another model, termed *rate theory*, equates drug-receptor activation with the kinetic rate of offset of drugs and describes activation in terms of kinetics rather than binding. A model termed the *inactivation model* mathematically bridges these two approaches and warrants discussion. Although protein allosterism, that property that views proteins as malleable structures with a spectrum of conformations, as opposed to rigid matrices, is not precluded with the foregoing models, cooperative protein effects are not specifically accommodated in the occupation, rate, and inactivation theories, as originally described. Therefore, a discussion of two-state theory as it applies to drug-receptor interaction will be included. It should be noted that the foregoing theoretical models will be considered not as viable candidates for the definitive description of the black box that is the receptor, but only as kinetic representations of the characteristic properties of drugs as measured in physiological systems. The nature of the characteristic drug constants is secondary to quantity, because this latter property has predictive value in a variety of biological systems.

In the following description of drug-receptor theory, frequent references are made to other chapters for more detailed analysis. The mathematical representations of drug-receptor interactions in the following pages are useful tools for classifying drugs and receptors, but they are based on a number of assumptions. It is hoped that discussions of these assumptions in later chapters will furnish the reader with a realistic measure of the level of confidence with which to ascribe experimentally derived parameters to theoretical constants.

## Occupation Theory

The evolution of occupation theory can be described by the historical development of the models proposed to explain the activation of a tissue by a drug. The first step in the process concerns the binding of the drug $A$ to the drug receptor $R$. It should be noted that the equations to follow assume that the concentration of drug in the receptor compartment (region immediately surrounding the receptors) rises instantaneously to the equilibrium concentration. It will be seen in subsequent chapters that failure of pharmacologic systems to adhere to this ideal situation is a major obstruction to quantitative classification of drug-receptor interactions. The consequences of failure to achieve receptor-compartment concentrations of drug instantaneously are most serious when studying the kinetics of drug-receptor interaction (Chapter 13), although steady-state analyses also are affected; concentration-time relationships are dealt with also in Chapter 4. Assuming that a concentration of drug $A$ is in the receptor compartment such that free diffusion controls access to the receptor $R$, the binding of $A$ to the receptor can be described by the equation

$$[A] + [R] \underset{k_2}{\overset{k_1}{\rightleftharpoons}} [A \cdot R]$$

where $k_1$ and $k_2$ are the association and dissociation rate constants, respectively, $[A \cdot R]$ is the concentration of drug-receptor complex, and $[R]$ is the concentration of free unbound receptor. The rate of change of drug-receptor complex $(\partial[A \cdot R]/\partial t)$ is

$$\partial[A \cdot R]/\partial t = k_1[A] \cdot [R] - k_2[A \cdot R] \tag{1.1}$$

and at equilibrium, $\partial[A \cdot R]/\partial t = 0$; thus,

$$k_1[A] \cdot [R] = k_2[A \cdot R] \tag{1.2}$$

It should be noted that the subsequent derivation makes the assumption that the concentration of drug $[A]$ is unaffected by receptor binding, i.e., the concentration of drug far exceeds the "concentration" of receptors. The consequence of failure to conform to this condition is dealt with in Chapter 7. Letting $[R_t]$, the total concentration of receptors, equal $[R] + [A \cdot R]$,

$$[A] \cdot [R_t] - [A] \cdot [A \cdot R] = (k_2/k_1)[A \cdot R] \tag{1.3}$$

Substituting $K_A = k_2/k_1$ and rearranging,

$$\frac{[A \cdot R]}{[R_t]} = \frac{[A]}{[A] + K_A} \tag{1.4}$$

This is one case of the Langmuir adsorption isotherm describing the adsorbence of substances onto surfaces (i.e., activated charcoal) applied by Clark to describe the binding of small molecules to cell membranes. Although Eq. 1.4 adequately describes drug-receptor binding curves obtained experimentally, it is not the only relationship capable of doing so. As put succinctly by Clark, "The chief disadvantage of Langmuir's formulae is that even the simplest of them provides a curve that can be fitted for considerable stretches by an embarrassingly large number of other formulae." Also, it should be noted that Eq. 1.4 is the special case in which one drug molecule binds to one receptor, more general binding isotherms are not bound by this restriction.

Assuming that the adsorption isotherm is an adequate approximation of the binding of a drug to a population of receptors, Eq. 1.4 shows that the fraction of receptors occupied by drug depends on the drug concentration and the equilibrium dissociation constant of the drug-receptor complex $(K_A)$. This latter parameter corresponds to the concentration of drug that binds to 50% of the available receptor population. Clearly, the lower this concentration (i.e., the smaller is $K_A$), the greater affinity the drug has for the receptor; the affinity is defined as the reciprocal of the equilibrium dissociation constant $(K_{affinity} = K_A^{-1})$. These are chemical terms and reflect the probability of the drug occupying the receptor at any given instant. Thus, a high affinity means a low equilibrium dissociation constant, or $k_1 \gg k_2$, a rate constant for onset (rate of approach of drug to the receptor) much greater than the rate constant for offset (rate of diffusion away from the receptor). The most important aspect of Eq. 1.4 is that it yields a parameter that is dependent on the relative rates of onset and offset of a particular drug for a particular receptor, and thus $K_A$ becomes a drug constant with a unique value for each type of pharmacologic receptor. In this sense, $K_A$ can be used to classify drugs and, as will be seen later, can be useful for predicting drug responses.

The graphic form of Eq. 1.4 and the much more common semilogarithmic graphic form are shown in Fig. 1.8. The experimentally determined concen-

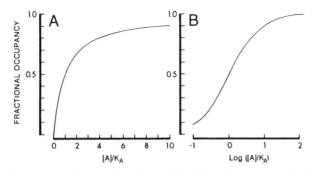

**FIG. 1.8.** The Langmuir adsorption isotherm. **A:** Relationship between fractional receptor occupancy (ordinate) and drug concentration, as a fraction of $K_A$ (abscissa). **B:** Semilogarithmic form of the same curve.

tration of a drug that occupies 50% of the available drug receptors is an important parameter, because it represents $K_A$. The semilogarithmic form of the Langmuir isotherm allows estimation of this quantity much more readily than the representation of $[A \cdot R]/[R_t]$ as a simple function of $[A]$. When the amount of bound ligand can be measured isotopically or gravimetrically (i.e., adsorption of a gas to a metal surface or chemical to activated charcoal), $K_A$ can be determined directly. However, when this binding process is linked to the production of a response that itself is the product of many saturable processes, $K_A$ is not easily determined, and null procedures are required (see Chapter 7).

The Langmuir adsorption isotherm provides a useful model for the binding of drugs to receptors, but at the time of Clark's analysis of drug responses, no adequate quantification of the ability of drugs to produce a response was available. Clark assumed that the response ($E_A$ as a fraction of the maximal response $E_M$) was directly proportional to the number of receptors occupied by drug:

$$\frac{E_A}{E_M} = \frac{[A \cdot R]}{[R_t]} \qquad [1.5]$$

Implicit in this relationship is the fact that complete receptor occupancy is required for maximal response. Although Clark recognized that the response was a result of two processes, the first that of "fixation" (binding) and a second that followed fixation, it was not until Ariëns (1) introduced the concept of intrinsic activity that this latter property was given a name and a quantitative scale.

Ariëns observed that even though tissues were exposed to a number of quarternary nitrogen compounds in concentrations that clearly exceeded the respective $K_A$ values (i.e., the receptors were saturated with the compounds), not all of the drugs produced the maximal response. This observation was not in accord with Eq. 1.5, where it is assumed that maximal receptor occupation yields a maximal response. To accommodate this finding, Ariëns introduced a proportionality factor termed *intrinsic activity* (denoted $\alpha$) and defined the response as

$$\frac{E_A}{E_M} = \frac{\alpha[A \cdot R]}{[R_t]} = \frac{\alpha \cdot [A]}{[A] + K_A} \qquad [1.6]$$

Thus, intrinsic activity was defined as that property of the agonist that produces the "effect per unit of pharmacon-receptor complex." Differences between this definition of $\alpha$, as given by Ariëns, and subsequent common usage of this term are discussed in Chapter 8. The limits of $\alpha$ are $\alpha = 1$ for full agonists, $\alpha = 0$ for antagonists, and $0 < \alpha < 1$ for agonists that are incapable of producing the maximal response even at full receptor occupation. This latter class of drugs Ariëns called "dualists," because they possessed the dual properties of producing responses and antagonizing responses to more powerful agonists. This treatment of drug responses still employed Clark's original assumption that the tissue response was linearly related to receptor occupancy. Therefore, maximal receptor occupancy for full agonists ($\alpha = 1$) was still required for maximal tissue response.

Stephenson, in his modeling of pharmacologic responses, eliminated this assumption with the introduction of a parameter called stimulus ($S$), defined as

$$S = \frac{e \cdot [A \cdot R]}{[R_t]} = \frac{e \cdot [A]}{[A] + K_A} \qquad [1.7]$$

where $e$ is dimensionless proportionality factor denoting the power of a drug to produce a response in a tissue. As can be seen from a comparison of Eqs. 1.6 and 1.7, Stephenson's stimulus is formally identical with response, as defined by Ariëns. The major difference was in the treatment of response; Stephenson assumed response to be some undefined function of stimulus, the only requirements being that it be monotonic and continuous:

$$\frac{E_A}{E_M} = f(S) = f\left[\frac{e \cdot [A]}{[A] + K_A}\right] \qquad [1.8]$$

Introduction of the function $f$ dissociates receptor stimulus and tissue response as directly proportional quantities. This expedient eliminates the necessity for the assumption that a maximal tissue response requires maximal receptor occupation by a drug. In addition to being a more versatile approach to the description of drug responses, this idea was more in accord with experimental evidence indicating that maximal tissue responses could be achieved at submaximal receptor occupancies. The ramifications of and nature of function $f$ in Eq. 1.8 will be dealt with in greater detail in Chapter 2, but it is clear from this model that drugs with different capacities to initiate a response (efficacy $e$) could produce equal responses by occupying different fractions of the receptor population. This is the basis for experimental measurement of relative efficacy and is an important tool in drug-receptor pharmacology (see Chapter 8).

As shown in Fig. 1.9A, changes in efficacy in the Stephenson model produce changes in location parameters and maxima of concentration-response curves. The function $f$ in Eq. 1.8 was taken to be a rectangular hyperbola (Fig. 1.9B), allowing for submaximal receptor occupancies to yield maximal responses. Therefore, changes in $e$ determine the locations of dose-response curves along the concentration axis (potency) as well as maximal responses. This conforms to later experimental results that demonstrate drug potency to be dependent not only on affinity but also on efficacy (see Chapter 8). This model accounted for the varying maxima obtained with a series of alkyl-trimethylammonium compounds in guinea pig ileum (Fig. 1.10A); the experimental data were modeled using experimental estimates of affinity (Fig.

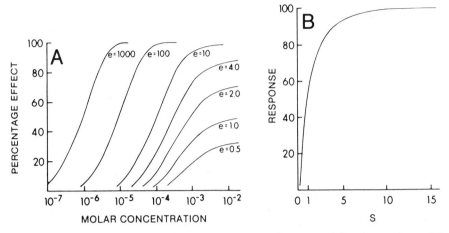

**FIG. 1.9.** Effects of changing efficacy on responses in terms of Stephenson's model. **A:** Dose-response curves to agonists of varying efficacies. Stimulus calculated with Eq. 1.7, and response taken from theoretical calibration curve $[R = S/(S + 1)]$ shown in **B**. (From ref. 25.)

1.10B). It should be noted that only the curve shown in Fig. 1.9B was used to calculate dose and response and to model the experimental data shown in Fig. 1.10A.

This model was revised further by Furchgott, who defined intrinsic efficacy ($\epsilon$) as

$$\epsilon = e/[R_t] \qquad [1.9]$$

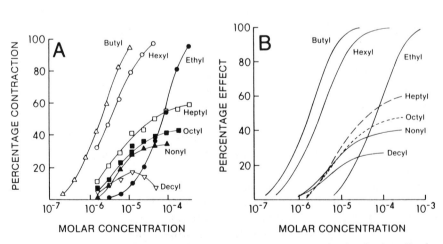

**FIG. 1.10.** Description of agonist response in terms of Stephenson's stimulus hypothesis. **A:** Concentration-response curves for a series of alkyltrimethylammonium compounds as spasmogens in guinea pig ileum. Names on curves refer to lengths of alkyl chains. **B:** Fitting of the data shown in A using experimentally derived $K_A$ values, estimates of efficacy, and the stimulus-response curve. (From ref. 25.)

where $[R_t]$ refers to the tissue concentration of receptors; $\epsilon$ is a quantal unit for the capacity of a drug to initiate a stimulus from one receptor. With this change, stimulus capacity was defined as a strictly drug-related term, whereas Stephenson's efficacy $e$ was a drug- and tissue-related term (i.e., a given drug could have different efficacies in different tissues). Equation 1.8 then is rewritten

$$\text{response} = f\left[\frac{\epsilon \cdot [R_t]}{1 + K_A/[A]}\right] \qquad [1.10]$$

This is the basic definition of a drug-mediated response in terms of occupation theory. There is an essential feature of Eq. 1.10 that is noteworthy: Drug-mediated responses in any given tissue depend on two tissue factors and two factors strictly related to drug-receptor interaction. The tissue factors are $[R_t]$, the density of drug receptors in the tissue, and $f$, the nature, and, more important, the efficiency of the functions converting receptor stimulus into tissue response. The drug-receptor–related parameters are $K_A$, the equilibrium dissociation constant of the drug-receptor complex, and $\epsilon$, the intrinsic efficacy of the drug for the receptor. The importance of these latter two parameters lies in the fact that they are unique for each drug-receptor interaction and do not depend on species, type of tissue, or type of response. Therefore, they can be and are used to classify drugs and drug receptors: accurate measurements of $K_A$ and relative intrinsic efficacies form the basis of receptor pharmacology.

**TABLE 1.2.** *General assumptions in occupation theory*

1. The interaction between a drug and a receptor is bimolecular and readily reversible.
2. A response results from equilibrium or steady-state (pseudo-equilibrium) occupation of receptors. In the presence of a competitive antagonist, there is equilibrium occupation of the receptors by the antagonist.
3. Either a graded response is obtained from each individual cell, or the tissue behaves as a syncytium.
4. A response results from a stimulus that is in turn proportional to the concentration of agonist-receptor complexes.
5. For any given tissue, a stimulus or response is independent of time; thus, the stimulus-response relationship is characteristic of the particular tissue.
6. The concentration of the unbound drug near the receptors can be measured or assumed to be equal to the concentration of unbound drug in the external solution bathing the tissue. Therefore, a negligible amount of drug is taken up by the tissue and receptors.
7. Specific irreversible drugs can inactivate some of the receptors without modifying the stimulus-response relationship.
8. The stimulus to any individual organ is the sum of the total number of agonist-receptor complexes. A maximal stimulus occurs when all of the receptors are occupied.
9. The occupation of one receptor does not affect the tendency of other receptors to be occupied.

Adapted from ref. 22.

Occupation theory provides a convenient model to quantify and predict drug-receptor interactions. The assumptions made to construct this model are important in that they form the frame of reference for the measured parameters; a compilation of these assumptions is shown in Table 1.2.

### The Operational Model of Drug Action

An alternative model of agonism that has theoretical and practical advantages over classical occupation theory in the description of drug action was introduced by Black and Leff (3). Termed the operation model, this approach describes agonism without the artificial proportionality factor, efficacy, required by occupation theory. Moreover, the parameter used to quantify agonism has a chemical definition and thus theoretically is experimentally accessible. The model originates with the experimental observation that most agonist dose-response curves are hyperbolic in nature. Therefore, if the agonist binding to the receptor is governed by mass action, then the function relating the quantity of agonist-receptor complex and drug response must either be linear or hyperbolic in nature as well. Specifically, let the response $E_a$ be a hyperbolic function of agonist concentration $[A]$:

$$E_a = \frac{[A] \cdot E_m}{[A] + b} \qquad [1.11]$$

where $b$ is a fitting constant and $E_m$ is the maximal tissue response, then agonist concentration can be rearranged to:

$$[A] = \frac{E_a \cdot b}{E_m - E_a} \qquad [1.12]$$

Similarly, Eq. 1.4, relating agonist concentration and the quantity of agonist receptor complex ($[A \cdot R]$), can be rearranged to:

$$[A] = \frac{[A \cdot R] \cdot K_A}{[R_t] - [A \cdot R]} \qquad [1.13]$$

Equating Eqs. 1.12 and 1.13 and rearranging:

$$E_a = \frac{[A \cdot R] \cdot K_A \cdot E_m}{[A \cdot R](K_A - b) + [R_t] \cdot b} \qquad [1.14]$$

In the case where $K_A < b$, infinite and negative values for tissue response ($E_a$) are allowed, therefore, this case has no physical application to drug-receptor kinetics. The other two possibilities allow for a linear (where $K_A = b$) or a hyperbolic (where $K_A > b$) relationship to exist between $E_a$ and $[A \cdot R]$. Since there are few examples of linear relationships between agonist concentration and tissue response, the operational model assumes a hyperbolic relationship between these quantities. Therefore, tissue response $E_a$ is redefined as a hyperbolic function of the agonist-receptor complex (i.e., the operational model defines constant $b$ in Eq. 1.11):

$$\frac{E_a}{E_m} = \frac{[A{\cdot}R]}{K_E + [A{\cdot}R]} \qquad [1.15]$$

where $K_E$ is the value of $[A{\cdot}R]$, which elicits half the maximal tissue response. Combining Eq. 1.15 with Eq. 1.4:

$$\frac{E_a}{E_m} = \frac{[R_t]{\cdot}[A]}{K_A{\cdot}K_E + ([R_t] + K_E)[A]} \qquad [1.16]$$

This equation is the essential one in the operational model. It defines the production of tissue response as a function of agonist concentration $[A]$, agonist binding to the receptor $K_A$, the total number of response-producing units (receptors $[R_t]$) and a fitting constant for the production of response from a given concentration of agonist-receptor complex $K_E$. This latter parameter has both receptor and tissue properties in that it incorporates the concept of intrinsic efficacy (i.e., the agonist-dependent property of receptor activation) *and* the various tissue-dependent processes that translate initial receptor stimulus to response. This feature of $K_E$ can be used to quantify relative agonist efficacy (see Chapter 8).

Black and Leff defined a transducer constant $\tau$ as ($[R_t]/K_E$) as a consolidation of agonism. This constant serves as a practical measure of efficacy (as defined by Stephenson in occupation theory) since response is directly proportional to its magnitude. With this parameter, Eq. 1.16 can be rewritten:

$$\frac{E_a}{E_m} = \frac{[A]{\cdot}\tau}{K_A + (\tau + 1){\cdot}[A]} \qquad [1.17]$$

It can be seen from this analysis that the production of response is modeled by two successive saturable hyperbolic functions. The first is the binding of the agonist to the receptor and the second is the operational "binding" of the agonist-receptor complex ($[A{\cdot}R]$) to a possible series of hyperbolic functions to produce response. These concepts are illustrated in Fig. 1.11, where the agonist binding curve and those relating $[A{\cdot}R]$ complex and $[A]$ to tissue response are shown.

It should be noted that response $E_a$ is expressed as a fraction of the total tissue response $E_m$, a parameter not necessarily observed as the maximal response to the agonist. This experimental measure is obtained as $[A]$ approaches infinity. Under these circumstances, the maximal response (termed $\alpha$) to a given agonist is obtained from Eq. 1.17 as:

$$\underset{(E_a \text{ as } [A] \to \infty)}{\text{asymptote}} = \frac{E_m\tau}{\tau + 1} \qquad [1.18]$$

Similarly, another important experimental parameter, the concentration of

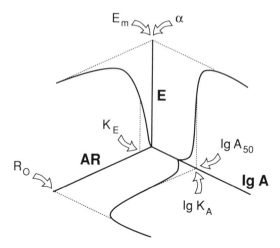

**FIG. 1.11.** Schematic diagram of the operational model of agonism. Shown is the interdependence of the agonist concentration and response (E), agonist concentration and the production of drug-receptor complex (AR), and the hyperbolic relationship between AR and response E. Parameters defined in Eqs. 1.16, 1.18, and 1.19. (From ref. 18.)

agonist that produces half the maximal response (termed the $A_{50}$), can be calculated from Eq. 1.17 as:

$$[A_{50}] = \frac{K_A}{1 + \tau} \qquad [1.19]$$

It can be seen from this equation that the location parameter for an agonist dose-response curve depends on the equilibrium dissociation constant of the agonist-receptor complex $(K_A)$ *and* the efficacy of the agonist in the particular tissue system $(\tau)$.

A specific form of the operational model is relevant to a large and important family of receptors that utilize a membrane-bound protein for the production of cellular response. These coupling proteins (G-proteins) utilize agonist-activated receptors to hydrolyze guanosine triphosphate (GTP), an essential cellular second messenger) for the production of cofactors for cellular function. Under these circumstances, the production of cellular response is proportional to the production of a ternary complex between the agonist, receptor, and G protein in the cell membrane. If response $(E_a/E_m)$ is directly proportional to the amount of ternary complex ($[A \cdot R \cdot T]$, where $[T]$ is the initial quantity of receptor-coupling protein), then Eq. 1.16 can be expressed as:

$$\frac{E_a}{E_m} = \frac{[R_t] \cdot [A]}{K_A \cdot K_{AR} + ([R_t] + K_{AR})[A]} \qquad [1.20]$$

where $K_{AR}$ is the equilibrium dissociation constant of the activated receptor/ G protein complex. This particular form of the operational model is relevant to the quantification of agonist intrinsic efficacy in binding and functional studies to be described in later chapters. Specifically it will be seen that when the dose-response curves of two agonists are compared within the same tissue, then the tissue-dependent aspects of $K_E$ cancel and only the receptor-specific aspects of efficacy for the two agonists are relevant (i.e., relative values of $K_{AR}$). For example, Fig. 1.12 shows dose-response curves to two β-adrenoceptor agonists, isoproterenol and prenalterol, in a variety of isolated tissue preparations. These dose-response curves are adequately fit by the

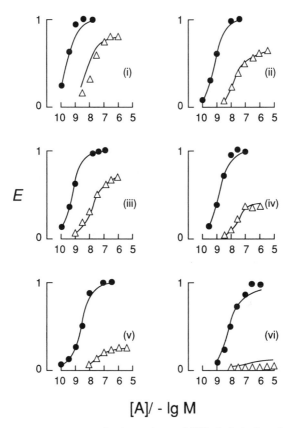

**[A]/ - lg M**

**FIG. 1.12.** Dose-response curves for isoproterenol (*filled circles*) and prenalterol (*open triangles*) in various tissues. Curves fit with operational model (Eq. 1.20) with respective $K_A$ values for isoproterenol and prenalterol of 0.2 μmol/L and 0.4 nmol/L and respective $K_{AR}$ values of 2.7 nmol/L and 0.5 μmol/L [$R_t$] was allowed to vary for each tissue (all values for [$R_t$] × 10$^{-6}$): **i:** Guinea pig trachea ([$R_t$] = 2.3), **ii:** rat left atrium ([$R_t$] = 0.85), **iii:** cat left atrium ([$R_t$] = 1.0), **iv:** cat papillary muscle ([$R_t$] = 0.33), **v:** guinea pig left atrium ([$R_t$] = 0.18), and **vi:** guinea pig extensor digitorum longus muscle ([$R_t$] = 0.06). (Experimental data from ref. 16 and curve fit from ref. 3.)

operational model across these tissue types with a conserved number of agonist-receptor constants. Specifically, the $K_A$ for isoproterenol is 0.2 μmol, $K_A$ for prenalterol = 0.04 μmol, $K_{AR}$ isoproterenol = 2.7 nM, $K_{AR}$ prenalterol = 0.5 μmol. The only tissue-dependent factor required to account for the range of agonist activity of these two agonists in these tissues is a variation of $[R_t]$ given in the figure legend.

In general, these analyses are valid only for the case in which agonist binding to the receptor and the production of agonist response in a tissue can be described by rectangular hyperbolae. When this is not the case experimentally, a modification of Eq. 1.16 is required to model data. Under these circumstances, a general logistic function can be utilized to model response production as a function of $[A]$:

$$\frac{E_a}{E_m} = \frac{[R_t]^n \cdot [A]^n}{[R_t]^n \cdot [A]^n + ([A] + K_A)^n K_E{}^n} \qquad [1.21]$$

When this form of the operational model is used, the observed maximal response of an agonist is given by:

$$\underset{(E_a \text{ as } [A] \to \infty)}{\text{asymptote}} = \frac{E_m \tau^n}{\tau^n + 1} \qquad [1.22]$$

and the concentration of agonist required for half maximal response is given by:

$$[A_{50}] = \frac{K_A}{(2 + \tau^n)^{1/n} - 1} \qquad [1.23]$$

The estimation of drug-related constants (i.e., $K_A$ and relative values of $\tau$) represents special experimental problems under the circumstance when tissue response is not a rectangular hyperbola of agonist concentration (i.e., when $\neq 1$ in Eq. 1.21). These cases are dealt with specifically in Chapters 7 (Agonist Affinity) and 8 (Efficacy).

In general, the operational model has the advantage of simplicity in that no *ad hoc* constants to account for agonism are required for the description of drug effect. Within the framework of this model, agonist action can be completely described in a given system by the parameters $K_A$, $[R_t]$, and $K_E$, one less than in standard occupation theory where agonism is described by $K_A$, $\epsilon$, $[R_t]$ and the function $f$, which defines the relationship between receptor occupancy and tissue response. Notably, most of the constants in the operational model are experimentally accessible (i.e., $K_A$, see Chapter 7; $[R_t]$, see Chapter 2; $K_E$, see Chapter 8 for the case in which $K_E = K_{AR}$). The measurement and interpretation of various constants for agonist and antagonist activity are described in later chapters in terms of standard occupation theory and the operational model.

### Rate Theory

An alternative model to explain the effects of drugs, based on the rates of onset and offset of drugs to and from receptors, was proposed by Paton; this model is referred to as rate theory. It was introduced as an alternative to occupation theory in light of the latter model's failure to account for a number of observations in experimental pharmacology. Specifically, Paton's model accounts for the general observation that antagonists act much more slowly than agonists and that the rates of offset of antagonists often are inversely proportional to their potencies. Also, occupation theory cannot account for a phenomenon observed in some experimental systems termed "fade," in which agonists produce peak but transient responses, followed by steady-state responses of lower magnitude; rate theory provides a convenient explanation for this observation, as well as a rationale for specific receptor desensitization. Perhaps the most attractive feature of rate theory, however, is the chemical definition of intrinsic efficacy (*vide infra*), strictly an operational proportionality constant in occupation theory.

Rate theory is based on the premise that it is not the occupation of the receptor by agonist, but rather the rate of drug-receptor combination, that produces the response. As put by Paton, "Instead of thinking of the receptor as, say, a note on an organ, such that as long as it is depressed a note is emitted, we think of it like a piano, one burst of sound and then silence." Thus, agonist activity depends on the rate of association ($V_f$) of [A] to [R], given by

$$V_f = \frac{k_1[A] \cdot [R]}{[R_t]} \qquad [1.24]$$

where $k_1$ is the rate of onset and $[R_t]$ is the total concentration of receptors. At equilibrium ($\partial[A \cdot R]/\partial t = 0$), and substituting for $k_1[A] \cdot [R]$ from Eq. 1.2,

$$V_{eq} = \frac{k_2[A \cdot R]}{[R_t]} \qquad [1.25]$$

where $V_{eq}$ is the rate of association at equilibrium. Substituting from Eq. 1.4,

$$V_{eq} = \frac{k_2}{1 + (K_A/[A])} \qquad [1.26]$$

Paton assumed that the response was the product of the velocity of agonist-receptor combination ($V_f$ for responses at any given time and $V_{eq}$ for responses at equilibrium) and a proportionality factor $\phi$ that reflected the processing of the receptor stimulus by the tissue. Thus, effect $E$ is given by

$$E = \phi \cdot V_{eq} \qquad [1.27]$$

The maximal response (when $[A] \gg K_A$) from Eqs. 1.26 and 1.27 reduces to $E_M = \phi k_2$; thus, the intrinsic efficacy of an agonist equals the rate of offset

of agonist from the receptor. Intuitively, this is logical if the response results
from agonist association with a free receptor; the more quickly the agonist
dissociates dictates greater availability of free receptors for further quantal
stimulation by association with the agonist molecules. Also, this accounts
for the slower activity of antagonists, because a low $k_2$ dictates a low capacity
for producing a response. Therefore, drugs with a slow rate of offset from
the receptor produce no response, but do bind to receptors (i.e., antagonists).
In fact, Paton demonstrated a positive correlation between potency and rate
of offset for a series of alkyltrimethylammonium compounds, showing that
the more potent a compound was, the more slowly it was washed off of the
receptors (Fig. 1.13).

There is a fundamental difference between occupation theory and rate
theory in the kinetics of agonist responses. If one could remove diffusion
limitations within a tissue (i.e., assume that the concentration of agonist
rises to the equilibrium value instantaneously) and observe the receptor-unit
equivalent of response (in the case of occupation theory, stimulus; for rate
theory, either response as Paton defined it in Eq. 1.27 or a stimulus that
precedes response), two different patterns would be observed. This can be
demonstrated by the respective equations determining receptor occupation
and rate of receptor occupation. Substituting $[R_t] = [R] + [A \cdot R]$, Eq. 1.1
can be rewritten as

$$\partial[A \cdot R]/\partial t = k_1[A] \cdot [R_t] - [A \cdot R](k_1[A] + k_2) \tag{1.28}$$

The solution for Eq. 1.28 is

$$-k_1[A][R_t](1 - e^{-(k_1[A]-k_2)t}) \tag{1.29}$$

Equating 1.28 and 1.29 and rearranging,

$$\frac{[A \cdot R_t]}{[R_t]} = \frac{[A]}{[A] + K_A}(1 - e^{-(k_1[A]+k_2)t}) \tag{1.30}$$

This is the equation defining receptor occupancy as a function of time, and
it defines the kinetics of the response in terms of occupation theory. The
generation of a stimulus by this equation is shown in Fig. 1.14A.

From Eq. 1.24, and letting $[R] = [R_t] - [A \cdot R]$,

$$V_f = k_1[A]\left(1 - \frac{[A \cdot R]}{[R_t]}\right) \tag{1.31}$$

Substituting from Eq. 1.30,

$$V_f = \frac{[A]}{[A] + K_A}(k_2 + k_1[A]e^{-(k_1[A]+k_2)t}) \tag{1.32}$$

Note that as $t \to \infty$ (equilibrium), Eq. 1.32 reduces to Eq. 1.25. This equation
defines the rate of receptor occupancy with time in terms of rate theory; a

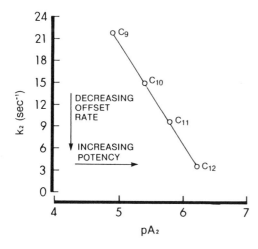

**FIG. 1.13.** Correlation between the rate constant for offset and potency. Offset (ordinate) for a series of alkyltrimethylammonium compounds from muscarinic receptors of guinea pig ileum and potency of these compounds as antagonists of responses mediated by muscarinic receptors ($pA_2$ = $-$log molar concentration that produces a twofold shift to the right for an agonist concentration-response curve as abscissa). Numbers on data points refer to numbers of carbons in alkyl chains. (Data from ref. 24.)

response (or stimulus) produced by an agonist under these conditions is shown in Fig. 1.14B. Clearly, the patterns of stimulation with these two schemes are different; occupation theory defines a gradual increase to a steady-state response, whereas rate theory predicts a transient peak response followed by a decline to a steady state ("fade"). Such a pattern is predicted for a range of concentrations from threshold to near maximal receptor occupancy (Fig. 1.15A). The pattern of responses shown in Figs. 1.14B and 1.15A was observed by Paton in guinea pig ileum with a series of alkyltrimethylammonium compounds (Fig. 1.15B); these experimental results supported the rate model. Whereas this pattern of responses was observed in this particular experimental system, there are many others in which such biphasic responses are not observed, and in fact the relationship of response to time resembles more what is seen in Fig. 1.14A. This fact has been cited as evidence against rate theory, but it should be kept in mind that there are reasons why the kinetics of response development may not demonstrate fade even within the

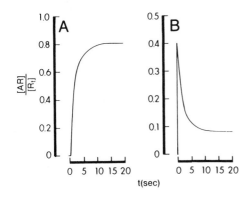

**FIG. 1.14.** Kinetics of receptor occupancy according to occupational theory **(A)** and rate theory **(B)**. For both curves, $[A]/K_A = 4$, $k_1 = 1$ $\mu M^{-1}$ $sec^{-1}$, $k_2 = 1$ $sec^{-1}$.

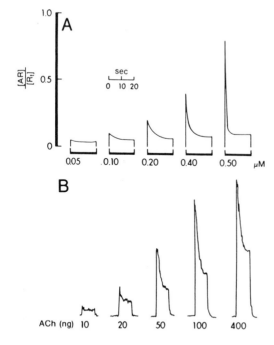

FIG. 1.15. Kinetics of receptor occupancy according to rate theory for a series of increasing concentrations of agonist. **A:** Responses calculated with Eq. 1.20. $[A] = 0.05$, 0.1, 0.2, 0.4, 0.5 μM; $k_1 = 1$ μM sec$^{-1}$, $k_2 = 0.1$ sec$^{-1}$. **B:** Data obtained in guinea pig ileum for acetylcholine. (From ref. 24.)

rate-theory model. The responses predicted by Eq. 1.32, with a series of agonist concentrations shown in Figs. 1.15A and 1.15B, demonstrate two features of this model: The phenomenon of fade is a minor event at low receptor occupancies, and the rate of decline from peak response greatly increases with increasing concentration. A comparison for Eq. 1.32 at $t = 0$ ($V_{peak}$) and $t \to \infty$ ($V_{eq}$) illustrates this latter fact; the magnitude of fade is given by:

$$\frac{V_{peak}}{V_{eq}} = \frac{[A] + K_A}{K_A} \qquad [1.33]$$

showing that the higher the concentration, the more one would expect to see fade.

Both of these features suggest situations in which fade may be so slight as to be unobserved. The first arises when the agonist is powerful and the stimulus-response mechanisms of the tissue are efficient, such that responses are achieved at very low receptor occupancies. The second arises with high concentrations of agonist at which fade is most likely to be observed; the rates of rise and fall of the peak response may far exceed the rate of diffusion of agonist into the receptor compartment, so that the fast peak is not observed. Considering these factors, the definitive test whether or not rate theory truly describes receptor activation probably will not depend on the kinetics of the response.

There is much to recommend rate theory as a model for drug-receptor interaction. Although there are substantial differences between the predictions of occupation theory and rate theory, these differences are difficult to demonstrate experimentally. The major problem is the preponderance of isolated-tissue test systems in which diffusion, not drug-receptor interaction, is rate-limiting. Also, it is possible that in some tissues the generation of a response from a stimulus is the rate-limiting step; thus, the kinetics of the response cannot be relied on to reflect receptor events.

A more detailed description of Paton's kinetic experiments with antagonists is given in Chapter 12.

### Receptor-Inactivation Theory

A receptor model put forth by Gosselin merits attention because it accommodates the major elements of both occupation theory and rate theory. Conceptually and mathematically, occupation theory and rate theory are two special cases of a receptor-inactivation theory. The model proposes that a drug $(A)$ binds to a receptor $(R)$ with a rate of onset $k_1$ and rate of offset $k_2$ to form a complex $(A \cdot R)$ and that this converts the receptor into an inactive form $R'$ incapable of binding or being activated by drug. The transition from $A \cdot R$ to $R'$ is governed by a rate constant $k_3$. The inactive form $R'$ then reverts to native receptor $R$ (capable of being activated), a process with a rate constant $k_4$ (Scheme 1.1). The stimulus intensity is seen as being proportional to the rate of receptor inactivation (rate of formation of $R'$), which is equal to $k_3[A \cdot R]$. This model views stimulation as a succession of quantal events (as does rate theory) and has most of the transient characteristics of rate theory, but because stimulus equals $k_3[A \cdot R]$, stimulus also depends on the number of occupied receptors (as does occupation theory).

It can be seen that if $k_3 \ll k_4$, no significant amounts of $R'$ accumulate (any $R'$ formed goes to $R$ as quickly as it is formed). If $k_3$ is the smallest rate constant (i.e., $k_2 \gg k_3 \ll k_4$), then kinetically the model will essentially describe occupation theory. If, however, $k_3$ is the largest rate constant ($k_3 \gg k_1, k_2, k_4$), it can be seen that no appreciable quantity of $[A \cdot R]$ appears,

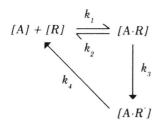

**SCHEME 1.1.** Schematic diagram of receptor interactions for receptor inactivation theory.

and the receiver can appear in either form $R$ or $R'$. Thus, the conversion from $R$ to $R'$ is controlled by $k_1$, a condition formally identical with that of rate theory.

Receptor inactivation, given the proper rate constants, predicts a transient peak response followed by a reduced steady state (fade). An example of the concentration $[A \cdot R]$ produced by a given concentration of drug $A$ as a function of time is given in Fig. 1.16A; the formation of $R'$ also is shown. The stimulus is proportional to $[A \cdot R]$; thus, a transient peak that decreases to a steady-state response is predicted. Like rate theory, receptor-inactivation theory predicts increasing fade with increasing dose (Fig. 1.16B). Also, receptor-inactivation theory describes a special circumstance in which fade

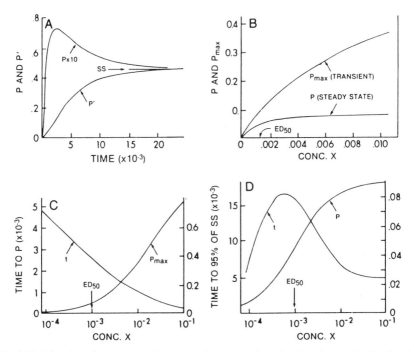

**FIG. 1.16.** Kinetics of responses in terms of receptor-inactivation theory. **A:** Production of $A \cdot R$ and $R'$ with time. Ordinate: Fractional values. Abscissa: Time in arbitrary units corresponding to rate constants. Curves calculated for $[A] = 10^{-3}$, $k_1 = 10^{-1}$, $k_2 = 10^{-4}$, $k_2 = 10^{-3}$, $k_4 = 10^{-4}$. $P$ and $P'$ refer to fractional concentrations of $A \cdot R$ and $R'$, respectively. SS refers to steady state. **B:** Values of $P$ at transient maximum and steady state at fixed concentrations of agonist. Rate constants as for part A. Note that the ratio of $P_{max}$ to $P$ increases with increasing concentration. **C:** Transient maximum and time to peak at given concentrations of agonist. $P_{max}$ curve same as in part B on a logarithmic scale of concentration. Note that the time to peak decreases with increasing transient contraction and concentration. **D:** Properties of the steady state. $P$ refers to the magnitude of the steady state as a function of concentration (abscissa), and $t$ refers to time to steady state. Note that, in contrast to the case for rate or occupation theory, $t$ is a biphasic function of concentration. (From ref. 11.)

would not be predicted, namely, when $(k_1[A] + k_2 + k_3 - k_4)^2 - 4k_3k_1[A]$ is equal to or does not substantially exceed zero. As with rate theory, there are difficulties in verifying this model experimentally on the basis of fade (*vide supra*).

Receptor-inactivation theory also predicts that the latent period between addition of drug and peak response decreases with dose (Fig. 1.16C); these kinetics differ from those of rate theory, which predict maximal stimulation at $t = 0$ (no latent period, compare Figs. 1.14B and 1.16A). This model also differs kinetically from occupation theory, which predicts that the rates of receptor occupation and production of stimuli increase with increasing doses of drug. Receptor-inactivation theory predicts a biphasic rate of change; the time required for attainment of steady states is greater in the region of the midpoint in the dose-response curve (i.e., low and high doses reach a steady state faster than intermediate doses [Fig. 1.16D]). Finally, receptor-inactivation theory predicts highly damped oscillations of stimuli. It can be seen from the previous discussion that although receptor-inactivation theory can be differentiated from both rate theory and occupation theory, the critical differences depend on kinetic behavior that most likely cannot be verified experimentally. All steady-state analyses are incapable of distinguishing receptor-inactivation, rate, and occupation theories.

Inactivation theory equates maximal receptor occupancy with $(k_3 \cdot k_4)/(k_3 + k_4)$. This quantity is formally identical with intrinsic efficacy. Table 1.3 shows the relationships between kinetic constants $k_3$ and $k_4$ and the expected resulting behaviors of drugs.

### Two-State Models

If one drug molecule binds to one receptor to generate a response, the binding reaction can be described by a simple hyperbola according to the Langmuir adsorption isotherm (Eq. 1.4). It has been demonstrated in some systems, however, that receptor activation follows a sigmoidal rather than hyperbolic relationship, thereby denoting cooperative binding. This suggests that the binding of drug molecules to receptors to produce a response is not

**TABLE 1.3.** *Classification of drugs according to receptor-inactivation theory*

| Type | $k_3$ | $k_4$ |
|------|-------|-------|
| Full agonist | Large | Very large |
| Partial agonist | Large | Large |
| Antagonist with transient excitatory effect and long persistence | Intermediate | Small |
| Reversible antagonist | Zero | $k_2 > 0$ |

From ref. 11.

an independent process and that the activation of the receptor by one drug molecule affects the subsequent activation by another. This type of behavior is difficult to demonstrate experimentally, because the index of binding, if response is studied, usually is a multivariate process, the nature of which determines the shape of the dose-response curve. However, there is a fundamental drug response that can be measured, namely, ionic-conductance changes in postsynaptic membranes, which may be directly proportional to formation of drug-receptor complexes. In such systems, experimental data have been accumulated that do not conform to a simple hyperbolic relationship between concentration and response. This observation of sigmoidicity has provided the experimental impetus for proposals of cooperative interactions between receptor subunits. Figure 1.17 shows GABA-induced conductance changes in the crustacean neuromuscular junction; a hyperbola, as would be defined by the Langmuir adsorption isotherm for the binding of a single drug to a single receptor, fails to fit the data points adequately. The sigmoidicity in this curve is evident. One way to explain these results is to postulate an interaction between the drugs and receptors such that the binding of one drug molecule affects the binding of another. This effect is called cooperativity. The particular models for drug-receptor interaction that conveniently incorporate cooperative effects are two-state models.

In general, two-state models describe a receptor population that exists in an equilibrium between two states, activated ($R$) and inactivated ($T$). Each receptor is thought to be made up of subunits termed protomers (the collection of protomers making up the receptor being an oligomer). The number ($n$) of protomers making up the receptor can vary from unity to any number, but each protomer is constrained to one of the two states, $R$ or $T$. The equilibrium describing the relative proportions of receptors in the $R$ and $T$ states is characterized by an equilibrium constant for the $T$-to-$R$ transition termed the "allosteric constant":

$$L = [T]/[R] \qquad\qquad [1.34]$$

In the case of ion channels, the $R$ state would correspond to the open channel, while the $T$ state would denote the closed channel. The stimulus is proportional to the number of open channels (receptors in the $R$ state); thus, in the absence of drug, the equilibrium $T \rightleftharpoons R$ would lie heavily to the left (i.e., most channels closed, $L$ large). In this scheme, drugs would produce responses by binding preferentially to the $R$ state, thereby shifting the equilibrium from $T$ toward $R$ (because total $R$ would be composed of free $R$ plus drug-bound $R$). A spectrum of possible fractional channel openings can be produced by drugs with affinities for both states of the receptor, because binding to the $T$ state competes for formation of the $R$ state. Two-state models are capable of explaining experimentally observed cooperativity in drug effects as well as the finding that the activated form of the receptor (open channel) seems to be the same for all drugs. Agonists do not appear to change ionic conductance

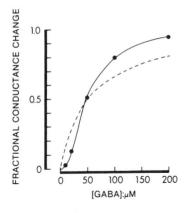

FIG. 1.17. Experimental sigmoidal concentration-response curve. Conductance change (ordinate) as a function of molar concentration of GABA (abscissa) in crustacean neuromuscular junction. *Broken line* indicates hyperbolic function with same $K_A$ according to the Langmuir adsorption isotherm with $N = 1$. (Data from ref. 26.)

by graded opening of channels, but rather by opening them for varying lengths of time.

In general, there are two possible multiple-subunit, two-state models: one in which the subunits are independent of each other, and the other in which they are not. An independent-subunit model describes a receptor made up of subunits, the conformation of each being independent of the conformations of its neighbors. The transition of the receptor from the $T$ form to the $R$ form depends on the transition of all protomers being in the $R$ conformation (Scheme 1.2). It should be noted that this model displays cooperativity with respect to drug-induced channel opening *without* allosteric interaction between the subunits (i.e., the binding of drug to one protomer has no effect on the binding to another in the same oligomer). Drugs have microscopic equilibrium dissociation constants for each protomer, and the consequence of binding shifts the equilibrium between the two states, increasing the fraction of total oligomers to the higher affinity state and therefore altering the macroscopic affinity of the protein for the drug. Thus, cooperativity is achieved without interaction between binding sites. The fraction of channels (each consisting of $n$ protomers) opened by a drug with a differential affinity for the $R$ state ($K_{AR}/K_{AT} = M$) is given by

$$\rho_{\text{open}} = \left[ \frac{1}{1 + L[(1 + M\alpha)/(1 + \alpha)]} \right]^n \qquad [1.35]$$

where $\alpha$ is a normalized drug concentration ($\alpha = [A]/K_{AR}$) and $L$ is the

$$T \underset{}{\overset{L}{\rightleftharpoons}} R$$

$$K_{AT} \updownarrow \qquad \qquad \updownarrow K_{AR}$$

$$A \cdot T \qquad \quad A \cdot R \qquad \textbf{SCHEME 1.2.}$$

allosteric constant. In such a system, the number of channels open in the absence of a drug is ($\alpha = 0$)

$$\rho_{\text{open}}(0) = \left(\frac{1}{1+L}\right)^n \qquad [1.36]$$

The maximal number of channels opened by a drug is given by ($\alpha \rightarrow \infty$)

$$\rho_{\text{open}}(\infty) = \left(\frac{1}{1+LM}\right)^n \qquad [1.37]$$

Thus, it can be seen that in systems heavily favoring closed channels ($L$ large), a drug with even a high selective affinity for the open channel may fail to open all of the channels. This may never become evident in drug responses, because there could be any number of specific relationships between maximal tissue response and fraction of open channels.

One of the most attractive features of this model is that it provides a chemical definition for intrinsic efficacy, that property of drugs that produces the response (in this case, converts receptors into the $R$ form). An antagonist would be defined as a drug that did not selectively bind to the $R$ form, but rather fixed the ratio $L$ by nonselectively binding to both the $T$ and $R$ states ($M = 1$). A partial agonist would bind preferentially to the $R$ state, but also to the $T$ state, thereby producing a partial shift in equilibrium toward $R$. A full agonist would be more selective for $R$ and would produce a greater shift of the equilibrium toward the $R$ state. In this scheme, a correlate for intrinsic efficacy as given by occupation theory is

$$\epsilon = \left(\frac{K_{AT}}{K_{AR}} - 1\right) = \left(\frac{1}{M} - 1\right) \qquad [1.38]$$

Inherent in two-state systems is a concept not found in occupation theory or rate theory, namely, negative efficacy. A drug with preferential affinity

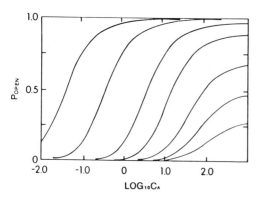

FIG. 1.18. Concentration-response curves calculated from independent-subunit model. $N = 4$, $L = 5.6$, $M =$ (from right to left) 0.063, 0.034, 0.017, 0.0048, 0.0013, 0.00013, 0.000013. Ordinate: Fraction of channels open. Abscissa: Logarithms of $\alpha$, where $\alpha$ refers to $[A]/K_{AR}$. (From ref. 6.)

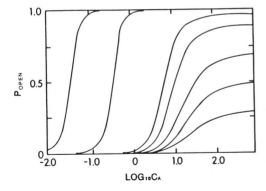

**FIG. 1.19.** Concentration-response curves calculated from dependent-subunit model. $N = 4$, $L = 1,000$, $M =$ (from right to left) 0.22, 0.18, 0.14, 0.10, 0.075, 0.0075, 0.00075. Ordinate: Fraction of channels open. Abscissa: Logarithms of $\alpha$, where $\alpha$ refers to $[A]/K_{AR}$. (From ref. 6.)

for the *T* state will close normally open channels and demonstrate a negative efficacy. The effects of a range of drugs with varying ratios of affinity for the *T* and *R* states (intrinsic efficacy) are shown in Fig. 1.18. It can be seen from these calculations that differential affinity for the *R* and *T* forms can produce changes in the locations and maxima of concentration-response curves to drugs. Comparison to Fig. 1.9A shows the similarity to changes in intrinsic efficacy in terms of occupation theory.

Another possible model is one in which the conformation of each protomer is dependent on that of its neighbor. Thus, if a drug binds to one protomer and constrains it to the *R* state, then the drug generates new high-affinity binding sites; this accounts for cooperativity. The equation for the fraction of open channels is

$$\rho_{\text{open}} = \frac{1}{1 + L[(1 + M\alpha)/(1 + \alpha)]^n} \qquad [1.39]$$

The effects of drugs with different relative efficacies for the *T* and *R* states (intrinsic efficacy) in terms of this model are shown in Fig. 1.19. As with the independent-subunit model (Fig. 1.18), the relative affinities for the *T* and *R* states can affect both the locations and the maxima of dose-response curves.

## SPECIFIC RECEPTOR MODELS

The major theme of this book is the classification of drugs and drug receptors for the prediction of therapeutic effects in humans. It is a tenet of this theme that drug receptors as recognition and transducing units are comparatively immutable with respect to organ type, tissue function, and pathological state when compared to other biochemical processes within cells that mediate function. There are numerous examples of dose-response behavior that deviates from simple Langmuir kinetics (i.e., complex dose-response curves). In some cases the deviations from simple drug receptor binding occur further on in the stimulus-response chain of cells and thus represent the complex interpretation of initially simple membrane interactions; these will be discussed further in Chapters 2 and 11. The modification of drug effect by cellular biochemical processes does not have an impact on receptor classification since the modifications usually are common for all agonists and antagonists and thus do not impart selectivity. There are exceptions to this generality where the receptor stimulus strength controls the initiation of biochemical reactions of differing threshold sensitivity. These effects can resemble receptor selectivity and are discussed in Chapter 11. Null methods usually employed to dissect receptor specific drug activity cancel stimulus-response modification of receptor signals.

In contrast, there are examples of where nonlangmuirian kinetics reflect

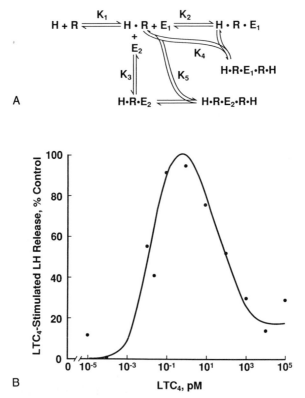

**FIG. 1.20.** Explicit model for the leukotriene $C_4$ ($LTC_4$)-mediated release of luteinizing hormone in anterior pituitary cells. **A:** Schematic diagram of a system in which a single receptor (R) binds a hormone (H) and interacts with two effector couplers ($E_1$ and $E_2$) to form active ternary complexes $H \cdot R \cdot E_1$ and $H \cdot R \cdot E_2$ and further to form two *inactive* dimer complexes $H \cdot R \cdot E_1 \cdot R \cdot H$ and $H \cdot R \cdot E_2 \cdot R \cdot H$. (From ref. 20.) **B:** Dose-response curve for $LTC_4$-mediated release of luteinizing hormone in anterior pituitary cell. (Data points from ref. 14 and modeled dose-response curve from ref. 20.) Parameters for simulation were $K_1 = 0.001$ pM$^{-1}$, $K_2 = 1000$ pM$^{-1}$, $K_3 = 30$ pM$^{-1}$, $K_4 = 0.1$ pM$^{-1}$, $K_5 = 0.003$ pM$^{-1}$.

events at the receptor and in these cases, drug behavior becomes receptor system specific and does involve receptor classification. For example, Hill coefficients of greater than unity for agonist dose-response curves in some ion channel systems reflect cooperativity at the receptor level. Under these circumstances, this becomes a property of the receptor and not simply a postreceptor modification of response by cellular processes. It can be useful to modify the existing theoretical receptor theories to describe aberrant drug behavior since this behavior may transcend tissue function, species, and pathology. A case in which a general receptor mechanism affects the description of drug effect in theoretical terms is the "floating receptor" (also called "mobile receptor") model in which an agonist-activated receptor diffuses in two dimensions in the cell membrane and collides with a transducing protein to form a ternary complex. This is a formalized part of the operational model of drug action and is extremely relevant to descriptions of agonism in functional (see Chapter 8) and radioligand (see Chapter 12) studies. In these cases it may be appropriate to extend classical receptor theory to describe dose-response curves since this extension may apply to other response systems as well.

There are receptor models that can describe complex dose-response curves as well. For example, Fig. 1.20A shows a model of a single receptor that interacts with two effector couplers to form active ternary complexes and further to produce two inactive dimers from the same ternary complexes. With this model, strikingly broad and even biphasic dose-response curves can be predicted. Figure 1.20B shows the experimental dose-response curve to leukotriene $C_4$ in anterior pituitary cells for the release of luteinizing hormone. The data span seven orders of magnitude and a complete range of response. The drawn dose-response curve was modeled using the scheme shown in Fig. 1.20A with a selected set of equilibrium dissociation constants.

It is important to define when postreceptor events modify the shapes of dose-response curves and when the curves reflect membrane receptor effects. While the complexity of such models limits their use as general descriptions of drug action, they can be extremely useful for hypothesis testing. Discerning receptor- versus nonreceptor-mediated divergences from ideal behavior is discussed more fully in Chapter 11.

## REFERENCES

1. Ariens, E. J. (1954): Affinity and intrinsic activity in the theory of competitive inhibition. *Arch. Int. Pharmacodyn. Ther.*, 99:32–49.
2. Ariens, E. J. (1964): *Molecular Pharmacology, Vol. 1.* Academic Press, New York.
3. Black, J. W., and Leff, P. (1983): Operational models of pharmacological agonist. *Proc. R. Soc. Lond. [Biol.]*, 220:141–162.
4. Buchheim, R. (1849): *Beitrage zur Arzneimmittellehre.* Voss, Leipzig.
5. Clark, A. J. (1937): General pharmacology. In: *Heffner's Handbuch d-exp. Pharmacol. Erg. band 4.* Springer, Berlin.

6. Colquhoun, D. (1973): The relationship between classical and cooperative models for drug action. In: *Drug Receptors*, edited by H. P. Rang, pp. 149–182. University Park Press, Baltimore.

7. Dohlman, H. G., Caron, M. G., and Lefkowitz, R. J. (1987): A family of receptors coupled to guanine nucleotide regulatory proteins. *Biochemistry*, 26:2657–2661.

8. Ehrlich, P. (1909): Veber den jetzigen Stand der Chemotherapie. *Berl. Dtsch. Chem. Ges.*, 42:17–47.

9. Furchgott, R. F. (1966): The use of β-haloalkylamines in the differentiation of receptors and in the determination of dissociation constants of receptor-agonist complexes. In: *Advances in Drug Research, Vol. 3*, edited by N. J. Harper and A. B. Simmonds, pp. 21–55. Academic Press, New York.

10. Furchgott, R. F. (1972): The classification of adrenoreceptors (adrenergic receptors). An evaluation from the standpoint of receptor theory. In: *Handbook of Experimental Pharmacology, Catecholamines, Vol. 33*, edited by H. Blaschko and E. Muscholl, pp. 283–335. Springer-Verlag, Berlin.

11. Gosselin, R. E. (1977): Drug-receptor inactivation: A new kinetic model. In: *Kinetics of Drug Action*, edited by J. M. Van Rossum, pp. 323–356. Springer-Verlag, Berlin.

12. Harms, H. H. (1976): Isoproterenol antagonism of cardioselective beta-adrenergic receptor blocking agents. A comparative study of human and guinea pig cardiac and bronchial beta-adrenergic receptors. *J. Pharmacol. Exp. Ther.*, 199:329–335.

13. Hollenberg, M. (1991): Structure activity relationships for transmembrane signalling: The receptor's turn. *FASEB J.*, 5:178–186.

14. Hulting, A.-L., Lindgren, J. A., Hokfelt, T., Eneroth, P., Werener, S., Patrono, C., and Samuelsson, B. (1985): Leukotriene $c_4$ as a mediator of luteinizing hormone release from rat anterior pituitary cells. *Proc. Natl. Acad. Sci. USA*, 82:3834–3838.

15. Karlin, A. (1967): On the application of a "plausible model" of allosteric proteins to the receptor for acetylcholine. *J. Theor. Biol.*, 16:306–320.

16. Kenakin, T. P., and Beek, D. (1980): Is prenalterol (HI33/80) really a selective beta-1 adrenoceptor agonist? Tissue selectivity resulting from differences in stimulus-response relationships. *J. Pharmacol. Exp. Ther.*, 213:406–412.

17. Kenakin, T. P., and Beek, D. (1982): In vitro studies on the cardiac activity of pernalterol for $\beta_1$-adrenoceptors: Measurement of agonist affinity by alteration of receptor number. *J. Pharmacol. Exp. Ther.*, 220:77–85.

18. Leff, P., Giles, P. H., Martin, G. R., and Wood, J. (1990): Estimation of agonist affinity and efficacy by direct, operational model-fitting. *J. Pharmacol. Meth.*, 23:225–237.

19. Leighton, H. J., Butz, K. R., and Parmeter, L. (1979): Effect of α-adrenergic agonists and antagonists on neurotransmission in the rat anococcygeus muscle. *Eur. J. Pharmacol.*, 58:27–38.

20. Leiser, J., Conn, M. P., and Blumm, J. J. (1986): Interpretation of dose-response curves for luteinizing hormone release by gonadotropin-releasing hormone, related peptides, and leukotriene $C_4$ according to a hormone/receptor/effector model. *Proc. Natl. Acad. Sci. USA*, 83:5963–5967.

21. MacKay, D. (1966): A new method for the analysis of drug-receptor interactions. In: *Advances in Drug Research, Vol. 3*, edited by N. J. Harper and A. B. Simmonds, pp. 1–19. Academic Press, New York.

22. MacKay, D. (1977): A critical survey of receptor theories of drug action. In: *Kinetics of Drug Action*, edited by J. M. Van Rossum, pp. 255–322. Springer-Verlag, Berlin.

23. Marshall, P. B. (1955): Some chemical and physical properties associated with histamine antagonism. *Br. J. Pharmacol.*, 10:270–278.

24. Paton, W. D. M. (1961): A theory of drug action based on the rate of drug-receptor combination. *Proc. R. Soc. Lond. [Biol.]*, 154:21–69.

25. Stephenson, R. P. (1956): A modification of receptor theory. *Br. J. Pharmacol.*, 11:379–393.

26. Takeuchi, A., and Takeuchi, N. (1967): Anion permeability of the inhibitory post-synaptic membrane of the crayfish neuromuscular junction. *J. Physiol. (Lond.)*, 191:575–590.

# 2

# Stimulus-Response Mechanisms

*Like a surrealist biochemical version of "The House That Jack Built"—this is the hormone that triggered the receptor that activated the adenylate cyclase that formed the cAMP that activated the protein kinase that phosphorylated the phosphorylase kinase that phosphorylated the glycogen phosphorylase that phosphorylated the glycogen that yielded the glucose that ended up in the bloodstream.*

—N. D. Goldberg, 1975

Whereas detailed models have been constructed to describe quantitatively the formation of the agonist-receptor complex and the production of the first consequence of that formation, namely, a biological stimulus, necessarily less generalization has been accorded to the production of the tissue response. This is partly because of the tremendous diversity of methods by which different organs process stimuli to produce responses and partly because of our lack of understanding of many of the processes involved. Fortunately, from the point of view of classification of drugs and quantification of drug effects, detailed knowledge of the processes that convert the receptor stimulus into the tissue response (stimulus-response mechanisms) is not necessary, because in many cases null methods cancel the impact of these processes on the translation of drug effects.

There are two tissue factors that control tissue responses, one related to the magnitude of total stimulus (receptor density) and one related to the transduction of total stimulus into response (to be described as a monotonic-increasing saturable function of stimulus, denoted $f$). Assuming that each agonist-receptor complex initiates quantal stimuli, there are at least three ways the magnitude of the stimulus from each receptor can be varied. First, the strength of the stimulus may vary with drug concentration, as would be expected of graded protein conformational changes due to agonist binding. Second, the quantal unit of stimulus may be uniform (i.e., as in a simple on/off switch), but the frequency of stimulation may vary with drug concentration (as per rate theory). Thus, for any given time period, one agonist may initiate quantal responses more frequently than another, thereby producing

*39*

a greater total stimulus. Third, the receptor may be activated for varying lengths of time. In this setting, for example, an ion channel can be open or closed, and one agonist may open the channel for a longer period of time than another, thereby producing greater stimulus. This could apply to agonists activating receptors that then bind to transducer proteins in the cell membrane, subsequently to produce ternary complexes. The longer the agonist is able to keep the receptor protein in a favorable conformation, the greater the probability of a fruitful collision (one leading to production of a ternary complex) in the lipid matrix of the cell membrane.

The total stimulus imparted to the tissue by a given concentration of agonist is the sum of the quantal stimuli from all responding units, namely, the activated drug receptors. The tissue then processes the total stimulus into a response. In electronic terms, the summed stimuli correspond to a preamplifier, and the tissue stimulus-response mechanisms constitute a power amplifier that intensifies the signal. There are two aspects to the power amplifier. The first is its inherent output (i.e., strength). Some tissues have efficient stimulus-response mechanisms that can amplify a weak stimulus into a large response; others have less efficient mechanisms, and therefore weak agonists produce no response. These latter tissues can be considered to have low-output amplifiers. A second aspect of the power amplifier is the volume control. Intrinsic to the various stimulus-response mechanisms are the cofactors, enzymes, and catalysts involved in the production of responses. Thus, usually there is an element of control within the limits of any given power amplifier. It is worth considering the contributions of receptor density and stimulus-response mechanisms to the total tissue response separately.

## RECEPTOR DENSITY: THE PREAMPLIFIER

The number of units (receptors) capable of producing stimuli in the organ clearly is a factor in the total stimulus imparted by any concentration of agonist. Thus, the activation of a single receptor by agonist binding yields a quantal amount of stimulation to the response-producing machinery of the cell. This stimulation may take a variety of forms, i.e., receptor occupation, the rate of receptor occupation, a shift in the equilibrium between receptor states. Assuming that the measurements of responses are made from defined response units (i.e., cells, collections of cells, and structured organs [see Chapter 3]), the total stimulus is the sum of the quantal receptor stimuli. Therefore, the higher the number of drug receptors $[R_t]$ is, the larger the receptor stimulus.

Receptor density can vary dramatically, even within a given tissue type. For example, in skeletal muscle end plates, the receptors for tetrodotoxin have a density of $10/\mu m^2$, whereas the density of acetylcholine receptors in the same tissue is several orders of magnitude higher ($10,000/\mu m^2$).

## BIOCHEMICAL MEASUREMENT OF RECEPTOR DENSITY

A common method of measuring receptor density involves radioligand binding experiments. Thus, the total specific radioactive ligand bound to the receptor per milligram of tissue protein yields a measure of receptor density. Although these methods clearly have been of significant value for quantification of receptor effects, caution must be exercised in interpreting radioligand binding data in terms of effects on responses. Examples can be found in which the receptor number correlates well with the tissue response; the relative potencies of oxotremorine on guinea pig and mouse ileum (8 to 1) parallel the numbers for muscarinic receptor densities in these two tissues (7.6 to 1). However, radioligand binding studies measure only receptor presence, whereas response is mediated both by receptor presence and by coupling to stimulus-response apparatus. Therefore, although correspondence between radioligand estimates of receptor density and the potencies of agonists may be found in some systems, it should not be expected. For example, Fig. 2.1 shows the correlation between density of binding sites for a radioligand thought to bind to β-adrenoceptors and the potency of isoproterenol in various tissues. The correlation for normal tissues is rather good ($T = 3.5$; degrees of freedom, d.f. $= 3$), but when animals are treated with reserpine, a drug that produces supersensitivity (increased stimulus-response coupling) to β-adrenoceptor agonists by postjunctional mechanisms (not involving receptor number), the correlation between receptor number and isoproterenol potency is poor. This demonstrates the superseding effects of receptor coupling on tissue sensitivity to agonists and the tenuous dependence of sensitivity on receptor density.

If the receptors measured by radioactive markers are not coupled to response mechanisms, serious dissimilarities can occur. For example, whereas extracellular β-adrenoceptors can be detected in fetal mouse hearts, no response can be elicited by β-adrenoceptor agonists until much later in the cycle of development. In rat uterus, the estrous cycle greatly affects the

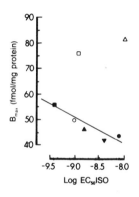

FIG. 2.1. Dependence of tissue sensitivity on receptor density. Ordinate: Maximal density of β-adrenoceptors in fmol/mg protein. Abscissa: Logarithms of molar concentrations of isoproterenol that produce half-maximal responses. Receptor density measured as binding sites for β-adrenoceptor radioligand [$^3$H]IHYP; sensitivity measured in isolated tissues. Data for normal rabbit left ventricle (●), guinea pig left ventricle (▼), guinea pig right atrium (▲), rat uterus (■), and reserpine-pretreated cat right atrium (○), cat left ventricle (□), and cat soleus muscle (△). Regression line for normal tissues $T = 3.5$, d.f. $= 3$, $p < 0.05$; all data $T = 0.25$, d.f. $= 5$, n.s. (Data from ref. 22.)

relative numbers of α- and β-adrenoceptors, but the response characteristics of this tissue do not coincide with the observed changes in receptor numbers (Table 2.1). It is known that for some receptors, a significant uncoupling of the drug recognition site and effector mechanism occurs during desensitization. Thus, radioligand binding experiments that measure receptor density overestimate the numbers of viable receptors capable of producing responses. The ability of receptor coupling to supersede the effects of receptor density is demonstrated in two tissues from the mouse: Whereas mouse thymus has 4.6 times more β-adrenoceptors than does mouse spleen, the spleen is 20 times more sensitive to β-adrenoceptor agonists.

A striking example of where cell ontogeny affects receptor presence and coupling capriciously is the rat cerebral cortex. Figure 2.2 shows the effect of development on cholinergic receptor number and maximal response to the cholinergic agonist carbachol. Whereas the receptor number increases steadily from day 2 to day 40, the maximal response does not follow but rather peaks at day 7. Therefore, receptor binding techniques measuring receptor presence would overestimate the functional importance of muscarinic receptors with development. The relative importance of receptor presence and coupling is dealt with more fully in Chapter 9.

The magnitude of the total tissue receptor number may have no relevance to the tissue response if cell-to-cell coupling is efficient and only small numbers of muscle cells need be activated for a tissue syncytial response. Drug uptake mechanisms can exacerbate this effect if they prevent complete penetration of drug into the tissue matrix and subsequently produce drug concentration gradients within tissues. Concentration gradients (discussed more fully in Chapter 5) often are functions of the routes of entry of drugs into a tissue. For example, theoretical considerations and experimental data indicate that a given concentration of norepinephrine penetrates only an outer shell of smooth-muscle cells in the rat vas deferens when the tissue is exposed

**TABLE 2.1.** *Effects of estrogen treatment on α-adrenoceptors of rabbit uterus*

|  | No treatment | Estradiol[a] treatment |
|---|---|---|
| Norepinephrine log $EC_{50}$[b] | $-6.53 \pm 0.06$ | $-6.52 \pm 0.6$ |
| Maximal response[c] (g) | $2.7 \pm 0.1$ | $2.9 \pm 0.2$ |
| $\alpha_2$-Adrenoceptor density[d] (fmol/mg protein) | $51 \pm 10$ | $291 \pm 38$ |

[a] 0.25 mg/kg$^{-1}$, estradiol valerate in peanut oil i.m. on days 1 and 3.
[b] Logarithm of molar concentration required to produce half-maximal response.
[c] Maximal isometric tension produced by norepinephrine.
[d] As measured by [$^3$H]dihydroergocryptine binding.
Data from Hoffman et al. (11.)

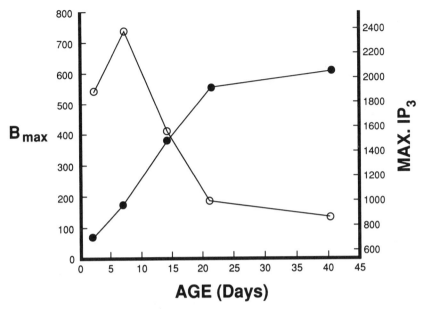

**FIG. 2.2.** The ontogenic effects of muscarinic receptor number and maximal response to carbachol in rat cerebral cortex. Abscissa: Age of rat in days. Right-hand ordinate: Maximal number of muscarinic receptors as measured by [$^3$H]$N$-methylscopolamine binding (•). Left-hand ordinate: Maximal production of inositol triphosphate [IP$_3$] by carbachol in cortical slices expressed as the percentage of basal (o). (From ref. 29.)

to this agonist in an organ bath *in vitro*. Under these circumstances, the conditions of the experiment (*in vitro* incubation with drugs) will bias the outcome of an experiment designed to test the effect of receptor number on tissue response. Specifically, incubation of rat vasa deferentia with the irreversible α-adrenoceptor-blocking agent phenoxybenzamine produces a disproportionately greater decrease in receptors involved in the production of a tissue response *in vitro*, as compared with total tissue receptor number (Fig. 2.3). In this experiment, the alkylating agent preferentially alkylates the outer layer of muscle cells most important to the tissue response; whereas the response depends on this outer core, the total receptor number reflects receptors throughout the tissue, many of which are not involved in contraction under *in vitro* conditions. Under these circumstances, the magnitude of the total tissue receptor density is not relevant to the magnitude of the stimulus imparted to the tissue by an agonist. In general, the ability of receptor coupling to "trump" changes in receptor density and the importance of the fractional tissue mass needed for responses make it hazardous to take radioligand binding data reflecting receptor density and attempt to extrapolate it to tissue responses.

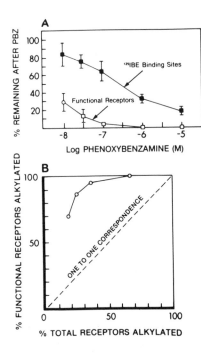

**FIG. 2.3.** Alkylation of total and functional receptors. **A:** Comparison of percentage of α-adrenoceptors after incubation of rat vas deferens with phenoxybenzamine in an organ bath. Ordinate: Percentage of α-adrenoceptors not alkylated by phenoxybenzamine. Abscissa: Logarithms of molar concentrations of phenoxybenzamine incubated with tissues for 10 min. Number of total tissue α-adrenoceptors as measured by radioligand binding of $^{125}$IBE (■) and functional α-adrenoceptors used for contraction *in vitro* (□). The latter quantities were measured by the method of Furchgott (see Chapter 7). **B:** Correlations between percentages of total receptors alkylated and functional receptors alkylated by phenoxybenzamine. Calculated from A. (Data from ref. 23.)

## RELATIONSHIP BETWEEN STIMULUS AND RESPONSE: THE POWER AMPLIFIER

It has long been known that the tissue response often is a nonlinear function of receptor occupancy. For example, insulin produces glucose oxidation in fat cells at receptor occupancies well below receptor saturation (Fig. 2.4). Although such a relationship was described in theoretical terms by Stephenson, studies with irreversible drug-receptor antagonists provided the first

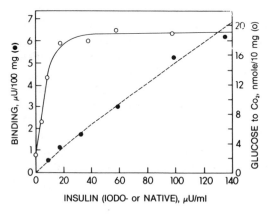

**FIG. 2.4.** Dependence of binding and rate of glucose oxidation on insulin concentration in fat cells. Ordinates: binding of iodoinsulin in μU/100 mg fat cells (●); rate of glucose metabolism by cells (○). Abscissa: Concentration of insulin in μU/mL. (From ref. 21.)

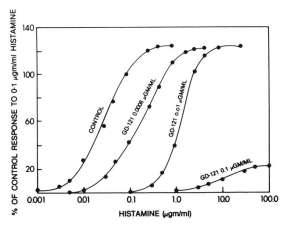

**FIG. 2.5.** Concentration-response curves for histamine on guinea pig ileum. Ordinate: Percentage of control response to 0.1 $\mu$g/mL$^{-1}$ histamine. Abscissa: Logarithms of concentrations of histamine. Responses before (control) and after irreversible alkylation of histamine receptors by GD-121. (From ref. 26.)

experimental data to suggest that the relationship between agonist-receptor occupancy and tissue response may not always be linear. Thus, irreversible alkylation of fractions of the available receptors resulted in a tissue that was still capable of producing the maximal response to powerful drugs (Fig. 2.5). The implication was that because a fraction of the available receptors was irreversibly inactivated and the tissue still produced the maximal response, only the remaining fraction of receptors was required to be activated to

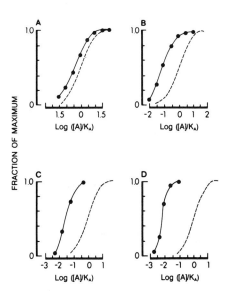

**FIG. 2.6.** Relationships between receptor occupancy and concentration-response curve. Ordinates: Fractional maximal response or receptor occupancy. Abscissae: Logarithms of molar concentrations of agonists normalized as fractions of the $K_A$. *Solid line* represents response; *broken line* represents calculated receptor occupancy. **A:** Phenylephrine in rabbit papillary muscle. (Data from ref. 33.) **B:** Norepinephrine in rabbit aorta. (Data from ref. 3.) **C:** Carbachol in guinea pig ileum. (Data from ref. 7.) **D:** Acetylcholine in guinea pig ileum. (Data from ref. 31.)

produce the maximal response. Thus, the irreversibly inactivated portion of the receptor population was "spare" or unnecessary for production of the maximal response. With the advent of null procedures to measure agonist-receptor equilibrium dissociation constants (see Chapter 7), further experimental evidence has accumulated that demonstrates disparities between tissue response and receptor occupancy (Fig. 2.6). Thus, it is clear that many tissues amplify receptor stimuli in the production of responses; this amplification is made evident in nonlinear stimulus-response curves.

## STIMULUS-RESPONSE CURVES AND "SPARE RECEPTORS"

For a great many drugs, a regression of percentage stimulus on percentage organ response is clearly nonlinear. Figure 2.7 shows such regressions for a range of cholinergic and adrenergic agonists in different tissues. The hyperbolic nature of these relationships illustrates a general phenomenon, namely, that many drugs are more powerful than they need be (at least when responses are measured *in vitro*), in that maximal responses can be produced with generation of submaximal stimuli (submaximal receptor occupancy). This phenomenon has been given the general name "receptor reserve" (spare receptors, spare capacity), but this term can be ambiguous from two standpoints. The first problem is one of definition. Under the condition of a nonlinear stimulus-response relationship (*vide infra*), the magnitude of the receptor reserve is dependent on the level of response measured. As originally defined, the receptor reserve is the fraction of the total receptor pool not required for a maximal tissue response. Figure 2.8 shows the relationship be-

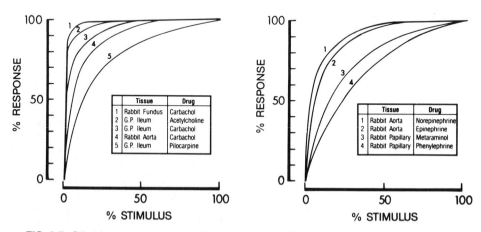

**FIG. 2.7.** Stimulus-response curves for muscarinic and α-adrenoceptor agonists in some tissues. Sources of muscarinic receptor data **(left):** 1, ref. 7; 2, ref. 31; 3 and 4, ref. 8. Sources of α-adrenoceptor data **(right):** 1 and 2, ref. 3; 3, ref. 32; 4, ref. 33.

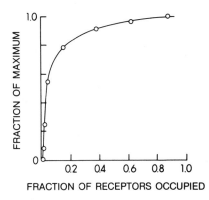

**FIG. 2.8.** Response of rabbit aorta to norepinephrine as a function of receptor occupancy. Ordinate: Response as a fraction of maximal response to norepinephrine. Abscissa: Fractional receptor occupancy. (From ref. 3.)

tween α-adrenoceptor occupancy for norepinephrine in rabbit aorta and response. It can be seen from this figure that virtually all of the receptors are required for maximal response (no receptor reserve as originally defined), but only 5% are required for half-maximal response. Thus, even though there is no receptor reserve for maximal response, there is a very large reserve for half-maximal response. Because of such ambiguities, it is more appropriate to refer to nonlinear stimulus-response relationships rather than receptor reserves. In cases in which quantification of "reserves" is useful, or, more correctly, quantification of efficiency of coupling, one approach is to compare the concentrations of agonist required for half-maximal response and half-maximal receptor occupancy. Unlike the reserve for maximal response, which is difficult to quantify experimentally, this ratio can be readily estimated by comparison of semilogarithmic occupancy-response and concentration-response curves. The magnitudes of the effective receptor reserves for the drugs and tissues in Fig. 2.6 are shown in Table 2.2. It will be seen

**TABLE 2.2.** *Effective receptor reserves for agonists in selected tissues*

| Tissue | Drug | $-\log EC_{50}$[a] | $-\log K_A$[b] | Reserve[c] |
|--------|------|------------------|---------------|-----------|
| Rabbit | Phenylephrine | 6.03 | 5.5 | 3.4 |
| Rabbit aorta | Norepinephrine | 7.9 | 6.47 | 21 |
| Guinea pig ileum | Carbachol | 6.5 | 4.92 | 38 |
| Guinea pig ileum | Acetylcholine | 7.23 | 5.1 | 398 |

[a] Negative logarithm of molar concentration producing half-maximal response.
[b] Negative logarithm of molar concentration producing half-maximal receptor occupancy.
[c] $K_A \div EC_{50}$; refers to the ratio between number of receptors in tissue and that needed for half-maximal response.
Data from graphs shown in Fig. 2.6.

in Chapter 8 that these quantities can be directly related to relative intrinsic efficacies of agonists.

Second, the term "receptor reserve" connotes a property of a tissue, when in fact the phenomenon is dependent on both the tissue and the drug. This is because it is the intrinsic efficacy of the drug that determines the response at any given receptor occupancy, not the number of receptors in the tissue. Figure 2.9 shows clearly the differences in receptor reserve in rat anococcygeus muscle for the $\alpha$-adrenoceptor agonists norepinephrine and oxymetazoline. Thus, whereas 95% of the receptors are spare with respect to production of a half-maximal response by norepinephrine, a somewhat greater percentage is required by oxymetazoline (87% are spare). Similarly, 30% are not needed for production of a tissue maximal response by norepinephrine, and 17% are extraneous with respect to a maximal response by oxymetazoline. Thus, to refer to a given tissue as having a cholinergic receptor reserve is not meaningful, because the tissue may have a reserve for acetylcholine, but not for the weaker muscarinic agonist pilocarpine; i.e., one drug's spare receptor is another drug's essential receptor.

It is also known that physiological conditions and pathological states can affect membrane receptor density. The changes in receptor number, transducer coupling protein levels, and sensitivity of stimulus-response mechanisms with aging have been studied for many tissue types. Pathology also can alter receptor number and tissue sensitivity to agonists. Figure 2.10 shows the response of human cardiac tissue to isoproterenol expressed as a function of receptor occupancy. As with the tissues shown in Fig. 2.7, the steeper the hyperbolic function is between occupancy and response, the more efficient the coupling is between the receptor and the stimulus-response mechanisms in the tissue. The data in Fig. 2.10 are taken from humans with progressively more severe conditions of congestive heart failure. Whereas nearly normal cardiac tissue has a significant effective receptor reserve for isoproterenol (filled circles), this collapses to a *linear* relationship in patients with severe (class IV) heart failure. This indicates a loss in the efficiency

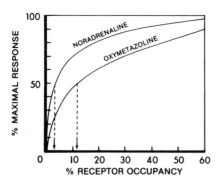

FIG. 2.9. Relative receptor reserve for norepinephrine and oxymetazoline in rat anococcygeus muscle. Ordinate: Response as a fraction of the maximal response to norepinephrine. Abscissa: Receptor occupancy as a fraction of maximal occupancy. (From ref. 14.)

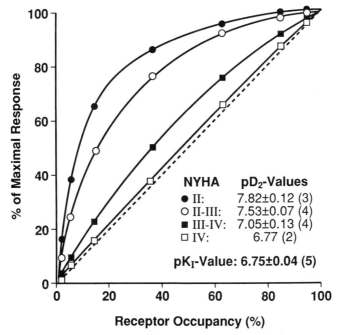

**FIG. 2.10.** Receptor occupancy versus tissue response for isoproterenol in human iso-lated, electrically driven right atria. Abscissa: Percentage of receptor occupancy for iso-proterenol. Ordinate: Positive inotropic response expressed as a percentage of the maxi-mal response to isoproterenol. Data from patients with aortic valve disease in various stages of heart failure: New York Heart Association (NYHA) class II heart failure (●), class II,III heart failure (○), class III,IV heart failure (■), and class IV heart failure (□). (From ref. 5.)

of receptor coupling of β-adrenoceptors with this disease. Such changes in receptor-coupling capability can cause pronounced changes in agonist sensi-tivity especially for low-efficacy agonists. In these cases agonist efficacy may become insignificant and leave only receptor antagonism. This would be problematic during therapeutic agonist treatment.

## INHERENT POWER OF STIMULUS-RESPONSE MECHANISMS

A range of isolated tissues containing pharmacologically identical drug receptors subserving the same type of response can vary dramatically in terms of sensitivities to drugs. For example, Fig. 2.11 shows the sensitivity of aorta to norepinephrine in four different species; a potency range of 390 is obtained. Clearly, one possible explanation for such effects concerns dif-ferences in receptor numbers; i.e., rat aorta may have 390 times the α-adre-noceptor-receptor density of guinea pig aorta. Another more subtle differ-ence may lie in the inherent amplification capabilities of the different tissues.

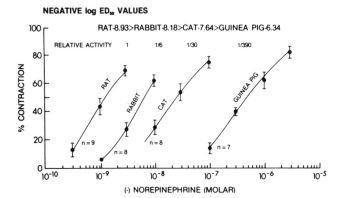

**FIG. 2.11.** Sensitivities of aortae from various species to norepinephrine. Ordinate: Contraction as a percentage of maximal contraction. Abscissa: Logarithms of molar concentrations of norepinephrine. (From ref. 27.)

The elements that determine the amplification factor relate to the nature of mechanisms, the saturability of each element in the mechanism, and the number of saturable elements in the total process. The concept of saturability is important to the amplification of receptor stimuli. If a given agonist-receptor complex modifies a second dynamic process, and if that process (or subsequent processes) becomes the rate-limiting step in the succession of mechanisms to the tissue response, then the concentration of agonist producing the half-maximal response will underestimate the true equilibrium dissociation constant of the agonist-receptor complex. Thus, the dose-response curve for the agonist will lie to the left of the occupancy-response curve; i.e., amplification occurs.

An interesting demonstration of differences in the way in which tissues process initial stimuli can be seen in cardiac tissue where calcium entry via gated calcium channels mediates cardiac contraction. Figure 2.12 shows the intracellular levels of calcium (as measured by the calcium-sensitive bioluminescent protein aequorin) and the isometric twitch contraction in four species of cardiac muscle. The diversity in the relationship between the relative strengths of the calcium signals and the tissue response across species is evident.

One saturable step produces nonlinearity in the stimulus-response relationship. More than one such step introduces a disproportionately greater degree of nonlinearity, because the amplified product of one step is further amplified by the succeeding steps. An example of such multiplicity is shown in Fig. 2.13. Clearly, the greater the number of saturable steps, the greater the amplification. An example of subsequent cellular processes producing sequential amplification can be found in the muscarinic responses of rabbit bladder. As shown in Fig. 2.14, the broken line denoting receptor occupancy by carba-

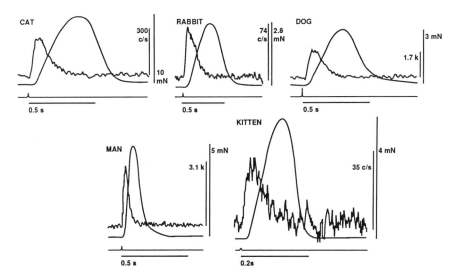

**FIG. 2.12.** Relationships between the intracellular calcium signals and mechanical responses of isolated right ventricular papillary muscles from various species. Levels of intracellular calcium (as measured by aequorin luminescence) shown as noisy tracings; mechanical isometric twitch contractions shown as smooth curves. Lower trace shows electrical stimulus artifact. All preparations stimulated at 1 Hz and equilibrated at 37°C. (From ref. 24.)

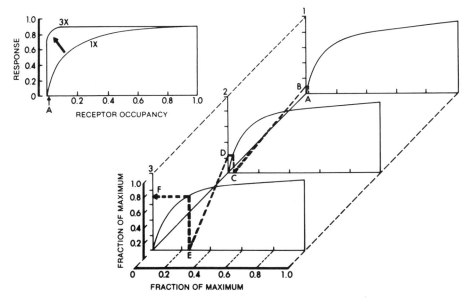

**FIG. 2.13.** Effects of sequential hyperbolic responses on overall response. Ordinate: Fraction of maximal response for each process. Abscissa: Molar concentration of substrate for each reaction. The product of each reaction becomes the starting material for the succeeding reaction. **Inset:** Relationship between concentration of starting material and overall end product; a threefold amplification occurs because of the series sequence of saturable nonlinear reactions.

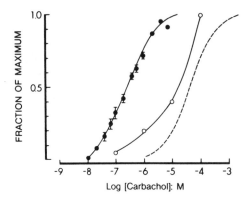

FIG. 2.14. Effects of carbachol on receptor occupancy, calcium uptake, and contractile response in rabbit bladder. Ordinate: Fraction of maximal response. Abscissa: Logarithms of molar concentrations of carbachol. Receptor occupancy in *broken line*: uptake of radioactive calcium (○, $N = 6$) and contractile response (●, $N = 8$). (Data from ref. 1.)

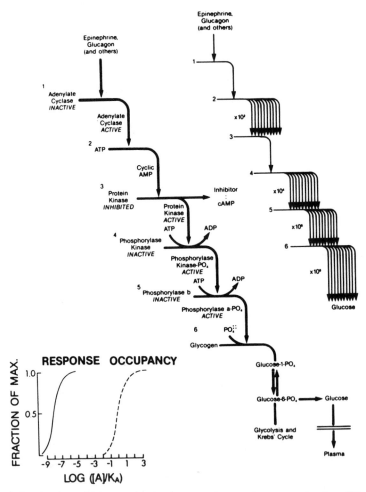

FIG. 2.15. Production of glucose by β-adrenoceptor or glucagon-receptor stimulation. **Inset:** A magnification factor of eight orders of magnitude is produced by the cascade of reactions. (From ref. 9.)

chol lies to the right of the curve denoting calcium uptake by the tissue. There is evidence that one of the first consequences of muscarinic receptor stimulation is entry of extracellular calcium ion. The concentration-response curve, response being the end product of the process mediated by the extracellular calcium, lies farther to the left of the calcium-uptake curve, demonstrating a further amplification. A very large amplification factor (i.e., eight orders of magnitude) can be achieved by a cascade of saturable steps. Figure 2.15 shows such a cascade that produces glucose by β-adrenoceptor- or glucagon-receptor stimulation.

In human neutrophils, activation of formyl peptide receptors results in formation of superoxide, and this response is blocked by activation of β-adrenoceptors. It has been shown that activation of one β-adrenoceptor results in a 100-fold increase in the GTPase activity of the $G_s$ coupling protein to that receptor and that each receptor may generate as many as 10,000 molecules of cyclic AMP (25). Thus, approximately 500 occupied β-adrenoceptors can completely block superoxide production generated by 50,000 occupied formyl peptide receptors in this tissue.

Not only can the receptors of different tissues from different species be coupled with varying efficiency, different cellular processes within even the same cell can be differentially coupled. For example, in guinea pig left atria, elevations of intracellular cyclic AMP produce positive inotropy (via calcium entry through calcium channels) and an increased rate of relaxation (via phosphorylation of the calcium pump on the sarcoplasmic reticulum). However, equilibration of atria with the membrane-permeable analogue dibutyl cyclic AMP shows that the relaxation response to this second messenger is four times more sensitive than the inotropic response (Fig. 2.16). The rele-

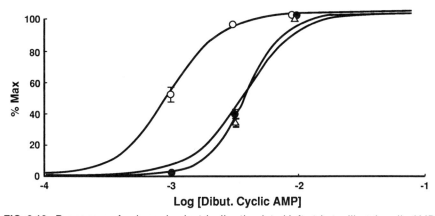

**FIG. 2.16.** Responses of guinea pig electrically stimulated left atria to dibutyl cyclic AMP. Ordinate: Response expressed as a percentage of the maximal response to forskolin in the same preparation. Abscissa: Logarithms of molar concentrations of dibutyl (Dibut.) cyclic AMP. Diastolic relaxation (o) and positive inotropy measured at peak time (•) and after 90 min (Δ) from nine atria. (From ref. 20.)

vance of such differential coupling to receptor classification and selective agonist responses is discussed in Chapter 11.

## Nature of Stimulus-Response Mechanisms

The complexity of stimulus-response mechanisms makes them difficult to delineate and study, but some mechanisms have been shown to amplify chemical signs. A fundamentally saturable process could occur at the site of drug-receptor interaction, namely, the cell membrane. If the hormone-receptor complex diffuses within the planar surface of the cell membrane and collides with a transducer protein to produce a ternary complex (and, subsequently, a response), then the equilibrium dissociation constant of the ternary complex can significantly affect the amplification factor of the stimulus-response mechanism; the molecular sequence is shown in Fig. 2.17A.

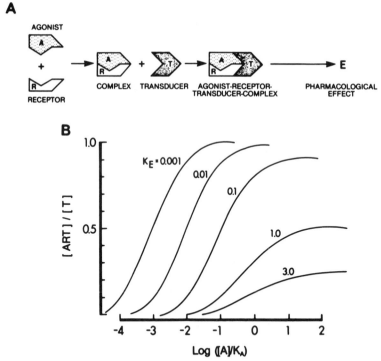

**FIG. 2.17.** Amplification by production of a ternary complex. **A:** Schematic of elements that compose the ternary complex of hormone, receptor, and transducer protein. (From ref. 4.) **B:** Dependence of production of a ternary complex on hormone concentration. Ordinate: Ternary complex as a fraction of maximum. Abscissa: Logarithms of molar concentrations of drug as fractions of $K_A$. Curves represent fractional production of ternary complex for designated equilibrium dissociation constants of transducer-protein-receptor complex ($K_E$). Calculated from Eq. 2.2.

Thus, the quantity of ternary complex ($[ART]$) can be calculated as

$$\frac{[ART]}{[T]} = \frac{[A \cdot R]}{[A \cdot R] + K_E} \qquad [2.1]$$

where $K_E$ is the equilibrium dissociation constant of the ternary complex and $[T]$ is the transducer protein complex. Calculation of $[A \cdot R]$ from Eq. 1.4 leads to

$$\frac{[ART]}{[T]} = \left[1 - K_E \left(1 + \frac{K_A}{[A]}\right)\right]^{-1} \qquad [2.2]$$

It can be seen from Eq. 2.4 that if $K_E$ is very low, large quantities of ternary complex will result from relatively small quantities of $[A \cdot R]$; Fig. 2.17B shows the amplifications for various ratios of $K_E/K_A$.

At the level of a single cell, amplification can occur if the product of an agonist-receptor complex serves as a cofactor or catalyst for some ongoing cellular process. Under these circumstances, one drug-receptor complex can yield a great deal of secondary product if that complex serves to activate an enzyme that has sufficient substrate. Another type of amplification can occur if the immediate product of the drug-receptor complex acts as a trigger for a further cascade, as in the production of a small amount of accumulated intracellular "trigger calcium" produced by inhibitors of $Na^+$-$K^+$ ATPase that cause release of far greater amounts of calcium from myocardial sarco-plasmic reticulum for cardiac contraction. In some cases, the drug-receptor complex serves as an activator for cellular enzymes such as adenyl cyclase, which then can produce a second messenger (cyclic AMP). One complex activating one enzyme then is capable of producing a relatively large quantity of cyclic AMP for the response. The entry of ions via channels opened by drugs suggests an analogous situation in which the intracellular ions may affect membrane potential and therefore subsequent channel opening and response. Parenthetically, under these circumstances, arithmetic summation of receptor stimuli may be invalid.

The production of a second messenger such as calcium, cyclic AMP, or cyclic GMP is a relatively common occurrence in physiological systems. By their very nature, such processes can lead to amplification. A simple model of production of a second messenger leads to the following relationship between the true $K_A$ that determines drug-receptor binding and the observed concentration producing a half-maximal response (apparent $K_A$):

$$K_{apparent} = \left[\frac{K/(\alpha \cdot R_t)}{[K/(\alpha \cdot R_t)] + 1}\right] \cdot K_A \qquad [2.3]$$

where $K$ is the equilibrium dissociation constant for the intracellular mediator and the intracellular receptor, $\alpha$ is a proportionality constant reflecting the size of the pool of intracellular messenger, and $R_t$ is the total number of extracellular receptors for the agonist. It can be seen from Eq. 2.3 that if the size of the intracellular messenger pool is large or the number of extracellular receptors is large relative to the equilibrium dissociation constant of the messenger for the site of activation, then the apparent $K_A$ will be substantially smaller than the true $K_A$; i.e., concentrations of agonist producing relatively small extracellular receptor occupancies will produce disparately large quantities of intracellular messenger and presumably correspondingly large tissue responses. The effects of decreasing values of $K/(\alpha \cdot R_t)$ (large pools or large extracellular receptor numbers with respect to the $K$ for intracellular activation) are shown in Fig. 2.18.

Stimulus amplification can occur directly at the receptor level in systems that possess a memory for the stimulus. For example, the insulin-dependent tyrosine kinase activity of insulin receptors remains even after insulin dissociates from the receptor, most likely because of autophosphorylation. Amplification also can occur for transducer protein-linked receptors. For example, some receptors activate G proteins to promote the exchange of guanosine diphosphate (GDP) for guanosine triphosphate (GTP). Once this occurs the G protein remains activated and able stimulate effectors until an intrinsic GTPase activity hydrolyzes the GTP back to GDP. This second step has a longer time span than most agonist-receptor interactions (ranging from 1 to 15 $\min^{-1}$), thereby bestowing a memory to the system for agonist activation. Under these circumstances, considerable amplification of a receptor signal can be achieved.

Tissues have two opposing needs for optimal efficiency, namely, to be able to respond to very low concentrations of agonist and also to have sensitive control of the time course of response (temporal responsiveness) (36). Stimulus-response mechanisms can control the sensitivity of systems to agonists and also the time course of drug effect. Tissues can be made sensitive to low concentrations of agonists by increasing the number of responding units (receptors). Temporal sensitivity (i.e., mechanisms to remove the stimulus when the agonist is removed from the receptor compartment) can be obtained

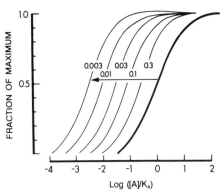

**FIG. 2.18.** Concentration-response curves for a drug that releases an intracellular second messenger. Ordinate: Receptor occupancy by *A* for the extracellular membrane receptor (*heavy line*) or production of intracellular second messenger as a fraction of the maximum. Abscissa: Logarithms of molar concentrations of *A* as fractions of $K_A$ for extracellular membrane receptor. Numbers on curves represent various values of $K/[\alpha \cdot R_t]$ (see Eq. 2.3).

by reducing the affinity of the agonist for the receptor. Thus, a neurotransmitter can be released into a restricted compartment (i.e., synaptic cleft) to achieve high local concentrations and act on a high density of receptors for which it has low affinity. For example, acetylcholine has a low affinity for the receptors in the frog neuromuscular junction, but the receptor density is extremely high (i.e., 20,000 receptors/$\mu m^2$). Clearly, a low affinity of the agonist for the receptor would decrease tissue sensitivity to the agonist, but amplification mechanisms in the cell can buffer the need for high agonist-receptor occupancy. Therefore, the activation of a small number of receptors could produce a large response. Such a system would be temporally sensitive since small changes in receptor occupancy would lead to larger changes in tissue response.

The sensitivity of systems can be enhanced by increasing the affinity of the agonist for the receptor (i.e., decrease the rate of offset of the agonist from the receptor). However, the cost of such increased sensitivity could be a loss of temporal responsiveness, i.e., when the transmitter is removed from the receptor compartment, the signal is not removed with it. A further drawback can be observed in receptor G-protein systems in which the agonist-activated receptor diffuses in the membrane to a transducer protein, which then carries the agonist message. If the agonist-receptor complex is long-lived, this increases the likelihood of unproductive collisions between activated receptors and already activated transducer proteins.

## SELECTIVE RECEPTOR COUPLING AND INTRACELLULAR COMPARTMENTALIZATION

An interesting and not well-understood area of receptor pharmacology is the apparent selective coupling of certain receptor populations to certain functions and the apparent compartmentalization of intracellular messenger pools. For example, the rat adipocyte contains two subtypes of $\beta$-adrenoceptor ($\beta_1$- and so-called "atypical" $\beta_3$-adrenoceptors). Most of the lipolytic response to the atypical $\beta$-adrenoceptor agonist BRL 37344 is mediated by only 15% of the total $\beta$-adrenoceptor mixture of $\beta_1$- and $\beta_3$-adrenoceptors. Thus, it appears that in this cell type a relatively small proportion of the total population selectively controls the cellular response. The selectivity appears to occur at the level of the second-messenger allocation. Figure 2.19A shows the lipolytic responses and cyclic AMP responses to isoproterenol and BRL 37344. From this figure it can be seen that BRL 37344 is a more potent lipolytic agonist but a less potent producer of intracellular cyclic AMP. Figure 2.19B shows that the cyclic AMP generated by activation of $\beta_3$-adrenoceptors (by BRL 37344) produces proportionately greater lipolysis than the cyclic AMP generated by activation of $\beta_1$-adrenoceptors (isoproterenol). Thus, it appears that one receptor population in this cell is more efficiently

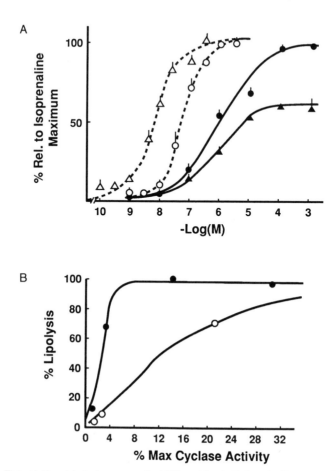

**FIG. 2.19.** The relationship between cyclic AMP and lipolysis in rat adipocytes. **A:** Lipolysis (o, ∆) and cyclic AMP production (•, ▲) in rat adipocytes and adipocyte ghosts. Data shown for isoproterenol (•, o) and the atypical β-adrenoceptor agonist BRL 37344 (▲, ∆). All data expressed as a percentage of the maximum to isoproterenol. Although BRL 37344 is a less potent and efficacious producer of cyclic AMP, it is a more potent lipolytic. **B:** The relative utilization of cyclic AMP by adipocytes as produced by isoproterenol (o) and BRL 37344 (•). The conversion of cyclic AMP into a lipolytic response is more efficient for BRL 37344 than for isoproterenol. (From ref. 12.)

coupled to the response mechanism than another at the level of the second messenger.

It can be assumed that the mobile receptors on the cell membrane have free access to coupling mechanisms and thereby transmit information to the cytosol. Second messengers such as cyclic AMP, cyclic GMP, and calcium are generated in the cytosol and utilized in biochemical processes. The simplest assumption to make would be that intracellular messengers freely diffuse within the cytosol and have access to all structures therein. However, cells are not empty spheres of cytosol but rather highly structured bodies with lattices and other structures within. Also, if there are removal mechanisms for the messengers present in the cell, then the relative proximity of these to the sites of messenger utilization may further compartmentalize the cell. This is shown schematically in Fig. 2.20A, where the two processes of cardiac inotropy and relaxation are depicted as the result of the effects of increased intracellular cyclic AMP emanating from a single pool. However, this second messenger diffuses throughout the cytoplasm where it is hydrolyzed by degradative mechanisms such as the enzyme phosphodiesterase. The extent of degradation is determined by the rate of diffusion in the catabolic compartment ($k_t$), the Michaelis-Menten constant for enzyme activation ($K_m$) and the maximal rate of cyclic AMP hydrolysis ($V_{max}$). For example, the differential equation for the presentation of the second messenger ($[C_b]$) to a compartment is given by:

$$\frac{d[C_b]}{dt}(+) = k_t([C_a] - [C_b]) \qquad [2.4]$$

However, within this compartment is a catabolic saturable removal process for the second messenger described by Michaelis-Menten kinetics:

$$\frac{d[C_b]}{dt}(-) = \frac{[C_b] \cdot V_{max}}{[C_b] + K_m} \qquad [2.5]$$

At steady-state, the respective rates of presentation and removal are equal (equate 2.4 and 2.5) and the concentration of second messenger in the compartment (as a multiple of the $K_m$ for removal, $[C_b]/K_m$) is given by:

$$[C_b]/K_m = \frac{1/2([C_b]/K_m - (V_{max}/k_t \cdot K_m) - 1)}{1/2\sqrt{(1 + (V_{max}/k_t \cdot K_m) - ([C_a]/K_m)^2 + 4[C_a]/K_m)}} \qquad [2.6]$$

From this equation it can be seen that differences in second-messenger concentration at the site of production ($[C_a]$) and site of utilization ($[C_b]$) can be produced by the combination of slow diffusion (small $k_t$) or a sensitive (low $K_m$) removal mechanism of high maximal rate (high $V_{max}$). These factors are encompassed by the magnitude of the term $V_{max}/K_m \cdot k_t$. Within the cytoplasm of a cell there could be selective diffusion barriers (i.e., nonuniform $k_t$ values for regions of the cytoplasm) and localized (perhaps membrane-bound) degradative enzymes. This would lead to different values of $V_{max}/K_m \cdot k_t$ throughout the cell with corresponding differences in $[C_b]/[C_a]$ in different regions of the cell. These differences in second-messenger concentration could lead to differences in cellular function. Figure 2.20B shows the relationship of $[C_b]$ to $[C_a]$ according to Eq. 2.8 for various values of $V_{max}/K_m \cdot k_t$. As can be seen from this figure, as the removal mechanism becomes capable of removing the messenger and thus depleting $[C_b]$, differences in second-messenger concentration at the site of production ($[C_a]$ and utiliza-

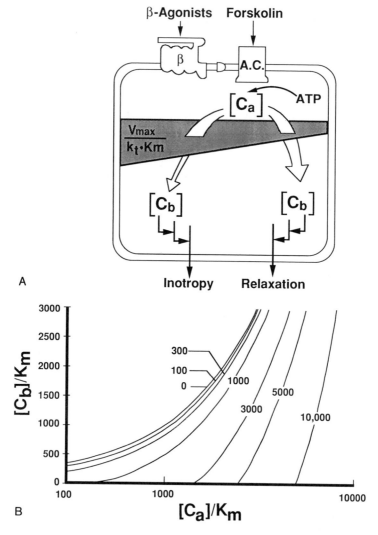

**FIG. 2.20.** A general model for the differential distribution of cyclic AMP concentrations within a cardiac cell. **A:** Cross-section of a cell showing the internal structure. **B:** Schematic depiction of a cardiac cell in which activation of membrane β-adrenoceptors or forskolin directly produces a focus of production of intracellular cyclic AMP (concentration $[C_a]$). Thus $[C_a]$ diffuses into the cytosol with a diffusion constant $k_t$ where it can be degraded by phosphodiesterase with specific $K_m$ and $V_{max}$ values. The impedance to a given concentration $[C_a]$ in the receptor compartment is directly proportional to $V_{max}/K_m \cdot k_t$. The concentrations of cyclic AMP $[C_b]$ participate in various biochemical processes such as inotropy and diastolic relaxation. **C:** Relationship between $[C_a]$ produced at the cell membrane and $[C_b]$ in the cytosol with various levels of $k_t/K_m \cdot V_{max}$ (shown next to the curves). Abscissa: Molar concentrations of $[C_a]$ expressed as fractions of the $K_m$ for degradation. (From ref. 20.)

tion ($[C_b]$) may occur. Also, there is a steeper relationship between $[C_a]$ and $[C_b]$ as removal becomes more important.

Such effective compartmentalization makes it difficult to equate total cell second-messenger levels and function. For example, β-adrenoceptor stimulation and consequent elevations in intracellular cyclic AMP in cardiac cells results in an inotropic response. However, prostaglandin $E_1$ is known to elevate intracellular cyclic AMP in cardiac muscle, but these elevations do *not* result in mechanical responses (10). It could be postulated that the relative locations of β-adrenoceptors and receptors for prostaglandin $E_1$ on the cell membrane result in different foci of cyclic AMP production and that cytoplasmic compartmentalization makes the prostaglandin-dependent cyclic AMP inaccessible to inotropic mechanisms.

## MATHEMATICAL APPROXIMATION OF STIMULUS-RESPONSE MECHANISMS

The nonlinear stimulus-response relationships found experimentally can be approximated mathematically. One of the most flexible relationships between occupancy and response is the general logistic function. The rationale for the use of this equation is based on the frequent observation that receptor occupancy and tissue response is linked by a hyperbolic function. Under these conditions, a general relationship between receptor occupancy (ρ) and tissue response ($R$) is given by:

$$R = \frac{\rho^n}{\rho^n + \beta} \qquad [2.7]$$

where β is a fitting parameter the magnitude of which is inversely proportional to the efficiency of receptor coupling to stimulus-response mechanisms. As can be seen from this equation, the lower the value of β, the steeper the relationship is between receptor occupancy and tissue response (i.e., the more efficient is receptor coupling).

It should be noted that there are two components to the parameter β, namely, a *tissue* component, which quantifies the efficiency of the various biochemical processes that link cellular response with the amount of receptor stimulus, and an *agonist* component, which is specific for the drug and characterizes the "power" of the drug to induce receptor stimulus. It is useful to differentiate these two aspects of agonism since the former can be a useful characterization of tissue systems (i.e., the efficiency of receptor coupling for a given tissue) and the latter can be a useful characterization of agonists (i.e., intrinsic efficacy [see Chapter 8]). It is worth considering these two aspects of stimulus-response coupling in terms of two commonly used drug-receptor theories, the operational model of drug action and occupation theory.

Within the framework of the operational model of drug action (Chapter 1), $\beta$ is equal to $\tau^{-1}$ where $\tau$ is the ratio $K_E/[R_t]$. The term $K_E$ is defined as the quantity of ternary complex required for half-maximal tissue response and $[R_t]$ is the total receptor density. The term $\beta$ is small when $[R_t]$ is large (i.e., the receptor density is high) or when little receptor stimulation is required to activate cellular response mechanisms (i.e., small $K_E$). The fitting parameter $n$ in Eq. 2.7 allows systems in which the dose-response curves to the agonist cannot be fit by the rectangular hyperbola (i.e., Hill coefficients less than or greater than unity). It can be seen that $K_E$ is a tissue *and* a drug-related parameter for agonism encompassing both the efficiency of the tissue in converting the receptor signal into a tissue response and the power of the agonist to produce the receptor signal. There are circumstances in which the drug-specific aspects of agonism can be further subdivided into a term $K_{AR}$, the equilibrium dissociation constant of the ternary complex for G protein–linked membrane receptors and a tissue factor. Under these conditions, the operational model could subdivide the tissue contribution to receptor coupling (defined as a term $K_E'$, the apparent dissociation constant of the summed hyperbolic functions relating the amount of ternary complex to tissue response) and $K_{AR}$. Thus, the term $K_E$ in Eq. 2.7 would equal $K_{AR} \cdot K_E'$.

In terms of receptor occupation theory, the fitting constant $\beta$ encompasses the various stimulus-response steps between receptor occupancy and tissue response, agonist efficacy, and receptor density. Within the term $\beta$ would be a purely tissue-related constant of receptor coupling (a fitting parameter denoted $\beta'$), which would be unique to the tissue and represent the efficiency of receptor coupling for *all* agonists in that tissue. The other tissue factor would be $[R_t]$. The drug-specific aspect of agonism would be described by the intrinsic efficacy ($\epsilon$) of the agonist. Therefore, the term $\beta$ in Eq. 2.7 would be defined as being equal to $\beta'/([R_t] \cdot \epsilon)$.

The importance of Eq. 2.7 is related to the ability of converting receptor occupancy, as defined by the Langmuir adsorption isotherm, into tissue response in a systematic manner. The magnitude of $\beta$ can be manipulated to define the relationship between receptor occupancy and tissue response and thus the power of agonists and tissues to convert drug-receptor complex formation into a cellular signal. There are two specific applications for Eq. 2.7 to experimental results. The first relates to the modeling of responses to a range of drugs in one tissue. In this case, single estimates of $\beta'$ and $n$ should be sufficient to model all agonist responses in a given tissue, provided that accurate estimates of $K_A$ and relative $\epsilon$ are known for the agonists. A classic example of this type of approach is the modeling of guinea pig ileal responses to trimethylammonium compounds by Stephenson. In this case, the rectangular hyperbola $[R = S/(S + 1)]$ in Stephenson's terminology was used as the model for the stimulus-response relationship (see Fig. 1.9B). This is a specific form of Eq. 2.7 where $n = 1$ and $S = \rho \cdot [R_t] \cdot \epsilon$. Therefore the term

$\beta$ in Eq. 2.7 is equal to $(\epsilon \cdot [R_t])^{-1}$. An example of this application is shown in Fig. 2.21.

Another application of the general logistic function (Eq. 2.7) is the characterization of the efficiency of stimulus-response mechanisms in various tissues. The implications of such an approach are considerable in view of the predictive value of constants characterizing the efficiency of receptor coupling in various organs. This, in turn, could be useful for predicting organ responses to partial agonists of low efficacies (see Chapter 8). Figure 2.22 shows data points for the agonist actions of isoproterenol and prenalterol on three different isolated tissues fit with curves predicted by assigning specific values of $\beta$ (Eq. 2.7) for each tissue. Under these circumstances, the greater amplification of stimuli in rat left atria, as compared to the guinea pig extensor digitorum longus, is reflected in the steeper occupancy-response curve for the former tissue (lower receptor occupancy yields large response); this is modeled by a lower value of $\beta$ (1.0 versus 20). Theoretically, the fitting parameter $\beta$ assigned to these tissues should reflect the response of these tissues to all $\beta$-adrenoceptor agonists, provided that $K_A$ (to determine receptor occupancy) and relative efficacy are known. The parameter $\beta$ simply sets the level of the power amplifier.

In terms of the operational model, the same approach to fitting a family of curves can be achieved by manipulating the magnitude of $\tau$. As shown in Fig. 1.12, the relative agonist effects of isoproterenol and prenalterol can be modeled by assuming a constant agonist-specific relative efficacy ($K_{AR}$ in terms of the production of a ternary complex of the $\beta$-adrenoceptor-occupied ternary complex) and varying the magnitude of $[R_t]$.

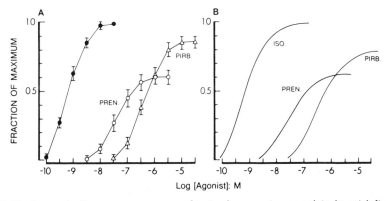

**FIG. 2.21.** Concentration-response curves for $\beta$-adrenoceptor agonists in rat left atria: experimental and calculated. Ordinate: Response as a fraction of the maximal response to isoproterenol. Abscissa: Logarithms of molar concentrations of agonists. **A:** Experimental data of Kenakin and Beek (18,19). **B:** Data in A calculated from experimental estimates of $K_A$ and relative efficacy and Eq. 2.7 setting $\beta = 0.01$. One estimate of $\beta$, a tissue constant, fits data for all three agonists. Experimental parameters: isoproterenol, $K_A = 0.02$ μM; prenalterol, $K_A = 79$ nM; pirbuterol, $K_A = 1$ μM; relative efficacies isoproterenol/prenalterol/pirbuterol $= 1/0.004/0.009$.

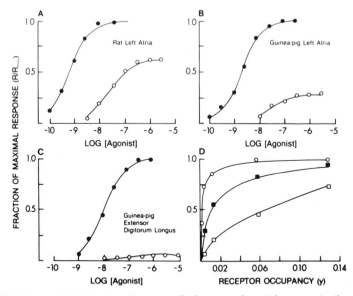

**FIG. 2.22.** General logistic function as a fit for experimental concentration-response curves. Ordinates: Response as a fraction of the maximal response to isoproterenol. Abscissae: **A–C,** logarithms of molar concentrations of drugs; **D,** fractional receptor occupancy for isoproterenol as calculated by Langmuir adsorption isotherm. Data points refer to isoproterenol (•) and prenalterol (o). Equation 2.7 was used to generate the theoretical stimulus-response curves shown in D for three tissues: rat left atria (o), $\beta = 1.0$; guinea pig left atria (■), $\beta = 3.5$; guinea pig extensor digitorum longus (□), $\beta = 20$. Data points and theoretically calculated concentration-response curves for tissues shown in A to C. (From ref. 17.)

## MANIPULATION OF STIMULUS-RESPONSE MECHANISMS: VOLUME CONTROL

Within any multifactorial stimulus-response cascade there is an element of control of the end product (response) in terms of availability of cofactors or control of feedback mechanisms. Thus, to a limited extent, tissue sensitivity to agonists can be manipulated. There are two aspects to this that are important to pharmacologists. The first concerns the veracity of data obtained *in vitro* in terms of correctly mimicking what is happening *in vivo*. For example, the binding affinity of β-adrenoceptor agonists can be changed considerably in biochemical experiments by the presence of GTP. This raises the question of possible differences in cellular levels of GTP *in vivo* and *in vitro* and corresponding differences in $K_A$ values for β-agonists measured *in vitro*. The second aspect of the manipulation of tissue sensitivity is the possible utility of the exercise for independently measuring agonist affinity and relative efficacy. Thus, it may be advantageous to modify the magnitude of agonist response in a tissue in order to measure either $K_A$ or $\epsilon$ independently (this will be dealt with more fully in Chapters 7 and 8).

There are three principles that can be used to manipulate the magnitude of a tissue response to a drug. The first is not involved with the stimulus-response mechanism and cannot be considered to involve the volume setting of the power amplifier. Specifically, the receptor density can be manipulated by a number of means to increase or decrease the receptor stimulus imparted to the tissue; this affects the strength of the preamplifier. The most commonly encountered principle involves the dynamic properties of receptors. Cells respond to the chronic level of hormonal (or drug) stimulation by controlling receptor number. Thus, if neurotransmission is interrupted, as, for example, by depletion of neuronal transmitter or denervation, the absence of stimulus triggers cellular mechanisms that increase receptor density. The same effect can be obtained by chronic exposure of tissues to antagonists that prevent neurotransmitters or hormones from imparting stimuli to the cell. Similarly, if stimulation is exceptionally intense, as, for example, during chronic exposure to agonist, this excess stimulation triggers receptor uncoupling and internalization, leading to a decrease in receptor density. This process is given the name "receptor regulation," with increases being referred to as "up-regulation," and decreases as "down-regulation." Chronic exposure to agonists or antagonists *in vivo* often can provide tissues with altered receptor densities.

Two other principles involved in the manipulation of responses have to do with volume setting of the power amplifier. One involves the availability of cofactors in the stimulus-response chain. For example, calcium is required for contraction, and, in general, the source of calcium can be extracellular or intracellular storage sites or both. In those tissues that utilize extracellular calcium for contraction, the control of calcium-ion concentration in the incubation medium can, within limits, control the sensitivity of the tissue to spasmogens. For example, the concentrations of extracellular calcium and/or magnesium greatly affect guinea pig ileal sensitivity to cholinergic agonists (Fig. 2.23). A second principle is inhibition of control mechanisms in the stimulus-response chain. For example, β-adrenoceptor agonists produce responses by elevating intracellular concentrations of the second messenger

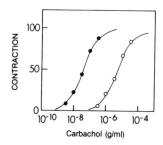

FIG. 2.23. Effects of calcium and magnesium on the dependence of the sensitivity of guinea pig ileum to carbachol. Ordinate: Contraction as a percentage of maximal response. Abscissa: Logarithms of concentrations of carbachol in $g/mL^{-1}$. Responses in the presence of 2.5 (○) and 1.5 mM (●) calcium ions. (From ref. 6.)

**A**

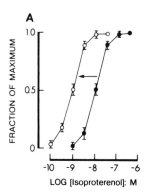

**B**

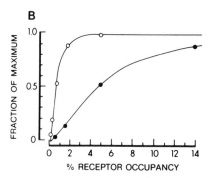

FIG. 2.24. Potentiation of responses of guinea pig papillary muscle to isoproterenol after iso-butylmethylxanthine (IMX). **A:** Concentration-response curves to isoproterenol. Ordinate: Response as a fraction of the maximal response. Abscissa: Logarithms of molar concentrations of isoproterenol. Responses in the absence (•, $N = 8$) and presence (o, $N = 12$) of IMX. **B:** Effects of IMX on occupancy-response curves. Ordinate: As for part A. Abscissa: Percentage receptor occupancy by isoproterenol. Curves in the absence (•) and presence (o) of IMX. (From ref. 19.)

cyclic AMP; a fine control of this mechanism is provided by concomitant destruction of this messenger by the enzyme phosphodiesterase. Therefore, inhibition of this control mechanism leads to a greater quantity of cyclic AMP per given receptor stimulus and a resulting increase in sensitivity to the agonist. Figure 2.24A shows the effects of phosphodiesterase inhibition on concentration-response curves for isoproterenol on guinea pig papillary muscle; a 10-fold potentiation is observed. Figure 2.24B shows the increased efficiency in stimulus-response coupling produced by the enzyme inhibition.

### REFERENCES

1. Anderson, G. F., and Marks, B. H. (1982): Spare cholinergic receptors in the urinary bladder. *J. Pharmacol. Exp. Ther.*, 221:598–603.
2. Ariëns, E. J., Beld, A. J., DeMiranda, J. F. R., and Simonis, A. M. (1979): The Pharacon-receptor-effector concept. A basis for understanding the transmission of information in biological systems. In: *The Receptors, A Comprehensive Treatise*, edited by R. D. O'Brien, pp. 33–91. Plenum Press, New York.
3. Besse, J. C., and Furchgott, R. F. (1976): Dissociation constants and relative efficacies of agonists acting on alpha adrenergic receptors in rabbit aorta. *J. Pharmacol. Exp. Ther.*, 197:66–78.

4. Black, J. W., and Leff, P. (1983): Operational models of pharmacological agonist. *Proc. R. Soc. Lond. [Biol.]*, 220:141–162.
5. Brown, L., Dieghton, N. M., Bals, S., Sohlman, W., Zerkowski, H-R., Michel, M. C., and Brodde, O-E. (1992): Spare receptors for β-adrenoceptor-mediated positive inotropic effects of catecholamines in human heart. *J. Cardiovasc. Pharmacol.*, 19:222–232.
6. Burgen, A. S. V., and Spero, L. (1968): The action of acetylcholine and other drugs on the efflux of potassium and rubidium from smooth muscle of the guinea-pig intestine. *Br. J. Pharmacol.*, 34:99–115.
7. Furchgott, R. F. (1967): The pharmacological differentiation of adrenergic receptors. *Ann. N.Y. Acad. Sci.*, 139:553–570.
8. Furchgott, R. F. (1978): Pharmacological characterization of receptors: Its relation to radioligand-binding studies. *Fed. Proc.*, 37:115–120.
9. Goldberg, N. D. (1975): Cyclic nucleotides and cell function. In: *Cell Membranes, Biochemistry, Cell Biology, and Pathology*, edited by G. Weissman and R. Claiborne, pp. 185–202. H. P. Publishing, New York.
10. Hayes, J. S., Brunton, L. L., and Mayer, S. E. (1980): Selective activation of particulate cAMP-dependent protein kinase by isoproterenol and prostaglandin $E_1$. *J. Biol. Chem.*, 255:5113–5119.
11. Hoffman, B. B., Lavin, T. N., Lefkowitz, R. J., and Ruffolo, R. R., Jr. (1981): Alpha adrenergic receptor subtypes in rabbit uterus: Mediation of myo-metrial contraction and regulation by estrogens. *J. Pharmacol. Exp. Ther.*, 219:290–295.
12. Hollenga, Ch., Brouwer, F., and Zaagsma, J. (1991): Relationship between lipolysis and cyclic AMP generation mediated by atypical β-adrenoceptors in rat adipocytes. *Br. J. Pharmacol.*, 102:577–580.
13. Kenakin, T. P. (1984): The relative contribution of affinity and efficacy to agonist activity. Organ selectivity of noradrenaline and oxymetazoline with reference to the classification of drug receptors. *Br. J. Pharmacol.*, 81:131–134.
14. Kenakin, T. P. (1986): Receptor reserve as a tissue misnomer. *Trends Pharmacol. Sci.*, 7: 93–95.
15. Kenakin, T. P. (1991): Drugs and receptors: An overview of the current state of knowledge. *Drugs*, 40:666–687.
16. Kenakin, T. P. (1992): Tissue response as a functional discriminator of receptor heterogeneity: Effects of mixed receptor populations on Schild regressions. *Mol. Pharmacol.*, 41: 699–707.
17. Kenakin, T. P., and Beek, D. (1980): Is prenalterol (H133/80) really a selective beta-1 adrenoceptor agonist? Tissue selectivity resulting from differences in stimulus-response relationships. *J. Pharmacol. Exp. Ther.*, 213:406–412.
18. Kenakin, T. P., and Beck, D. (1984): Relative efficacy of prenalterol and pirbuterol for $β_1$-adrenoceptors: Measurement of agonist affinity by alteration of receptor number. *J. Pharmacol. Exp. Ther.*, 229:340–345.
19. Kenakin, T. P., and Beek, D. (1984): The measurement of the relative efficacy of agonists by selective potentiation of tissue responses: Studies with isoprenaline and prenalterol in cardiac tissue. *J. Auton. Pharmacol.*, 4:153–159.
20. Kenakin, T. P., Ambrose, J. R., and Irving, P. E. (1991): The relative efficiency of beta adrenoceptor coupling to myocardial inotropy and diastolic relaxation: Organ-selective treatment for diastolic dysfunction. *J. Pharmacol. Exp. Ther.*, 257:1189–1197.
21. Kono, T., and Barham, F. W. (1971): The relationship between the insulin-binding capacity of fat cells and the cellular response to insulin. *J. Biol. Chem.*, 246:6210–6216.
22. Mattsson, H., Hedberg, A., and Carlsson, E. (1983): Intrinsic sympathomimetic activity of the partial agonist prenalterol in relation to beta adrenoceptor interaction in various tissues in vitro. *J. Pharmacol. Exp. Ther.*, 224:654–661.
23. Minneman, K. P., and Abel, P. W. (1984): Relationship between $α_1$-adrenoceptor density and functional response of rat vas deferens. Studies with phenoxybenzamine. *Naunyn Schmiedebergs Arch. Pharmacol.*, 327:238–246.
24. Morgan, J. P., and Morgan, K. G. (1984): Calcium and cardiovascular function. *Am. J. Med.*, 142:33–46.
25. Mueller, H., Weingarten, R., Ransnas, L. A., Bokoch, G. M., and Sklar, L. A. (1991): Differential amplification of antagonistic pathways in neutrophils. *J. Biol. Chem.*, 266: 12939–12943.

26. Nickerson, M. (1956): Receptor occupancy and tissue response. *Nature*, 178:697–698.
27. Patil, P. N., Fudge, K., and Jacobowitz, D. (1972): Steric aspects of adrenegic drugs. XVIII. α-Adrenergic receptors of mammalian aorta. *Eur. J. Pharmacol.*, 19:79–87.
28. Roach, P. J. (1977): Functional significance of enzyme cascade systems. *Trends Biochem. Sci.*, 2:87–90.
29. Rooney, T. A., and Nahorski, S. R. (1987): Postnatal ontogeny of agonist and depolarization-induced phosphoinositide hydrolysis in rat cerebral cortex. *J. Pharmacol. Exp. Ther.*, 243:333–341.
30. Ruffolo, R. R., Jr. (1982): Review: Important concepts of receptor theory. *J. Auton. Pharmacol.*, 2:277–295.
31. Sastry, R., and Cheng, H. C. (1972): Dissociation constants of D- and L-lactoylcholines and related compounds at cholinergic receptors. *J. Pharmacol. Exp. Ther.*, 180:326–339.
32. Sheys, E. M., and Green, R. D. (1972): A quantitative study of alpha adrenergic receptors in the spleen and aorta of the rabbit. *J. Pharmacol. Exp. Ther.*, 180:317–325.
33. Siegl, P. K. S., and McNeill, J. H. (1982): Antagonism with dibenamine, D-600, and Ro 3-7894 to estimate dissociation constants and receptor reserves for cardiac adrenoceptors in isolated rabbit pupillary muscles. *Can. J. Physiol. Pharmacol.*, 60:1131–1137.
34. Stephenson, R. P. (1956): A modification of receptor theory. *Br. J. Pharmacol.*, 11:379–393.
35. Strickland, S., and Loeb, J. N. (1981): Obligatory separation of hormone binding and biological response curves in systems dependent upon secondary mediators of hormone action. *Proc. Natl. Acad. Sci. U.S.A.*, 78:1366–1370.
36. Taylor, C. W. (1990): The role of G-proteins in transmembrane signalling. *Biochem. J.*, 272: 1–13.

# 3

# Drug Response Systems

*Although this may seem a paradox, all exact science is dominated by the idea of approximation.*

—BERTRAND RUSSELL (1872–1970)

### DRUG RESPONSE: LEVELS OF MEASUREMENT

When considering drug actions, various levels of responses can be measured. For example, the hemodynamic improvement, as reflected in the reduction in heart size, the improved renal function, and the reversal of pulmonary edema in congestive heart failure, is the clinical response to a cardiotonic drug. Although this is the desired end product, it is difficult to classify and quantitate the primary response to the drug. This is because the changes in pathological and physiological states (i.e., changes according to the Frank-Starling relationship) and neuronal (sympathetic tone) and hormonal (renin-angiotensin system) reflexes greatly modify the primary drug response. Each of these factors introduces biological variation, and thus accurate quantification becomes more difficult. From the point of view of classifying, both qualitatively and quantitatively, the effects of drugs, the minimal convenient response system is required. Figure 3.1 shows various possible levels at which drug effects can be studied, along with some advantages and disadvantages of each. The choice of the best system in which to test drugs depends on the type of information required. In general, the object of many pharmacologic experiments is prediction of the integrated human responses to a drug at minimal cost with respect to expenditure of effort and resources, and with maximal accuracy. As shown in Fig. 3.1, the types of preparations range from the simplest (biochemical measurements on receptors in membrane fragments) to the most complex (*in vivo* experiments in animals with intact reflex mechanisms). Clearly, for a clinician, the most complex system is optimal, because the effects of neural, hormonal, and autoregulatory reflex mechanisms are important to the overall clinical effects of a drug. However,

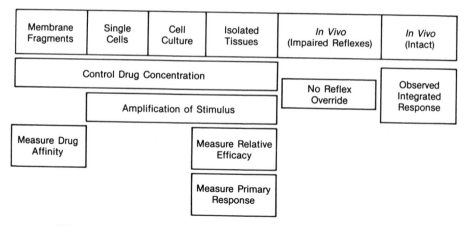

**FIG. 3.1.** Theoretical advantages of various response systems for drugs.

in terms of determining the primary effects of drugs, such complexity is not only costly from the point of view of resources but also detrimental in terms of possible inaccuracy. This is because the various special problems associated with *in vivo* experimentation (pharmacokinetics, reflex mechanisms, absorption) can modulate, potentiate, or otherwise obscure the primary response. Chapter 13 discusses how these factors, obfuscations to the pharmacologist interested in drug classification, can be utilized constructively in the drug development process to produce organ-selective drugs.

## SYSTEMS FOR THE STUDY OF DRUG AND RECEPTOR INTERACTION

Drug-receptor interaction can be studied either by radioligand binding or measurement of response in functional systems. There are generally three types of systems *in vitro*, with variants of each, in which such studies can be carried out. They are biochemical preparations of receptors either as soluble proteins or in membrane fragments (natural or reconstituted), whole cells (either as a single cell, in aggregates, tissue slices, cell cultures, surrogate expression systems), or isolated tissues. Another variant overlaid on these techniques is the study of drug effect in human versus animal sources. Clearly, the study of drugs with human receptors for the prediction of therapeutic effects has obvious advantages, but in many cases human tissue is not available. In these instances receptors from animal sources must be used, raising an ever-present question as to the applicability of the resulting data to human systems. In some cases, there is evidence that such data correlate well with human receptor data. For example, Fig. 3.2 shows the correlation between equilibrium dissociation constants of antagonist-receptor com-

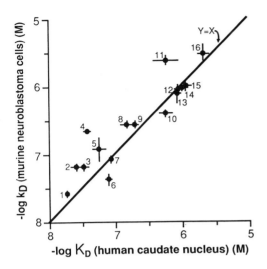

**FIG. 3.2.** Equilibrium dissociation constants for antidepressants and related compounds in human brain muscarinic receptors and muscarinic receptors in murine neuroblastoma cells. 1, imipramine; 2, desipramine; 3, protriptyline; 4, doxepin; 5, amitriptyline; 6, amoxapine; 7, maprotiline; 8, trimipramine; 9, nortriptyline; 10, clomipramine; 11, mianserin; 12, butriptyline; 13, iprindole; 14, 2-OH-imipramine; 15, 3-Cl-2-OH-imipramine; 16, didesmethylimipramine. (From ref. 21.)

plexes for a series of antidepressants measured in human caudate nucleus and murine neuroblastoma cells (clone N1E-115). Although encouraging, such correlations can never ensure that animal and human systems will be identical for all drugs studied. The unequal weight of negative evidence should be considered in the testing of drugs in uncharacterized test systems. Thus, if two receptors are slightly different, it would still be possible for the binding profiles of a number of ligands to be identical for the two receptors. This identity would not indicate that the two receptors were the same (i.e., it is not possible to prove a hypothesis, only to disprove it). The discernment in binding with one ligand might constitute evidence that the receptors were different and thus the evidence with a single ligand would greatly outweigh the apparent agreement of data with a large number of ligands. For example, Table 3.1 shows the equilibrium dissociation constants for four $\alpha_2$-adrenoceptor antagonists for $\alpha_2$-adrenoceptors cloned from mouse and human genes and expressed in COS-7 cells. The receptors cloned from the human genes (human $\alpha_2$-C4 and human $\alpha_2$-C10 receptors) and a mouse gene (mouse M$\alpha_2$-4H receptor) have indistinguishable affinity for atipamezole and yohimbine.

**TABLE 3.1.** *Equilibrium dissociation constants of $\alpha_2$-adrenoceptor antagonists for human and mouse $\alpha_2$-adrenoceptor subtypes expressed in COS-7 cells*

| Antagonist | Human $\alpha_2$-C4 | Mouse M$\alpha_2$-4H | Human $\alpha_2$-C10 |
|---|---|---|---|
| Atipamezole | 3.6 ± 0.4 | 1.6 ± 0.02 | 2.9 ± 0.2 |
| Yohimbine | 3.1 ± 0.1 | 3.8 ± 0.8 | 3.4 ± 0.6 |
| Prazosin | 121.1 ± 10.4 | 97.3 ± 17.7 | 2,034 ± 350.4 |
| Idazoxan | 52.3 ± 7.7 | 9.8 ± 0.7 | 12.2 ± 3.7 |

From ref. 32.

Therefore, reliance on data with these two antagonists would not distinguish these receptors. However, data with prazosin and idazoxan show human $\alpha_2$-C10 and human $\alpha_2$-C4 to be different. Interestingly, the creation of chimeric mouse and human receptors indicates that a *single* residue in the fifth transmembrane domain of the $\alpha_2$-adrenoceptor accounts for interspecies variation between receptors in mouse and humans (32).

Direct observation of drug interactions with receptors can be made with radioligand binding experiments. In some cases, the agreement between isolated tissue experiments and radioligand binding experiments is quite good. For example, Fig. 3.3A shows the correlation between the binding affinity of 60 muscarinic antagonists (measured in rat cerebral cortex) and their affinity as blockers of muscarinic contraction in guinea pig ileum. Other systems do not agree as well. Figure 3.3B shows the affinity of $\beta$-adrenoceptor antagonists for $\beta$-adrenoceptors in rat adipocytes as measured in binding experiments and as blockers of isoproterenol-stimulated adenylate cyclase. In this case there is no correlation between the functional data and the binding data. The major advantage of radioligand binding experiments is the fact that the binding of drug to receptors can be viewed directly, thus allowing the direct measurement of ligand affinity. However, there also are membrane systems in which agonist response can be measured. For example, receptor-mediated, G-protein activation can be assayed by measuring receptor-stimulated steady-state GTPase activity or binding of GTP (or GTP$\gamma$S) binding.

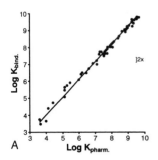

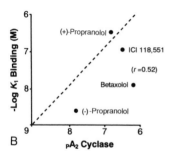

**FIG. 3.3.** Correlations between estimates of antagonist equilibrium dissociation constants measured in binding and functional studies. **A:** Correlation for 60 muscarinic antagonists for binding to rat cerebral cortex membranes and antagonism of contraction of guinea pig ileal contraction. (From ref. 3.) **B:** Differential effects of antagonists in rat adipose tissue when measured with binding and functional techniques. Estimates of the pA$_2$ of $\beta$-adrenoceptor antagonists as inhibitors of $\beta$-adrenoceptor ligand binding ([$^{125}$I]cyanopindolol) as ordinates and blockade of adenylate cyclase activation by isoproterenol as abscissae. (From ref. 6.)

Some possible disadvantages of radioligand binding studies include the potential for artifacts stemming from the biochemical preparation of membranes and the lack of radioactive ligands for some receptors. Especially when dealing with agonists, there are differences in the interaction of ligands with receptors at low versus high receptor occupancies and radioligand experiments sometimes may view drug-receptor binding from a different vantage point than functional studies. In the latter, powerful cellular amplification of signals generated by low receptor occupancies may produce a situation in which the measurable scale for agonist effect is observed at low receptor occupancies in functional systems and at high receptor occupancies in the corresponding binding system. Measuring drug parameters from these two vantage points sometimes can lead to differences between binding and functional studies. In addition, the lack of cellular components in biochemical binding experiments (i.e., GTP) may change the binding of ligands from what is operable in the intact system. In spite of these potential problems, the convenience and simplicity of radioligand binding have made this technique extremely valuable in the study of drugs and drug receptors, and a great deal of data regarding the mechanism of action of drugs has been obtained from its use. Chapter 12 deals with the use of drug-receptor models in the description of ligand-binding phenomena.

## CELL CULTURE AND THE EXPRESSION OF RECEPTORS IN SURROGATE SYSTEMS

Drug-receptor interaction also can be studied in cultured cells. A major advantage of this approach is that human cell lines can be used. Cell culture techniques offer the potential to measure physiological responses to agonists in systems in which the response may be amplified from the initial stimulus produced at the membrane level. Also, a more physiological estimate of drug-receptor interaction may be obtained. For example, with sealed cells containing GTP accessible to G proteins, the affinity of an agonist may be considerably lower than that measured in broken cell membrane preparations (see Chapter 7). This may be more physiologically representative of agonist affinity than what is obtained in membrane preparations. If receptor processes such as desensitization are to be studied, a whole-cell system offers a more physiological readout. However, caution must be used in the study of receptor events in living cells. For example, Fig. 3.4 shows the rapid decrease in binding of the muscarinic receptor agonist carbachol in intact rat cerebellar cells due to desensitization. This effect is not seen in membranes from the same cells (Fig. 3.4). This could be important in binding studies in which reactions are equilibrated for a set time period to achieve a steady state without a constant readout of reaction product.

There are potential variations in receptor systems studied in cell culture.

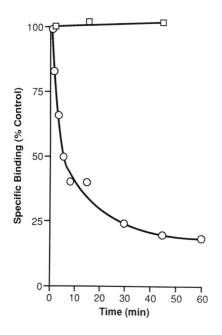

**FIG. 3.4.** Time course for loss of carbachol binding, as measured by carbachol displacement of [³H]QNB, in intact cerebellar cells (○) and membranes from the same cells (□). (From ref. 33.)

One significant variation can be the level of receptor expressed in the cell at different cell passages. For example, Table 3.2 shows the 200-fold difference in the level of β-adrenoceptor expression in transformed Chinese hamster fibroblasts. Figure 3.5A shows the receptor levels for 5-HT$_{1A}$ receptors in polyclonal NIH-3T$_3$/5-HT$_{1A}$ cells from passage 1 to 32. Figure 3.5B shows the corresponding maximal response to 5-HT as an inhibitor of cyclic AMP

**TABLE 3.2.** *[¹²⁵I]CYP Binding in transfected and nontransfected CHW cells: levels of β-adrenoceptor*

| Cell line | n | $B_{max}$ (pmol/mg) |
|---|---|---|
| CHW[a] | 3 | 0.042 ± 0.007 |
| CTF-40 | 4 | 0.084 ± 0.023 |
| CTF-17 | 5 | 0.43 ± 0.09 |
| CTF-33 | 4 | 0.97 ± 0.08 |
| CTF-39 | 5 | 2.93 ± 0.64 |
| CTF-31 | 13 | 3.18 ± 0.34 |
| CTF-23 | 14 | 3.55 ± 0.43 |
| CTF-21 | 7 | 5.08 ± 0.76 |
| CTF-37 | 3 | 8.39 ± 1.45 |
| CTF-36 | 14 | 8.42 ± 1.28 |
| A431 | 6 | 1.25 ± 0.2 |

From ref. 7.
[a] Nontransfected.

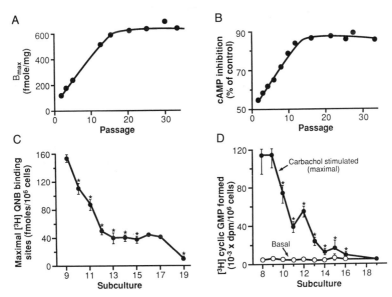

**FIG. 3.5.** Variations in receptor density and response in cell culture systems. **A:** Maximal receptor density (in fmol/mg protein) of 5-HT$_{1A}$ receptors in polyclonal NIH-3T$_3$/5-HT$_{1A}$ cells as a function of cell passage number. **B:** Maximal inhibition of cyclic AMP produced by 5-HT in the cells shown in A. (Data for A and B from ref. 57.) **C:** Density of muscarinic receptors as measured by [$^3$H]QNB binding with various subcultures of N1E-115 cells. **D:** Maximal responses to the muscarinic agonist carbachol in various subcultures of N1E-115 cells. (Data for C and D from ref. 36.)

formation in the same cells. Figure 3.5C shows the density of muscarinic receptors with different subcultures of N1E-115 cells; the corresponding decrease in the activity of the muscarinic agonist carbachol in the same cells is shown in Fig. 3.5D. The basal activity of the response system is not changed during this period. This type of data shows that the passage number of a given cell culture may be critical to both the type and magnitude of a receptor signal.

A powerful technique becoming increasingly available to pharmacologists studying receptor mechanisms is the genetic expression of receptors in surrogate cell systems. Discussion of the techniques used to detect and isolate the genetic material that codes for a given receptor, the transfection of that material into a host cell, and the promotion of receptor expression are beyond the scope of this monograph and constitute a large and sophisticated technology. In general, given an amino acid sequence for a receptor, an oligonucleotide probe can be constructed of nucleic acids known to code for the amino acid sequence that will bind to the appropriate DNA region on the gene coding for the whole receptor. This probe then can be used to scan cDNA libraries to detect the appropriate DNA, which then can be isolated. The DNA can be amplified by polymerase chain reaction techniques and then inserted into a vector, which will allow entry of the genetic material into a host cell. These vectors also can contain promoters that, when activated, will force the surrogate cell to express the receptor protein. Also, vectors can contain other genetic material to code for markers that will enable selection of the successfully transfected cells. For example, a phleomycin-resistance gene can be introduced into the vector. Phleomycin treatment of the whole cell colony (transfected and nontransfected cells) would then kill the non-transfected cells. This would allow further culture of a pure population of the successfully transfected cells. These techniques can be immensely powerful in that pure populations of receptors can be expressed in cell membranes for pharmacologic analysis. The following discussion will assume that the transfection and expression process preceding the pharmacologic analysis has been correct (i.e., no translational errors have occurred) and that a correct amino acid sequence for the desired receptor is present in the surrogate cell system membrane. The pharmacologic analysis of drug-receptor interactions under these circumstances is still subject to the constraints discussed in other chapters. However, there are also a number of other factors unique to expression systems that should be considered.

The first potential problem stems from the fact that the correctly expressed receptor often is placed in an alien environment (when compared to a cell that naturally expresses the receptor). Therefore, if posttranslational events (i.e., such as receptor glycosylation) are important to the tertiary structure of the receptor and if these amenities are not available in the surrogate cell, then differences may result. Another potential difference can be the lipid environment of the receptor once it enters the cell membrane. It is well-known that the tertiary structure of many proteins can be dependent on the lipid constitution of the membrane. For example, Table 3.3 shows the effects of phospholipid concentration in membranes reconstituting purified muscarinic receptors. The apparent affinity of oxotremorine changes by a factor of 7 with a fourfold difference in the phosphatidylcholine content of the membranes. The fact that the affinity does not change in the presence of GTP indicates that the differences lie in the interaction of the oxotremorine-activated receptor and the G-protein coupler. Differences can occur for antagonists as well. Table 3.4 shows that a 7.5- to 9-fold difference in the affinity

**TABLE 3.3.** *Effect of phospholipid concentration on the interaction of $G_o$ with muscarinic receptors*

| Phosphatidylcholine (mg) | $K_d - GTP$ (nM) | $K_d + GTP$ (μM) |
|---|---|---|
| 0.12 | 7.4 | 8.9 |
| 0.24 | 20 | 8.9 |
| 0.48 | 50 | 8.9 |

From ref. 23.

**TABLE 3.4.** *Effects of phospholipids or antagonist affinity*

| Environment | [³H]QNB (pM) | | Pirenzepine atrium (nM) |
|---|---|---|---|
| | Cerebrum | Atrium | |
| Native mAChR, intact membrane | 44 ± 5 | 43 ± 5 | 790 ± 30 |
| Inserted mAChR | | | |
| PrBCM-treated cerebral membrane | 44 ± 6 | 59 ± 7 | 980 ± 63 |
| PrBCM-treated atrial membrane | 78 ± 11 | 72 ± 13 | 1,275 ± 143 |
| CHS | 70 ± 13 | 81 ± 12 | 220 ± 34 |
| CHS:PC (80:20) | 74 ± 17 | 82 ± 25 | 440 ± 73 |
| CHS:PC (50:50) | 75 ± 21 | 81 ± 28 | 830 ± 80 |
| CHS:PC (20:80) | 130 ± 26 | 140 ± 19 | 1900 ± 138 |
| PC[a] | 530 ± 75 | 590 ± 65 | 13,500 ± 1,290 |
| CHS:PC:PI (4:48:48)[b] | 170 ± 33 | 240 ± 53 | 5,200 ± 270 |
| Isolated mAChR (digitonin) | 330 | 380 | 690 |

From ref. 2.
[a] Egg L-α-phosphatidylcholine.
[b] PI, soybean L-α-phosphatidylinositol.
mAChR, muscarinic acetylcholine receptor; PrBCM, propyl benzylcholine mustard; CHS, cholesteryl hemisuccinate; PC, porcine cerebrum.

of the muscarinic antagonist [³H]quinuclidinylbenzylate ([³H]QNB) when measured in natural membranes from porcine cerebrum and atrium and after purification and removal of lipid. In contrast, no significant effect was seen with pirenzepine, another muscarinic antagonist (Table 3.4). Reinsertion of the solubilized receptor into native membranes in which the existing receptors were previously inactivated by alkylation indicated a complete reversal of the effect, thus indicating that the difference in the affinity for [³H]QNB was caused by the membrane. When the purified receptor was inserted into lipid vesicles of various lipid composition, an array of affinities was observed.

One of the most important aspects of the expression of receptors in surrogate systems is the fact that the true profile of activity of some drugs and perhaps some receptor systems may require natural integrated systems to be correctly interpreted. Figure 3.6 shows an array of possible interactions

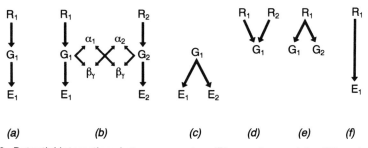

**FIG. 3.6.** Potential interactions between receptors (R), coupling proteins (G), and effector systems (E) in cell membranes. (From ref. 52.)

between seven transmembrane receptors, transduction coupling proteins, and effector systems in physiological systems. One simple system is a single receptor $(R)$ linked through a single coupling protein $(G)$ to a single effector $(E_1)$ in the membrane. A more complex scenario would be two receptors, each binding to separate transduction proteins. When the transducers are activated, they generate interchangeable $\beta\gamma$ subunits, which can cross over the signal transduction process of each receptor to its effector ($b$ in Fig. 3.6). Alternatively, a single receptor-activated transducer could interact with more than one effector ($c$), two receptors could compete with a single transduction protein ($d$) or a single receptor could divide its time between two or more G proteins ($e$; see Chapter 8 for examples of this). Finally, a receptor may interact directly with an effector without an intervening transduction protein ($f$). There is an increasing number of examples of these interactions occurring and modifying drug activity in physiological systems. If such interactions are important to the activity of a given drug, then a correct representation of that activity may not be made if all of the players are not present or are not present in the correct stoichiometry in the system. If the receptor were not a solitary actor, it could be likened to placing Hamlet on an empty stage and expecting the grandeur of Shakespeare to result. Such potential problems are obvious for agonists that promote the formation of ternary complexes between receptor, agonist, and transducer proteins.

Different receptor/G-protein ratios have been shown to occur in various cellular clones and these varying ratios can, in turn, have consequences to the measurement of ligand affinities. Table 3.5 shows data from cloned murine fibroblast B82 cells. As the number of muscarinic receptors increases in each clone, the percentage of high-affinity sites decreases. Since all of the transfected clones originated from the same patient B82 line, the G-protein levels should be similar; therefore, the clones shown in Table 3.5 represent

**TABLE 3.5.** *Binding parameters for $M_1$ muscarinic receptors in a series of transfected B82 cells*

| Clone | $B_{max}$ (fmol/$10^6$ cells) | [$^3$H]QNB $K_d$ (pM) | $K_H$ ($\mu$M)[b] | Carbachol[a] | |
| | | | | % H[c] | $K_L$ ($\mu$M)[d] |
|---|---|---|---|---|---|
| LK3-1 | 12 ± 0.98 | 100 | 7.7 | 100 | |
| LK3-4 | 18 ± 1.5 | 110 | 1.9 | 43 ± 7.3 | 46 |
| LK3-6 | 30 ± 4.4 | 97 | 3.8 | 68 ± 10 | 34 |
| LK3-7 | 96 ± 15 | 150 | 5.8 | 62 ± 12 | 41 |
| LK7-2 | 140 ± 19 | 150 | 7.1 | 47 ± 10 | 53 |
| LK3-3 | 240 ± 15 | 160 | 4.8 | 40 ± 7.6 | 45 |
| LK3-8 | 260 ± 48 | 190 | 2.4 | 42 ± 5.9 | 53 |

From ref. 37.
[a] Displacement of [$^3$H]QNB by carbachol.
[b] Equilibrium dissociation constant of carbachol with high-affinity site.
[c] Percentage of sites apparently in the high-affinity form.
[d] Equilibrium dissociation constant of carbachol with low-affinity site.

varying levels of receptor to G-protein ratios. It would be predicted that increases in the amounts of G protein, relative to receptor, should favor the formation of ternary complexes and thus increase the likelihood of observing a high-affinity site in binding studies. This has been shown experimentally in reconstituted systems (see Table 7.2). The data in Table 3.5 are consistent with this prediction as well. This effect can have consequences to the observation of affinity of ligands with efficacy (either positive or negative) or the potency of ligands in displacing ligands with efficacy. The possible precoupling of receptors to G proteins in such systems further complicates the interactions. Figure 3.7A shows ligand saturation curves for a hypothetical agonist in systems of varying receptor/G-protein ratios. The ordinate scale of

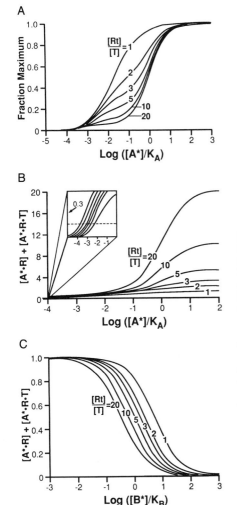

FIG. 3.7. Variations in binding curves for efficacious ligands in systems with varying receptor/G-protein levels. **A:** Saturation binding curves for a radioactive ligand with $K_1 = K_2 = 0.01$ (where $K_1$ and $K_2$ refer to the equilibrium dissociation constants of the drug receptor and ternary complex, respectively), $[T] = 1.0$ and $[R_t] =$ (for each curve reading right to left) 1, 2, 3, 5, 10, and 20. Ordinate scale normalized to a fraction of the maximal radioactivity bound. **B:** Simulation shown in A on an absolute scale where the ordinates are the actual relative amounts of radioactivity bound. **Inset** shows the lower part of the abscissal axis expanded and the relative location on the x-axis of ligand concentrations producing a constant level of specific binding. **C:** Curves for the displacement of a constant level of specific binding for the ligand shown in A and B by an antagonist with low intrinsic efficacy ($K_{B1} = 1$; $K_{B2} = 0.1$). Displacement curves for systems with $[R]/[T]$ ratios (from left to right) of 20, 10, 5, 3, 2, and 1.

this figure has been normalized to illustrate the complex curves obtained as the ratio of receptor to G protein decreases. Figure 3.7B shows the same data with an absolute scale (showing the actual relative levels of radioactive species) along with an inset expansion of part of the curves to show the relative locations of low levels of radioactive binding. A standard practice in radioligand-binding studies is to work at constant low levels of bound radioactivity to simplify comparison of displacement curves. If this were to be done for this ligand in this series of systems, the displacement curves for a nonradioactive, low-efficacy ligand, shown in Fig. 3.7C would be observed. Thus, a 16-fold variation in potency in the displacing ligand would be observed in systems with receptor/G-protein ratios varying from 20 to 1.

The ratio of receptors to coupling proteins can be critical to the magnitude and even the type of responses observed with agonists. Figure 3.8 shows the effects of varying expression levels of $\alpha_2$-C10 receptors in transfected Chinese hamster ovary (CHO) cells. At a receptor expression level of 0.3

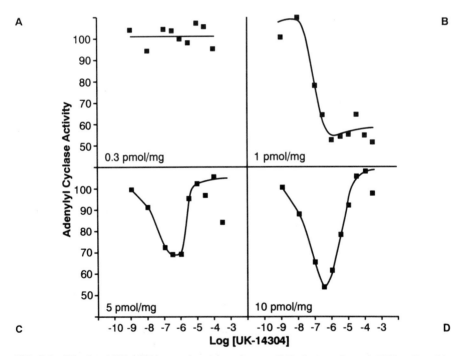

**FIG. 3.8.** Effects of UK-14304 on adenylyl cyclase activity in transfected CHO cells with different expression levels of $\alpha_2$-C10 receptors. Membranes prepared from CHO cells expressing 0.3 **(A)**, 1.0 **(B)**, 5 **(C)**, and 10 **(D)** pmol/mg $\alpha_2$-10 receptors. A: The $\alpha_2$-adrenoceptor agonist produces no effects on adenylyl cyclase activity in membranes with 0.3 pmol/mg. B: At the 1-pmol/mg receptor levels, UK-14304 produced inhibition of adenylyl cyclase, which became a biphasic response (C) at expression levels of 5 pmol/mg. D: The biphasic response was more pronounced at 10 pmol/mg. (From ref. 20.)

pmol/mg in the membranes, no effect on adenylyl cyclase is produced by the $\alpha_2$-adrenoceptor agonist UK-14304 (Fig. 3.8A). However, at a higher expression level (1 pmol/mg), a concentration-dependent decrease in adenylyl cyclase activity is observed with UK-14304 (Fig. 3.8B). This agonist response to UK-14304 can be eliminated by inactivation of the receptor coupler $G_i$ protein by prior treatment of the cells with pertussis toxin (see Fig. 3.9B). If $\alpha_2$-C10 receptors are expressed at a higher level in CHO cells (5 pmol/mg), then a biphasic adenylyl cyclase response is obtained (Fig. 3.8C). The increase in adenylyl cyclase activity is eliminated by inactivation of the receptor coupler $G_s$ protein prior treatment of the cells with cholera toxin (Fig. 3.9C). The biphasic response is more pronounced at an expression level of 10 pmol/mg (Fig. 3.8D). These data show that the $\alpha_2$-C10 receptor, when expressed in CHO cells is abie to couple to two G proteins with differing sensitivity dependent on the expression level. In general, the magnitude and even type of response produced by agonists in surrogate expression systems may be dependent on the expression level of receptors in cells.

In view of the known interactions of agonists with coupling proteins, the most reliable receptor classification is thought to come from studies with antagonists. However, the definition of a true antagonist is critical to the correct classification of drugs and drug receptors in expression systems. In common usage, an antagonist is defined as a ligand that does not produce a measurable response in a physiological system and blocks the effects of an agonist in that system. By *implication* this leads to the mechanistic description of that ligand only binding to the receptor and not taking part in further interactions of the receptor with other membrane-bound species. However, with the discovery of ligands with negative efficacy that destabilize ternary complex formation, the mere observation of no response cannot be relied on to define a simple antagonist. For example, Fig. 3.10 shows that reconstitu-

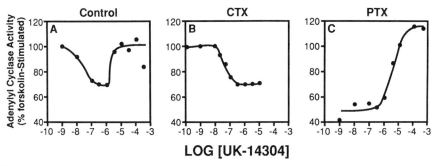

**LOG [UK-14304]**

**FIG. 3.9.** Simultaneous interaction of the $\alpha_2$-C10 receptor with two G proteins in transfected CHO cells. Response to UK-14304 in normal transfected CHO cells **(A)** and those incubated with 20 μg/mL cholera toxin (CTX) **(B)** to decrease $G_s$-protein coupling, or 500 ng/mL pertussis toxin (PTX) **(C)** to inactivate $G_i$-protein coupling. (From ref. 20.)

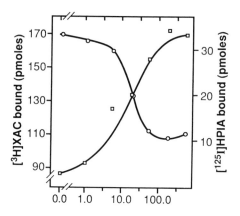

**FIG. 3.10.** Effects of added G proteins in a reconstituted system of adenosine $A_1$ receptors on the binding of an agonist ($[^{125}I]$HPIA) and an antagonist, xanthine amine congener ($[^3H]$XAC). (From ref. 43.)

tion of purified bovine brain adenosine $A_1$ receptor with G proteins shows characteristic increased agonist binding. However, of note is the fact that *decreased* antagonist binding also can be shown. If a ligand changes a receptor to alter subsequent binding to coupling proteins, then the observed affinity of that ligand will be subject to the relative quantities of receptors and coupling protein present in the membrane.

Receptors have affinity for G proteins and will spontaneously form complexes with them in cell membranes given the correct stoichiometry. Figure 3.11 shows graphically that a spontaneous activation of GTPase can be achieved in a reconstituted system of $D_1$ dopamine receptor upon addition of graded amounts of $G_{i2}$ protein. Therefore, as receptors are expressed in

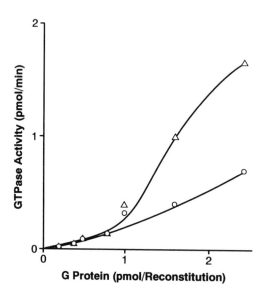

**FIG. 3.11.** Spontaneous activation of $G_{i2}$ protein upon reconstitution with $D_2$ dopamine receptor. Curves for $G_{i2}$ protein reconstituted with $\approx$75 fmol $D_2$ dopamine receptor alone (o) and in the presence of dopamine (Δ). (From ref. 44.)

surrogate systems at various densities, the tendency for spontaneous receptor/G-protein coupling to occur will vary. This could affect ligands that alter equilibria between receptors and G proteins, whether they are agonists or negative-efficacy antagonists (see Fig. 3.10 and Chapter 8 for examples). A further complication arises if the receptor is capable of coupling with more than one type of G protein (as in the example shown in Fig. 3.8). There are numerous other examples of such receptor promiscuity in reconstituted and natural membrane systems (see Chapter 8), opening the possibility that absence of a key G protein or the introduction of an otherwise absent G protein in a given expression system may seriously alter the observed affinity of agonists or other ligands in that system. A negative antagonist could alter the balance of preexisting equilibria between receptors and coupling proteins, thereby producing complex binding phenomena. Under these circumstances the composition of the expression system could be critical to its observed affinity. These ideas are discussed more fully in Chapters 8, 9, and 12.

Given the potential complexities of the correct assembly of a measuring system for the activity of drugs and classification of receptors, it is worth critically evaluating the available data comparing cell expression systems and those from other sources. One of the most accessible data bases is the one for the muscarinic receptor in which the genes for five human subtype receptors have been cloned and expressed in various cell systems. Table 3.6 shows binding data for the affinity of four selective muscarinic antagonists for the five muscarinic receptor subtypes expressed in various cells. In most cases, the data are consistent with less than a three- to fivefold difference in affinities for any given antagonist for the subtypes. However, there are exceptions such as the affinity of atropine in mammalian kidney cells (HEK) and other expression systems for m1 and m2 receptors. Although such divergence may indicate differences in binding conditions, the fact that no difference was observed with m3 receptors might suggest a more specific and perhaps systematic problem. The uniformly lower estimates for the affinity of pirenzepine in these cells and the fact that complex binding curves (i.e., high- and low-affinity states) were selectively obtained for AFDX-116 suggest that this expression system may confer special properties to the receptors. Subtypes of $\alpha_1$-adrenoceptors also have been expressed in various systems (Table 3.7). In some cases the data agree strikingly, as for the $\alpha_{1C}$-adrenoceptors expressed in COS-7 and HeLa cells with WB4101. In other cases such as the rat $\alpha_{1A}$-adrenoceptor in kidney tissue and COS-7 cells for WB4101 and hamster $\alpha_{1B}$-adrenoceptors in COS-7 and HeLa cells for prazosin, significant differences can be found. Human $\beta_2$-adrenoceptors also have been cloned and expressed in cell systems (Table 3.8). The affinity of the radioligand [$^{125}$I]cyanopindolol is consistent in these studies as is the affinity of betaxolol and ICI 118,551. However, there are significant differences with propranolol. Similarly, the affinities of selective antagonists for $\alpha_2$-adrenoceptors expressed from human clones in COS-7 cells are consis-

**TABLE 3.6.** *Affinity of antagonists for muscarinic receptor subtypes from human genes expressed in various cell types*

| Antagonist | Cell | Receptor | | | | | Ref. |
|---|---|---|---|---|---|---|---|
| | | m1 | m2 | m3 | m4 | m5 | |
| Atropine | CHO | 9.3 | 9.0 | 9.0 | 9.2 | 8.8 | 1 |
| | CHO | 9.7 | 8.8 | 9.8 | 8.7 | 9.7 | 4 |
| | Oocytes | 9.4 | 8.8 | | | | 7 |
| | Murine fibroblasts | 9.3 | 9.0 | | | | 8 |
| | HEK | 8.5 | 7.8 | 9 | | | 9 |
| Pirenzepine | CHO | 8.1 | 6.6 | 6.8 | 7.5 | 6.8 | 1 |
| | CHO | | 6.0 | | | 7.0 | 2 |
| | CHO | | 6.0 | 6.7 | | | 4 |
| | COS-7 | | 6.3 | | 7.8 | | 3 |
| | CHO | 8.2 | 6.6 | 6.9 | 7.4 | 7.0 | 5 |
| | Oocytes | 8.0 | | | | | 6 |
| | Murine fibroblasts | 7.8 | | | | | 8 |
| | HEK | 6.3 | 4.9 | 5.9 | 5.6 | | 9 |
| | CHO | | 6.6 | 6.9 | 7.4 | 7.0 | 10 |
| AFDX-116 | CHO | | 6.6 | 6.1 | 6.4 | 5.5 | 3 |
| | CHO | 5.9 | 6.7 | 6.1 | | 5.5 | 4 |
| | HEK | 7.3/5.2 | 7.7/6.1 | 6.5/6 | 5.6 | | 9 |
| Himbacine | Murine fibroblasts | 7.0 | 7.8 | | | | 8 |
| | CHO | 7.0 | 8.0 | 7.0 | 8.0 | 6.3 | 5 |
| 4-DAMP | Murine fibroblasts | 8.7 | 8.1 | | | | 8 |
| | CHO | 9.2 | 8.4 | 9.3 | 8.9 | 9.0 | 5 |

Affinity expressed as $-\log K_i$ for displacement.

1. Bolden, C.; Cusack, B., and Richelson, E. (1992): *J. Pharmacol. Exp. Ther.*, 260: 576–580.
2. Bonner, T. I., Young, A. C., Brann, M. R., and Buckley, N. J. (1988): *Neuron*, 1:403–410.
3. Bonner, T. I., Buckley, N. J., Young, A. C., and Brann, M. R. (1987): *Science*, 237: 527–532.
4. Buckley, N. J., Bonner, T. I., Buckley, C. M., and Brann, M. R. (1989): *Mol. Pharmacol.*, 35:469–476.
5. Dorje, F., Wess, J., Lambrecht, G., Tacke, R., Mutschler, E., and Brann, M. R. (1991): *J. Pharmacol. Exp. Ther.*, 256:727–733.
6. Fukuda, K., Higashida, H., Akiba, I., Maeda, A., Mishina, M., and Numa, S. (1987): *Nature*, 327:623–625.
7. Kubo, T., Fukuda, K., Mikami, A., et al. (1989): *Nature*, 323:411–416.
8. Lai, J., Nunan, L., Waite, S. L., Ma, S-W., Bloom, J. W., Roeske, W. R., and Yamamura, H. I. (1992): *J. Pharmacol. Exp. Ther.*, 262:173–180.
9. Peralta, E. G., Ashkenazi, A., Winslow, J. W., Smith, D. H., Ramachandran, J., and Capon, D. J. (1987): *EMBO J.*, 119:3923–3929.
10. Wess, J., Lambrecht, G., Mutschler, E., Brann, M. R., and Dorje, F. (1991): *Br. J. Pharmacol.*, 102:246–250.

tent, with the exception of data for WB4101 (Table 3.9). The trend in the available data is general agreement with some exceptions. The question then is how to interpret the exceptions. As with the data for mutant receptors shown in Table 3.1, one could take the view that negative data (i.e., affinities that do not match) should be weighted more heavily than consistent data and

**TABLE 3.7.** *Affinity of α-adrenoceptor antagonists for $\alpha_1$-adrenoceptors expressed in cell lines*

| Receptor | Cell | WB4101 | $K_i$ (nM) Prazosin | Phent. | Indor | Coryn | Ref. |
|---|---|---|---|---|---|---|---|
| $\alpha_{1A}$-Adrenoceptors | | | | | | | |
| Rat | COS-7 | 2 | | | | | 1 |
| | Kidney[a] | 0.1 | | | | | 2 |
| $\alpha_{1B}$-Adrenoceptors | | | | | | | |
| Rat | COS-7 | 29 | 0.6 | 340 | 226 | 517 | 1 |
| | Kidney | 5.1 | | | | | 2 |
| Hamster | COS-7 | 8.5 | 0.3 | 155 | 84 | 640 | 3 |
| | COS-7 | 10 | 2.5 | 300 | | | 4 |
| | COS-7[b] | 5.9 | 0.3 | 82 | | | 6 |
| | HeLa | 12 | 0.11 | | | | 5 |
| $\alpha_{1C}$-Adrenoceptors | | | | | | | |
| Bovine | COS-7 | 0.68 | 0.37 | 15.3 | | 142 | 1 |
| | COS-7 | 0.6 | 0.3 | 5 | 6 | 78 | 3 |
| | HeLa | 0.7 | 0.06 | | | | 5 |

[a] Radioactive ligand [$^{125}$I]HEAT (m2-{β-(4-hydroxy-3-[$^{125}$I]iodophenyl)ethylaminomethyl}-tetralone).
[b] Radioactive ligand [$^3$H]prazosin.
Phent., phentolamine.
1. Lomasney, J. W. S., Cotecchia, S., Lorenz, W., et al. (1991): *J. Biol. Chem.,* 266: 6365–6369.
2. Klijn, K., Slivka, S. R., Bell, K., and Insel, P. A. (1990): *Mol. Pharmacol.,* 39:407–413.
3. Schwinn, D. A., Lomasney, J. W., Lorenz, W., et al. (1990): *J. Biol. Chem.,* 265: 8183–8189.
4. Cotecchia, S., Schwinn, D. A., Randall, R. R., Lefkowitz, R. J., Caron, M. G., and Kobilka, B. K. (1988): *Proc. Natl. Acad. Sci. U.S.A.,* 85:7159–7163.
5. Schwinn, D. A., Page, S. O., Middleton, J. P., et al. (1991): *Mol. Pharmacol.,* 40:619–626.
6. Perez, D. M., Piascik, M. T., and Graham, R. M. (1991): *Mol. Pharmacol.,* 40:876–883.

that they might indicate posttranslational differences in expressed receptors or differences in receptor environment that are made manifest in the observed affinity of selected drugs. However, another equally plausible hypothesis is that the expression systems may be indicating special properties of certain antagonists (e.g., negative efficacy). This idea is supported by expres-

**TABLE 3.8.** *p$K_i$ Estimates of β-adrenoceptor antagonists for the human $\beta_2$-adrenoceptor expressed in cell lines*

| Cell line | CYP | Betax. | ICI 118,551 | Prop. | Ref. |
|---|---|---|---|---|---|
| Mouse B82 | 10.3 | 7.0 | 8.5 | 8.6 | 1 |
| CHW | 9.9 | 6.22 | 8.6 | | 2 |
| Mouse B82 | 10.7 | | | 9.66 | 3 |

CYP, [$^{125}$I]cyanopindolol; Betax., betaxolol; Prop., propranolol.
1. Fraser, C. M., Chung, F-Z., and Venter, J. C. (1987): *J. Biol. Chem.,* 262:14843–14846.
2. Bouvier, M., Hnatowitch, M., Collins, S., et al. (1988): *Mol. Pharmacol.,* 33:133–139.
3. Chung, F-Z., Wang, C-D., Potter, P.C., Venter, J. C., and Fraser, C. M. (1988): *J. Biol. Chem.,* 263:4052–4055.

**TABLE 3.9.** *Affinities of α-adrenoceptor antagonists for α₂-adrenoceptors expressed in COS-7 cells*

| Antagonist | $\alpha_2$-C4[a] | | $\alpha_2$-C10[b] | |
|---|---|---|---|---|
| | Ref. 1 | Ref. 2 | Ref. 1 | Ref. 2 |
| Yohimbine | 0.93 | 0.3 | 1.6 | 0.5 |
| Phentolamine | 33 | 12.7 | 4.1 | 10 |
| Prazosin | 41 | 10.7 | 302 | 1800 |
| WB4101 | 0.94 | 0.3 | 7.8 | 0.9 |

[a] Human gene for $\alpha_2$-adrenoceptor on chromosome 4.
[b] Human gene for $\alpha_2$-adrenoceptor on chromosome 10.

1. Regan, J. W., Kobilka, T. S., Yang-Feng, T. L., Caron, M. G., Lefkowitz, R. J., and Kobilka, B. K. (1988): *Proc. Natl. Acad. Sci. U.S.A.,* 85:6301–6305.
2. Bylund, D. B., Blaxall, H. S., Iversen, L. J., Caron, M. G., Lefkowitz, R. J., and Lomasney, J. W. (1992): *Mol. Pharmacol.,* 42:1–5.

sion data that are consistent, except for a select few, with a series of antagonists. In any case, the critical question is whether surrogate expression systems will reflect drug affinity accurately as it will be operative therapeutically. It is premature to make judgments, but the tremendous promise of receptor expression in surrogate systems offers advantages often not available in natural tissue systems. For example, a pure population of receptors can be expressed in a membrane and the drug affinity for a single receptor type can be determined. It is always possible that in natural tissues, a mixture of receptor subtypes is present and the observed affinity is for an amalgam of binding affinities. In fact, receptor expression in cells offers the opportunity to determine which natural tissue systems most closely resemble pure receptor populations. Table 3.10 shows the affinity of a selection of

**TABLE 3.10.** *Affinities of α-adrenoceptor antagonists for α₂-adrenoceptors expressed in COS-7 cells and those found in HT29 cells*

| Antagonist | HT29 cells | | COS-C10[a] | |
|---|---|---|---|---|
| | $K_i$ (nM) | Slope[b] | $K_i$ (nM) | Slope |
| Rauwolscine | 0.44 | | 0.32 ± 0.02 | 1.05 |
| Yohimbine | 0.65 | | 0.5 ± 0.02 | 1.38 |
| WB4101 | 1.27 ± 0.03 | 1.23 | 0.91 ± 0.03 | 1.01 |
| BAM 1303 | 1.43 ± 0.08 | 1.03 | 0.39 ± 0.03 | 1.16 |
| Phentolamine | 4.22 ± 0.64 | 0.91 | 4.1 ± 0.3 | 1.07 |
| Spiroxatrine | 8.3 ± 1.6 | 0.94 | 5.5 ± 0.8 | 1.21 |
| Raubasine | 8.9 | | 6.4 ± 0.3 | 1.1 |
| Aukammigine | 104 ± 10 | 1.14 | 71 ± 7 | 0.91 |
| ARC-239 | 171 | | 131 ± 16 | 0.98 |
| Chlorpromazine | 253 ± 22 | 1.05 | 78 ± 10 | 1.08 |
| Prazosin | 316 | | 302 ± 18 | |

[a] Human gene for $\alpha_2$-adrenoceptors on chromosome 10.
[b] Slope of displacement curve.
From ref. 12.

α-adrenoceptor antagonists for human $\alpha_2$-adrenoceptors expressed in COS cells and the naturally occurring $\alpha_2$-adrenoceptors found in HT29 cells. The close agreement indicates that HT29 cells appear to have a pure population present in the membrane. An added possible bonus of this type of study is the ability to select potentially different antagonists. For example, the threefold difference for chlorpromazine, although small, is larger than for the other antagonists. This may suggest that chlorpromazine binding is more complex than that operative for the other antagonists.

In general, the new technology of receptor expression and reconstitution of membrane systems offers the potential to construct and thereby understand the complexities of ligand-receptor binding and activation.

## ISOLATED TISSUES

This monograph deals primarily with classification of the molecular properties of drugs. It should be noted that because the global effects of drugs *in vivo*, with respect to reflex and central control, cannot be predicted in isolated tissues, often the effects of drugs in the central nervous system or on the mechanisms controlling inflammatory responses cannot be quantified in this way. In these cases, whole-animal models are essential, and isolated tissues play a minimal role.

In general, the independent variable from which all drug classification data are obtained is *drug concentration*, and it is from this parameter that the dependent variable, *drug response*, is obtained. Therefore, it is of paramount importance that accurate estimates of the independent variable (drug concentration at the receptor) be available from which to calculate drug affinity and efficacy. The system of maximal complexity in which this can be done with any measure of confidence is the isolated tissue. Tissue structure and drug-removal processes within isolated tissues often can severely modulate drug concentrations at the receptor, but there are procedures designed to first detect and then overcome these obstacles; discussion of these problems will be found in Chapters 4 and 5. In view of these procedures, it is not unreasonable to assume that the drug concentration at the receptor can be controlled and that reliable independent variables can, for the most part, be obtained in isolated tissues.

Another prime consideration is the prediction of responses. As seen in Chapter 2, organs often greatly amplify receptor stimuli to generate responses. It is unlikely that *in vivo* these responses are further amplified. Therefore, the isolated tissue will usually be the simplest unit capable of generating the magnitude of response to be expected *in vivo*. Because biochemical systems lack amplification mechanisms, agonists of low intrinsic efficacy that produce responses in tissues often do not generate biochemical responses, and function rather as antagonists in subcellular membrane systems. For example, the low-efficacy partial agonist prenalterol produces powerful changes in cardiac state (tachycardia and positive inotropy). How-ever, increases in cyclic AMP, the initial intracellular messenger responsible for these responses, cannot be detected biochemically (Fig. 3.12). These data indicate that the increased level of cyclic AMP is too low to measure biochemically, but sufficient for the amplification systems in the myocardial cell to produce a response. Therefore, the agonist effects of prenalterol seen *in vitro* and *in vivo* (in animals and humans) would not have been predicted in a biochemical system that measured increases in cyclic AMP in this tissue.

Isolated tissues have been used pharmacologically for a number of years, and much experience with these systems has been reported in the scientific literature. The procedures for isolated-tissue experimentation usually are simple and cost-effective, and most isolated tissues are amenable to experi-ments utilizing the single most important concept in experimental pharmacol-ogy, namely, the null procedure. Dealt with more fully in Chapter 6, null procedures allow the state of the tissue to be determined before and after an intervention. For example, the sensitivity of a tissue to an agonist can be determined with a concentration-response curve. Thus, a series of dependent variables (responses) is obtained for a given series of independent variables (agonist concentrations). The agonist then is removed by washing the tissue with fresh bathing medium; this allows removal of the agonist from the recep-tor compartment and a return of the tissue to the predrug state. The tissue then can be equilibrated with an antagonist, and after a sufficient period of time, the concentration-response curve for the agonist can be repeated. In null procedures, it is *assumed* that the repeated challenge to the agonist in the absence of an intervention (i.e., antagonist) would have generated the original control concentration-response curve. Experimentally, this can be verified, and all experiments using this approach must conform to this restric-tion. Therefore, the null hypothesis contends that the state of the tissue (sensitivity to agonist) *has not changed* in the time period during which antagonist was introduced into the organ bath. If a change of state (sensitiv-ity) is observed (i.e., if the null hypothesis is disproved), then the change of state can be attributed to the intervention (presence of the antagonist), and

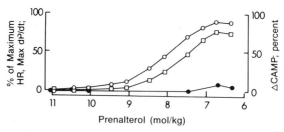

**FIG. 3.12.** Effects of prenalterol on heart rate (○), cardiac contractility (maximal $dP$/dt, □), and myocardial cyclic AMP levels (●) in anesthetized cats. (From ref. 26.)

by comparing equal tissue states (equal responses), the extent of the impact of such interventions can be quantified. The control of drug concentration in the receptor compartment and the resilience of isolated-tissue systems to repeated stimulation allow this rather rigorous procedure to be successful. This, in turn, forms the basis for quantification of responses to drugs and determination of the fundamental properties of drugs. In this way, isolated tissues offer simple, convenient, and reliable test systems.

The choice of which isolated tissue to use is based on what information is required. In general, there are three settings for pharmacologic experiments. The first historically has been the use of isolated tissues for bioassay, in which the types and magnitudes of responses to unknown materials allow identification and quantification. The second uses the tissue as a response system for study of the magnitude of the pharmacologic effect. The third relates to the use of tissues to predict therapeutic effects in humans.

### Bioassay

Because isolated tissues can be exquisitely sensitive amplifiers of agonist stimuli and because a stimulus is dependent on, among other things, drug concentration, it follows that tissues can be used to detect and quantify drugs in biological fluids. The process of identification and quantification of biologically active substances by measurement of tissue responses has been given the name "bioassay." In these procedures, various isolated tissues for which responses can be measured are superfused with fluid (i.e., blood); the type and magnitude of the response can be used to identify the biologically active components in the fluid (Fig. 3.13). Identification of the substance can be achieved by judicious choice of tissues; for example, the rat colon is very sensitive to angiotensin, but relatively insensitive to other substances normally found in the circulation; thus, this tissue is useful in the detection of this autacoid. Concentration-response curves for known concentrations of substances can be obtained, thereby calibrating the tissues with respect to magnitude of response versus concentration of substance. In this way, the concentration of biologically active substance in the fluid can be estimated.

With the advent of sophisticated chemical (i.e., high-pressure liquid chromatography) and biochemical (radioimmunoassay) techniques that are capable of identifying and quantifying biologically active substances, the need for isolated tissues for bioassays is diminishing. However, in terms of the discovery of unknown substances that function as mediators in physiological and/or pathophysiological states, isolated tissues still are valuable tools. The utilization of blood vessels in bioassays for endothelium-derived relaxing factor (EDRF) is an example. Thought to be released by a number of substances from the fragile layer of endothelial cells lining the lumen in blood vessels, EDRF may be an important mediator of lumen diameter. This sub-

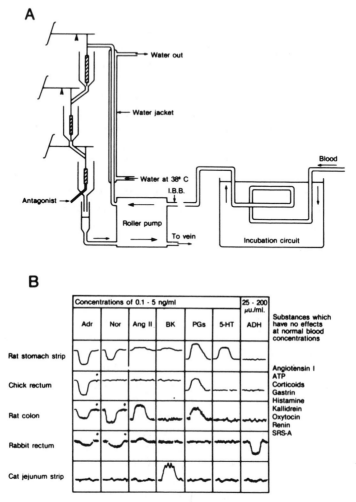

**FIG. 3.13.** Superfusion cascade experiment for bioassay. **A:** Blood (or other nutrient fluid to be analyzed) is pumped through a warming jacket (37°C) and allowed to superfuse a series of isolated organs, the movements of which are detected by transducers. The fluid is collected in a reservoir and may be recirculated. **B:** Reactions of some blood-bath organs to various endogenous substances to be found in the circulation. Adr, epinephrine; Nor, norepinephrine; Ang II, angiotensin II; BK, bradykinin; PGs, prostaglandins; 5-HT, 5-hydroxytryptamine; ADH, vasopressin. (From ref. 54.)

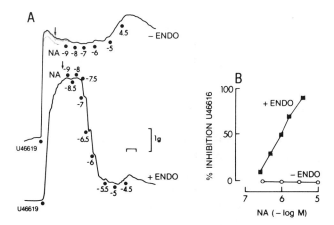

**FIG. 3.14.** Bioassay for EDRF. **A:** Relaxation of precontracted (UK-46,619, 10 nM) pig circumflex coronary artery produced by norepinephrine (NA; negative numbers refer to logarithms of molar concentrations) in artery with intact endothelium (+ENDO); preparation with endothelium removed (−ENDO) shows no relaxation to NA. **B:** Cumulative concentration-response curves to norepinephrine showing relaxation only in preparations with intact endothelium (+ENDO). (From ref. 14.)

stance is unstable, with a very short half-life. However, EDRF produces relaxation of blood vessels, and the various mechanisms that release this substance can be studied through this pharmacologic response; in effect, the blood vessel provides a bioassay for EDRF (Fig. 3.14).

### Tissues as Mirrors of Drug Actions

There is a large body of data suggesting that the drug receptors studied in animals correspond to those in humans (see Table 1.1). Also, there is considerable evidence to show that drug receptors are the same, with respect to interaction with drugs, neurotransmitters, and hormones, across species, organs, and types of tissues. Therefore, it follows that studies of drug interactions with drug receptors can be carried out on any tissue suitable for *in vitro* experimentation; the tissue can be considered to be primarily a response amplifier for the drug receptor. From this point of view, studies of the α-adrenoceptors in rabbit aorta become relevant to prediction of effects on the α-adrenoceptors in guinea pig atria. Given this latitude, the pharmacologist can tailor the type of response system to specific needs. Two factors become useful variants in the choice of isolated tissue used for experimentation: the magnitude of the amplification factor for receptor stimuli, and the capability for manipulation of the amplification. As shown in Fig. 2.11, tissues can vary dramatically in terms of sensitivity to agonists. When weak, low-efficacy agonists are used, differences in stimulus amplification can translate into a spectrum in which an efficiently coupled tissue generates a response to the agonist and a poorly coupled tissue generates no response, and in fact the weak "agonist" then functions as an antagonist of more powerful agonists (see Fig. 11.8). This can be advantageous in that the affinity of the low-efficacy agonist can more easily be measured in a tissue that generates no response to the weak agonist. Alternatively, if the intrinsic efficacy or antagonist is to be quantified, a tissue with a powerful stimulus-response apparatus will be more appropriate to increase the amplification of the low-level stimulus. There are circumstances in which the magnitude of the response to an agonist may need to be manipulated. Such control is more easily achieved in some tissues than in others. For example, because the guinea pig ileum is dependent on extracellular calcium for contraction, control of the calcium concentration in the fluid bathing the tissue subsequently can control responses to spasmogens (drugs producing contraction) (see Fig. 2.23). On the other hand, rabbit aorta primarily utilizes intracellular calcium stores for contractions mediated by some spasmogens; thus, the manipulation of extracellular calcium would have little effect on contractile responses in this tissue.

### Tissues as Predictors of Therapeutic Effects

If an antihypertensive drug reduces blood pressure by blockade of $\alpha$-adrenoceptors, it is reasonable to quantify the blocking potency in isolated tissues and predict therapeutic potency in humans. In this case, the fundamental property of the drug can be quantified in any tissue containing $\alpha$-adrenoceptors, and the parameters obtained can be applied globally to these same receptors in human blood vessels. However, there are examples of therapeutic effects that cannot be effectively quantified in this way, either because the nature of the therapeutically useful event is not known or because it is too complex a process to be easily predicted from a simple isolated-tissue assay. In some of these cases there have been specialized isolated-tissue systems to predict therapeutic effects and still retain the advantages of isolated-tissue experimentation. These will be dealt with later in this chapter.

## TISSUE VIABILITY AND STABILITY

The two primary prerequisites for isolated-tissue preparations are viability and stability. Thus, the tissues must be isolated and placed in life-support systems by procedures that do not damage viability, and the needs of these organs must be met to ensure stability with respect to organ function over the course of the experiment. The first consideration is the source of the isolated tissue.

## Sources of Tissues

Tissues can be obtained from animals or humans. There are three basic subsets of animals from which tissues can be obtained: healthy inbred laboratory animals, genetically special animals, and animals pharmacologically or surgically altered for specific purposes. The first subset represents by far the largest source of isolated tissues in pharmacology. In general, homogeneous species of animals matched for strain, age, and weight are used for pharmacologic experiments. The control of factors such as age and weight does much to ensure tissue homogeneity and subsequent reproducibility of isolated-tissue experiments.

There are genetically specialized animal species that are very useful in certain pharmacologic settings. For example, it is postulated that the failing human myocardium responds substantially better to digitalis than does healthy human myocardium. This suggests a need for animal models of congestive heart failure for more predictive testing of potential treatments for this disease. In this instance there is a hereditary cardiomyopathic strain of Syrian hamster (UMX7.1) that can be used as a model for heart failure, and myocardial tissue from this species could be valuable in predicting effects in human failing hearts. Figure 3.15 shows the lower cardiac performance and increased end-diastolic pressure (indicating failure of the ventricle to empty completely, a hallmark of ventricular failure) in Syrian hamsters versus normal golden hamsters. There are genetic strains of animals available (e.g., spontaneously hypertensive rats as a model for human primary hypertension) for many disease states that allow for specialized isolated-tissue experimentation.

Another way of obtaining specialized isolated tissues is by surgical or chemical manipulation. For example, in dogs, surgical creation of an atrioventricular fistula (a shunt between the abdominal aorta and vena cava is produced, thereby introducing a state of volume overload to the intact myocardium) yields a heart in failure after a period of 56 days. Figure 3.16A shows

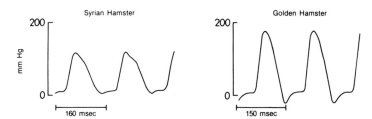

**FIG. 3.15.** Intraventricular pressure tracings for myopathic hamster (Syrian) and normal hamster (golden) hearts. Syrian hamster demonstrates low myocardial performance characteristic of failing hearts. (From ref. 45.)

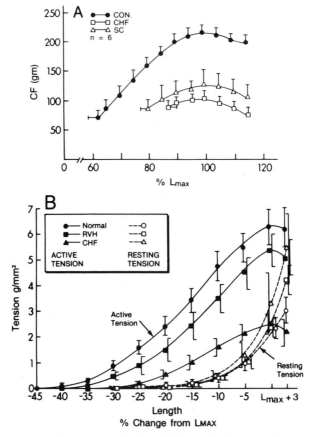

**FIG. 3.16.** Animal models of congestive heart failure. **A:** Mean length–contractile-force (active tension) curves for dog hearts in control state (CON), during congestive heart failure with patent aortocaval shunt (CHF), and after shunt closure (SC). All points for CHF and SC significantly depressed from control. (From ref. 38.) **B:** Length-tension curves for papillary muscles from normal (•), hypertrophied (■), and failing (▲) cat right ventricles. Open symbols show resting tension; filled symbols show actively developed tension. Note the significant depression of active tension generated by tissues from cats with congestive heart failure. (From ref. 47.)

the depressed length-versus-contractile-force curves obtained in hearts put into failure by volume overload. The state of myocardial failure precludes the sizable increased contractile-force response to increased length seen in healthy hearts. Under these circumstances, the heart cannot respond adequately to changes in volume. Isolated tissues from such animals can be useful for predicting drug effects in failed myocardium. For example, ventricular failure can be produced in cats by chronic pulmonary artery obstruction; the papillary muscles from these hearts demonstrate no differences with respect to passive tension, but a greatly reduced capacity to generate active tension when compared with tissue from normal hearts (Fig. 3.16B).

In addition to surgical manipulation, chronic drug treatments can be used to manipulate physiological states of organs. A classic example of this is treatment of rats with diethylstibestrol to achieve a state of estrus; because the estrous cycle greatly alters the responsiveness of rat uterus to drugs, homogeneity with respect to this variable is essential.

Whereas animals are widely used for the testing of drugs, isolated tissues may be obtained from humans as well. Typically, tissues can be obtained as by-products of surgical procedures (e.g., human atrial appendages from coronary bypass operations) or by rapid postmortem acquisition. In both of these settings, the question of tissue viability is paramount. Compromise on this prerequisite can occur because of damage incurred during handling of tissue, because of the period of time that elapses before adequate life support can be given to the tissue, or because the organ often is diseased to begin with. These factors must be considered when testing drugs on such tissues and using the resultant data to predict responses in humans.

### Preservation of Viability

In general, the aim of isolated-tissue experimentation is to isolate an organ in its normal functioning state and to be able to quantify and control drug concentration. Implicit is the assumption that the organ is in a physiological state comparable to that in the whole animal. It is in this realm that the years of empirical experimentation in isolated-tissue research are valuable, because much effort has been expended (and results documented) to find the particular ideal *in vitro* conditions for each specific type of isolated tissue. Although it is difficult to know that the *in vitro* state of the tissue exactly corresponds to *in vivo* function, conditions can be defined that will produce a stable and viable tissue suitable for the testing of drug effects. There are two aspects to this. One relates to the prediction of responses in humans, and here a question usually remains as to the accuracy of predictions in isolated tissues. The other aspect relates to the use of tissues as amplifiers of drug stimuli. In terms of homogeneous and stable test systems for drugs and the use of tissues for classifying drugs, *in vitro* conditions can be explicitly defined that will allow for an acceptable degree of reproducibility (*vide infra*).

Work by pioneers such as Tyrode (1878–1930), Ringer (1835–1910), and Krebs (1900–1981) has established the ionic compositions for nutrient solutions (which now bear their names) for isolated-tissue experimentation. Over the years, these solutions have been modified for individual tissues, reflecting the spectrum of ionic needs for various organs in the body. The osmolarity of the bathing medium must be controlled, as changes in this factor can affect the size of the extracellullar space and the volume of muscle cells. Figure 3.17 shows the effects of changing the nutrient-solution tonicity on the extracellular space in guinea pig teniae coli. The pH of the nutrient solution is important from the standpoint of tissue viability, as well as the correct ionization of drugs with respect to extracellular fluid *in vivo*. Temperature is another important variable, because it can greatly affect tissue basal activity and responsiveness to drugs. For example, rat uterus produces erratic spontaneous contractions at a temperature of 37°C and thus cannot readily be used as a preparation for the study of drugs. However, reduction of the temperature to room temperature yields a regularly contracting tissue suitable for *in vitro* experimentation. Reduction of the bath temperature also can be useful to reduce basal levels of tissue oxygen consumption, thereby diminishing the risk of anoxia and tissue death; this factor is particularly important in studies on myocardial tissue.

The ion content, osmolarity, pH, and temperature of the bathing solution can be controlled for each type of isolated-tissue preparation. However, a more variable factor in the control of tissue viability is adequate delivery of oxygen to the tissue. This is because oxygenation depends on factors that vary with respect to experimental apparatus (i.e., the partial pressure of oxygen in the bathing medium) and to tissue requirements (oxygen consumption and thickness of the tissue). The partial pressure of oxygen at a depth $X$ (measured from the outer surface) in a flat tissue (wall thickness, $T$), to be denoted $Po_{2(wall)}$, relative to the partial pressure of oxygen in the medium surrounding the tissue $Po_{2(bath)}$, is given by

$$\frac{Po_{2(wall)}}{Po_{2(bath)}} = 1 - \frac{V_{O_2}}{120S \cdot D} \frac{T \cdot X - X^2}{Po_{2(bath)}} \qquad [3.1]$$

where $V_{O_2}$ is tissue oxygen consumption, $S$ is the solubility coefficient of oxygen in the medium, and $D$ is the diffusion coefficient of oxygen within the wall. From this equation it can be seen that if tissue oxygen consumption

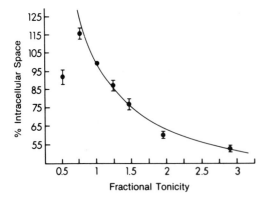

FIG. 3.17. Effect of nutrient-solution tonicity on intracellular space and smooth-muscle cell volume of guinea pig teniae coli. Hypertonicity of Krebs (sucrose added) expressed as a multiple of normal tonicity. Volume (ordinate) of intracellular space expressed as percentage of value in normal solution. (From ref. 8.)

is high or diffusion into the tissue is slow (low $D$), $Po_{2(wall)}$ could be less than $Po_{2(bath)}$, and a concentration gradient of oxygen across the thickness of the wall could develop. This would be more pronounced for thick rather than thin preparations (large $T$). This has two possible consequences for isolated-tissue experiments. The first is that the tissue may have a $Vo_2$ or thickness $T$ that precludes adequate basal oxygenation. Figure 3.18A shows the $Po_{2(bath)}$ required to produce maximal contractile tensions in some arterial prepara-

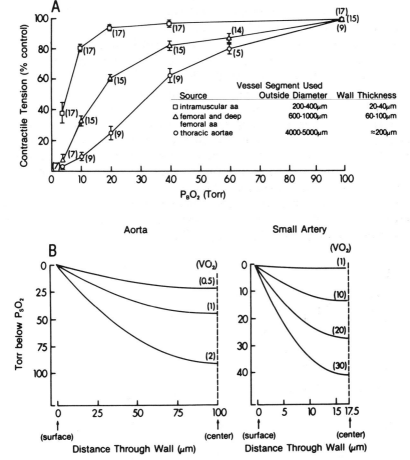

**FIG. 3.18.** Oxygenation of vascular smooth muscle. **A:** Relationship between partial pressure of oxygen in organ bath (P$_{BO2}$) and contraction to $10^{-7}$ M epinephrine for three different sizes of arteries (helical strips). Preparations with thinnest walls were least depressed by hypoxia. **B:** Calculated oxygen gradients within walls of rabbit aorta and small arteries. Isopleths were calculated from Eq. 3.1 and indicate that as oxygen consumption (V$_{O2}$) increases, a concentration gradient for oxygen develops within the wall, and a central core of the arterial wall becomes hypoxic (ordinate reflects the decrease in oxygen tension in the arterial wall versus oxygen tension in the organ bath). (From ref. 13.)

tions. It can be seen from this figure that the thickness of the arterial wall greatly affects adequate oxygenation. The other possibility is that, whereas oxygenation is adequate for basal tissue activity, the oxygen supply is not adequate for increased activity (i.e., production of a tissue response). Therefore, when $V_{O_2}$ increases, an oxygen gradient develops in the tissue that compromises the magnitude of the response to a drug. This is illustrated in Fig. 3.18B, where the oxygen concentration gradients through the walls of rabbit aortae and small arteries have been calculated at various oxygen consumptions. Note how in the aorta, a fourfold increase in oxygen consumption produces a striking concentration gradient for oxygen. These factors are particularly important for tissues of high oxygen consumption, such as the heart. Using equations similar to Eq. 3.1, a "critical thickness" for a preparation can be calculated beyond which it would be expected that a hypoxic core of cells would be present in the tissue.

Another factor in the delivery of oxygen to tissues is $S$, the solubility of oxygen in the medium. Because most experiments are conducted in aqueous nutrient solutions, this is a constant factor. However, in thick preparations (usually myocardium), blood perfusion has been utilized for organ preservation. The increased capacity of blood to carry oxygen greatly reduces the negative term in Eq. 3.1 and prevents oxygen concentration gradients from developing in thick preparations. Figure 3.19 shows that, whereas Krebs-perfused canine coronary artery does not respond to calcium chloride, blood-perfused artery demonstrates contraction; these data may reflect differences in oxygen-carrying capacity in the bathing media.

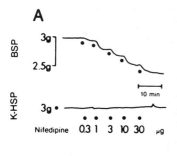

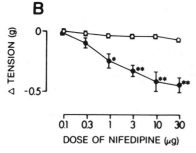

FIG. 3.19. **A:** Responses to calcium of canine coronary artery perfused with blood (BSP) or Krebs-Henseleit solution (K-HSP). **B:** Dose-response curves to calcium in blood-perfused (•) and Krebs-Henseleit-perfused (o) preparations. $*p < 0.05$, $**p < 0.01$, statistical significance from Krebs-perfused solutions. (From ref. 34.)

In general, although empirical methods and techniques are available to preserve tissue viability, criteria still are required to reject or accept isolated tissues as suitable systems for the study of drug effects. In some cases, an adequate scale of basal activity is available on which to base an opinion on tissue viability. For example, Fig. 3.20 shows transmembrane electrical potentials ($E_m$) for 363 cells from 36 canine saphenous veins; the normal distribution allows some degree of prediction of the significance of differences between resting membrane potentials for any given preparation of vein and the population of saphenous veins. Thus, if a tissue were found to have an $E_m$ of 38 mV (outside the 95% confidence limits of the mean $E_m$ for saphenous vein), this probably would indicate that the particular preparation could not be regarded as a normal representative of the population and therefore should be rejected.

More commonly, such indicators of basal activity are not available, and responses to drugs fulfill this discriminatory role. Figure 3.21A shows the concentrations of isoproterenol required to produce half-maximal relaxation in guinea pig trachea, and Fig. 3.21B shows the concentrations of histamine required to produce half-maximal contraction in the same tissue. These distributions are approximately normal and allow for 95% confidence limits to be calculated for the concentrations of isoproterenol or histamine required for the half-maximal response in this tissue. Therefore, if the sensitivity of any given guinea pig tracheal preparation did not fall within the 95% confidence limits, there would be only a 5% probability that the tissue represented the population. If this tolerance was unacceptable to the experimental procedure, this tissue could be rejected. This becomes a factor only when the

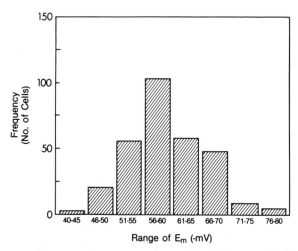

**FIG. 3.20.** Frequency histogram for transmembrane electrical potentials ($E_m$) for 363 cells recorded from 36 canine saphenous veins. (From ref. 35.)

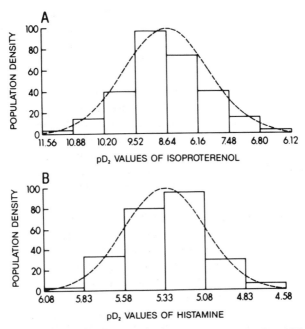

**FIG. 3.21.** Sensitivity of guinea pig tracheae to isoproterenol (**A**, $N = 128$) and histamine (**B**, $N = 75$). Sensitivity quantified as the negative logarithm of the molar concentration of agonist producing half-maximal response (pD₂). Ordinates are population densities (percentage of population per 0.25 interval of pD₂ value). Gaussian density functions derived from the mean pD₂ values; the area under the curve is equal to the area of the histograms. (From ref. 19.)

particular isolated tissues are required to be a representative sample of the population for prediction of therapeutic effect. In terms of internal comparisons of drugs on the same tissue, the absolute sensitivity of the tissue to drugs may not be a prime consideration. This is because there are a number of factors that cause differences in tissue sensitivities that are not due to differences in tissue viabilities. These include differences in efficiencies of coupling of stimulus-response mechanisms, ages of animals, and receptor densities and will be considered in the next section of this chapter. Because of the variances in tissue sensitivity introduced by these factors, tests of homogeneity should be applied more to the sample of preparations used for a defined study rather than to the entire population. For example, if a comparison to determine drug potency is to be carried out on a set of 20 guinea pig tracheae, and these come from 20 strain-, age-, and weight-matched animals, it is possible that the sensitivities of these tissues may be outside the 95% confidence limits of the population but still be internally homogeneous. Under these circumstances, the tissues provide valid comparisons with each other and are valuable for *in vitro* study.

### Tissue Stability

Another prime consideration in isolated-tissue experimentation is the requirement that the preparation be stable throughout the course of the experiment. As previously pointed out, null procedures that utilize a tissue as its own control (i.e., comparison between tissue states before and after a given intervention) tacitly assume stability. It is imperative that the basal state or sensitivity to drugs of the tissue not change during the course of the experiment. Usually, "control" experiments, in which tissue sensitivity is monitored in the absence of the intervention, are carried out either before or concomitant with the experimental procedure. Figure 3.22A shows responses of rat vasa deferentia to phenylephrine obtained with an interval of 80 min between curves. Figure 3.22B shows the relaxant effects of isoproterenol on human bronchial smooth muscle before and after a 2-hr equilibration period. In general, various isolated tissues have different "stability windows" with respect to agonists: these must be determined for each experiment.

In view of possible random spontaneous changes in tissue sensitivity, concurrent control experiments can be critical to the evaluation of experiments aimed at drug and drug-receptor classification. The ideal situation is one in which the control tissue shows no changes in sensitivities to drugs over the

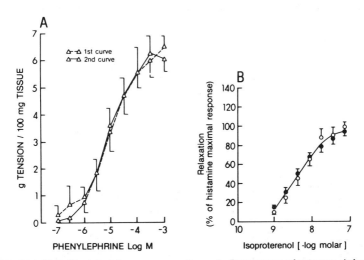

**FIG. 3.22.** Stability of isolated-tissue preparations. **A:** Responses of rat vasa deferentia to phenylephrine. Ordinate: Contraction in grams of tension per 100 mg tissue. Abscissa: Negative logarithms of molar concentrations of phenylephrine. Interval between first and second curve was 80 min. (From ref. 16.) **B:** Responses of human isolated bronchial smooth muscle to isoproterenol. Ordinate: Relaxation of histamine contraction expressed as a percentage of the maximal response. Abscissa: Negative logarithms of molar concentrations of isoproterenol. Second curve (o) obtained 2 hr after initial curve (•). (From ref. 41.)

time course of the experiment. In the event that a change is observed, the experimenter is left to decide whether to "correct" for fluctuations in sensitivity observed in the control tissue. If the changes in sensitivity result from changes in tissue viability, a theoretically interesting question arises whether a correction factor can be applied to the experiment. The rationale for such a factor is that the tissue samples are homogeneous enough to assume that the magnitude of the change in sensitivity observed in the control tissues is the same as in the experimental tissues. The possible hazard of such reasoning is clear, and, in practice, significant changes in the sensitivities of control tissues suggest technical problems, and the experiment should be repeated. This point is discussed further in Chapter 6.

## HOMOGENEITY OF ISOLATED TISSUES

A factor that could be relevant to the effective use of isolated tissues is the possible variation in tissue sensitivity to a drug with respect to the anatomy of the preparation. For example, Fig. 3.23 shows the general decline in the sensitivity of ring preparations of rabbit aorta to a variety of spasmogens as the tissues are taken from regions at differing distances from the aortic arch. Clearly, comparison of preparations from regions 1 and 7, with respect to drug effects, could yield quite erroneous results. In some cases, receptor density can be shown to be the causative factor. As discussed in Chapter 2,

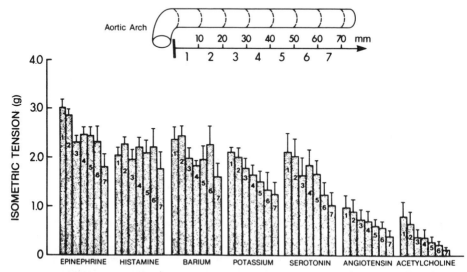

**FIG. 3.23.** Maximal responses to various agonists in different segments of rabbit descending thoracic aortae. Aortae were cut into spiral strips, and each strip cut into seven segments corresponding to orientation from aortic arch shown at top. (From ref. 1.)

the magnitude of a tissue response can be greatly affected by the number of responding units (receptors) available on the cell membrane to respond to the drug. Thus, if receptor density varies with the anatomical source of the tissue preparation, the sensitivity to drugs will parallel this variation. For example, the relative densities of α-adrenoceptors and β-adrenoceptors vary with the anatomy of the rabbit urinary bladder. Thus, whereas the bladder base has a greater density of α-adrenoceptors than does the bladder body (Fig. 3.24A), the reverse pattern is observed for β-adrenoceptors (Fig. 3.24B). These differences in receptor densities are reflected in the more powerful α-adrenoceptor-mediated responses obtained in the bladder base (Fig. 3.25A) and the more powerful β-adrenoceptor-mediated responses in the bladder body (Fig. 3.25B). If drugs activate both receptor types, the

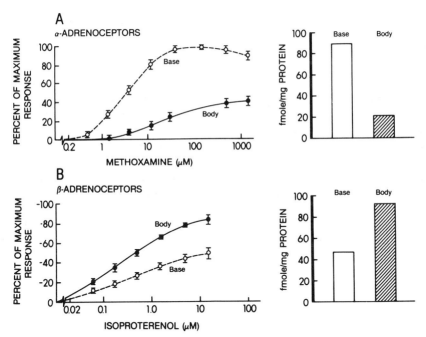

**FIG. 3.24.** Relationships between receptor densities and responses of rabbit urinary bladder base and body. **A:** Concentration-response curves to the α-adrenoceptor stimulant methoxamine. Ordinate: Contraction expressed as percentage of the maximal increase in tension in bladder base (Δ 1,600 mg over basal). Abscissa: Concentrations of methoxamine in micromoles (logarithmic scale). Histograms show the relative densities of [³H]dihydroergotamine-binding sites assumed to be α-adrenoceptors. The larger number of α-adrenoceptors in the bladder base parallels the larger response in methoxamine. **B:** Concentration-response curves to the β-adrenoceptor stimulant isoproterenol. Ordinate: Relaxation as a percentage of basal muscle tone. Abscissa: Concentrations of isoproterenol in micromoles (logarithmic scale). Histograms show the relative densities of [³H]dihydroalprenolol-binding sites assumed to be β-adrenoceptors. As for A, the receptor density parallels the magnitude of response. (From ref. 31.)

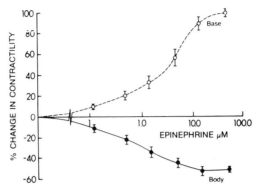

**FIG. 3.25.** Responses of rabbit urinary bladder to epinephrine. Ordinate: Contraction (0 to 100) expressed as percentage to maximal contractile response obtained in bladder base, relaxation (0 to −60) as percentage of basal tone. Abscissa: Concentrations of epinephrine in micromoles (logarithmic scale). Epinephrine stimulates α-adrenoceptors to produce contraction and β-adrenoceptors to produce relaxation. The opposite total responses of bladder base (α > β) and body (β > α) reflect the receptor predominances shown in Fig. 3.24. (From ref. 31.)

resulting organ response to the drug can be complex. For example, epinephrine activates both α- and β-adrenoceptors, producing urinary bladder contraction and relaxation, respectively. The relative populations of these two receptors cause epinephrine to have totally dissimilar tissue responses in the bladder base and body (Fig. 3.25); clearly, tissue strips from this organ could well be heterogeneous with respect to anatomy and responses to adrenergic drugs. These types of complications can increase with the complexity of the tissue. For example, pupil diameter is controlled by an α-adrenoceptor-mediated contraction of the iris sphincter, a β-adrenoceptor-mediated relaxation of the iris sphincter, and an α-adrenoceptor effect on the iris dilator. These three components can be observed separately in the effects of isoproterenol on pupil diameter in the guinea pig (Fig. 3.26).

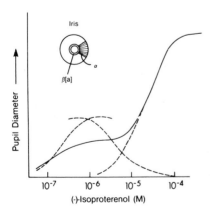

**FIG. 3.26.** Ocular responses to isoproterenol in guinea pigs. The initial response reflects β-adrenoceptor-mediated relaxation of the sphincter; the antagonistic second phase is the α-adrenoceptor constrictor component on the sphincter. The major dilation (third component) reflects α-adrenoceptor effects on the iris dilator. (From ref. 40.)

Another source of heterogeneity among samples of isolated tissues concerns the ages of the animals. Usually this would not present a problem with respect to a given series of acute experiments, because a sample of age-matched animals could be used. However, if this variable is not controlled, then dissimulations may arise when experiments are duplicated over long periods of time or when different laboratories wish to compare data. Figure 3.27A shows the differences in sensitivities of tracheae for young ($118 \pm 7$ g), middle-aged ($417 \pm 9.5$ g), and old ($757 \pm 23.2$ g) guinea pigs; a 4.5-fold difference in sensitivities is observed. Figure 3.27B shows the effects of age on rabbit aortic responses to sodium nitrite. The effects of age on drug responses can be quite dramatic, as in the increased responses of rat mesenteric

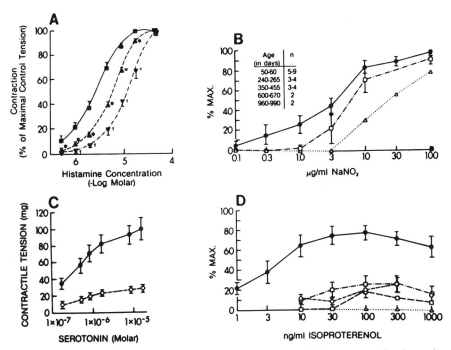

**FIG. 3.27.** Effects of age on responses of tissues to drugs. **A:** Responses of guinea pig tracheae to histamine. Ordinate: Contractions as percentages of maximal contraction. Abscissa: Logarithms of molar concentrations of histamine. Tissues from young (■, $N = 10$), middle-aged (▲, $N = 28$), and old (▼, $N = 8$) guinea pigs. (From ref. 9.) **B:** Responses of rabbit aortae to sodium nitrite. Ordinate: Relaxation as a percentage of induced contraction to histamine. Abscissa: Logarithms of molar concentrations of sodium nitrite. Tissues from rabbits 50 to 60 days old (●), 350 to 455 days old (□), and 960 to 990 days old (△). (From ref. 22.) **C:** Responses of helically cut rat mesenteric artery to serotonin. Ordinate: Contractile tension in milligrams. Abscissa: Logarithms of molar concentrations of serotonin. Tissues from rats 3 to 5 weeks old (○) and 9 to 13 weeks old (●). (From ref. 15.). **D:** Responses of rabbit aortae to isoproterenol. Ordinate and abscissa as for B. Tissues from rabbits 50 to 60 days old (●), 240 to 265 days old (○), 350 to 455 days old (□), and 600 to 670 days old (□). (From ref. 22.)

artery to serotonin with increased age (Fig. 3.27C). In this instance, a period of only 4 weeks produced significant differences in responsiveness. A similar effect can be seen in rabbit aorta, in which significant relaxation to isoproterenol was produced only in rabbits aged 50 to 60 days (Fig. 3.27D).

In general, anatomical location and animal maturity should be kept homogeneous to avoid possible heterogeneity of drug effects.

## QUANTIFICATION OF TISSUE RESPONSES

In pharmacologic analyses it is important that experimental conditions be maximized for accurate measurements of the drug-dependent variable of tissue response. There are factors separate from considerations of tissue viability and stability that are relevant to the measurement of responses. In general, a response can be thought of as any change in the state of the tissue. Responses can be quantified as contraction, relaxation, or a change in the frequency or magnitude of basal activity; some commonly measured responses are shown in Fig. 3.28. This figure shows that responses can be measured as sustained contractions (Fig. 3.28A), inhibition of twitch contraction (Fig. 3.28B), transient contraction (Fig 3.28C), or sustained relaxation of induced contraction (Fig. 3.28D). For a reliable response scale to be obtained, the tissue must be placed in a state optimal for detection and measurement of state changes. A fundamental tool in this process, at least for isolated muscular tissue, is the length-tension curve. If a muscle is stretched, it will resist force with a passive tension related to the elastic properties of the tissue. Muscle also contracts to a stimulus and thus is able to generate an active tension. The dependence of the magnitude of the active tension, the dependent variable of interest in pharmacologic experiments, on the basal resting tension placed on the muscle is defined by the length-tension curve for the muscle (Fig. 3.29A). As can be seen in Fig. 3.29A, if the resting tension on the muscle is too low, little active tension will be detected. Similarly, if the resting tension is too great, the active tension diminishes; the optimal experimental condition is the tissue length ($L_{max}$) at which the active tension is maximal. It is important to define this point for each type of isolated tissue and equilibrate preparations at this basal length. Muscle contraction can be quantified in terms of isometric tension generated or isotonic shortening at a constant load. Figure 3.29B shows the effect of resting load on the degree of isotonic shortening obtained in canine trachea; as resting load is increased (resting and total tension increase), the capability of the muscle to shorten (lateral distance between curves 1 and 3) diminishes.

Determination of length-tension relationships may be critical when comparing tissues in different physiological or pathophysiological states. For example, blood vessels from spontaneously hypertensive rates or hyperlipidemic rabbits often are compared with those from normal animals in attempts

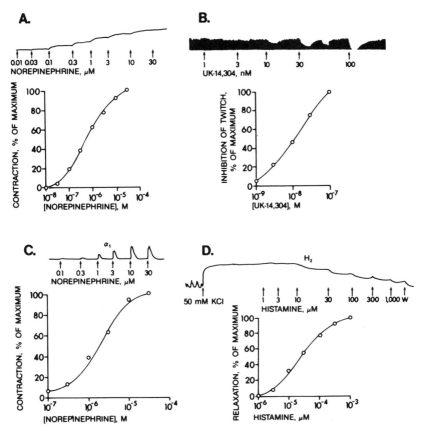

**FIG. 3.28.** Responses of isolated tissues to drugs. Ordinates: Responses as percentages of the maximal response to the agonist. Abscissae: Molar concentrations of drugs (logarithmic scale). **A:** Contraction of guinea pig aorta to norepinephrine. Sustained contractions allow cumulative addition of norepinephrine. **B:** Inhibition of electrically induced twitch contraction in guinea pig ileum by UK-14304. Electrical field stimulation produced uniform twitch contractions of this tissue due to released acetylcholine. UK-14304 inhibits the release of acetylcholine by a presynaptic mechanism, thereby inhibiting twitch contraction. **C:** Contraction of rat vas deferens to norepinephrine. Contractile responses are not sustained in this preparation; therefore, transient responses to drug stimulation are obtained. Under these circumstances, cumulative addition of agonist (as for A) is not feasible, and agonist must be removed from the bath by washing after every response. **D:** Relaxation of rat uterus by histamine. This tissue must be precontracted with a spasmogen (i.e., KCl) to produce an elevated contractile tone so that relaxation to agonist can be observed. Histamine is added cumulatively. (From ref. 42.)

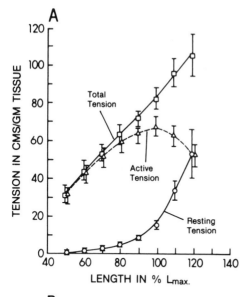

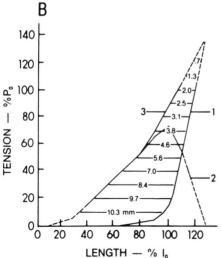

**FIG. 3.29.** Length-tension curves for isolated tissues. **A:** Canine bronchial smooth muscle. Ordinate: Tension as a percentage of the maximal active tension. Abscissa: Length of tissue as percentage of $L_{max}$, the length at which maximal active tension is obtained. As the tissue is stretched, resistance to lengthening generates passive resting tension (o). At various muscle lengths, the maximal increase in tension to electrical stimulation was recorded (□). The active tension generated by the contractile elements of the muscle is calculated by subtraction of the total and resting tensions (▽). Note how as the muscle is stretched excessively (beyond $L_{max}$), total tension is nearly completely generated by the elastic elements of the tissue (resting tension), and the preparation becomes incapable of producing active tension in response to electrical stimulation. (From ref. 49.) **B:** Isotonic tissue shortening in canine tracheae. Ordinate: Muscle tension as percentage of mean active tension from a large sample of isometric experiments. Abscissa: Muscle length as percentage of $L_{max}$. Numbers refer to resting tension (1), total tension (3), and active tension (2). Horizontal lines joining curves 1 and 3 refer to the shortening that the muscle is capable of at the various afterloads shown on the ordinate. Note that as the load increases, the tissue is less able to shorten. (From ref. 51.)

to study the effects of these pathological conditions on vessel reactivity to drugs. It is important in these studies to correct for differences in vessel thickness and muscle mass, because these factors may produce artifactual differences in reactivities to drugs. Figure 3.30 shows the active tension generated by mesenteric arteries from large and small rats (vessels of different muscle masses). It is clear that the correct resting tensions for generation of optimal active tensions are different for the two arteries. Therefore, if both types of arteries were to be placed at the $L_{max}$ for arteries from small rats (resting tension of 800 mg), the active tension produced by arteries from large rats would seriously underestimate the true tension-generating capacity of these tissues.

It is important to consider technical problems in the measurement of tissue responses. For example, contractile responses from small arteries often are difficult to measure because of the low magnitude of active tension. In these cases, spiral strips can be used to increase the muscle mass from which recordings can be made. Thus, a helix cut along the spiral configuration of the smooth-muscle cells theoretically produces a continuous chain of cells oriented for longitudinal contraction (Fig. 3.31A). However, deviation of the pitch of the helix from the true orientation of the smooth-muscle cells can produce serious differences in the responses of helical preparations to spasmogens. Figure 3.31B shows the effects of pitch on generated tension with respect to the angle used to cut a helical strip. The extremes of the possible orientations illustrate an interesting paradox: Whereas a drug that produces contraction of smooth-muscle cells also contracts a circumferential-ring preparation of rabbit aorta, it also produces paradoxical relaxation of a longitudinal aortic preparation (Fig. 3.31C), probably because the contraction of the muscle cells produces lengthening of the artery. It is clear from such data that considerable heterogeneity, with respect to muscle response, can be introduced by variances in the preparation of helical muscle strips. An alternative is to use ring preparations of blood vessels suspended between hooks. Such preparations avoid geometric problems and are simple to use, but also are subject to greater heterogeneity with respect to receptor

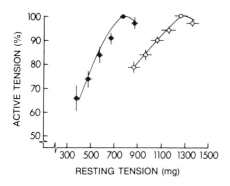

**FIG. 3.30.** Resting tension versus active tension in arteries of different dimensions. Ordinate: Active tension normalized as percentage of maximal active tension. Abscissa: Resting tension placed on the tissue. Mesenteric arteries from small (•, 200 to 250 g, age 2 to 3 months) and large (○, 600 to 700 g, age 6 to 8 months) rats. Wall thicknesses for mesenteric arteries from small rats ($0.18 \pm 0.02$ mm) and large rats ($0.21 \pm 0.01$ mm). (From ref. 58.)

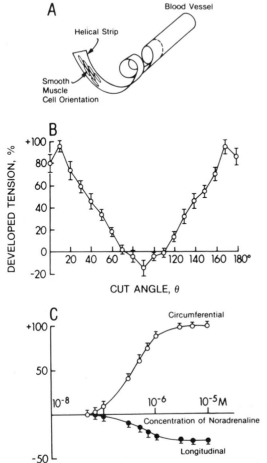

**FIG. 3.31.** Effect of helical pitch on responses of spiral strips of blood vessels to drugs. **A:** Schematic of spiral-strip preparation. **B:** Effect of angle of cut on maximal responses of femoral arteries to norepinephrine (100 μM). Abscissa: Pitch of the helical cut in degrees. Positive values indicate contraction, negative values relaxation. **C:** Responses of rings (circumferential contraction, o) and longitudinal preparations (•) of femoral artery to norepinephrine (abscissa, logarithmic scale). (B and C from ref. 39.)

density (see Fig. 3.22). A most useful approach to the quantification of responses of small blood vessels is the measurement of perfusion pressure. Thus, the artery is placed on a cannula and perfused through the lumen in an organ bath at a constant flow. The perfusion pressure is monitored, and provided that the artery produces the highest resistance to flow, pressure is proportional to the caliber of the lumen. Thus, spasmogens that constrict the arterial wall produce increases in perfusion pressure. Such preparations can be valuable for measurement of responses in preparations normally too small for mechanical measurement of contraction. For example, Fig. 3.32 shows α-adrenoceptor-mediated increases in coronary perfusion pressure in guinea pig hearts produced by a range of agonists. Such concentration-response curves would be exceedingly difficult to obtain accurately in isolated guinea pig coronary artery because of the small diameter of the vessels, but by using

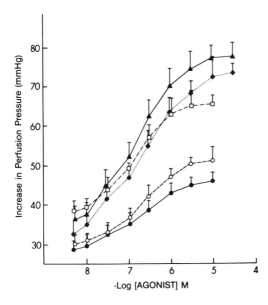

**FIG. 3.32.** Responses of guinea pig coronary circulation to α-adrenoceptor agonists. Ordinate: Increases in perfusion pressure (above basal) of Langendorf isolated perfused guinea pig hearts. Abscissa: Negative logarithms of molar concentrations of agonists added to perfusate. Increased pressure indicates increases in coronary vascular resistance. Responses to norepinephrine (Δ, NE; $N = 16$), clonidine (□, CLO; $N = 17$), α-methylnorepinephrine (♦, α-MeNE; $N = 16$), BHT-920 (○, BHT; $N = 3$), and phenylephrine (●, PHE; $N = 15$). (From ref. 17.)

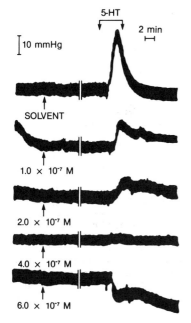

**FIG. 3.33.** Vascular perfusion pressure of guinea pig isolated stomach. Blood vessels of the stomach perfused at a constant flow rate with oxygenated Krebs-Henseleit solution; changes in perfusion pressure indicate vasoconstriction (increased pressure) or vasorelaxation (decreased pressure) of small resistance vessels. Responses to serotonin (12.5 ng/mL$^{-1}$ over 5-min infusion) in the absence (solvent) and presence of various concentrations of the serotonin antagonist ketanserin (added at *arrow*). (From ref. 56.)

the whole heart as a conduit organ for the vessels, reliable responses can be obtained. Figure 3.33 shows similar responses in a perfused guinea pig stomach; the perfusion pressure is controlled by microvessels far too small to be used under normal *in vitro* conditions, but reliable responses can be obtained by whole-organ perfusion.

## SPECIALIZED PREPARATIONS

Isolated tissues also can be used to predict therapeutic responses. There are cases in which electronic manipulation of response measurements can increase the amount of information gained from an isolated tissue. For example, the β-adrenoceptor agonist isoproterenol increases the strength of contraction of electrically stimulated guinea pig left atria (Fig. 3.34A). A concentration-response curve can be obtained that will quantify this response and

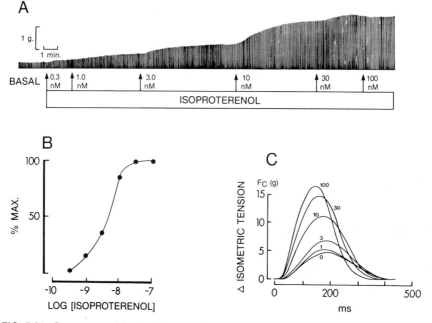

**FIG. 3.34.** Responses of isolated myocardium to isoproterenol. **A:** Dynograph tracing of electrically induced twitch contraction of guinea pig left atria. Increased strength of isometric contraction is produced by isoproterenol. **B:** Concentration-response curve for data in A. Ordinate: Increases in contraction (over basal) as percentages of maximal increase (to 100 nM isoproterenol). Abscissa: Logarithms of molar concentrations of isoproterenol. **C:** High-speed oscilloscope tracings of electrically stimulated twitch contractions of guinea pig papillary muscles. These twitch contractions are qualitatively the same as seen in A, except that the time scale is greatly expanded. Note how isoproterenol increases the rates of rise and fall of the contraction and shortens the duration of contraction, in addition to increasing twitch height. Numbers next to curves refer to isoproterenol concentrations (nmol/L). (C from ref. 18.)

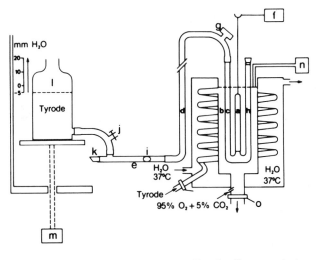

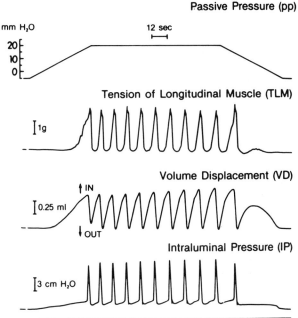

FIG. 3.35. Apparatus for studying gastrointestinal peristalsis. **Top:** One end of the ileum (a) is placed over an opening in U-tube (c, h); the other end is tied shut and connected to the isometric transducer (f); this records longitudinal contractions. Pressure in the tubing apparatus and ileum is measured by a pressure transducer (g). Gradual lifting of the pressure bottle (l) with the servomotor (m) increases pressure in the ileum and produces radial distention. This distention in turn activates sensory receptors in the ileum resulting in coordinated contractions and relaxations. These rhythmic movements produce expulsion of fluid from the ileum, and the resulting volume displacement moves an air bubble (i) in the glass tube (e). The movement of the bubble reflects volume displacement and is measured by an ultrasonic transit-time device (k). **Bottom:** Induction of peristaltic reflex. The passive pressure is increased linearly by raising the pressure bottle (*top tracing*). The respective tracings from bottom to top reflect readings from transducers g, k, and f, respectively. (From ref. 55.)

can be used for drug and drug-receptor classification (Fig. 3.34B). However, more information about the pharmacologic effects of isoproterenol on the heart can be obtained from this same type of experiment by further analysis of the twitch response. Figure 3.34C shows high-speed scans of the myocardial twitch response of a guinea pig papillary muscle to isoproterenol; these data reveal that in addition to increasing the strength of contraction, isoproterenol increases the rates of rise and fall of contraction and diminishes the twitch duration. Although this information is not necessary from the point of view of drug-receptor classification, it is helpful if the aim of the experiment is to predict the therapeutic effect of isoproterenol on the heart. In some instances the information desired may require specialized isolated tissues. For example, it is difficult to predict the effects of a drug on cardiac performance (output) based on studies of isolated muscle, because changes in strength, rate of contraction, and relaxation, as well as other factors, have complex effects on contractile function that may differ in systole and diastole. Under these circumstances, more complex preparations, such as the isolated working-heart preparation, may better predict therapeutic effects. This approach can be used for more complex responses that involve more than one physiological mechanism. Figure 3.35 shows a preparation of isolated intestine that can be used to study gastrointestinal peristalsis; this response involves muscle and nerves and is best studied in such intact preparations.

## REFERENCES

1. Altura, B. M., and Altura, B. T. (1970): Heterogeneity of drug receptors in different segments of rabbit thoracic aorta. *Eur. J. Pharmacol.*, 12:44–52.
2. Berstein, G., Haga, T., and Ichiyama, A. (1989): Effect of lipid environment on the differential affinity of purified cerebral and atrial muscarinic acetylcholine receptors for pirenzepine. *Mol. Pharmacol.*, 36:601–607.
3. Birdsall, N. J. M., Hulme, E. C., Keen, M., Stockton, J. M., Pedder, E..K., and Wheatley, M. (1987): Can complex binding phenomena be resolved to provide a safe basis for receptor classification? In: *Receptor Biochemistry and Methodology, Vol. 6, Perspectives on Receptor Classification*, edited by J. W. Black, D. H. Jenkinson, and V. P. Gerskowitch, pp. 61–71. Alan R. Liss, New York.
4. Blinks, J. R. (1965): Convenient apparatus for recording contractions of isolated heart muscle. *J. Appl. Physiol.*, 20:755–757.
5. Blinks, J. R., and Koch-Weser, J. (1963): Physical factors in the analysis of the actions of drugs on myocardial contractility. *Pharmacol. Rev.*, 15:531–599.
6. Bojanic, D., Jansen, J. D., Nahorski, S. R., and Zaagsma, J. (1985): Atypical characteristics of the β-adrenoceptor mediating cyclic AMP generation and lipolysis in the rat adipocyte. *Br. J. Pharmacol.*, 84:131–137.
7. Bouvier, M., Hnatowitch, M., Collins, S., Kobilka, B. K., Deblasi, A., Lefkowitz, R. J., and Caron, M. G. (1988): Expression of human cDNA encoding the $\beta_2$-adrenergic receptor in Chinese hamster fibroblasts (CHW): Functionality and regulation of the expressed receptors. *Mol. Pharmacol.*, 33:133–139.
8. Brading, A. F., and Setekleiv, J. (1968): The effect of hypo- and hypertonic solutions on volume and ion distribution of smooth muscle of guinea pig taenia coli. *J. Physiol. (Lond.)* 195:107–118.

9. Brink, C., Duncan, P. G., Midzenski, M., and Douglas, J. S. (1980): Response and sensitivity of female guinea-pig respiratory tissues to agonists during ontogenesis. *J. Pharmacol. Exp. Ther.*, 215:426–433.

10. Bristow, M. R., Ginsburg, R., Strosberg, A., Montgomery, W., and Minobe, W. (1984): Pharmacology and inotropic potential of forskolin in the human heart. *J. Clin. Invest.*, 74:212–223.

11. Broadley, K. J. (1979): The Langendorff heart preparation—reappraisal of its role as a research and teaching model for coronary vasoactive drugs. *J. Pharmacol. Methods*, 2:143–156.

12. Bylund, D. B., Blaxall, H. S., Iversen, L. J., Caron, M. G., Lefkowitz, R. J., and Lomasney, J. W. (1992): Pharmacological characteristics of $\alpha_2$-adrenergic receptors: Comparison of pharmacologically defined subtypes with subtypes identified by molecular cloning. *Mol. Pharmacol.*, 42:1–5.

13. Chang, A. E., and Detar, R. (1980): Oxygen vascular smooth muscle contraction revisited. *Am. Physiol. Soc.*, 238:H716–H728.

14. Cocks, T. M., and Angus, J. A. (1984): Endothelium-dependent modulation of blood vessel reactivity. In: *The Peripheral Circulation*, edited by S. Hunyor, J. Ludbrook, J. Shaw, and M. McGrath, pp. 9–21. Elsevier, Amsterdam.

15. Cohen, M. L., and Berkowitz, B. A. (1974): Age-related changes in vascular responsiveness to cyclic nucleotides and contractile agonists. *J. Pharmacol. Exp. Ther.*, 191:147–155.

16. Cordellini, S., and Sannomiya, P. (1984): The vas deferens as a suitable preparation for the study of $\alpha$-adrenoreceptor molecular mechanisms. *J. Pharmacol. Methods*, 11:97–107.

17. Decker, N., and Schwartz, J. (1984): Postjunctional alpha-1 and alpha-2 adrenoceptors in the coronaries of the perfused guinea-pig heart. *J. Pharmacol. Exp. Ther.*, 232:251–257.

18. Diederen, W., and Weisenberger, H. (1981): Studies on the mechanism of the positive-inotropic action of AR-L 115 BS, a new cardiotonic drug. *Arzneimittelforschung*, 31:177–182.

19. Douglas, J. S., Ridgway, P., and Brink, C. (1977): Airway responses of the guinea pig in vivo and in vitro. *J. Pharmacol. Exp. Ther.*, 202:116–124.

20. Eason, M. C., Kurose, H., Holt, B. D., Raymond, J. R., and Liggett, S. B. (1992): Simultaneous coupling of $\alpha_2$-adrenergic receptors to two G-proteins with opposing effects. *J. Biol. Chem.*, 267:15795–15801.

21. El-Fakahany, E., and Richelson, E. (1983): Antagonism by antidepressants of muscarinic acetylcholine receptors of human brain. *Br. J. Pharmacol.*, 78:97–102.

22. Fleisch, J. H., Maling, H. M., and Brodie, B. B. (1970): Beta-receptor activity in aorta. *Circ. Res.*, 26:151–162.

23. Florio, V. A., and Sternwies, P. C. (1989): Mechanisms of muscarinic receptor action and $G_o$ in reconstituted phospholipid vesicles. *J. Biol. Chem.*, 264:3909–3915.

24. Gaddum, J. H. (1953): Bioassays and mathematics. *Pharmacol. Rev.*, 5:87–134.

25. Ginsburg, R., Bristow, M. R., Billingham, M. E., Stinston, E. B., Schroeder, J. S., and Harrison, D. C. (1983): Study of the normal failing isolated human heart: Decreased response of failing heart to isoproterenol. *Am. Heart J.*, 106:535–540.

26. Hedberg, A., Carlsson, E., Fellenius, E., and Lundgren, B. (1982): Cardiostimulatory effects of prenalterol, a beta-1 adrenoceptor partial agonist, in vivo and in vitro. *Naunyn Schmiedebergs Arch. Pharmacol.*, 318:185–191.

27. Hill, A. V. (1928): Diffusion of oxygen and lactic acid through tissues. *Proc. R. Soc. Lond.* [*Biol.*], 104:39–96.

28. Hooker, C. S., Calkins, P. J., and Fleisch, J. H. (1977): On the measurement of vascular and respiratory smooth muscle response in vitro. *Blood Vessels*, 14:1–11.

29. Kenakin, T. P. (1984): The classification of drugs and drug receptors in isolated tissues. *Pharmacol. Rev.*, 36:165–222.

30. Krebs, H. A. (1950): Body size and tissue respiration. *Biochim. Biophys. Acta*, 4:249–269.

31. Levin, R. M., and Wein, A. J. (1979): Distribution and function of adrenergic receptors in the urinary bladder of the rabbit. *Mol. Pharmacol.*, 16:441–448.

32. Link, R., Daunt, D., Barsh, G., Chruscinski, A., and Kobilka, B. (1992): Cloning of two mouse genes encoding $\alpha_2$-adrenergic receptor subtypes and identification of a single amino acid in the mouse $\alpha_2$-C10 homolog responsible for an interspecies variation in antagonist binding. *Mol. Pharmacol.*, 42:16–17.

33. Maloteaux, J-M., Gossuin, A., Pauwels, P. J., and Laduron, P. M. (1983): Short-term disappearance of muscarinic cell surface receptors in carbachol-induced desensitization. *FEBS Lett.*, 156:103–107.
34. Matsumoto, Y., Inui, J., and Hashimoto, K. (1984): Different responses of the isolated canine coronary artery superfused with blood or Krebs-Henseleit solution. *Naunyn Schmiedebergs Arch. Pharmacol.*, 327:156–158.
35. Matthews, W. D., McCafferty, G. P., and Grous, M. (1984): Characterization of alpha adrenoceptors on vascular smooth vein. *J. Pharmacol. Exp. Ther.*, 231:355–360.
36. McKinney, M., Stenstrom, S., and Richelson, E. (1984): Muscarinic responses and binding in a murine neuroblastoma clone (N1E-115): Selective loss with subculturing of the low-affinity agonist site mediating cyclic GMP formation. *Mol. Pharmacol.*, 26:156–163.
37. Mei, L., Lai, J., Yamamura, H. I., and Roeske, W. R. (1989): The relationship between agonist states of the $M_1$ muscarinic receptor and the hydrolysis of inositol lipids in transfected murine fibroblast cells (B82) expressing different receptor densities. *J. Pharmacol. Exp. Ther.*, 251:90–97.
38. Newman, W. H., Webb, J. G., and Privitera, P. J. (1982): Persistence of myocardial failure following removal of chronic volume overload. *Am. Physiol. Soc.*, 243:H876–H883.
39. Ohashi, T., and Azuma, T. (1980): Paradoxical relaxation of arterial strips induced by vasoconstrictive agents. *Blood Vessels*, 17:16–26.
40. Patil, P. N., and Ruffolo, R. R., Jr. (1980): Evaluation of adrenergic alpha- and beta-receptor activators and adrenergic alpha- and beta-receptor blocking agents. In: *Adrenergic Activators and Inhibitors, Part I*, edited by L. Szekeres, pp. 89–134. Springer-Verlag, Berlin.
41. Raffestin, B., Cerrina, J., Boullet, C., Labat, C., Benveniste, J., and Brink, C. (1985): Response and sensitivity of isolated human pulmonary muscle preparations to pharmacological agents. *J. Pharmacol. Exp. Ther.*, 233:186–233.
42. Ruffolo, R. R., Jr. (1984): Use of isolated, physiologically responding tissues to investigate neurotransmitter receptors. In: *Monographs in Neural Sciences, Vol. 10*, edited by M. M. Cohen, pp. 53–84. S. Karger, Basel.
43. Schutz, W., and Freissmuth, M. (1992): Reverse intrinsic activity of antagonists on G protein-coupled receptors. *Trends Pharmacol. Sci.*, 13:376–380.
44. Senogles, S. E., Spiegel, A. M., Pardrell, E., Iyengar, R., and Caron, M. (1990): Specificity of receptor G-protein interactions. *J. Biol. Chem.*, 265:4507–4514.
45. Sievers, R., Parmley, W. W., James, T., and Wikman-Coffelt, J. (1983): Energy levels at systole vs. diastole in normal hamster hearts vs. myopathic hamster hearts. *Circ. Res.*, 53:759–766.
46. Sonnenblick, E. H. (1965): Determinants of active state in heart muscle: Force, velocity, instantaneous muscle length, time. *Fed. Proc.*, 24:1396–1409.
47. Spann, J. F., Jr., Buccino, R. A., Sonnenblick, E. H., and Braunwald, E. (1967): Contractile state of cardiac muscle obtained from cats with experimentally produced ventricular hypertrophy and heart failure. *Circ. Res.*, 21:341–354.
48. Staff of the Department of Pharmacology, University of Edinburgh. (1968): *Pharmacological Experiments on Isolated Preparations*. Livingston, London.
49. Stephens, N. L., Kroeger, E., and Mehta, J. A. (1969): Force-velocity characteristics of respiratory airway smooth muscle. *J. Appl. Physiol.*, 26:685–692.
50. Stephens, N. L., Meyers, J. L., and Cherniack, R. M. (1968): Oxygen, carbon dioxide, $H^+$ ion, and bronchial length-tension relationships. *J. Appl. Physiol.*, 25:376–383.
51. Stephens, N. L., and Van Niekerk, W. (1977): Isometric and isotonic contractions in airway smooth muscle. *Can. J. Physiol. Pharmacol.*, 55:833–838.
52. Taylor, C. W. (1990): The role of G proteins in transmembrane signalling. *Biochem. J.*, 272:1–13.
53. Tyrode, M. V. (1910): Mode of action of some purgative salts. *Arch. Int. Pharmacodyn. Ther.*, 20:205–210.
54. Vane, J. R. (1969): The second Gaddum memorial lecture. The release and fate of vasoactive hormones in the circulation. *Br. J. Pharmacol.*, 35:209–242.
55. Van Neuten, J. M., and Fontaine, J. (1976): In vitro pharmacology: Study of the peristaltic reflex and other experiments on isolated tissues. In: *Synthetic Antidiarrheal Drugs*, edited by W. Van Bever and H. Lal, pp. 114–132. Marcel Dekker, Basel.
56. Van Neuten, J. M., Janssen, P. A. J., Van Beek, J., Khonneux, R., Verbeuren, T. J., and

Vanhoute, P. M. (1981): Vascular effects of ketanserin (R 41 468), a novel antagonist of 5-HT$_2$ serotonergic receptors. *J. Pharmacol. Exp. Ther.*, 218:217–230.
57. Varrault, A., Journot, L., Audiger, Y., and Bockaert, J. (1992): Transfection of human 5-hydroxytryptamine$_{1A}$ receptors in NIH-3T$_3$ fibroblasts: Effects of increasing receptor density on the coupling of 5-hydroxytryptamine$_{1A}$ receptors to adenylyl cyclase. *Mol. Pharmacol.*, 41:999–1007.
58. Wyse, G. D. (1980): On the "normalization" of active developed force of isolated helical strips of muscular and elastic arteries for variation in wall thickness. *J. Pharmacol. Methods*, 4:313–326.
59. Zannad, F., Graham, C. W., and Aronson, J. K. (1982): The effects of digoxin and dopamine on the oxygen consumption, lactate production and haemodynamic performance of an isolated, perfused, working guinea-pig heart. *Eur. J. Pharmacol.*, 81:263–271.

# 4

---

# Diffusion

Diffusion of a drug to the receptor can be an important factor in isolated-tissue experiments in two situations. The first relates to the removal of drug from the receptor compartment by a chemical or physiological mechanism. If such a process occurs, then the tissue response is mediated by the flux of the drug concentration at the receptor; this flux is controlled by the magnitude of the rate of drug removal and the magnitude of the rate of drug delivery; this latter process is controlled by diffusion. Therefore, diffusion becomes important in the production of a response. The second situation arises when temporal processes (e.g., kinetics of drug actions, desensitization) are studied. In view of these effects, a discussion of the process of drug delivery to the receptor is warranted.

## DIFFUSION TO THE TISSUE SURFACE

In an isolated-tissue experiment, the tissue is incubated, perfused, or superfused with a physiological salt solution; drugs added to the bathing medium reach the receptor compartment (the region near the receptors) by bulk diffusion. Diffusion is a random process. If a volume of bathing medium were to be divided into an infinite number of opposing horizontal surfaces stacked together, the equations of random Brownian motion would dictate the probability of movement of a drug molecule from one surface to another. This is reflected by the fact that in two opposing surfaces, in one of which the number of drug molecules is greater than in the other, equal fractions of drug molecules will cross into the opposing surface. However, because one surface has a greater number of molecules than the other, a net flow of molecules to the surface of lower concentration will occur. Thus, concentration gradients provide the driving force behind bulk diffusion. The equations describing diffusion from a point source can be solved with computer techniques or resistance-capacitance analogs of electrical circuits; these calculations have relevance to conditions in which diffusion calculations are important to drug concentrations (i.e., iontophoretic application of drug to a small

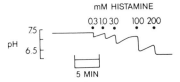

mM HISTAMINE

FIG. 4.1. Changes in organ-bath pH after addition of small volumes (0.1 mL) of histamine HCl solutions. Volume of organ bath 17 mL. Rapid decrease in pH indicates the speed of mixing of added solution and gassed solution in the organ bath. (From ref. 9.)

area of cell membrane by a micropipette). In organ-bath experiments, provided that mixing is adequate, the diffusion from a point source (tip of a pipette or syringe dispensing a drug solution into the medium) is much faster than diffusion into tissues. Experiments have shown that conductance changes across electrodes placed in organ baths occur within 50 msec of injection of potassium into the bath. Figure 4.1 shows the immediate changes in organ-bath pH produced by high concentrations of histamine added to an organ bath containing a pH electrode. The changes actually are greater than shown, because the buffering capacity of the solution begins immediately to counter the decreased pH of the solution. Generally it is unlikely that diffusion of drug within the organ bath will be a rate-limiting step; the following calculations will assume that the medium bathing the tissue is an infinite reservoir of drug at constant concentration.

In the case of tissues perfused or superfused with solution, the rate of drug delivery may be important. If drug is delivered to the receptor compartment ($V$) at a rate $Q$, and it is assumed that the concentration of drug rises instantaneously to concentration $[A]$ at $t = 0$, the concentration in the receptor compartment with time $[A_t]$ is given by

$$[A_t] = [A](1 - e^{-(Q/V)t}) \qquad [4.1]$$

It can be seen that if the flow rate $Q$ is low and the volume of the receptor compartment large, then a considerable time will be required for equilibration of the drug with the receptor compartment (Fig. 4.2). If there is a mechanism

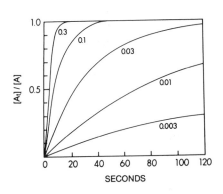

FIG. 4.2. Rates of equilibration of receptor-compartment concentrations of drug to perfusate concentrate with various rates of perfusion. Ordinate: Concentration of drug in the receptor compartment at time $t$ ($[A_t]$) as a fraction of the concentration perfusing the tissue ($[A]$). Abscissa: Time in seconds. Numbers next to curves refer to ratios of flow rate to effective volume of receptor compartment ($Q/V$). Note that as the receptor-compartment volume is large (i.e., large area of tissue required to be perfused by the conduit vessel) or $Q$ small (low flow rate), a considerable time delay is produced between when a given concentration is perfused into the organ and when that concentration reaches the receptors. Curves calculated with Eq. 4.1.

removing the drug from the receptor compartment, then $Q$ can directly affect the steady-state concentration (flux) of drug at the receptor and hence the response. The situation becomes more complicated when a bolus injection is the source of the drug in perfusion or superfusion experiments. This is because the drug is diluted en route to the tissue (according to Fick's second law of diffusion) and reaches the surface of access to the receptor compartment in a heterogeneous concentration dependent on the path length of perfusion and $Q$. Thus, [A] in Eq. 4.1 becomes a biphasic function of $t$; the relationship between the concentration of $A$ injected into the perfusion system and [A] in the receptor compartment then becomes complex and difficult to predict. For this reason, steady-state perfusion as opposed to bolus injection is preferable when quantitative information about concentration fluxes of drugs (i.e., importance of uptake mechanisms) is required.

## CHEMICAL EFFECTS ON CONCENTRATION GRADIENTS

Because concentration gradients provide the driving force for bulk diffusion, any process that affects the concentration of a drug in the organ bath will affect the rate of diffusion into the tissue. This is true also of processes within the tissue, but this present discussion will focus on processes in the bathing medium surrounding the tissue. There are two processes that possibly could affect drug concentration in the organ bath: chemical degradation (i.e., photolysis, chemical transformation) and adsorption to surfaces.

Some drugs are notoriously unstable in physiological salt solutions unless precautions are taken. For example, catecholamines such as epinephrine and norepinephrine are quickly degraded by molecular oxygen, the process being accelerated by traces of heavy metals, alkaline pH, and ultraviolet light. Addition of antioxidants such as ascorbate ion or ethylenediaminetetraacetic acid (EDTA) to complex the traces of heavy-metal ions greatly increases the stability of catecholamines in solution. Figure 4.3A shows the inhibition of norepinephrine oxidation by ascorbate and EDTA in physiological salt solution.

Another possible source of drug removal is adsorption to surfaces. This phenomenon has been characterized for many drugs (usually basic in chemical nature) and specifically can be a problem with peptides and polypeptides. Figure 4.3B shows the adsorption of histamine to a glass surface; in this case, a complex formation between heavy-metal ions may be important, because EDTA prevents the adsorption. Other approaches found to be useful for various drugs have been the use of plastic surfaces, siliconization of glassware, and addition of bovine serum albumin to the medium. Adsorption to surfaces can further be a complication if drugs adsorb during one experiment and leech into the bathing medium from the pool of adsorption sites in another. Such effects necessitate impeccable cleaning of apparatus between experiments when dealing with drugs of high potency.

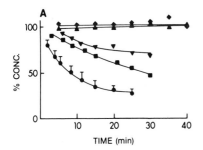

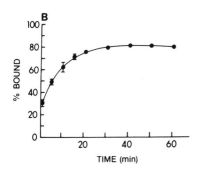

**FIG. 4.3.** Removal mechanisms for drugs in organ baths. **A:** Chemical degradation of norepinephrine in physiological salt solution. Ordinate: Percentage of an initial concentration of norepinephrine (312 nM). Abscissa: Time in minutes. Incubation in physiological saline at 37°C (●, $N = 4$), 32°C (■, $N = 3$), 27°C (▼, $N = 3$), and 37°C in the presence of ascorbic acid 113.6 μM (▲, $N = 3$) or EDTA 54.1 μM (♦, $N = 3$). (From ref. 8.) **B:** Adsorption of histamine to a glass surface. Ordinate: Percentage of solution of 4 ng/mL$^{-1}$ radioactive histamine bound to glass surface. Abscissa: Time in minutes. By 40 min, 80% of the histamine in solution is bound to the glass surface. (From ref. 19.)

The forthcoming discussion will assume that the drug in the bathing medium is at an infinite and constant concentration with respect to the receptor compartment. Given this, the path of a drug molecule into the core of an isolated tissue can be calculated. The first obstacle the drug encounters is the unstirred water layer that surrounds any solid mass in a fluid.

## UNSTIRRED WATER LAYERS

When a solid body such as an isolated tissue is placed in a well-stirred liquid, the body is surrounded by a layer of static liquid in which transfer of solute (drug) occurs only by diffusion and thermal convection; concentration gradients do not play a role in solute transfer. Referred to as boundary-layer effects by physical chemists, the effects of unstirred water layers have been studied since the turn of the century (11). Unstirred water layers are regions of slow laminar flow parallel to the tissue-medium interface; thus, if diffusion in the organ bath and in the tissue is rapid, the unstirred water layer can be rate-limiting with respect to access of the drug to the receptor.

Just how effective unstirred water layers can be as diffusion barriers can be seen from kinetic studies of uptake processes in tissues. Figure 4.4 shows the effects of varying thicknesses of the unstirred layer (δ) on an active transport process modeled after the active uptake of substances across intestinal mucosa. It can be seen that an unstirred layer of 400 μm introduces a

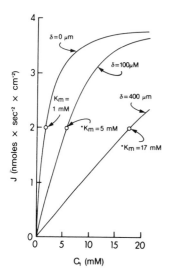

**FIG. 4.4.** Effects of unstirred water layers on active-transport kinetics. Ordinate: Rate of flux with $J_{max} = 4$ nmol sec$^{-1}$ cm$^{-1}$, $K_m = 1$ mM, $D = 0.5 \cdot 10^{-5}$ cm$^2$ sec$^{-1}$. Abscissa: Concentration of substrate. Curves calculated for $\delta = 0$, 100, and 400 $\mu$m; a 17-fold increase in the apparent $K_m$ is observed in the presence of an unstirred layer of 400 $\mu$M. (From ref. 24.)

17-fold increase in the observed Michaelis-Menten constant for the uptake process and can greatly reduce uptake kinetics. The thickness of an unstirred water layer determines to what extent it can function as a diffusion barrier in isolated-tissue experiments. The half-time required for a solute to diffuse to the tissue surface through an unstirred water layer of thickness $\delta$ is

$$t_{1/2} = a_v \delta^2 / D \qquad\qquad [4.2]$$

where $D$ is the solute diffusion coefficient in free solution and $a_v$ is a proportionality constant that in the absence of serious volume-flow effects approximates to 0.38. It can be seen from Eq. 4.2 that the importance of an unstirred water layer as a diffusion barrier depends on its thickness and on the diffusion coefficient of the medium. Although this latter factor usually is assumed to be constant in most experiments, stabilization of water molecules into a latticelike structure by proteins in the cell membrane may produce hydration shells that in turn may introduce heterogeneity in $D$, the diffusion coefficient of solute in the medium. It has been shown that the viscosity of the medium also affects the thickness of the unstirred layer. Stirring the bulk solution reduces the thickness of the unstirred layer and subsequently its effect on diffusion. Figure 4.5A shows the effects of stirring on the thickness of the unstirred water layer for rabbit jejunum; an effective reduction of 200 $\mu$m was achieved. Figure 4.5B shows how mixing can affect the kinetics of active transport of D-glucose in rabbit jejunum and correct the distorted Michaelis-Menten kinetics produced by the absence of stirring. These data indicate that efficient mixing in the organ bath can be important to effective diffusion of drugs into tissues.

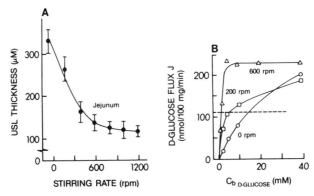

**FIG. 4.5.** Effects of stirring on unstirred water layers. **A:** Effects of stirring on the thickness of the unstirred water layer on rabbit jejunum. Ordinate: Thickness of unstirred water layer in micromoles. Abscissa: Bulk stirring rate in revolutions per minute. **B:** Effects of stirring on kinetics of active transport of D-glucose in rabbit jejunum. Ordinate: Uptake of glucose in nmol 100 mg$^{-1}$ min$^{-1}$. Abscissa: Concentration of D-glucose in millimoles. Stirring corrects the distorted Michaelis-Menten kinetics and decreases the observed Michaelis-Menten constant ($K_m$) of the uptake process. (From ref. 1.)

Mixing of a physiological salt solution in the organ bath usually is achieved by vigorous oxygenation. It should be noted that, whereas efficient stirring is important to diffusion, invaginations and microfolds and macrofolds in the tissue surface provide regions of unstirred water layers that effectively cannot be overcome by organ-bath mixing. Such folding of epithelia greatly increases the effective unstirred water layer for a given tissue.

## DIFFUSION INTO TISSUES

To reach the receptor compartment, drugs must diffuse from the surface toward the center of the tissue; this process follows Fick's second law of diffusion, which relates concentration with respect to time ($\partial[A]/\partial t$) in terms of a diffusion coefficient in the tissue $D'$ and the second derivative of $[A]$ with respect to spatial coordinates that depend on the shape of the tissue. Thus,

$$\partial[A]/\partial t = D' \cdot \nabla^2[A] \qquad [4.3]$$

This equation has different specific forms for diffusion into different geometric shapes. The equation for diffusion of a constant concentration of drug $[A]$ at the surface of a plane sheet of thickness $l$ diffusing into the sheet is given by

$$\frac{\partial[A]}{\partial t} = D' \cdot \frac{\partial^2[A]}{\partial x^2} \qquad [4.4]$$

where $x$ is the distance into the tissue. A graphic solution has been given for Eq. 4.3 by Crank (5), and it can be useful to predict the penetration of solutes into tissues (the shape of which can be approximated by a plane sheet); the graphic solution is shown in Fig. 4.6. The numbers adjacent to the curves refer to values of $D' \cdot t/l^2$, and substitution of experimentally derived diffusion coefficients in tissues ($D'$) and thicknesses of various tissues ($l$) allows estimates of drug penetration with time for any given drug and tissue. It should be noted that these calculations are made with the model of the plane sheet as a membrane dividing a solution of drug concentration $[A]$ and one in which $[A] = 0$. Usually both faces of the tissue are exposed to drug solution, and the penetration of drug depicted in Fig. 4.6 occurs from each face; in this case, tissue thickness should read $2l$, and $x$ refers to depth toward the center of the tissue, not to the other face.

The diffusion of a drug into a cylinder of radius $r$ is given (5) by

$$\frac{\partial[A]}{\partial t} = \frac{1}{r}\frac{\partial}{\partial r}\, r \cdot D'\, \frac{\partial[A]}{\partial r} \qquad [4.5]$$

The graphic solution for this equation is given in Fig. 4.7.

Last, the penetration of a drug into the center of a sphere is given (5) by

$$\frac{\partial[A]}{\partial t} = D' \cdot \left(\frac{\partial^2[A]}{\partial r^2} + \frac{2}{r}\frac{\partial[A]}{\partial r}\right) \qquad [4.6]$$

where $r$ is the radius of the sphere. The graphic solution for Eq. 4.5 is shown in Fig. 4.8.

It had been pointed out as early as 1928 by A. V. Hill that the diffusion rates of experimental substances were substantially slower in tissues. Figure 4.9 shows the decreased rates of diffusion for a wide variety of substances

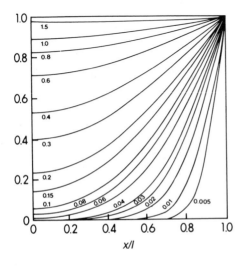

**FIG. 4.6.** Diffusion of a drug into a plane sheet. Ordinate: Concentration of drug at depth $x$ ($[A_x]$) as a fraction of concentration at the tissue surface ($[A_o]$). Abscissa: Depth ($x$) into the tissue as a fraction of tissue thickness ($l$). Numbers next to curves refer to values of $D \cdot t/l^2$; assuming $D = 6.73\ 10^{-6}$ cm$^2$/sec$^{-1}$ (diffusion coefficient of glucose in free solution) in a plane sheet of thickness 1 mm, $[A_x]/[A_o]$ at $t/l = 0$ for $D \cdot t/l^2 = 0.3$ is 0.4; this means that 40% of the surface concentration reaches the inner core after 111 sec. This figure represents a plane sheet exposed to drug only on one surface. (From ref. 5.)

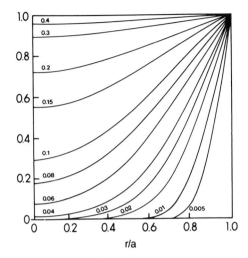

**FIG. 4.7.** Diffusion of a drug into a cylinder. Ordinate: Concentration of drug at a radial depth $r$ ([$A_r$]) as a fraction of the surface concentration ([$A_o$]). Abscissa: Radial depth $r$ as a fraction of radius $a$. Numbers next to curves refer to values of $D \cdot t / r^2$. (From ref. 5.)

into skinned frog muscle fibers as compared with water; in general, there is an abundance of evidence to show that solutes diffuse more slowly into the matrix of an organ. The reason for this relates to the three-dimensional structure of tissues. The diffusional coefficient in free solution ($D$) measures the random rate of travel by a straight path; if obstructions are encountered, a longer total path to achieve the same linear movement results. Thus, the distance traversed by a drug molecule in a given volume of tissue is longer when the drug must diffuse around a muscle cell. Figure 4.10A shows the array of muscle cells into which drugs must diffuse to penetrate the wall of the cat coronary artery. Figure 4.10B shows the ratio of extracellular space

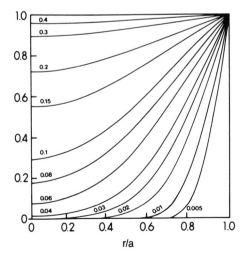

**FIG. 4.8.** Diffusion of a drug into a sphere. Ordinate: Concentration of drug at a radial depth $r$ ([$A_r$]) as a fraction of the surface concentration ([$A_o$]). Abscissa: Radial depth $r$ as a fraction of the radius of the sphere ($a$). Numbers next to curves refer to values of $D \cdot t / r^2$. (From ref. 5.)

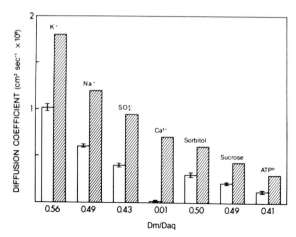

**FIG. 4.9.** Diffusion coefficients at 20°C in single-skinned muscle fibers (*hatched bars*) and in water (*open bars*). Number of experiments above each error bar (standard error of the mean); the ratio of the diffusivity in muscle to that in water ($D_m/D_{aq}$) is given beneath each pair of bars. (From ref. 12.)

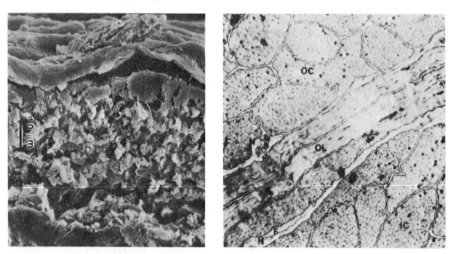

**FIG. 4.10.** Structure of tissues. **A:** Scanning electron micrograph of a cross section of cat coronary artery. The top layer of endothelial cells covers a dense array of muscle cells. (Courtesy of F. Greenstein, Department of Toxicology, Burroughs Wellcome Co., Research Triangle Park, NC). **B:** Electron micrograph of vas deferens musculature showing inner circular (IC); outer longitudinal (OL), and outer circular (OC) layers. The spaces between muscle-cell layers are small, ranging from 3 to 10 μm, and contain collagen and small nerve bundles. (From ref. 13.)

to cellular volume in guinea pig vas deferens; for contraction of this preparation to occur, drugs must penetrate past the circular muscle layers (OC, IC) to the longitudinal muscle. It should be noted that the effective volume of the extracellular space can be altered by physical factors such as resting tension or orientation and thus can be variable between tissues. Also, the contractile state can alter effective extracellular space; this could be a factor within any given experiment as a tissue contracts and relaxes.

A proportionality factor can be used to accommodate slower diffusion in the extracellular space of a tissue:

$$D' = D/\lambda^2 \qquad [4.7]$$

where $D'$ and $D$ are the diffusion coefficients in the tissue and free solution, respectively, and $\lambda$ is defined as the *tortuosity factor*. Values of $\lambda$ can be determined for various tissues; for instance, the tortuosity factor for cat papillary muscle (13) is 1.44. Figure 4.11 shows the penetration of a drug into a cylindrical tissue 1 mm in diameter after 110 sec. The various curves represent different tortuosity factors. When $\lambda = 1.0$, there is no impedance, and diffusion identical with that in free solution is observed; after 110 sec, 71% of the surface concentration penetrates to the core of the tissue. As the tortuosity factor increases, diffusion occurs more slowly; for example, for a cylinder of $\lambda = 1.9$, only 10% of the surface concentration penetrates to the core of the tissue by 110 sec. For greater tortuosity factors, only an outer shell of the cylinder is penetrated by drug after 110 sec (i.e., $\lambda = 3.9$).

The calculations in Fig. 4.11 illustrate the penetration of a molecule with a rate of diffusion in free solution equal to that of glucose. This rate of diffusion depends on the viscosity of the medium ($\eta$) and the radius of the

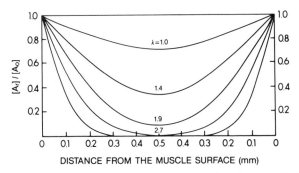

**FIG. 4.11.** Effect of tortuosity factor on penetration of a drug into a cylindrically shaped isolated tissue. Ordinate: Concentrations of drug at point $r$ ($[A_r]$) as fractions of the concentration at the surface of the muscle ($[A_o]$). Abscissa: Radial distance from the surface of the muscle into the center of a cylinder 1 mm in diameter. Penetration of drug after 110 sec, assuming a diffusion coefficient in free solution of glucose ($6.73 \cdot 10^{-6}$ cm$^2$ sec$^{-1}$) calculated for tortuosity factors of 1.0 (free solution, no impedance to permeation) and increasing resistance of $\lambda = 1.4, 1.9, 2.7,$ and 3.9.

diffusing molecule ($r_D$) according to the Stokes-Einstein equation:

$$D = \frac{kT}{6\pi\eta \cdot r_D}$$                    [4.8]

where $k$ is Boltzmann's constant, and $T$ is absolute temperature. It can be seen from this equation that drugs of different molecular radii will have different diffusion characteristics. Figure 4.12 shows the penetration of isoproterenol (molecular weight = 211) into cat papillary muscle (1-mm diameter, $\lambda$ = 1.44) obtained after 154 sec and the penetration of polymeric isoproterenol (molecular weight = 12,800) after 173 sec. The slower penetration of the polymer relates to a reduced diffusion coefficient and highlights possible drug-related differences in diffusion. In addition to accounting for geometric effects on diffusion, tortuosity factors provide a general correction for other disparities encountered when studying drug diffusion in tissues and that in free solution. The equations describing free diffusion into structures assume an isotropic medium (structure and diffusion properties at any one point are the same in all directions), whereas structured tissues may have anisotropic properties (different diffusion properties in different directions). In general, the tortuosity factor can be an important parameter in calculations of drug diffusions into tissues, because calculations using diffusion coefficients in free solution will always overestimate drug penetration.

A useful approximation for the rate of drug diffusion into a tissue has been given by Waud (21) and relates the rate of entry to a resistance term ($R_e$):

$$\frac{\partial[A]}{\partial t_{in}} = \frac{[A_o] - [A_i]}{R_e}$$                    [4.9]

where $[A_o]$ and $[A_i]$ refer to the drug concentrations in the medium and in the receptor compartment, respectively. The magnitude of $R_e$ relates to the tortuosity and should be relatively constant for a given tissue type and range

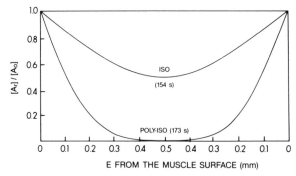

**FIG. 4.12.** Effect of molecular radius on diffusion. Ordinate and abscissa as for Fig. 4.11. Penetration of isoproterenol (ISO) after 154 sec and polymeric isoproterenol (POLY-ISO) after 173 sec. (Adapted from ref. 18.)

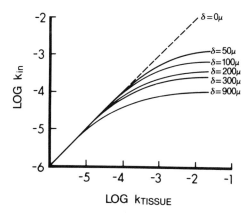

**FIG. 4.13.** Permeation constants for drugs in tissues with unstirred water layers. Ordinate: Logarithms of permeation constants for drugs into tissue covered by an unstirred water layer (cm sec$^{-1}$). Abscissa: Permeation of drug (cm sec$^{-1}$) into tissue without unstirred layer ($\delta = 0$). Numbers next to curves refer to thicknesses of unstirred layers in micrometers. Note how unstirred layers become important as barriers to drug permeation only when $k_{\text{tissue}}$ is high (i.e., low-tortuosity within the tissue).

of drugs of comparable molecular weights. One variable between experiments may be the thickness of the unstirred layer, because this depends on surface characteristics of the tissue and mixing in the organ bath. The total resistance is given by

$$R_{e\text{Total}} = R_{e\text{Tissue}} + (\delta/D) \qquad [4.10]$$

Using Eq. 4.10 and converting resistance $R_e$ into a permeation constant $k_{\text{in}}$ ($1/R$),

$$k_{\text{in}} = \frac{k_{\text{tissue}}}{1 + (k_{\text{tissue}} \cdot \delta/D)} \qquad [4.11]$$

It can be seen that in tissues with low tortuosity factors (high permeation constant $k_{\text{tissue}}$), a thick unstirred layer (large $\delta$) may contribute substantially to the total permeation of drug into the tissue ($k_{\text{in}}$) and that the importance of unstirred layers is proportional to the rate of permeation of drug into the tissue (Fig. 4.13). The permeation approximation utilizing $k_{\text{in}}$ will be used extensively in Chapter 5 to relate the importance of diffusion and uptake processes to drug responses.

## MEMBRANE VERSUS AQUEOUS APPROACH OF DRUGS TO RECEPTORS

The preceding discussions have assumed that all drugs approach the receptor through the aqueous phase in the extracellular compartment. There are examples of drugs (i.e., the calcium channel blocking dihydropyridines) that bind to their membrane receptors in a two-stage process, namely, a dissolution into the lipid bilayer and then a two-dimensional diffusion process to a binding site on the protein within the lipid bilayer. The two alternative models (aqueous approach and membrane approach) are shown schematically in Fig. 4.14A.

There is a considerable body of evidence available to support the membrane approach of some drugs such as dihydropyridines to calcium channels. For example, in patch-clamp experiments in which the dihydropyridine is

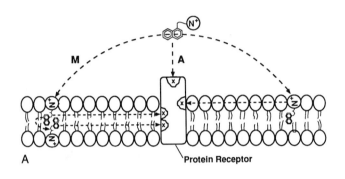

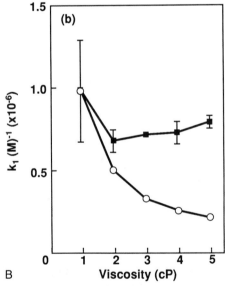

**FIG. 4.14.** Aqueous and membrane approaches for a drug to a membrane-bound receptor. **A:** The direct approach is through the aqueous phase to a hydrophilic part of the receptor. Two membrane approaches are shown. One is through the hydrophilic region (*right side*) or a hydrophobic region (*left side*). Also illustrated is the fact that the drug could diffuse to the inner monolayer and rearrange its position for a favorable approach to the receptor. (From ref. 17.) **B:** The effect of changing viscosity on the rate of binding of [³H]nimodipine to cardiac sarcolemmal membranes. Ordinate: Rate constant for binding. Abscissa: Viscosity expressed as a multiple of normal aqueous viscosity. ○, the predicted effects for a purely aqueous approach of the drug to the receptor; the experimental data (■) show the relative insensitivity of binding rate on viscosity. (From ref. 7.)

added to the medium outside the patch isolated for recording, drug responses are observed (10). It can be concluded that the drug dissolves into the membrane outside the patch and then diffuses laterally along the bilayer to the calcium channel. It is known that some drugs such as propranolol and dihydropyridines partition into the lipid bilayer in *specific* orientations, suggesting a more complex phenomenon than simple dissolution into bulk lipid. Another line of evidence to show that drugs may partition into the membrane before binding to receptors is the sensitivity or lack of sensitivity of drug diffusion to receptor-compartment aqueous viscosity. Since this type of drug diffusion consists of a two-stage process, namely, the aqueous diffusion of the drug molecule to the surface of the lipid membrane followed by the two-dimensional translation of the drug molecule through the lipid membrane to the receptor, perturbation of the aqueous phase should have limited effects on overall diffusion. If the approach of a drug to the receptor is solely through the aqueous phase (e.g., see Fig. 4.14A), then the viscosity of this aqueous phase should have predictable effects on the rate constant for diffusion. However, if part of the diffusion process is independent of the aqueous phase (i.e., within the lipid membrane), then aqueous viscosity is less important. Figure 4.14B shows the effect of changing viscosity on the rate constant for diffusion of [$^3$H]nimodipine in cardiac sarcolemmal membranes. The circles show the predicted effect of viscosity if this drug depended only on the aqueous phase for diffusion (i.e., a fivefold increase in viscosity should produce a fivefold decrease in the rate constant for diffusion). The squares show the relative insignificance of viscosity on the diffusion of nimodipine in this membrane preparation. These data support a membrane approach of this drug to the sarcolemmal receptors.

A general equation to describe two-dimensional approaches of drugs to receptors has been given by Rhodes et al. (17). Thus, the mean time of a drug molecule to fruitful collision with a receptor site is the sum of the time required for aqueous diffusion (in three-dimensional space, denoted $\tau_3$) and that required for translation in two-dimensional space within the lipid (denoted $\tau_2$). The total diffusion time ($\tau_{32}$) is given by:

$$\tau_{32} = \tau_3 + \tau_2$$

$$= \frac{c^3}{3bD_3} + \frac{b_2}{D_2} (\log (4b^2/a^2) - 1) \qquad [4.12]$$

where $a$ is the receptor radius, $b$ is the radius of a lipid membrane vesicle containing the receptor, $c$ is the radius of a sphere in solution containing one receptor, $D_3$ is the diffusion coefficient of the ligand in the aqueous media, and $D_2$ is the lateral-diffusion coefficient of the ligand within the lipid bilayer. It should be noted that Eq. 4.12 is derived for circular objects in a plane and that often this does not approximate noncircular molecules that require specific orientation to bind effectively to receptors. To accommodate this

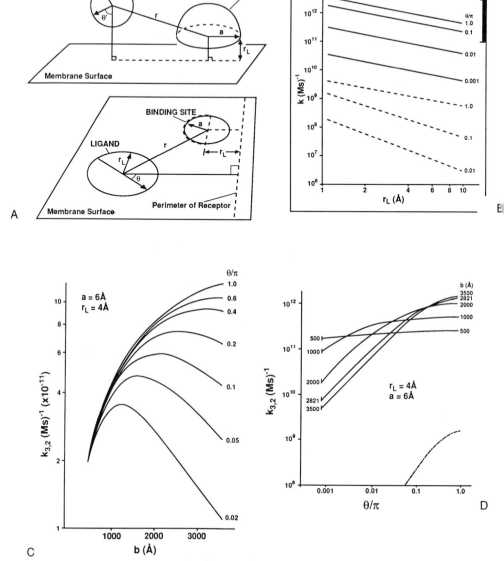

**FIG. 4.15.** Two-dimensional diffusion for drugs using the membrane approach. **A:** Schematic diagram of elements involved in the approach of an isotropic drug molecule through the aqueous phase either to a receptor or the membrane (*upper part*) and then, once the membrane (approximated as a circle), the approach to a receptor within the membrane (*lower part*). **B:** Rate of diffusion of drugs approaching the receptor through the aqueous phase (*broken lines*) and in a two-stage process through the membrane (*solid lines*). The various lines are for isotropic (i.e., spherical [$\theta/\pi = 1$]) drugs and anisotropic (i.e., ellipsoid) drugs ($\theta/\pi = 0.1$ to 0.001). **C:** Dependence of membrane approach diffusion rate on vesicle radius. **D:** Dependence of membrane approach diffusion rate on acceptance angle $\theta$ (anisotropy). (From ref. 17.)

effect, an angle $\theta$ is defined that describes the orientation of the ligand relative to the binding site for a fruitful (i.e., pharmacologically relevant) collision. Thus ligands can be essentially *isotropic* (approximating a sphere) and able to initiate fruitful collisions at many angles of approach (high $\theta$) or be anisotropic and thus highly restrictive in the orientation required for fruitful collisions (low $\theta$). For anisotropic bodies, the diffusion time in the two-dimensional plane of the lipid ($\tau_2$) must be divided by a probability term that describes the orientation of the ellipsoid to the active site of the target. This probability ($P_2$) is given by

$$P_2 = \frac{\theta}{\pi} + [1 - (\theta/\pi)] \frac{2D_R}{\pi D_2} \frac{2a^2}{} \qquad [4.13]$$

where $D_R$ relates to the mean angular displacement of the drug in a given time and $D_2$ is the diffusion coefficient in two dimensions. Thus, Eq. 4.12 for anisotropic bodies is modified to $\tau_{32} = \tau_3 + \tau_2/P$. The relative approaches in three- and two-dimensional space for these interactions are shown schematically in Fig. 4.15A. The rates of diffusion of drugs of varying anisotropy, either through the aqueous phase (broken lines) or the membrane (solid lines), are shown in Fig. 4.15B. As can be seen from this figure, the membrane approach is considerably faster. Figure 4.15C shows the rate constant for membrane-approach diffusion for drugs of various magnitudes of anisotropy (i.e., restricted approach angles from that of a uniform sphere) as a function of vesicle size (i.e., particle of membrane-containing receptors and utilized for drug binding). In this sense, the vesicle size approximates the field open per receptor in the cell membrane and relates to receptor density on the cell surface. The biphasic nature of these curves illustrates the two effects of increasing vesicle size. The first is that the first-step aqueous approach time for diffusion of the drug to the membrane surface decreases (i.e., there is a larger initial target for dissolution into the membrane). However, once the drug is dissolved into the membrane, larger vesicles make it less probable that the drug will find a receptor. This effect decreases $k_{3,2}$. This latter effect is most pronounced with highly anisotropic drugs and less important for drugs that can orient to the receptor site from a wider variety of approach angles. This effect is further shown in Fig. 4.15D where the rate of membrane approach diffusion is shown as a function of ligand acceptance angle (i.e., anisotropy of the drug) for vesicles of differing size. The shape of the drug (relative to the angle of the approach to the receptor site) becomes important for larger vesicles but relatively unimportant for smaller ones. It should be noted that the total size of the drug ligand plays a minor role in the rate of diffusion through the membrane.

The above discussion contains several tacit assumptions that should be considered. First, it is assumed that the depth to which the drug penetrates the membrane favors productive collisions with the receptor site. The interactions of drugs with heterogeneous lipid biological membranes is known to be very specific and not well approximated by simple lipid/aqueous partition models (see Chapter 5). Therefore, it is possible that certain drugs dissolve into membranes to an *unfavorable* depth thus precluding fruitful interactions. Also, drugs may "flip-flop" between bilayer faces even when they are specifically positioned in the membrane. Thermal "bobbing" and rotation within the membrane also may disrupt otherwise fruitful collisions. It is also assumed that the receptor is in a uniform reactive state during the diffusion process. This may not be the case if only one of two or more receptor conformations are differentially more reactive to the drug. Finally, the possibility of multiple collisions in lateral space is not considered in these calculations.

In general it can be seen from Fig. 4.15B that a membrane pathway approach of a drug to a receptor can be a faster process (up to three orders of magnitude) than an aqueous one. One reason for this disparity is that the initial target for the drug in the aqueous phase is very large (the total cell membrane). Theoretical calculations (2) indicate that if a drug collides with a surface, it is likely to collide with that surface more than once before drifting away into the aqueous phase. Specific binding within the membrane orients the drug for binding to the receptor, therefore the loss in dimensionality (from three to two dimensions) leads to an increase in the probability of binding. This can be an advantage for receptors of low density. In general, two-dimensional membrane diffusion for lipid-soluble drugs should be considered as a possibility when studying the kinetics of binding to receptors.

## CELL-TO-CELL COUPLING

The preceding discussion has been concerned with penetration of drug from the organ bath into the drug-receptor compartment. An unknown factor in the relationship between the amount of drug that has penetrated into the tissue and the magnitude of tissue response is the quantity of tissue that needs to be activated to produce a syncytial tissue response. As shown in Fig. 2.2, in rat vas deferens the number of receptors mediating the total tissue response is considerably less than the total tissue receptor concentration; this could indicate that only an outer shell of muscle cells mediates the total tissue response *in vitro*. A dominant factor in this relationship is the extent of cell-to-cell coupling in the tissue. Kinetic experiments indicate that diffusion is not sufficiently rapid to account for the kinetics of response in many blood vessels and cardiac muscle, suggesting rapid myogenic propagation. One mechanism of myogenic propagation may relate to a morphological site for low-resistance pathways between muscle cells termed a *nexus*. Thus, drug activation of one cell may well activate another cell if that cell is joined via a nexus. Figure 4.16 shows schematic representations of three types of smooth muscle: type A, in which cells are individually innervated and few low-resistance pathways (nexuses) exist; type B, in which innervation does not extend to every cell and more "coupled cells" are found; type C, in

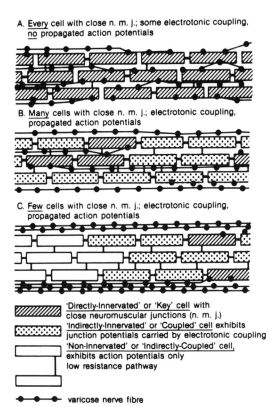

A. Every cell with close n. m. j.; some electrotonic coupling, no propagated action potentials

B. Many cells with close n. m. j.; electrotonic coupling, propagated action potentials

C. Few cells with close n. m. j.; electrotonic coupling, propagated action potentials

'Directly-Innervated' or 'Key' cell with close neuromuscular junctions (n. m. j.)

'Indirectly-Innervated' or 'Coupled' cell exhibits junction potentials carried by electrotonic coupling

'Non-Innervated' or 'Indirectly-Coupled' cell, exhibits action potentials only low resistance pathway

varicose nerve fibre

**FIG. 4.16.** Three types of smooth muscle with various types of intercellular coupling. (From ref. 4.)

which there is a highly developed system of intercellular couplings. It would be predicted that fewer numbers of muscle cells would need to be activated by a drug to produce a syncytial response in type C muscle than type A muscle. In view of the unknown relationship between fractional muscle cell activation and tissue response, it is difficult to assess the relative importance of drug permeation into tissues and the speed of penetration on the magnitude and kinetics of response.

### REFERENCES

1. Barry, P. H., and Diamond, J. M. (1984): Effects of unstirred layers on membrane phenomena. *Physiol. Rev.*, 64:763–872.
2. Berg, H. C., and Purcell, E. M. (1977): Physics of chemoreception. *Biophys. J.*, 20:193–219.
3. Burgen, A. S. V. (1966): The drug-receptor complex. *J. Pharm. Pharmacol.*, 18:137–149.
4. Burnstock, G. (1970): Structure of smooth muscle and its innervation. In: *Smooth Muscle*, edited by E. Bülbring, A. F. Brading, A. W. Jones, and T. Tomita, pp. 1–69. Edward Arnold, London.
5. Crank, J. (1975): *The Mathematics of Diffusion*, ed. 2. Clarendon Press, Oxford.
6. Cuthberg, A. W., and Dunant, Y. (1970): Diffusion of drugs through stationary water layers

as the rate limiting process in their action of membrane receptors. *Br. J. Pharmacol.*, 40: 508–521.

7. Herbette, L. G., Vant Erve, Y. M. H., and Rhodes, D. G. (1989): Interaction of 1,4 dihydro-pyridine calcium channel antagonists with biological membranes: Lipid bilayer partitioning cold occur before drug binding to receptors. *J. Mol. Cell Cardiol.*, 21:187–201.

8. Hughes, I. E., and Smith, J. A. (1978): The stability of noradrenaline in physiological saline solutions. *J. Pharm. Pharmacol.*, 30:124–126.

9. Kenakin, T. P., and Beek, D. (1982): A quantitative analysis of histamine $H_2$-receptor-mediated relaxation of rabbit trachea. *J. Pharmacol. Exp. Ther.*, 220:353–357.

10. Kokubun, S., and Reuter, H. (1984): Dihydropyridine derivatives prolong the open state of the Ca channels in cultured cardiac cells. *Proc. Natl. Acad. Sci. U.S.A.*, 81:4824–4827.

11. Krnjevic, K., and Mitchell, J. F. (1960): Diffusion of acetylcholine in agar gels and in the isolated rat diaphragm. *J. Physiol. (Lond.)*, 153:562–572.

12. Kushmerick, M. J., and Podolsky, R. J. (1969): Ionic mobility in muscle cells. *Science*, 166: 1297–1298.

13. Lane, B. P., and Rhodin, J. A. G. (1964): Cellular interrelationships and electrical activity in two types of smooth muscle. *J. Ultrastruct. Res.*, 10:470–488.

14. Nernst, W. (1904): Theorie der reaktions-geschwendigkeit in heterogenen systemen. *Z. Phys. Chem.*, 47:52–55.

15. Page, E. (1962): Cat heart muscle in vitro. *J. Gen. Physiol.*, 46:201–213.

16. Page, E., and Bernstein, R. S. (1964): Cat heart muscle in vitro. V. Diffusion through a sheet of right ventricle. *J. Gen. Physiol.*, 47:1129–1140.

17. Rhodes, D. G., Sarmiento, J. G., and Herbette, L. G. (1985): Kinetics of binding of mem-brane-active drugs to receptor sites: Diffusion-limited rates for a membrane bilayer ap-proach of 1,4 dihydropyridine calcium channel antagonists to their active site. *Mol. Pharma-col.*, 27:612–623.

18. Venter, J. C. (1978): Cardiac sites of catecholamine action: Diffusion models for soluble and immobilized catecholamine action on isolated cat papillary muscles. *Mol. Pharamcol.*, 14:562–574.

19. Verburg, K. M., and Henry, D. P. (1984): Binding of histamine by glass surfaces. *Agents Actions*, 14:633–642.

20. Watson, S. P. (1983): Rapid degradation of [$^3$H]-substance P in guinea-pig ileum and rat vas deferens in vitro. *Br. J. Pharmacol.*, 79:543–552.

21. Waud, D. R. (1968): On diffusion from a point source. *J. Pharmacol. Exp. Ther.*, 159: 123–128.

22. Waud, D. R. (1968): Pharmacological receptors. *Pharmacol. Rev.*, 20:49–88.

23. Waud, D. R. (1969): A quantitative model for the effect of a saturable uptake on the slope of the dose-response curve. *J. Pharmacol. Exp. Ther.*, 167:140–141.

24. Wilson, F. A., and Dietschy, J. M. (1974): The intestinal unstirred layer: Its surface area and effect on active transport kinetics. *Biochim. Biophys. Acta*, 363:112–126.

# 5

## Concentrations of Drugs in the Receptor Compartment

*The . . . ignorance about the concentration of agonist in equilibrium with receptors and about the relation between receptor activation and tissue response makes the chemical interpretation of concentration-response relations an illusion.*
—Sir James Black, 1976

Fine control of hormone and neurotransmitter concentrations in normally functioning organs is achieved by a delicate balance of secretion and reuptake or degradation (i.e., norepinephrine released from neurons is rapidly and efficiently taken back up into neurons; acetylcholine released from cholinergic nerves is degraded by acetylcholinesterase in the synaptic cleft, and the resulting choline taken back up into the nerve). These processes can be remarkably efficient, especially in terms of reducing a drug concentration in the receptor compartment within the matrix of the tissue. This, in turn, can be completely dissimilating with respect to accurate measurement of dependent variables in tissues and subsequent drug and drug-receptor classifications. In radioligand binding, studies of cells in culture or tissue homogenates, adsorption to surfaces, proteolytic enzymatic degradation, and solvation of drugs into lipid membranes also can seriously affect the concentration of the drug in the medium immediately accessible to the receptor. As seen from the discussion in Chapter 1, all estimates of drug affinity and efficacy depend on an accurate value for $[A_i]$, the concentration of drug in the receptor compartment. This must necessarily be assumed to be equal to the concentration of the drug added to the bathing medium, but if a removal or sequestration process is active during the process of diffusion, then the concentration of the drug at the receptor can be considerably less. Clearly, under these circumstances, accurate calculation of drug-receptor parameters is impossible. This chapter discusses the effects of removal processes (and release processes) on drug concentrations, the factors that add to or detract from their importance, and the conditions necessary for their inhibition.

## DRUG REMOVAL FROM THE RECEPTOR COMPARTMENT

Drug-removal mechanisms in tissues generally are driven by active processes either directly (transport process into the tissue) or indirectly (passive diffusion into the tissue driven by a concentration gradient produced by active degradation in the tissue). For modeling purposes, Michaelis-Menten kinetics will be assumed for the removal mechanism. Thus, the rate of removal ($J$) of drug ($[A_i]$) from the receptor compartment is given by

$$J = \frac{[A_i] \cdot J_{max}}{[A_i] + K_m} \qquad [5.1]$$

where $K_m$ is the Michaelis-Menten constant for removal (equilibrium dissociation constant for complex between drug and site of drug removal), and $J_{max}$ is the maximal rate of removal. A useful variant of Eq. 5.1 for isolated tissues is one in which the rate of removal is expressed in terms of the amount of drug leaving the receptor compartment in a given time (i.e., moles per second). Thus, Eq. 5.1 can be rewritten

$$J_{out} = \frac{[A_i] \cdot J_{max} \cdot V}{[A_i] + K_m} \qquad [5.2]$$

where $V$ is the volume of the tissue.

Unlike the situation for well-mixed enzyme reactions in homogenates, the availability of substrate ($[A_i]$) could be a dominating factor for uptake in a structured tissue. It should be stressed that a response is produced by the *residual* amount of drug in the receptor compartment and thus depends on the rate of removal and the rate of delivery into the receptor compartment; the receptors interact with a flux of drug entering from the organ bath by diffusion and leaving into a storage pool (or being degraded). Therefore, it is not meaningful to consider the effects on the response of a removal mechanism only in terms of the kinetic parameters of the removal mechanism; the importance of an uptake process in a tissue is incontrovertibly linked to the rate of diffusion into the receptor compartment. This latter factor is conveniently modeled by the permeation approximation

$$J' = k([A_o] - [A_i]) \qquad [5.3]$$

where $[A_o]$ and $[A_i]$ are the concentrations of drug in the organ bath and receptor compartment, respectively, and $k$ is a diffusion constant (the reciprocal of $R$ in Eq. 4.8). For isolated tissues, an entry rate in terms of moles per second is useful; thus, Eq. 5.3 can be rewritten

$$J_{in} = k_{in}([A_o] - [A_i]) \cdot S \qquad [5.4]$$

where $S$ is the surface area of the tissue. The parameter $k_{in}$ is the permeation constant discussed in Chapter 4. It should be noted that Eq. 5.4 is an approximation that simplifies concomitant diffusion and uptake in a tissue matrix in terms of two compartments separated by a diffusion barrier of permeability proportional to $k_{in}$, a simplified model that nevertheless can be useful for predicting the effects of diffusion and geometry on drug responses.

When a drug is added to the organ bath, it diffuses quickly to the surface of the tissue and subsequently into the tissue at a rate dependent on the thickness of the unstirred layer, the geometric shape of the tissue ($V/S$ ratio), and the tortuosity factor. The drug diffusing into the receptor compartment also is removed by the removal mechanism; thus, a steady state is achieved where $J_{in} = J_{out}$; combining Eqs. 5.2 and 5.4, the following equation can be derived (6) to calculate the concentrate of drug in the receptor compartment ($[A_i]$) for a given concentration in the organ bath ($[A_o]$):

$$[A_i] = -\tfrac{1}{2}\{-[A_o] + K_m + (J_{max}/k_{in})\,(V/S)\}$$
$$+ (\tfrac{1}{4}\{- [A_o] + K_m + (J_{max}/k_{in})\,(V/S)\}^2 + K_m \cdot [A_o])^{1/2} \qquad [5.5]$$

It can be seen from inspection of Eq. 5.5 that a variety of circumstances could cause $[A_i]$ to be considerably less than $[A_o]$ at a steady state (pseudo-equilibrium); i.e., a *constant* deficit of $[A_i]$ with respect to the organ-bath concentration could be achieved at the receptor. Under these circumstances, only a fraction of the drug added to the organ bath will find its way to the receptor, and the response will depend on the magnitude of this fraction. It is worth considering the factors that affect the magnitude of the fraction reaching the receptor compartment.

### Factors Controlling Removal of Drugs

A schematic representation of diffusion into the receptor compartment is shown in Fig. 5.1, where the volume of fluid in the receptor compartment represents the concentration of drug, and time is in arbitrary but equal periods $T_1, T_2, \ldots, T_n$. It is assumed that the volume of the organ bath is infinite with respect to the receptor compartment and that the concentration of drug on addition to the organ bath rises to $[A_o]$ instantaneously at $T_o$. Both of these approximations are reasonable in light of the usual relative volumes of tissues and organ baths and relative rates of diffusion in free solution and in tissues. Figure 5.1 shows the movement of fluid (drug) from the bath, through an unstirred layer (U.L.), and into the tissue compartment, which contains diffusion barriers representing a tortuosity factor. At $T_1$, fluid begins to flow through the diffusion barrier of the unstirred layer and into the tissue compartment. At $T_n$, equilibrium has been achieved; the only difference between the levels of fluid in the two compartments is their temporal relationship (i.e., there is a time lag between filling in the bath and tissue compart-

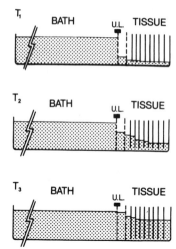

**FIG. 5.1.** Schematic diagram of temporal relationship between concentrations of drug in tissue bath and tissue. The tissue bath is assumed to be infinite in relation to tissue volume. The tissue compartment is separated from the bath by a diffusion barrier (unstirred layer [U.L.]) and contains within it diffusion barriers representing tortuosity. The level of fluid represents concentration of drug; $T_1$ to $T_n$ are arbitrary units of time. Note that, whereas filling of the tissue compartment is slower, the bath concentration eventually is attained within the tissue.

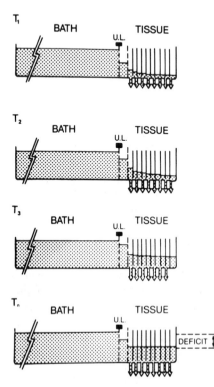

**FIG. 5.2.** Schematic diagram for temporal relationship between concentrations of drug in tissue bath and tissue, with an active removal process denoted by flow of fluid out of the tissue compartment (assumptions as for Fig. 5.1). Note that as for Fig. 5.1, the filling of the tissue compartment lags behind that in the bath compartment. But also, because of the active removal process from the tissue and diffusion barriers between the two compartments, a steady-state pseudoequilibrium can be reached in which the level of fluid in the tissue compartment is always lower than that in the organ-bath compartment.

*140*

ments). Figure 5.2 shows a removal process in the tissue compartments such that fluid exists from the tissue as well as flowing into it. Although there is still the temporal effect on filling (tissue filling lags behind bath-compartment filling), a steady state may be reached whereby the level in the tissue is always less than the level in the bath. There are several factors that exacerbate the magnitude of the deficit of drug in the tissue compartment. These are shown in Fig. 5.3 as they relate to Eq. 5.5. First, if access to the tissue compartment is hindered, an uptake process will have more of an effect on the fluid level; a thick unstirred layer (Fig. 5.3B) or large $V/S$ ratio (Fig. 5.3C) could produce a larger deficit in drug concentration between the bath and the tissue (compare with Fig. 5.3A). If mobility of drug within is hindered (high tortuosity factor), a removal mechanism could produce a greater deficit in drug concentration (Fig. 5.3D). The tortuosity and thickness of the un-

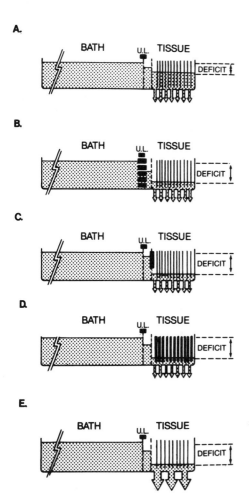

FIG. 5.3. Schematic diagrams for filling of the receptor compartment from an infinite-volume organ-bath compartment. Effects of various conditions. **A:** Control state, an active uptake process represented by movement of fluid out of the tissue compartment (see Fig. 5.2). **B:** Effects of an increased diffusion barrier between the organ-bath compartment and tissue compartment in the form of a thick unstirred layer (U.L.); this impedes the rate of flow between compartments and thus leads to a greater steady-state deficit of fluid (drug concentration) between compartments. **C:** Effects of a large $V/S$ ratio. In this case, the smaller surface area with respect to a larger tissue volume can be approximated by a limitation of the geometric area of access to the tissue compartment. This impedes flow into the compartment and increases drug deficit in the tissue. **D:** In this case, impedance into the tissue compartment is normal, but once within the tissue, flow is severely hindered (high λ). Therefore, the uptake process can exert a more pronounced effect on the steady-state level of fluid in the tissue compartment. **E:** The uptake process is exceedingly active; thus, flow out of the tissue compartment is very rapid with respect to flow into the compartment. The result is a larger deficit of drug at the receptor.

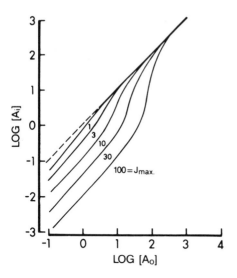

**FIG. 5.4.** Concentrations of drug at the receptor ([$A_i$]; ordinate) as functions of organ-bath concentrations of drug ([$A_o$]; abscissa) in a tissue with a removal process for the agonist. Effects of different maximal rates of removal (see Eq. 5.5). *Broken line* denotes no active removal process ([$A_o$] = [$A_i$]); $K_m$ = 1; $k_{in}$ = 1; $V/S$ = 1.

stirred layer relate to $k_{in}$, the permeation factor for drug into the tissue. Last, if the maximal rate of uptake ($J_{max}$) is high, a large deficit also can be produced (Fig. 5.3E). The relative magnitudes of the parameters describing these factors determine the magnitude of the deficit in drug concentration in the receptor compartment. The effects of changes in $J_{max}$ ($K_m$, $k_{in}$, $V/S$ constant) on the concentration of drug in the receptor compartment ([$A_i$]) as

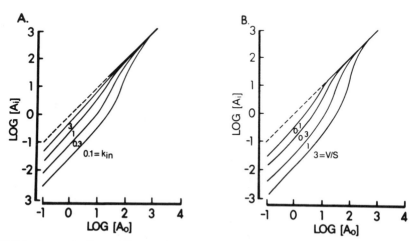

**FIG. 5.5.** Concentrations of drug at the receptor ([$A_i$]; ordinate) as functions of organ-bath concentrations of drug ([$A_o$]; abscissa) in a tissue with a removal process for the agonist. Effects of different **(A)** permeation constants ($k_{in}$) and **(B)** volume-to-surface rations ($V/S$) (see Eq. 5.5). *Broken line* indicates no active removal ([$A_o$] = [$A_i$]). A: $J_{max}$ = 10; $K_m$ = 3; $V/S$ = 1. B: $J_{max}$ = 30; $K_m$ = 1; $k_{in}$ = 1.

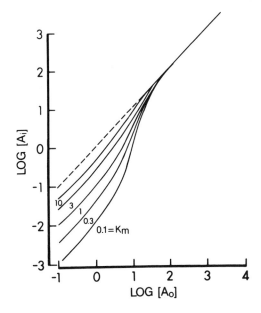

**FIG. 5.6.** Concentrations of drug at the receptor ($[A_i]$; ordinate) as functions of organ-bath concentrations of drug ($[A_o]$; abscissa) in a tissue with a removal process for the agonist. Effects of different Michaelis-Menten constants ($K_m$) for removal (see Eq. 5.5). *Broken line* indicates no active removal ($[A_o] = [A_i]$); $J_{max} = 10$; $k_{in} = 1$; $V/S = 1$.

compared with that in the bath ($[A_o]$) are shown in Fig. 5.4; the magnitude of the deficit and the concentration range at which the effects of removal are overcome (uptake saturated) are dependent on $J_{max}$. Qualitatively, the same effects are produced by changes in permeation ($k_{in}$, Fig. 5.5A) or volume-to-surface ratio ($V/S$, Fig. 5.5B). Last, the effects of changes in the Michaelis-Menten constant ($K_m$) for the removal process on receptor-compartment concentrations of drug are shown in Fig. 5.6; in this case, as $K_m$ increases, the concentrations of $[A_o]$ needed to overcome removal also increase, but the magnitude of the deficit decreases.

## Saturability of Uptake

Although the relative rates of diffusion into and removal out of the receptor compartment of drug can combine to produce a deficit of drug at the receptor, the importance of this deficit to the response depends on the relative dominance between these two processes. Most removal processes are saturable, thereby producing a concentration-dependent effect on tissue responses. If the concentrations of drug ($[A_o]$) are much greater than the $K_m$ for the removal process, this process will effectively be saturated and cease to influence receptor-compartment concentrations of the drug significantly. The $K_m$ for uptake processes is measurable biochemically and theoretically; because the organ-bath concentration of a drug is known, it should be possible to predict at what point a removal process will become saturated and thus will not influence the concentration of the same drug in the receptor compartment. However, the biochemical $K_m$ for an active process measured in a well-mixed solution can be considerably less than the effective $K_m$ in a structured tissue. Under these circumstances, the concentration of drug needed to saturate the removal process when the drug diffuses from the surface of the tissue can be much greater than that required in the tissue; i.e., an uptake process can be more difficult to saturate when present in a structured matrix with restricted diffusion than in a homogeneous biochemical reaction. For example, the effective $K_m$ for hydrolysis of acetylcholine by the enzyme acetylcholinesterase in a structured tissue is much greater than the $K_m$ in a homogenized preparation of the enzyme (7). One reason for this is the unstirred layer surrounding tissues. When such layers separate the bathing medium from a tissue that contains a removal process, there can be a decrease in concentration across the unstirred layer. Thus, the concentrations of drug at the surface ($[A_s]$) of the tissue and in the organ bath ($[A_o]$) are related by the following equation:

$$\frac{[A_s]}{[A_o]} = \left(1 + \frac{J_{max}}{K_m \cdot D} \cdot \frac{\delta}{\lambda^2}\right)^{-1} \qquad [5.6]$$

It can be seen from this equation that if the uptake process is of high maximal velocity (large $J_{max}$), or if the unstirred layer is thick (large $\delta$), a considerable concentration gradient can occur across the unstirred layer. However, if diffusion within the tissue is poor (high $\lambda$), the effect of the unstirred layer is minimized.

As seen in Fig. 4.4, the effective velocity of an active process in a tissue can be greatly decreased by the presence of an unstirred layer. One method of determining the point at which an active process is saturated is by measuring when the observed velocity is maximal ($J = J_{max}$); this occurs when $[A_i] \gg K_m$ (see Eq. 5.1). In the presence of an unstirred layer, the substrate concentration must be elevated considerably higher than the true $K_m$ to achieve $J_{max}$ (saturate the transport system). The effective increase in the $K_m$ for a removal process in a structured tissue covered by an unstirred layer of thickness $\delta$ is given by

$$\frac{K'_m}{K_m} = 1 + \frac{\delta \cdot J_{max}}{D \cdot K_m} \qquad [5.7]$$

where $K'_m$ is the effective $K_m$ of the uptake process with respect to saturability of the process by organ-bath concentrations of drugs, $K_m$ is the true $K_m$, and $D$ is the diffusion coefficient in free solution. This equation illustrates that it is more difficult to saturate a removal process with bath concentrations when the unstirred layer is thick ($\delta$ large), as expected, but also when $J_{max}$ is high. Therefore, unstirred layers generally should have greater effects on the saturability of a removal process if that process has a high capacity for removal (when the deficit of drug in the receptor compartment is large).

Another reason why active processes are difficult to saturate in structured organs is related to concentration gradients of substrates within tissues. If a drug must diffuse through a matrix of removal sites to reach the receptor, the concentration of drug becomes depleted as the drug passes through the tissue. Under these circumstances, there may be a saturating concentration of drug at the muscle surface, but a concentration considerably less than saturating at the tissue core. The relationship between the concentration of drug at the tissue surface ($[A_o]$) and that at a point $x$ in the tissue ($[A_x]$) when $[A_o] \gg K_m$ (apparently saturating concentration in the organ bath) is given by

$$[A_x] = [A_o] - \frac{J_{max}}{n \cdot D'} (l^2 - x^2) \qquad [5.8]$$

where $D'$ is the diffusion coefficient for drug in the tissue, $l$ is the thickness of the tissue, $x$ is the distance from the center, and $n = 2, 4,$ or $6$ for a slice, cylinder, or sphere, respectively. If it is assumed that $10 \cdot K_m$ is a saturating concentration, the surface concentration required to saturate the process at the core of the tissue ($x = 0$) is given by

$$[A_o] \geq 10 \cdot K_m + \frac{J_{max} \cdot \lambda^2 l^2}{n \cdot D} \qquad [5.9]$$

where $D$ is the diffusion coefficient for the drug in free diffusion, $\lambda$ is the tortuosity factor, and $n$ refers to the coefficients for Eq. 5.8. It can be seen that if the removal process is avid (high $J_{max}$), if the tissue is thick (large $l$), or if diffusion into the matrix of the tissue is slow (high tortuosity factor $\lambda$), the concentration of drug in the organ bath may have to exceed the true $K_m$ of the removal process by a considerable factor to saturate the process in the core of the tissue. For these reasons, the concentration of drug in the organ bath cannot easily be related to the saturability of a removal process in an isolated tissue.

## Concentration Gradients Within Tissues

As seen from Eq. 5.8, a concentration gradient of drug within a tissue can develop even when the surface concentration of drug exceeds the $K_m$ of the drug-removal process. The development of these concentration gradients is more likely at concentrations of drug that do not saturate the uptake process, and such concentrations are quite likely to be pharmacologically relevant with respect to the production of a response. The concentration of drug at any point in a tissue ($[A_x]$) relative to the surface concentration ($[A_o]$) can be calculated with the equations of Green (11). For a tissue slice of thickness $l$,

$$\frac{[A_x]}{[A_o]} = \frac{\cosh\{[J_{max}/(K_m \cdot D)] \cdot \lambda x\}}{\cosh\{[J_{max}/(K_m \cdot D)] \cdot \lambda l\}} \qquad [5.10]$$

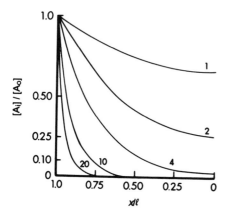

FIG. 5.7. Concentration gradients for an agonist penetrating into a tissue slice with various capabilities to remove the agonist from the extracellular space. Ordinate: Concentration of drug at point $x$ ($[A_x]$) as a fraction of the surface concentration (concentration of agonist in the organ bath $[A_o]$). Abscissa: Penetration into the tissue slice, depth $x$ into the slice, as a fraction of the diameter of the slice $l$. Concentration gradients calculated from Eq. 5.10, with $(J_{max}/K_m \cdot D)^{1/2}$ equal to the numbers next to the respective curves. (From ref. 11.)

where $x$ is the distance to the center plane of the tissue slice. The concentration gradients for drugs in tissue slices having removal mechanisms for the drugs of varying capacities and varying penetrabilities to drugs by diffusion are shown in Fig. 5.7.

The corresponding equation for a cylinder is

$$\frac{[A_x]}{[A_o]} = \frac{I_0\{[J_{max}/(K_m \cdot D)] \cdot \lambda x\}}{I_0\{[J_{max}/(K_m \cdot D)] \cdot \lambda r\}} \quad [5.11]$$

where $r$ is the radius of the cylinder and $I_0(x)$ is the hyperbolic Bessel function. The equation for a sphere is

$$\frac{[A_x]}{[A_o]} = \frac{r}{x} \cdot \frac{\sinh\{[J_{max}/(K_m \cdot D)] \cdot \lambda x\}}{\sinh\{[J_{max}/(K_m \cdot D)] \cdot \lambda r\}} \quad [5.12]$$

where $r$ is the radius of the sphere.

## EFFECTS OF REMOVAL MECHANISMS ON DRUG RESPONSES

Up to this point, the discussion has been confined to the combined effects of diffusion and drug-removal mechanisms on the concentrations of drugs in tissues and specifically within the receptor compartment. A steady-state deficit of drug in the receptor compartment can have profound effects on the observed magnitude of a drug response. This, in turn, can completely dissociate the values for the concentration in the organ bath and that actually present at the receptor; the removal process prevents the full concentration in the bath from reaching the receptors. Because the magnitude of a tissue response is dependent on the concentration of drug at the receptor, the drug will appear to be less potent than it actually is. This is illustrated in Fig. 5.8 for a tissue with a removal mechanism of characteristics $(J_{max} \cdot V)/(S \cdot k_{in} \cdot K_m)$

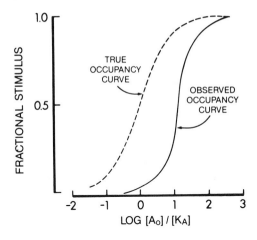

**FIG. 5.8.** Difference between actual and observed agonist occupancy curves in a tissue with a removal mechanism that produces a 30-fold deficit of agonist between the bath and receptor compartments. Ordinate: Fraction of maximal receptor occupancy multiplied by intrinsic efficacy to give fractional stimulus. Abscissa: Logarithm of molar concentration of agonist added to the organ bath as a multiple of the $K_A$ for the agonist for the receptor. The agonist appears to be 30 times less potent than it actually is.

= 30. The experimentally observed concentration-response curve is displaced considerably to the right of the receptor-occupancy curve. Such displacements of concentration-response curves can be totally misleading with respect to the potencies of agonists. For example, Fig. 5.9A shows the relative potencies of two agonists for the same receptor. One agonist, norepinephrine, is avidly taken up into nerve endings, whereas the other, methoxamine, is not. In a tissue with an active neuronal uptake mechanism, such as the rat anococcygeus muscle, methoxamine is more potent than norepineph-

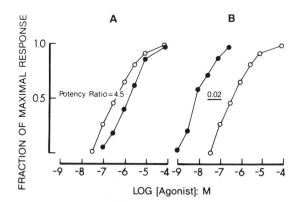

**FIG. 5.9.** Relative potencies of norepinephrine (●) and methoxamine (○) in the presence (**A**, untreated) and absence (**B**, cocaine) of an uptake process for norepinephrine. Ordinate: Response as a fraction of maximal response. Abscissa: Logarithm of molar concentration of agonist. In the rat anococcygeus muscle, a tissue with a powerful uptake process for norepinephrine, but not methoxamine, methoxamine has a higher potency. This relative potency is a product of the uptake process, and when this is neutralized by cocaine, the true relative potency can be observed; norepinephrine is considerably more potent than methoxamine. (Data from ref. 28.)

rine. However, this order of potency is artificial, because only a fraction of the concentration of norepinephrine added to the organ bath reaches the receptors. When this uptake process is inactivated, the true relative potencies of norepinephrine and methoxamine are observed (Fig. 5.9B); this demonstrates the power of uptake mechanisms to obscure the true responses of agonists.

Clearly, accurate measurement of drug potency and subsequent calculation of drug-receptor parameters depend on accurate location parameters for concentration-response curves. It follows that uptake processes for drugs must be effectively neutralized before accurate drug and drug-receptor classification can take place. As the previous discussion indicates, the temporal behavior of responses does not indicate the presence of agonist-uptake processes; i.e., a steady-state response can be achieved that is identical with an equilibrium state between drug and receptors, but these are in fact pseudoequilibria (Fig. 5.2). However, a blocker of the uptake process can unveil an otherwise undetectable pseudoequilibrium steady-state response. Figure 5.10A shows responses of rat anococcygeus muscle to norepinephrine; this tissue avidly removes norepinephrine from the receptor compartment by

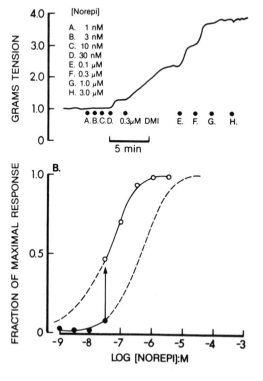

FIG. 5.10. Effects of an uptake process on a steady-state response. **A:** Contraction of rat anococcygeus muscle to norepinephrine. At D (30 nM), a 0.3-g steady-state contraction is produced. Addition of a blocking agent for norepinephrine uptake (0.3 μM DMI) eliminates the steady-state deficit of norepinephrine produced by the removal of this agonist by nerves and elevates receptor-compartment concentrations of norepinephrine. This is reflected in the increased response. **B:** The data in A plotted as concentration-response curves that demonstrate sensitization of the tissue to the agonist by uptake blockade. (From ref. 24.)

uptake of this catecholamine into nerves. At a steady-state response (point D), a constant level of response is obtained that outwardly resembles an equilibrium between the concentrations of drug in the organ bath and in the receptor compartment. In fact, it is really an equilibrium between the receptors and the fraction of the organ-bath drug concentration that can escape removal by neuronal uptake, and thus it is a pseudoequilibrium between the total bath concentration and receptors. This can be made evident by blockade of the uptake process; in Fig. 5.10A it can be seen that addition of a blocker of neuronal uptake (desmethylimipramine [DMI]), a drug that has no inherent agonist property, produces an increased response to the same concentration (D) of agonist. This increased response is due to the effects of removal of the uptake-dependent drug deficit. Figure 5.10B shows that blockade of the uptake process eliminates the deficit of agonist and effectively potentiates the tissue to the effects of the agonist. The magnitude of the potentiation reflects the importance of the uptake process as a modulator of agonist-receptor concentrations in the receptor compartment. Thus, a blockade of a powerful removal process or a moderate or avid removal process in concert with poor diffusion results in large potentiations of responses, whereas inhibition of weak removal mechanisms leads to small potentiations of responses.

Pharmacologically, the magnitude of potentiation to an uptake blocker (inhibitor of a removal process) can be used (within limits) as an indicator of the importance of uptake mechanisms and the relative importance of various factors associated with uptake and diffusion; in essence, isolated tissues can provide bioassays for the residual concentrations of drug that reach the receptor compartment. For example, Fig. 5.11 shows the effects of $V/S$ ratios on the sensitivity of guinea pig papillary muscles to norepinephrine. As noted in Fig. 5.5B, the larger the $V/S$ ratio, the more effect a given uptake process will have on the agonist concentration in the receptor compartment (see also Eq. 5.5). The greater the importance of a removal process, the smaller will be the fraction of the agonist concentration added to the organ bath that will

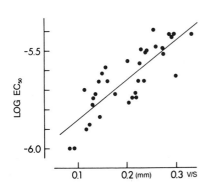

FIG. 5.11. Sensitivity of guinea pig papillary muscle to norepinephrine as a function of $V/S$ ratio. Ordinate: Logarithms of the molar concentrations of norepinephrine that produce half-maximal responses in guinea pig papillary muscles. Abscissa: Measured volume-to-surface ratios for papillary muscles. The positive correlation indicates that muscles with smaller volume-to-surface ratios are more sensitive to norepinephrine (i.e., less deficit of agonist is produced by uptake). The larger is $V/S$, the more effect the uptake mechanism can exert on norepinephrine diffusing into the tissue (see Fig. 5.3C), and the larger concentration deficit; this latter factor is reflected in the lower sensitivity of these muscles to norepinephrine. (From ref. 6.)

reach the receptors, and thus the lower the apparent sensitivity of the tissue (compare the curves in Fig. 5.8). Figure 5.11 illustrates the negative correlation between guinea pig papillary muscle sensitivity to norepinephrine and $V/S$. The previous sections of this chapter deal with the various geometric and diffusion factors that can affect the concentration of agonist in the receptor compartment. The study of organ sensitization to substrate agonists (agonists removed from the receptor compartment by a removal process) illustrates an additional aspect of diffusion and uptake, namely, the relative geometry of the site of agonist removal and receptors.

## Relative Geometry of Receptors and Uptake Sites

If the drug must diffuse past the site of removal in order to reach the receptors (i.e., if the removal mechanism becomes a diffusional barrier), the uptake process will have a greater effect on the magnitude of the drug response than if the receptors and uptake sites are in parallel. Figure 5.12A shows an effect of the relative geometry of uptake sites and receptors mediating responses. When the entry of histamine is constrained to one surface of a rabbit aortic strip by an artificial barrier, differences in the effects of uptake processes (in this case, metabolizing enzymes and uptake into muscle) can be observed. Interpretation of these data strictly in terms of differences in diffusion is complicated, however, by the possibility of differential muscle-cell sensitivity to histamine and cell-to-cell coupling, but nevertheless does illustrate a further level of complexity in the production of tissue responses by drugs added to bathing solutions. It would also be predicted that the proximity of the site of agonist removal to the receptor would be relevant to the importance of an uptake process. Figure 5.12B illustrates the relationship between tissue sensitization to norepinephrine after blockade of neuronal uptake and the width of the neuromuscular interval. These data show that when the nerve varicosity (site of removal) and postsynaptic membrane (receptor) are in close proximity, uptake severely modulates the production of responses, as illustrated by large tissue sensitizations after blockade of neuronal uptake. The effects of neuronal blockade are much less striking at large neuromuscular intervals.

## Effects of Uptake Inhibition on Responses

The restricted diffusion in tissues, the ability of tissues to actively metabolize drugs, and the geometric relationships between these factors can combine to yield striking differences between the true and observed potencies of drugs. These differences in observed and actual agonist activities can take different forms. For example, if stimulus-response coupling is efficient, such that agonist concentrations do not effectively approach the $K_m$ of the uptake

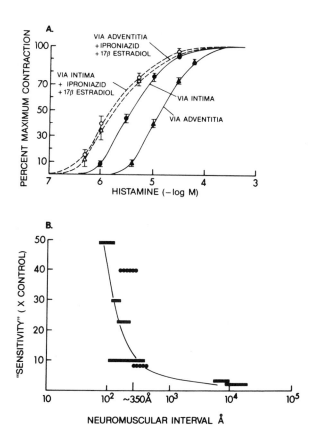

**FIG. 5.12.** Effects of the relative geometry of uptake and receptor sites. **A:** Ordinate: Contractions of rabbit aortae to histamine as fractions of the maximal response to histamine. Abscissa: Logarithms of molar concentrations of histamine. The entry of histamine was restricted to one surface of the muscle strip by a diffusion barrier, and responses were obtained in the presence and absence of inhibitors for metabolizing mechanisms for histamine. When the removal mechanisms are neutralized (+ iproniazid and 17β-estradiol), the sensitivity of the muscle to histamine does not depend on the surface from which the histamine diffuses (*broken lines*). However, in the presence of the removal mechanisms, the diffusion path greatly affects the deficit of histamine at the receptor. When entry is restricted to the adventitial side of the artery, the removal mechanism has a greater effect on the concentrations of histamine needed to produce responses than when entry is restricted to the intimal side. (From ref. 29.) **B:** Ordinate: Potentiations of responses of various tissues to norepinephrine produced by blockade of neuronal uptake. Abscissa: Distances in angstroms between the muscle (receptors) and nerves (sites of uptake) in these tissues. The fact that tissues with low neuromuscular intervals (nerves close to the muscle) demonstrate large potentiations to norepinephrine after uptake blockade indicates that the close proximity of the uptake sites to the receptors may be related to the ability of the removal mechanism to modulate receptor-mediated responses. In tissues in which the nerves are far from the receptors ($10^4$ Å), neuronal uptake is relatively unimportant, as demonstrated by the low magnitude of sensitization after uptake blockade. (From ref. 34.)

process, then a parallel shift of the agonist concentration-response curve to the right will be produced by an uptake process. Figure 5.13A shows a 350-fold deviation from the true potency of adenosine in guinea pig trachea caused by tissue uptake and degradation of this agonist. A different effect on an agonist response can be produced by a removal mechanism if the agonist is of low efficacy and must activate a large portion of the muscle to produce responses. Figure 5.13B show the striking increases in observed responses to the low-efficacy agonists inosine and 3-deoxyadenosine after blockade of tissue uptake processes. In these cases, not only a sinistral displacement of the concentration-response curve is produced, but also an increased maximal response.

A depression of the maximal response can be produced by a tissue removal mechanism, even for powerful agonists of high efficacy, if the uptake process is very active, tissue diffusion is restricted, and cell-to-cell coupling is poor. Under these circumstances, the agonist may not be capable of penetrating to and activating a sufficient quantity of muscle to produce the true maximal tissue response. Figure 5.14 shows a calculated concentration gradient for norepinephrine penetrating the wall of rat vas deferens. It was assumed that the surface concentration was nonsaturating with respect to tissue uptake;

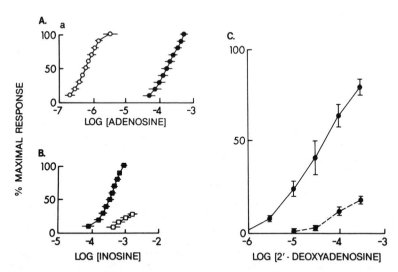

**FIG. 5.13.** Potentiation of tissue responses to agonists for adenosine receptors by adenosine-uptake blockers. Ordinates: Responses expressed as percentages of the maximal response; **A** and **B**, relaxation of spontaneous tone; **C**, inhibition of electrically evoked muscle twitch. Abscissae: Logarithms of molar concentrations of agonists. A: Responses of guinea pig trachea to adenosine in the absence (•) and presence (o) of the uptake blocker dipyridamole (0.5 μM). B: Responses of guinea pig trachea to inosine in the absence (■) and presence (□) of dipyridamole (0.5 μM). (A and B from ref. 30.) C: Responses of guinea pig ileum to 2′-deoxyadenosine in the absence (*broken line*) and presence (*solid line*) of dipyridamole (0.2 μM). (From ref. 27.)

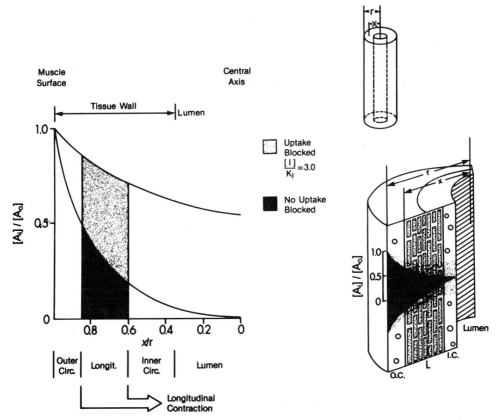

**FIG. 5.14.** Concentration gradients for norepinephrine in rat vas deferens. Graph shows the concentration of norepinephrine at a point $x$ in the wall ($[A_x]$) as a fraction of the organ-bath concentration ($[A_o]$). Abscissa: Fractional distance away from the central axis of the tissue (see schematic). Response is obtained only from the middle layer of longitudinal smooth muscle. Section of vas deferens indicates the concentration gradients schematically. For these calculations, it was assumed that $(J_{max}/K_m \cdot D)^{1/2}$ was 50 (see Eq. 5.10). (From ref. 21.)

thus, the hyperbolic Bessel function (Eq. 5.11) was used to calculate the concentration gradient. It can be seen that if the longitudinal response is measured, only 32% of the longitudinal muscle layer is exposed to norepinephrine; partial inhibition of the neuronal uptake mechanism (presence of an uptake blocker at three times the concentration required for half-maximal blockade; $[I]/K_I = 3$) diminishes the concentration gradient and increases the quantity of longitudinal muscle exposed to norepinephrine to 76%. If the amount of muscle activated in the absence of uptake blocker is insufficient for maximal response, the effect of the uptake blocker will be to increase the magnitude of the response, i.e., to potentiate responses to norepinephrine. Whether this type of effect translates to an increase in the maximal response of the tissue to the agonist depends on the relative capabilities of the removal mechanisms, the efficiency of cell-to-cell coupling, and the propensity for tissue desensitization to high concentrations of agonist.

It would be assumed that at extremely high concentrations ($[A_o] \gg K_m$), uptake would be saturated and no effective concentration gradients would occur; under these circumstances, at high agonist concentrations the maximal tissue response would be achieved in any case, and blockade of uptake should not increase the maximal response to any agonist. However, this assumes that uptake can effectively be saturated by concentrations of agonist added to the organ bath, and as seen in Eq. 5.9, an avid uptake process in a tissue with poor diffusion characteristics (high tortuosity factor) covered with a thick unstirred layer may require, depending on the $K_m$ of the uptake process, unrealistically high (and perhaps unachievable) concentrations of agonist at the muscle surface to saturate the uptake process at the core of the tissue. If saturation of the uptake process is attempted with high organ-bath concentrations of agonist, the outer layers of muscle are exposed to supramaximal concentrations of agonist, inviting the possibility of rapid de-

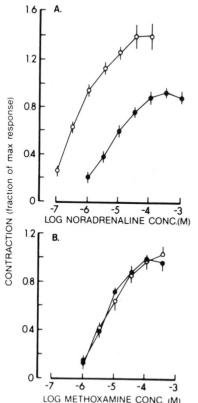

**FIG. 5.15.** Effects of cocaine on responses of rat vas deferens to **(A)** norepinephrine and **(B)** methoxamine. Ordinates: Fractions of maximal contraction before uptake blockade. Abscissae: Logarithms of molar concentrations of agonist. Responses in the absence (•) and presence (o) of cocaine (10 μM); bars represent SEM. (From ref. 21.)

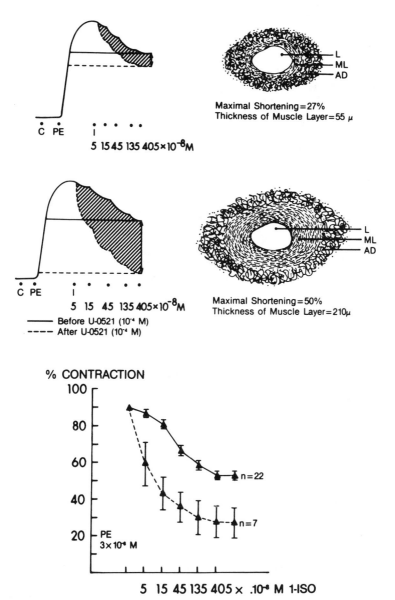

**FIG. 5.16.** Relaxation of precontracted canine saphenous vein by isoproterenol. **Top:** Responses in the absence (*solid line*) and presence (*broken line*) of U-0521, an inhibitor of the catecholamine-metabolizing enzyme catechol-*O*-methyl transferase. Curves are shown from thin-walled (*upper*) and thick-walled (*lower*) preparations. L, lumen; ML, muscular layer; AD, adventitia. **Bottom:** Mean concentration-response curves for isoproterenol relaxation of canine saphenous vein before (*solid line*) and after (*broken line*) U-0521. (From ref. 13.)

sensitization and subsequent diminished responses from these muscle cells. Under these circumstances, it is possible that an avid removal mechanism in a tissue could prevent observation of the true maximal response to an agonist. Figure 5.15A shows the increase in the maximal response to norepinephrine in rat vas deferens produced by blockade of the neuronal uptake mechanism for this agonist by cocaine; no such potentiation is observed for methoxamine, an agonist for the same receptor that is not a substrate for the uptake process (Fig. 5.15B).

As noted previously, the thickness of the muscle ($V/S$ ratio) can greatly affect diffusion characteristics and the subsequent effects of uptake on the drug concentration in the receptor compartment. In addition to affecting muscle sensitivity to agonists (demonstrated in Fig. 5.11), if the uptake and diffusional characteristics of a muscle severely restrict agonist penetration, $V/S$ ratios can affect maximal responses as well. Figure 5.16 shows the effects of inhibition of the degrading enzyme catechol-$O$-methyl transferase (COMT) on responses of canine saphenous vein to isoproterenol. The effects of uptake inhibition result in a larger increased maximal response in thick tissues as opposed to thin tissues.

It is clear that a variety of conditions can produce profound differences between concentrations of drugs in the organ bath and those producing responses at the receptor. Under these circumstances, a dissociation between dependent (response) and independent (concentration) variables can result that often precludes meaningful pharmacologic experiments. Therefore, it is of enormous practical importance that such nonequilibrium conditions be detected and neutralized.

## EFFECTIVE INHIBITION OF DRUG-REMOVAL PROCESSES

In general, quantitative pharmacologic experimentation requires a true equilibrium between organ-bath concentrations of drugs and receptors, and in order to achieve this, inhibition of drug-removal processes is necessary. It is a problem to know when such a drug-removal process is effectively eliminated because pseudoequilibrium steady states (drug removed from the receptor compartment) so closely resemble true equilibrium. There are two methods of eliminating an uptake process in a tissue. One can be utilized only in certain circumstances and involves removing or destroying the sites of removal. For example, neuronal uptake of catecholamines in a tissue can be neutralized by physical removal of the neural plexus in some tissues or by chemical destruction of nerves by *in vitro* or *in vivo* administration of 6-hydroxydopamine. By far the more widely applicable approach is inhibition of drug-removal mechanisms by introduction of an inhibitor ($I$) of the uptake process that has affinity for the site of removal (denoted $K_I$, where this is the equilibrium dissociation constant of the inhibitor-removal-site complex). It is possible to predict the relationship between the approach to true equilibrium (i.e., complete blockade of the uptake process) and the concentration of uptake inhibitor required to achieve this condition in certain circumstances; these calculations illustrate tenets that apply to the practical design of *in vitro* experiments.

The simplest case is that in which the concentration of drug in the receptor compartment ($[A_i]$) is nonsaturating with respect to the uptake process ($[A_i]$ $\ll K_m$). In view of the efficiency of stimulus-response mechanisms, the fact that in many cases only fractions of a tissue need be activated by agonist for full response (cell-to-cell coupling), and the observed displacement of concentration-response curves to the left of occupancy-response curves, this may be a valid condition for many experimental situations (i.e., some agonists act at very low concentrations). The effects of agonist removal on concentration-response curves need to be considered before the effects of uptake inhibition. By equating Eqs. 5.2 and 5.4, the following relationship between the concentration of drug in the organ bath ($[A_o]$) and that in the receptor compartment ($[A_i]$) can be derived:

$$\frac{[A_o]}{[A_i]} = y = \frac{J_{max}(V/S)}{k_{in} \cdot K_m} \cdot \left(1 + \frac{[A_i]}{K_m}\right)^{-1} + 1 \qquad [5.13]$$

This equation predicts the maximal deficit any removal process can have on an organ-bath concentration of agonist. Thus, when there is no uptake ($J_{max} = 0$), $[A_o] = [A_i]$, and the total amount of drug added to the organ bath diffuses to the receptors. When the concentration of agonist is very high, such that uptake is saturated ($[A_i] \gg K_m$), then $[A_o] \rightarrow [A_i]$, and again little deficit between bath and receptor-compartment concentrations will be observed. The maximal deficit predicted by Eq. 5.13 also becomes the maximal degree of sensitization of the tissue to the agonist after complete inhibition of the uptake process ($J_{max} = 0$, or $[A_i] \gg K_m$). In subsequent discussion, it will be useful to refer to this maximal sensitization as a reference point; it will be denoted by $y$.

Some interesting effects of diffusion and geometry are illustrated by Eq. 5.13 as well. It is reasonable to assume that because receptors are pharmacologically uniform over species and tissues, the same is true for uptake processes (i.e., the neuronal uptake process for catecholamines in one tissue will be the same as in another). However, it does not follow that the effects of a given type of uptake process on receptor-compartment concentrations of drugs will be uniform from tissue to tissue or even within the same tissue. This is because there is tissue variation with respect to the synergy among uptake, diffusion, and geometric factors. Therefore, it cannot be assumed that because an uptake process has no appreciable effect on a concentration-response curve to an agonist in one tissue, it will not have an effect in another. Figure 5.17 shows the effects a given uptake process ($J_{max}$ constant) can

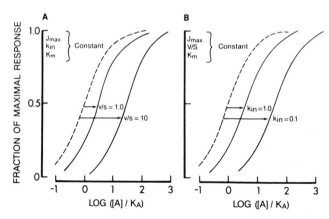

**FIG. 5.17.** Effects of geometric configuration and/or rate of drug permeation on sensitivities of tissues with identical uptake mechanisms for the agonist. *Broken line* denotes agonist potency in the absence of the uptake mechanism. Effects of a 10-fold increase in *V/S* **(A)** and a 10-fold decrease in $k_{in}$. In each case, the uptake characteristics are identical, but the effects of the uptake mechanism on agonist potency differ.

have on concentration-response curves in tissues with different diffusion or geometric characteristics. The capricious behavior of the effects of uptake processes producing pseudoequilibria in some tissues and not others poses a considerable practical problem for pharmacologic studies aimed at drug and drug-receptor classification.

### Effects of Partial Uptake Inhibition

Assuming that the uptake process follows Michaelis-Menten kinetics, the relationship between the rate of removal and a concentration of competitive inhibitor ($[I]$) for the uptake process is given by

$$J_{out} = \frac{[A_i] \cdot J_{max} \cdot V}{[A_i] + K_m(1 + [I]/K_I)} \qquad [5.14]$$

where $V$ is the volume of the tissue. At a pseudoequilibrium steady state ($J_{in} = J_{out}$), Eq. 5.14 can be equated with Eq. 5.3 to yield

$$[A_i] = \frac{[A_o'] (1 + [A_i]/K_m + [I]/K_I)}{(1 + [A_i]/K_m + [I]/K_I + J_{max})(V/S)/(k_{in} \cdot K_m)} \qquad [5.15]$$

where $[A_o']$ refers to the concentration of agonist in the organ bath in the presence of the uptake inhibitor. In the absence of an uptake inhibitor, Eq. 5.13 can be rearranged to yield $[A_i]$, and if it is assumed that equal responses emanate from equal concentrations of agonist at the receptor, then Eqs. 5.13 and 5.15 can be equated to yield the ratio of organ-bath concentrations required to produce equal responses in the presence and absence of an uptake inhibitor [$I$]:

$$\frac{[A_o]}{[A_o']} = \frac{y(1 + [A_i]/K_m + [I]/K_I)}{y(1 + [A_i]/K_m + [I]/K_I)} \qquad [5.16]$$

The ratio $[A_o]/[A_o']$ refers to the organ-bath concentrations that produce a given response in the absence ($[A_o]$) and presence ($[A_o']$) of uptake inhibition. Because the uptake inhibitor enables a larger fraction of the bath concentration to activate the receptors, $[A_o']$ will be less than $[A_o]$, and $[A_o]/[A_o']$ will quantify the tissue sensitization to the agonist (i.e., the potentiation of response produced by [$I$]). It will be convenient to refer to this sensitization (potentiation of the agonist) as $x$ ($[A_o]/[A_o'] = x$).

Inspection of Eq. 5.16 shows that the degree of potentiation is not independent of the relationship of the receptor concentration of agonist and the $K_m$ for removal ($[A_i]/K_m$). As pointed out earlier in this section, there are various pharmacologic circumstances in which it can be assumed that $[A_i] \ll K_m$ and that $[A_i]/K_m \rightarrow 0$; this is the simplest case to consider. Under these circumstances, Eq. 5.15 reduces to

$$\frac{[A_o]}{[A_o']} = x = \frac{y(1 + [I]/K_I)}{y + [I]/K_I} \qquad [5.17]$$

This equation illustrates that, as expected, the degree of tissue sensitization to an agonist is dependent on how completely the uptake process is inhibited (denoted by the magnitude of the ratio $[I]/K_I$); thus, when $[I] \gg K_I$, $x \rightarrow y$ (the maximal sensitization). However, Eq. 5.17 also illustrates another point less intuitively apparent, namely, the fact that the larger the maximal effect of the uptake process ($y$), the greater ($[I]/K_I$) must be to completely block the process; in short, it becomes more difficult to block the effects of a removal process if that process has large effects on agonist concentrations in the receptor compartment. Figure 5.18A shows the effects of a given concentration of uptake blocker in two tissues, one in which uptake is less important than in the other (tissue I, $y = 5$; tissue II, $y = 50$). Note that the concentration of uptake blocker adequate to completely block the effects of uptake in tissue I only partially blocks the effects of uptake in tissue II. The theoretical relationship between the degree of blockade of drug removal and the maximal effects of removal is shown in Fig. 5.18B. Experimental data for the effects of cocaine as a blocker of neuronal norepinephrine uptake in various tissues are shown in Fig. 5.18C. These curves illustrate the fact that concentrations of uptake blocker adequate for one tissue may not be adequate for another and therefore cannot be extrapolated from tissue to tissue. The predictions of Eq. 5.17 and the relationship shown in Fig. 5.18B show the quantitative relationships between sensitization and uptake inhibition.

It is useful to know the concentration of uptake inhibitor that will effectively neutralize the removal process. In view of the differences between transport processes in homogenates and structured tissues, an estimate of $K_I$

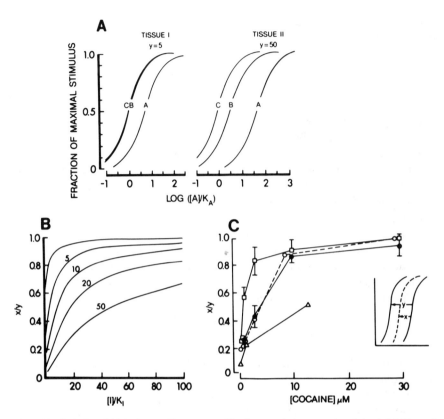

**FIG. 5.18.** Relationship between tissue sensitization and degree of uptake inhibition. **A:** In the absence of an uptake mechanism, the sensitivities of tissues I and II to the agonist are shown by curve C. In tissue I, uptake produces a fivefold deficit of agonist at the receptor; thus, the observed curve is A. In tissue II, the uptake mechanism produces a larger effect (50-fold), and the observed curve is A. In the presence of a concentration of uptake inhibitor 30 times the $K_i$ for uptake inhibition ($[I]/K_i = 30$), tissue I is nearly completely sensitized (curve B; uptake neutralized), but tissue II is not (curve B). (From ref. 27.) **B:** Relationship between sensitization ($x$) as a fraction of the maximal sensitization ($y$) and concentration of uptake inhibitor ($[I]$ as a multiple of the $K_i$). Numbers next to the curves refer to the maximal sensitization. Note that $[I]/K_i = 20$ produces nearly maximal sensitization if uptake effects are small ($y = 2$), but only 30% maximal sensitization if uptake produces a large effect on observed potency ($y = 50$). **C:** Experimental data showing fraction of maximal sensitization of tissues to norepinephrine (ordinate) produced by cocaine (abscissa). Guinea pig left atria ($\square$, $y = 5$, $N = 20$), trachea ($\bullet$, $y = 11$, $N = 15$), right atria ($\bullet$, $y = 13$), trachea ($\triangle$, $y = 36$). (B and C from ref. 20; data for right atria from ref. 32; data for trachea ($y = 36$) from ref. 8.)

obtained biochemically is not meaningful for predicting what concentration of an uptake inhibitor is adequate to completely block a removal process in a tissue. One practical method is to note the concentration at which tissue sensitization to the agonist is maximal. Figure 5.19A shows the theoretical sensitization to an agonist produced by inhibition of a removal mechanism that causes a 30-fold deficit of agonist at the receptor (with respect to the concentration in the organ bath). It can be seen from these calculations that the magnitude of sensitization decreases with constant incremental increases in uptake inhibition as the maximal sensitization ($y$) is approached. This is also demonstrated by the hyperbolic relationship of $x/y$ and $[I]/K_I$ shown in Fig. 5.18B. Figure 5.19B shows the sensitization of guinea pig trachea to norepinephrine produced by cocaine. At a concentration of 100 μM cocaine, essentially complete sensitization is observed; at this point the removal process may be assumed to be effectively neutralized. Unfortunately, this approach assumes that the uptake blocker is specific and has no other property that will affect the location of the concentration-response curve. This assumption should be verified experimentally, because complete inhibition of a powerful uptake process may require a high concentration of uptake blocker (i.e., $[I]/K_I \geq 300$ [Fig. 5.18B]). In the case of cocaine potentiation of norepinephrine in trachea, control experiments with salbutamol indicated that cocaine had no effects on curves for an agonist that was not a substrate for uptake but activated the same receptor (Fig. 5.19C).

In general, verification of assumed selectivity for uptake blockers is essential. It could be argued theoretically that if an uptake blocker possesses the structural requirements for interference with agonist binding to the site of uptake, it is not inconceivable that it also possesses characteristics for binding to the agonist receptor. Thus, an uptake blocker may possess affinity

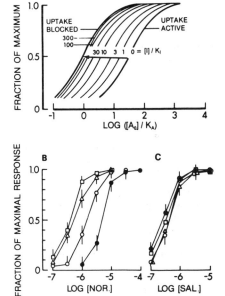

**FIG. 5.19.** Relationship between concentration of uptake inhibitor and tissue sensitization. **A:** Theoretical concentration-response curves in a tissue with an uptake process producing a 30-fold deficit of agonist at the receptor ($y = 30$). In the absence of an uptake inhibitor, observed potency is represented by the *heavy curve* marked uptake active. Increasing concentrations of uptake inhibitor ($[I]/K_I > 0$) produce shifts of the curve to the left until ultimately the heavy curve marked uptake blocked is obtained. As $[I]/K_I \to \infty$, the incremental magnitude of the sensitization becomes smaller. **B:** Sensitization of guinea pig trachea to norepinephrine produced by cocaine. Fractional relaxation (ordinate) in the absence, (•, $N = 16$) and presence of cocaine 1 μM (○, $N = 4$), 10 μM (△, $N = 4$), and 100 μM (□, $N = 16$). Abscissa: Logarithms of molar concentrations of norepinephrine; bars represent SEM. **C:** Effect of cocaine on tracheal responses to salbutamol, an agonist that is not a substrate for norepinephrine uptake, but activates norepinephrine receptors. All symbols as for B, except abscissa shows logarithms of molar concentrations of salbutamol. (B and C from ref. 22.)

for the uptake site (equilibrium dissociation constant $K_I$) and the receptor (equilibrium dissociation constant $K_{BI}$). The ratio of these binding constants will be denoted $\phi$, where $\phi = K_{BI}/K_I$. Under these circumstances, the uptake blocker will shift concentration-response curves to the left (sensitization) by uptake inhibition and concomitantly (depending on the magnitude of $\phi$) will shift curves to the right by receptor blockade. Experimentally, underestimation of the true magnitude of sensitization will be observed. Under these circumstances, the sensitization to the agonist is given by

$$x = \frac{y(1 + [I]/K_I)}{(y + [I]/K_I)(1 + [I]/K_I \cdot \phi)} \qquad [5.18]$$

It can be seen from Eq. 5.18 that if the inhibitor for the uptake process has appreciable blocking properties for the receptor ($\phi > 0$), then $x$ will not approach $y$ at any concentration of $I$, and maximal sensitization will not be achievable. Figure 5.20 shows the remarkable degree of selectivity ($\phi \geq 10^4$) required of an uptake blocker for complete sensitization to be observed. Under these circumstances, a control experiment that detects and quantifies any other properties of the uptake inhibitor such as receptor blockade should be carried out. One method to do this is to observe the effects of the uptake inhibitor on responses to an agonist not subject to uptake by the removal process; this can be used as a correction factor. The ramifications of this effect for receptor and drug classifications by agonist potency ratios will be discussed in Chapter 11.

### Estimation of $K_I$ for Uptake Inhibition

The $K_I$ for an uptake inhibitor obtained biochemically may have little relevance to the concentration required to inhibit the uptake process in a structured tissue. However, an *effective* $K_I$ for potentiation of agonist responses

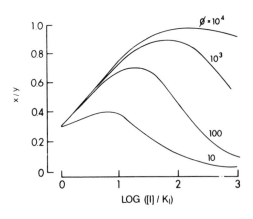

**FIG. 5.20.** Sensitization of tissues produced by uptake blockers with secondary receptor-blocking properties. Ordinate: Sensitization ($x$) as a fraction of maximal sensitization ($y$). Abscissa: Logarithms of molar concentrations of uptake blocker as multiples of $K_I$. Numbers next to curves refer to $\phi$, the relative affinity for uptake and receptor sites. For example, $\phi = 100$ means that $K_{BI}/K_I = 100$; the uptake blocker has 100 times the affinity for uptake sites as receptors. Under these conditions, only 68% of the maximal sensitization will be achievable with this uptake blocker. (From ref. 20.)

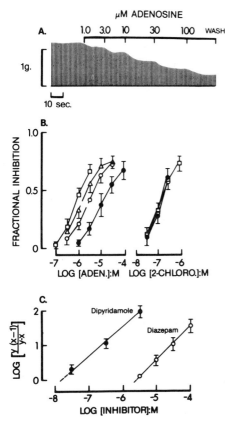

FIG. 5.21. Potentiation of adenosine-induced myocardial depression by adenosine-uptake blockers. **A:** Concentration-dependent depression of electrically stimulated twitch contraction of guinea pig left atria produced by adenosine. **B:** Concentration-response curves for adenosine and 2-chloroadenosine, an agonist for the same receptor that is not a substrate for the adenosine-uptake mechanism. Ordinate: Fractional depression of basal twitch tension. Abscissa: Logarithms of molar concentrations of adenosine or 2-chloroadenosine. Responses in the absence (•, $N = 6$) and presence of diazepam 10 μM (○, $N = 5$), 30 μM (△, $N = 4$), and 100 μM (□, $N = 5$). **C:** Regression according to Eq. 5.19 for calculation of $K_I$ for adenosine-uptake inhibitors. Data for diazepam (○, $N = 15$) and dipyridamole (•, $N = 8$). Bars represent standard errors. (From ref. 23.)

can be calculated from observed tissue sensitization to an agonist. Thus, Eq. 5.17 can be rearranged into a logarithmic form to yield the following equation:

$$\log\left[\frac{y(x - 1)}{y - x}\right] = \log[I] - \log K_I \qquad [5.19]$$

It can be seen from this equation that comparisons of various sensitizations ($x$) to an agonist obtained with various concentrations of $I$ can be related to the maximal sensitization ($y$) to yield a straight line with intercept $-\log K_I$. Figure 5.21A shows the agonist response in guinea pig atria to adenosine; in Fig. 5.21B it can be seen that these responses are potentiated by diazepam, an inhibitor of adenosine uptake in this tissue. For this method to be of value, the observed sensitization ($x$) must be corrected for other nonuptake-related effects of the uptake inhibitor (e.g., receptor blockade). In Fig. 5.21B it can be seen also that diazepam had no effects on the sensitivity of atria to 2-chloroadenosine, an adenosine-receptor agonist that is not removed by the uptake process. Therefore, no corrections for the adenosine-receptor effects were required. Figure 5.21C shows the regression for sensitization of guinea pig atria to adenosine produced by diazepam and another inhibitor of adenosine uptake, dipyridamole. These regressions indicate that irrespective of the biochemically derived $K_I$ for these blockers of adenosine uptake, in this tissue the effective $K_I$ for inactivation of adenosine is 2.5 μM for diazepam and 15.8 nM for dipyridamole.

### The Condition $[A_i] \nless K_I$ and Agonist Concentration Gradients

The previous discussion dealt with the situation in which $[A_i] \ll K_m$. If this condition is not met, then the slope of the concentration-response curve will depend on the magnitude of the concentration of agonist relative to the $K_m$ for uptake. This is evident from inspection of Eq. 5.5; Fig. 5.22A shows the effects of $V/S$ on the location and slope of concentration-response curves in a tissue with an agonist-removal process. In this figure it can be seen that as large ratios of $V/S$ produce large deficits of agonist in the receptor compartment, the necessarily large concentrations of agonist needed to overcome these deficits have differential effects on the slopes of the concentration-response curves. Figure 5.21B shows the correlation of slope with $V/S$, further illustrating the interrelationship of the magnitude of the effect of uptake and the slope of the concentration-response curve if the concentration of agonist is not considerably lower than the $K_m$ for uptake. Under these circumstances, potentiation of an agonist response becomes more difficult

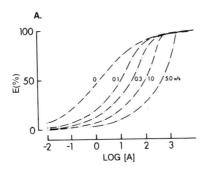

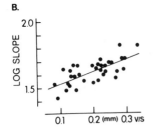

**FIG. 5.22.** Effects of tissue geometry and subsequent importance of uptake on slopes of concentration-response curves ($[A_o] \nless K_m$). **A:** Calculated concentration-response curves (parameters arbitrary) with increasing $V/S$ ratios (from Eq. 5.5). **B:** Experimentally observed slopes of concentration-response curves for norepinephrine in guinea pig papillary muscles of different $V/S$ ratios. (From ref. 6.)

to quantify in a uniform manner. Further complications arise when inhibition of the removal process alters the concentration gradient for an agonist in a tissue in which the response is limited by the quantity of muscle equilibrated with the agonist. Under these circumstances, Eq 5.17 cannot be used to predict sensitization to an agonist. Methods for calculation of the theoretical effects of muscle recruitment on drug responses require a number of assumptions about the avidity of uptake ($J_{max}$, $K_m$), the ease of diffusion ($\delta$, $\lambda$), and notably the fraction of muscle required for maximal response, and no general solution to this problem is applicable.

## AGONIST-INDUCED RELEASE OF ENDOGENOUS SUBSTANCES

The previous discussion was concerned with the effects of tissue removal mechanisms on drug responses. The opposite effect, namely, tissue-related augmentation of responses, can be equally obstructive to quantitative drug-receptor studies. The most common setting for this condition is agonist-induced release of endogenous agonist in a tissue, usually in the form of release of neuronal transmitter. Under these circumstances, the effects of the released substance could physiologically inhibit or augment the direct effects of the agonist; in either case, the true potency of the agonist will not be observed. The relationship between the concentration of direct agonist and the released substance (to be referred to as the *indirect* agonist) released by the direct agonist is dependent on the affinity of the direct agonist for the site of release and the size of the pool of indirect agonist from which release can occur. Assuming that an agonist [A] releases an indirect agonist [AI] from a pool $\theta$ (given arbitrary units of concentration), the fractional receptor occupancy ($\rho_{AI}$) for the response-producing entity (the indirect agonist AI) is given by

$$\rho_{AI} = \left[ 1 + \frac{K_{AI}}{\theta}\left( 1 + \frac{K_A}{[A]} \right) \right]^{-1} \qquad [5.20]$$

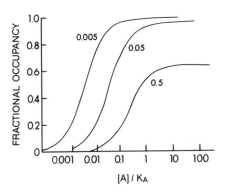

FIG. 5.23. Effects of an agonist that releases an endogenous (indirect) agonist in a tissue. Ordinate: Fractional receptor occupancy of the indirect agonist on receptors that subserve responses. Abscissa: Concentration of the releasing agent as a multiple of the equilibrium dissociation constant for the site of release (logarithmic scale). Effects of different effective values for the size of pool from which release takes place: $K_I/\theta = 0.005, 0.05$, and $0.5$. (Data from ref. 3.)

where $K_{AI}$ and $K_A$ are the equilibrium dissociation constants for the indirect agonist for the receptor and for the releasing agent $[A]$ for the site of release, respectively. It is evident from inspection of Eq. 5.20 that the magnitude of the maximal response depends on the relative values of $K_{AI}$ and $\theta$; i.e., if the pool is large (high $\theta$), receptor occupancy will be maximal, but if the pool is small or the affinity of the indirect agonist is low (high $K_{AI}$), full receptor occupancy may never be achieved (Fig. 5.23). The relative importance of the release of an indirect mechanism therefore depends on these two factors. Detection of this possibly misleading effect will be discussed in Chapter 9.

## ADSORPTION OF DRUGS TO SURFACES

A number of drugs bind to surfaces of vessels used in experiments (e.g., glass organ baths, glass filters in radioligand-binding experiments, storage vials; see also Chapter 4). Peptides are especially prone to adsorption to surfaces and where this occurs, serious differences in the assumed concentration of drug in the medium and the actual concentration can result. The adsorption of a drug to a binding site such as a surface can be approximated by the equations used to describe chemical antagonism. Thus, the collection of surface adsorption sites can be approximated by a "concentration" $[B]$ (with number of binding sites $n$) of chemical antagonist, which essentially removes a drug $[A]$ from the receptor compartment. Under these circumstances, the ratio between the drug-bound ($[A_{bound}]$) and total drug concentration ($[A_{total}]$) is:

$$\frac{[A_{bound}]}{[A_{total}]} = \left(1 + \frac{K_B'}{n \cdot [B]} + \frac{[A]}{n \cdot [B]}\right)^{-1} \qquad [5.21]$$

where $K_B'$ is the equilibrium dissociation constant of the adsorption site-drug complex. Figure 5.24 shows the effects of various amounts of adsorption on

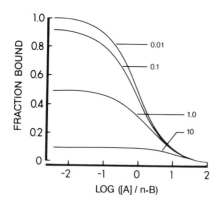

FIG. 5.24. Effects of binding of agonist $[A]$ to adsorption sites ($B$) on the fraction of agonist bound. Ordinate: Fraction of $[A]$ bound to the sites of adsorption. Abscissa: Logarithms of ratios $[A]$ to $B$. Numbers on curves represent values of $K_B' \cdot n$. Calculated from Eq. 5.21.

the fractional bound agonist as a function of the ratio of molar concentration of adsorption sites and agonist. This figure demonstrates the predicted effects of adsorption, namely, that when the agonist concentration is low and number of adsorption sites high, a great deal of agonist is bound, and little is free in solution; for a saturable binding process, high concentrations of agonist saturate the adsorption site binding and little effect on the free agonist concentration is observed. The actual free concentration of agonist $[A_{free}]$ for any total concentration $[A]$ and molar concentration of adsorption sites $[B]$ is:

$$[A_{free}] = \frac{K'_B}{2} \cdot \left\{ \left( \frac{[A]}{K'_B} - \frac{n \cdot [B]}{K'_B} - 1 \right) \right.$$

$$\left. + \left[ \left( 1 + \frac{n \cdot [B]}{K'_B} - \frac{[A]}{K'_B} \right)^2 + \frac{4[A]}{K'_B} \right]^{1/2} \right\} \qquad [5.22]$$

The fractional receptor occupancy of an agonist in the presence of a number of adsorption sites is given by:

$$\rho = \left( 1 + \frac{K_A \, (n \cdot [B] + K'_B + [A])}{[A] \cdot (K'_B + [A])} \right)^{-1} \qquad [5.23]$$

where $K_A$ is the equilibrium dissociation constant for the agonist-receptor complex. This equation predicts that, provided the binding is saturable, adsorption will always be surmountable. However, the relative agonist affinity for the receptor and the sites of adsorption will affect the behavior of agonist-occupancy dose-response curves in the presence of adsorption. Specifically, if the affinity of the agonist for the adsorption site is greater than that for the receptor $(K_A/K'_B > 1)$, then the concentration of agonist required to saturate the adsorption sites may be submaximal with respect to receptor binding. Under these circumstances, low doses of agonist will be affected more than

TABLE 5.1. Effects of surface pretreatments on adsorption of [³H]β-endorphin

| Filters presoaked in standard buffer[a] containing 0.1% of | cpm[b] |
|---|---|
| Lysine | 68,269 ± 2,639 |
| Arginine | 56,764 ± 710 |
| Bovine serum albumin | 42,563 ± 8,396 |
| Choline chloride | 2,142 ± 517 |
| Polylysine[c] | 192 ± 40 |
| Myelin basic protein | 172 ± 7 |

From ref. 7.
[a] Tris buffer (50 mM, pH 7.4) containing 0.01% Triton X-100.
[b] Counts per minute of radioactive [³H]β-endorphin.
[c] Molecular weight 15,000.

high doses, and a steepening of the dose-response curve may be observed (Fig. 5.25A). Alternatively, if the agonist affinity for the receptors is greater ($K_A/K_B' < 1$), parallel shifts in the dose-response curve will be observed (Fig. 5.25B).

Adsorption to surfaces can be a serious practical problem, both in functional and radioligand-binding experiments. There are methods to treat sur-

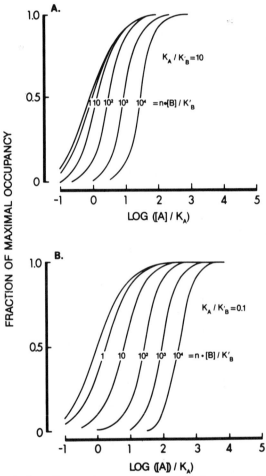

**FIG. 5.25.** Effects of adsorption on dose-response curves for an agonist. Ordinates: Agonist-receptor occupancy expressed as fractions of maximal occupancy. Abscissae: Logarithms of molar concentrations of agonist as multiples of $K_A$. Numbers on curves refer to values of $n \cdot [B]/K_B'$, where $[B]$ is the effective molar concentration of adsorption sites for agonist $[A]$, and $K_B'$ is the equilibrium dissociation constant of the agonist-adsorption site complex. **A:** Affinity of the agonist for the sites of adsorption is 10 times greater than the affinity for receptors. **B:** Affinity of agonist for adsorption sites is 0.1 times the affinity for receptors.

faces to reduce adsorption that can be useful. For example, radioactive β-endorphin is known to bind to the glass filters used for radioligand-binding experiments. However, as shown in Table 5.1, pretreatment of filters with a number of substances reduces this adsorption to as much as 0.000025% of that seen without treatment.

## CONCENTRATIONS OF DRUGS IN MEMBRANES

Some drugs are very lipid soluble and essentially concentrate into the lipid bilayer of plasma membranes. This can have two practical consequences to receptor classification by quantitative means where the knowledge of the concentration of drug in the receptor is a prerequisite. First, if the diffusion path of the drug to the receptor is via the lipid membrane (see Chapter 4), then the concentration of drug in the "receptor compartment" will most probably be severely underestimated if the aqueous phase concentration is used. Second, the drug in the lipid membrane can act as a depot for leaching into the aqueous phase. This latter effect is also discussed in Chapter 10 for alkylating drugs.

A common scale to determine possible lipid-membrane dissolution of drugs is to partition the drug into an octanol/buffer system and then to measure the

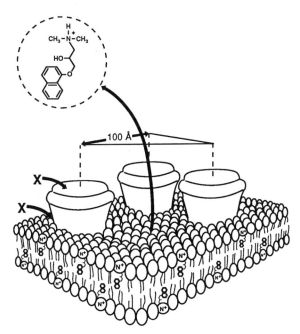

**FIG. 5.26.** The solvation of propranolol into the lipid membrane of cardiac sarcoplasmic reticulum. (From ref. 14.)

**TABLE 5.2.** *Partition coefficients*

| Drug[a] | Biological membranes | Octanol/buffer[b] |
|---|---|---|
| Bay P 8857 | 125,000 | 42 |
| Nisoldipine | 6,000 | 38 |
| Nimodipine | 5,000 | 730 |
| Propranolol | 200 | 18 |
| Acetylcholine | 32 | 0.003 |
| Timolol | 16 | 0.7 |
| Ethanol | 3 | 0.6 |

From ref. 15.

[a] Bay P 8857, nisoldipine, and nimodipine are dihydropyridine calcium antagonists; propranolol and timolol are β-adrenoceptor antagonists.

[b] 150 mM NaCl, 10 mM Tris/Cl, pH 7.2.

relative amounts in the aqueous and organic layer. This assumes that the behavior of an anisotropic substance such as a drug molecule will be identical in an isotropic bulk solvent system and a chemically anisotropic lipid bilayer. However, cell membranes are known to vary in their lipid content and makeup and may have several different domains (e.g., hydrophilic, hydrophobic, exofacial, and cytofacial leaflets) and these cannot effectively be approximated by bulk solvent systems. This is especially true of the region of the hydrocarbon core/water interface of the lipid bilayer. Also, some drugs are known to interact *selectively* with lipid membranes (see Chapter 4) and thus bind to certain regions within the bilayer. For example, Fig. 5.26 shows the binding of propranolol to the lipid membrane of cardiac sarcoplasmic reticulum. In this case, propranolol resides within a defined region and does not rotate and diffuse freely within the total lipid matrix.

The chemical differences between biological lipid membranes and bulk solvent systems make the latter unreliable predictors of drug concentrations in the membrane. For example, Table 5.2 shows the partition coefficients of some drugs in biological membranes and an octanol/buffer system. As can be seen from these data, membrane concentration does not correlate well with the bulk solvent. The concentration in the lipid bilayer can be calculated by expressing the amount of drug as a function of the total lipid content in the bilayer. This shows that striking concentration effects can be achieved by membrane dissolution. Table 5.3 shows the disparities between the aque-

**TABLE 5.3.** *Lipid/drug molar ratios*

| Drug | Aqueous concentration (mole) | Lipid/drug (mole/mole) | Membrane concentration (mole) |
|---|---|---|---|
| Bay P 8857 | $2.7 \times 10^{-8}$ | 330 | $2.8 \times 10^{-3}$ |
| Nisoldipine | $3.2 \times 10^{-8}$ | 4,300 | $2.2 \times 10^{-4}$ |
| Nimodipine | $1.5 \times 10^{-8}$ | 32,100 | $2.9 \times 10^{-5}$ |

From ref. 16.

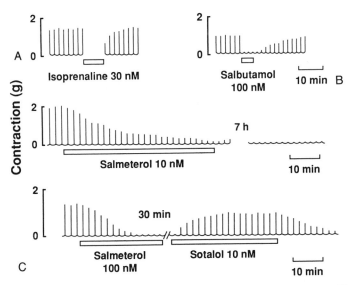

**FIG. 5.27.** Kinetics of onset and offset of salmeterol in guinea pig trachea. **A:** Electrically stimulated contractions of guinea pig superfused trachea; onset and offset of relaxation by β-adrenoceptor activation with isoprenaline. (From ref. 18.) **B:** Onset of relaxation by salbutamol. Tissue is perfused with *agonist-free* media for 7 hr with no reversal of relaxation. **C:** Reversal of salmeterol-induced β-adrenoceptor activation by the β-adrenoceptor antagonist sotalol. Upon removal of sotalol and with no further salmeterol added, the relaxation returns. (From ref. 1.)

ous and lipid concentrations of some drugs. If the path to the receptor is via the lipid bilayer, then these concentrations can have profound effects on receptor binding kinetics and steady states. In view of the selective binding of some drugs to confined regions of the lipid membrane, these could *still* be underestimations of the concentrations of drug brought into contact with the receptor.

The solvation of drugs in lipid membranes can be a source of loss from the aqueous receptor compartment or a sink for replenishment to the receptor compartment. Alternatively, drugs may anchor into a bilipid membrane in a particular orientation and be highly accessible to the receptor (see Chapter 4). Persistent binding of drugs can be quite dramatic as demonstrated by the extraordinary kinetics of the β-adrenoceptor antagonist salmeterol (1). A persistent *biological* effect can be shown for this agonist that is consistent with a nearly irreversible binding to a site near the receptor with diffusible access to the receptor. Figure 5.27 shows contractions of guinea pig electrically stimulated superfused trachea; this preparation is extraordinarily stable and demonstrates reproducible contractions for periods of 8 to 10 hr. Fast-acting β-adrenoceptor agonists such as salbutamol have an onset and offset of relaxant action on this preparation on the order of minutes (Fig. 5.27B).

In contrast, the long-acting $\beta_2$-adrenoceptor agonist salmeterol produces essentially irreversible relaxation of this preparation despite superfusion with agonist-free media for 7 hr (Fig. 5.27C). This long-lasting receptor activation is readily reversible by a competitive antagonist such as sotalol (Fig. 5.27C), but the intriguing finding is the *reestablishment* of receptor occupancy by salmeterol upon removal of the antagonist (Fig. 5.27C). This suggests that salmeterol is fixed in location near the receptor and can access the receptor from a sink or an anchor in the tissue. Such effects can be useful clinically for a long duration of action (1,18).

## CONCENTRATION AS A DETERMINANT OF SELECTIVITY *IN VIVO*

Clearly the concentration of drug in the receptor compartment is more subject to the effects of restricted diffusion and various degradation, uptake, and removal mechanisms in the whole organism than *in vitro*. In view of this, assumptions must be made as to the correspondence between the concentrations entering the access system to the relevant organ and the concentrations presented to the receptor after distribution and degradation. These necessary assumptions are a caveat to the application of *in vivo* data to molecular mechanisms at the receptor level. The quantification of agonism often involves the attempted measurement of simultaneous organ effects in the same body to determine agonist selectivity *in vivo*. Clearly, the receptor compartment concentrations of agonist may differ because of differences in diffusion access to the organ and rate of removal out of the receptor compartment. Under these circumstances, the kinetics of agonist response in two organs may depend more on the kinetics of agonist delivery in the respective receptor compartments and less on agonist selectivity.

The first-order kinetic models for drug concentration in the receptor compartment used for isolated tissues may be used as an approximation *in vivo*. Thus a steady-state infusion of drug into an *in vivo* system approximates the "infinite" pool of agonist in the organ bath and the receptor-compartment concentration depends on the relative rate of entry of drug into the organ perfusion system (and the potential obstacles to free diffusion) and the relative rate of removal (i.e., degradation, excretion). Assuming a common central pool of agonist (i.e., plasma steady-state concentration) and identical rates of diffusion and removal in all organs, the relative potency of agonists would not be influenced by kinetics because a constant error in potency for each agonist would be produced. However, if the rate of diffusion into and out of the receptor compartments for various organs were *not* constant for different agonists, then apparent selectivity might be observed, which does not depend on affinity or intrinsic efficacy. The potential problems with this type of selectivity is that the complex mechanisms that produce organ selective differences in agonist concentration may not be expected to be constant across animal test systems and humans.

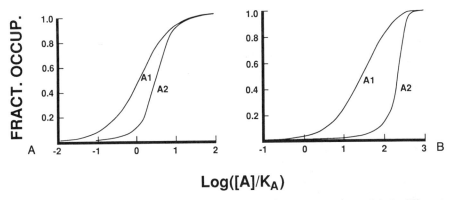

**Log([A]/$K_A$)**

**FIG. 5.28.** The effect of removal processes on the relative potency of agonists in different organs of the same *in vivo* system. The relative potency of an agonist relatively resistant to ($K_m$ for A1 = 10) and sensitive to ($K_m$ for A2 = 0.3) an agonist removal mechanism. Ordinates: Fractional receptor occupancy. Abscissae: Logarithms of molar concentrations of agonist expressed as fractions of the equilibrium dissociation constant of the agonist receptor complex. **A:** Relative potency in tissue I with relatively uninhibited access into the receptor compartment ($J_{max}/k_{in}$ = 30, V/S = 0.1). Potency ratio A1/A2 = 2.5. **B:** Relative potency in tissue II with restricted diffusion ($J_{max}/k_{in}$ = 30, V/S = 10). Potency ratio A1/A2 = 8. (From ref. 25.)

Figure 5.28 shows the relative potencies of two agonists A1 and A2 in the *same in vivo* system with the same central compartment doses of agonist as calculated with Eq. 5.5. One agonist is more sensitive to a removal process than the other (i.e., $K_m$ for A1 = 10, $K_m$ for A2 = 0.3) and tissue I has a relatively weak removal system due to uninhibited diffusion into the receptor compartment. Given these conditions the relative potency of A1/A2 is 2.5 (Fig. 5.28A). In contrast tissue II has a substantial barrier to diffusion into the receptor compartment but the same removal process. Under these circumstances the relative potency of A1/A2 = 8 (Fig. 5.28B). From these data it would appear that A2 was 3.2 times more selective for tissue I than for tissue II. The important feature of these data is the fact that the apparent selectivity stems not from ligand-receptor-related properties but rather from V/S ratios of the two organs (see Eq. 5.5). If this selectivity is observed in an animal test system, which is presumed to predict like selectivity in humans, then a costly dissimulation could occur if the same differences in V/S are not operable in humans.

## REFERENCES

1. Ball, D. I., Brittain, R. T., Coleman, R. A., Denyer, L. H., Jack, D., Johnson, M., Lunts, L. H. C., Nials, A. T., Sheldrick, K. E., and Skidmore, I. F. (1991): Salmeterol, a novel, long-acting β2-adrenoceptor agonist: Characterization of pharmacological activity in vitro and in vivo. *Br. J. Pharmacol.*, 104:665–671.

2. Black, J. W. (1976): Histamine receptors. In: *Receptors and Cellular Pharmacology, Vol. 1,* edited by E. Klüge, pp. 3–16. Pergamon Press, Oxford.
3. Black, J. W., Jenkinson, D. H., and Kenakin, T. P. (1981): Antagonism of an indirectly acting agonist: Block by propranolol and sotalol of the action of tyramine on rat heart. *Eur. J. Pharmacol.,* 65:1–10.
4. Chin, J. H., and Goldstein, D. B. (1981): Membrane-disordering action of ethanol: Variation with membrane cholesterol content and depth of the spin label probe. *Mol. Pharmacol.,* 19: 425–431.
5. Ebner, F. (1981): The positive inotropic effect of ( − )-noradrenaline and ( ± )-isoprenaline after chemical sympathectomy: Evidence in favour of differences at a postsynaptic site. *Naunyn Schmeidebergs Arch. Pharmacol.,* 316:8–18.
6. Ebner, F., and Waud, D. R. (1978): The role of uptake of noradrenaline for its positive inotropic effect in relation to muscle geometry. *Naunyn Schmeidebergs Arch. Pharmacol.,* 303:1–6.
7. Ferrar, P., and Li, C. H. (1980): β-Endorphin: Radioreceptor binding assay. *Int. J. Peptide Protein Res.,* 16:66–69.
8. Foster, R. W. (1967): The potentiation of responses to noradrenaline and isoprenaline in guinea pig isolated tracheal chain preparation by desipramine, cocaine, phentolamine, phenoxybenzamine, guanethidine, metanephrine and cooling. *Br. J. Pharmacol. Chemother.,* 31:418–427.
9. Furchgott, R. F. (1972): The classification of adrenoceptors (adrenergic receptors). An evaluation from the standpoint of receptor theory. In: *Handbook of Experimental Pharmacology, Catecholamines, Vol. 33,* edited by H. Blaschko and E. Muscholl, pp. 283–335. Springer-Verlag, New York.
10. Goldstein, A. (1949): The interactions of drugs and plasma proteins. *Pharmacol. Rev.,* 1: 102–165.
11. Green, A. L. (1976): The kinetics of enzyme action and inhibition in intact tissues and tissue slices, with special reference to cholinesterase. *J. Pharm. Pharmacol.,* 28:265–274.
12. Green, A. L., Lord, J. A. H., and Marshall, I. G. (1978): The relationship between cholinesterase inhibition in the chick biventer cervicis muscle and its sensitivity to exogenous acetylcholine. *J. Pharm. Pharmacol.,* 30:426–431.
13. Guimaraes, S., Azevedo, I., Cardoso, W., and Oliveira, M. C. (1975): Relation between the amount of smooth muscle of venous tissue and the degree of supersensitivity to isoprenaline caused by inhibition of catechol-*O*-methyl transferase. *Naunyn Schmeidebergs Arch. Pharmacol.,* 286:401–412.
14. Herbette, L., Katz, A. M., and Sturtevant, J. M. (1983): Comparisons of the interaction of propranolol and timolol with model and biological membrane systems. *Mol. Pharmacol.,* 24:259–269.
15. Herbette, L., Chester, D. W., and Rhodes, D. G. (1986): Structure analysis of drug molecules in biological membranes. *Biophys. J.,* 49:91–94.
16. Herbette, L., Vant Erve, Y. M. H., and Rhodes, D. G. (1989): Interaction of 1,4 dihydropyridine calcium channel antagonists with biological membranes: Lipid bilayer partitioning could occur before drug binding to receptors. *J. Mol. Cell. Cardiol.,* 21:187–201.
17. Homan, R., and Pownall, H. J. (1988): Transbilayer diffusion of phospholipids: Dependence on headgroup structure and acyl chain length. *Biochim. Biophys. Acta,* 938:155–166.
18. Jack, D. (1991): A way of looking at agonism and antagonism: Lessons from salbutamol, salmeterol, and other β-adrenoceptor agonists. *Br. J. Clin. Pharmacol.,* 31:501–514.
19. Kalsner, S. (1976): Sensitization of effector responses by modification of agonist disposition mechanisms. *Can. J. Physiol. Pharmacol.,* 54:177–187.
20. Kenakin, T. P. (1980): Errors in the measurement of agonist potency-ratios produced by uptake processes: A general model applied to β-adrenoceptor agonists. *Br. J. Pharmacol.,* 71:407–417.
21. Kenakin, T. P. (1980): On the importance of agonist concentration-gradients within isolated tissues. Increased maximal responses of rat vasa deferentia to ( − )-noradrenaline after blockade of neuronal uptake. *J. Pharm. Pharmacol.,* 32:833–838.
22. Kenakin, T. P. (1981): A pharmacological method to estimate the $pK_f$ of competitive inhibitors of agonist uptake processes in isolated tissues. *Naunyn Schmeidebergs Arch. Pharmacol.,* 316:89–95.

23. Kenakin, T. P. (1982): The potentiation of cardiac responses to adenosine by benzodiazepines. *J. Pharmacol. Exp. Ther.*, 222:752–758.

24. Kenakin, T. P. (1986): Tissue and receptor selectivity: similarities and differences. In: *Advances in Drug Research, Vol. 15*, edited by B. Testa, pp. 71–109. Academic Press, New York.

25. Kenakin, T. P. (1992): The study of drug-receptor interaction in in vivo systems. In: *The In Vivo Study of Drug Action*, edited by C. J. van Boxtel, N. H. G. Holford, and M. Danhof, pp. 1–15. Elsevier Science, Amsterdam.

26. Kenakin, T. P., and Beek, D. (1981): The measurement of antagonists potency and the importance of selective inhibition of agonist processes. *J. Pharmacol. Exp. Ther.*, 219: 112–120.

27. Kenakin, T. P., and Leighton, H. J. (1984): Pharmacological estimation of potencies of agonists and antagonists in the classification of adenosine receptors. In: *Methods in Pharmacology. Methods Used in Adenosine Research, Vol. 6*, edited by D. M. Paton, pp. 213–237. Plenum, New York.

28 Leighton, H. J. (1982): Quantitative assessment of the pre- and postsynaptic alpha-adrenoceptor antagonist potency of amitriptylene. *J. Pharmacol. Exp. Ther.*, 220:299–304.

29. Pascual, R., and Bevan, J. A. (1980): Asymmetry of consequences of drug disposition mechanisms in the wall of the rabbit aorta. *Circ. Res.*, 46:22–28.

30. Satchell, D. (1984): Purine receptors in trachea: Studies with adenosine deaminase and dipyridamole. *Eur. J. Pharmacol.*, 102:545–548.

31. Smithson, K. W., Millar, D. B., Jacobs, L. R., and Gray, G. M. (1981): Intestinal diffusion barrier: Unstirred water layer or membrane surface mucous coat? *Science*, 214:1241–1244.

32. Trendelenburg, U. (1968): The effect of cocaine on the pacemaker of isolated guinea pig atria. *J. Pharmacol. Exp. Ther.*, 161:222–231.

33. Trendelenburg, U. (1972): Supersensitivity in peripheral organs. In: *Receptors for Neurotransmitters and Peptide Hormones, Vol. 21*, edited by G. Pepeu, M. J. Kuhar, and S. J. Enna, pp. 99–105. Raven Press, New York.

34. Verity, M. A. (1971): Morphologic studies of vascular neuroeffector apparatus. In: *Physiology and Pharmacology of Vascular Neuroeffector Systems*, edited by J. A. Bavan, R. F. Furchgott, R. A. Maxwell, A. P. Somlyo, pp. 2–12. Karger, Basel.

35. Waud, D. R. (1969): A quantitative model for the effect of a saturable uptake on the slope of the dose-response curve. *J. Pharmacol. Exp. Ther.*, 167:140–141.

36. Wilson, F. A., and Dietschy, J. M. (1974): The intestinal unstirred layer: Its surface area and effect on active transport kinetics. *Biochim. Biophys. Acta*, 363:112–126.

# 6

## Analysis of Dose-Response Data

*If your experiment needs statistics, you ought to have done a better experiment.*
—LORD ERNEST RUTHERFORD, 1871–1937

*There are three kinds of lies: lies, damned lies, and statistics.*
—MARK TWAIN, 1835–1910

The views expressed in the quotations at the beginning of this chapter are extreme in that they presuppose that statistics *obscure* the obvious. It is true that statistics, if allowed to do so, can have nearly magical effects on the conclusions drawn from experiments; the power of the statement of probability less than or equal to an arbitrary figure can be overemphasized. However, statistical procedures also can function as a powerful equalizer in terms of reducing (or even eliminating) bias and introducing uniform criteria for studying differences that cannot easily be assessed by the investigator. The test of possible validity of hypotheses by statistical procedures can be tested by organized methods. In pharmacologic studies of drugs and drug receptors, such (unbiased) methods are essential; as stated by Bertrand Russell in 1935, "it is undesirable to believe a proposition when there is no grounds whatever for supposing it true." Statistics can provide an extremely useful tool for pharmacologists interested in drug and drug-receptor classification provided that two prerequisites are met: The tools must be used within the limits of their validity, and the limitations of the conclusions must be recognized.

To a large extent, statistics are concerned with the study of error. There are two types of errors: those lacking in accuracy (systematic errors) and those lacking in precision (random errors). Statistics can be helpful in dealing with random errors. In pharmacologic experiments designed to quantify drug effects, the two general problems are estimation of a true value by imprecise methods and measurement of a variable value with accurate methods. Two ways of dealing with the variability observed are to reduce it and to analyze it statistically.

In general, statistics deal with measurements of central tendencies and variabilities and the use of these to quantify the probability of real differences. The general problem is one of prediction of the scatter of some function predicted by calculation with observations using the internal evidence of a limited number of experiments. A hypothesis is formed (on the basis of evidence and perhaps a little imagination), and the consequences are deduced and tested experimentally. Evaluation of the data is centered on the null hypothesis, which assumes that differences between groups are attributable entirely to random variation. It should be noted, however, that statistical methods never prove anything, but only quantify a probability of obtaining a given result by random chance. The interpretation of the meaning of this probability is left to the experimenter. For instance, statistics can be used to calculate the probability that two groups of data are different to a level of confidence of 95% (i.e., there is a 5% chance that the groups are not different and that the observed difference still arose by random chance). Therefore, the certainty of conclusions reached by the experimenter must always be tempered with the knowledge that a given probability exists that the conclusions could be false; i.e., there is a 5% chance that the conclusions reached by the experimenter are false. As put succinctly by Finney (8) "the experimenter can assert conclusions about the treatments tested only insofar as he is prepared to take the responsibility for asserting that the bias is nonexistent or trivial."

## EXPERIMENTAL DESIGN

A major determinant of the cost, with respect to effort and resources, of an experiment, the ability of the experiment to effectively address a hypothesis, and the type of statistics to be utilized in data analysis is the experimental design. In general, a design determines the selection of treatments, the units of measurement, and the rules by which the treatments are allocated; a proper experimental design can greatly increase the accuracy-versus-effort ratio. Proper randomization is a key factor in experimental design. If the findings from a limited sample are to be applicable to the general population, care must be taken that the sample be as representative of the population as possible. For example, it would be hazardous to quantify agonist potency on atria from genetically myopathic hamsters and expect the values to be representative of all hamsters; a genetic bias would be introduced into the experiment. More subtle bias can be introduced if factors such as animal age, weight, and strain are ignored. Many such factors can be neutralized with minimal effort.

It is important that treatment groups be as homogeneous as possible. Strict randomization of treatment groups for small samples may lead to nonhomogeneous groups, in which case stratification of groups may be necessary. For example, if atrial sensitivity to agonists is to be quantified in a sample of rats and random selection of six of the rats happens to produce a sample of the six most obese and inactive animals of the population, it may be necessary to choose two lean and active animals to balance the sample. Clearly, stratification and randomization are dichotomous principles, and too much stratification would introduce bias into the experiment. The criteria for selection of subjects must be rigidly defined, with the understanding that the more rigid the criteria, the less generally applicable may be the findings.

Pharmacologic experiments concerned with tissue response are time dependent; that is, response is a function of agonist concentration *and* time. This can be more important for some types of preparations than for others; i.e., some preparations are extraordinarily stable and provide constant responses for given doses of agonist over long periods of time, whereas other tissues demand stringent preequilibration periods and have relatively short "stability windows" thereafter. The concept of a control response (i.e., tissue sensitivity in the absence of a given intervention) in pharmacologic studies is very important. If the effects of a given intervention are to be determined effectively, the predicted tissue sensitivity in the absence of the intervention must be known.

One approach to this problem allows a tissue to function as its own control, in that the sensitivity to an agonist can be measured more than once. In the absence of an intervention, the estimates of sensitivity should not be significantly different (see Fig. 3.22). If multiple assays are carried out concomitantly, one may be used to monitor random or systematic changes in tissue sensitivity. In the ideal situation, corrections to assays based on the control assay are not required (i.e., the assays are suitably rapid, and the tissues adequately stable). Often this does not occur, and "corrections" to experimental assays are applied in accordance with changes observed in the control tissues. For example, if two agonists are being compared in one tissue and the control tissue indicates that a twofold loss of sensitivity has occurred between the testing of the first agonist and second agonist, the potency of the second agonist can be assumed to be twice that observed. The reasoning for this adjustment is that a systematic error diminishes the tissue sensitivity by a factor of two during the course of the experiment. This procedure depends on the assumption that the changes in sensitivity in a series of isolated tissues occur at the same rate; this is an assumption for which there is no theoretical basis. For example, assume that a tissue suffers a gradual loss of sensitivity to an agonist because of inadequate delivery of nutrients to muscle cells; assume also that cell death follows a simple exponential function according to $P_{cell} = e^{-kt}$, where $P_{cell}$ is the percentage of muscle cells left viable, $k$ is a time constant for cell loss, and $t$ is time. It would be expected that because $k$ depends on nutrient and oxygen delivery versus demand, the rate constants for cell loss could differ considerably between tissues. Figure 6.1A shows the time courses of cell loss in two tissues with different rate

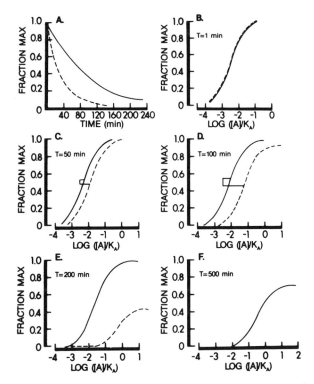

**FIG. 6.1.** Comparison of potencies of an agonist in two tissues with different rates of degeneration. **A:** Time course for cell loss assuming a simple exponential function of cell death. Fraction max = $e^{-kt}$. Abscissa: Time in minutes. *Solid line, k* = 0.01 sec$^{-1}$; *broken line, k* = 0.03 sec$^{-1}$. **B–F:** Sensitivities of the two tissues to an agonist, assuming response = stimulus/(stimulus + 0.003) and stimulus = $[R_t](1 + K_A/[A])^{-1}$. The graphs depict the responses in the two tissues, with $[R_t]$ corresponding to the changes determined in A. It can be seen that by 500 min, one tissue fails to respond to the agonist, whereas the other is capable of producing 70% of the control response.

constants $k$ for cell death; Fig. 6.1B–F show the sensitivities of the tissues to a given agonist assuming cell viability according to the relationships shown in part A. It can be seen that the rates of loss of sensitivity to the agonist in the two tissues are quite different and that correction for this to either tissue according to changes observed in the other would be meaningless. This problem could arise even if the control tissue showed no change in sensitivity; it still would not be clear whether or not the experimental tissues experienced a change in sensitivity.

Wherever possible, a crossover design should be applied to this problem. In this type of experiment, the tissue sensitivity is tested with the same agonist on the same tissue. Thus, if two agonists, $A$ and $B$, were to be compared in a given tissue, a sequential assay of potency for $A$, then $B$, and then a repeat for $A$, in which no change in tissue sensitivity to $A$ occurred over the time course of the experiment, would indicate no significant systematic error. A more satisfactory approach to comparing the potencies of two agonists in one tissue with a crossover design is by randomized dosing according to a Latin square ($2 \times 2$, $3 \times 3$, or $k \times n$ assays).

In general, a Latin square can be used to balance experimental factors (order of treatment, etc.) such that they do not influence the outcome of the experiment. For example, assume four treatments ($A$ to $D$) to be tested in four organ baths (1 to 4) on 4 consecutive days (I to IV); the following order could be constructed:

| | Day | | | |
|---|---|---|---|---|
| Bath | I | II | III | IV |
| 1 | $A$ | $B$ | $C$ | $D$ |
| 2 | $D$ | $A$ | $B$ | $C$ |
| 3 | $C$ | $D$ | $A$ | $B$ |
| 4 | $B$ | $C$ | $D$ | $A$ |

Each successive row has been rotated one treatment. Now, random ordering of rows and columns (i.e., columns to 4231 and then rows to 1423) leads to the following Latin square:

| | Day | | | |
|---|---|---|---|---|
| Bath | I | II | III | IV |
| 1 | $D$ | $B$ | $C$ | $A$ |
| 2 | $A$ | $C$ | $D$ | $B$ |
| 3 | $C$ | $A$ | $B$ | $D$ |
| 4 | $B$ | $D$ | $A$ | $C$ |

Note that each treatment is carried out in each organ bath and on each day.

There are situations in which such randomized assays are not practical (e.g., the time course for response is too long), but if responses to separate doses can be obtained conveniently, a randomized order of administration will be optimum. These assays as used for the measurement of agonist potency ratios are discussed specifically in Chapter 11. Another factor is the choice of the control tissue to be used for quantification of temporal changes (changes due to the time course of the experiment). If many preparations from one tissue can be obtained (e.g., a series of rings from one blood vessel), the choice of control should be randomized. Often tissues come in pairs (e.g., vasa deferentia, anococcygeus muscles), in which case one can be used for the experiment and one to control for temporal changes.

There are cases in which a crossover design is not practicable and treated tissues must be compared with untreated tissues (as opposed to a treated tissue being compared with itself before the treatment). The variability in such experiments is increased, but because this variability usually is random, proper statistical procedures can be helpful in data analysis. In these cases, a randomized block design (i.e., Latin square) is essential.

Clearly, accuracy can be increased by replication, but the advantage of doing large numbers of experiments to attain accuracy should be weighed against the cost and effort involved. It should be noted that the error of the mean is proportional to the square root of the number of measurements. For example, to reduce the error inherent in nine experiments by a factor of two, *36* (not 18) experiments must be done. There quickly comes a point at which replication attempts to reduce error are futile. A benefit of a balanced experimental design (i.e., $n_1 = n_2$) is that the multiplicative factor $(1/n_1 + 1/n_2)$ for the variance is minimum when $n_1 = n_2$.

Once a properly randomized experimental design has been implemented (with strict prior criteria for choice of subjects, treatments, and order), the data must be analyzed without bias, and the confidence level of a conclusion quantified. The following statistical procedures are helpful in this process.

## MEASURES OF CENTRAL TENDENCY AND VARIABILITY

Two important concepts in science are central tendency and variability; that is, What is the most representative estimate of a value, and what is the variability (error) inherent in the measurement? This latter value dictates the confidence with which we can consider the measurement of central tendency to be a true representative of the population mean. There are three general types of estimates of central tendency: the median (the statistic that divides the sample into two equally sized groups), the mode (the most commonly occurring value), and the mean (the sum of values divided by the number of values). The most widely used value in drug-receptor studies is the mean. A frequently used estimate of the variation of a mean is the standard error (SE). This is calculated by

$$\text{SE}(x) = \left[ \frac{n\sum x^2 - (\sum x)^2}{n^2(n-1)} \right]^{1/2} \qquad [6.1]$$

The standard error can be used to predict a confidence limit for a given mean; the statistic used in this procedure is $t$. The statistic $t$ is the difference between a normally distributed variable and the population mean divided by the standard deviation of the variable from a sample. Devised by Gosset (who published under the pseudonym of Student), the distribution of $t$ is most useful in predicting the frequency of small samples. Values of $t$ for a given level of confidence (e.g., 95% or 99%) can be found in tables (Appendix 1) for given degrees of freedom (calculated $n - 1$); the confidence limits are calculated as $\pm t \cdot \text{SE}(x)$. For example, if a sample mean is calculated to be

7.1, with a standard error of 0.8 for eight samples, the 95% confidence limits of this mean will be $t_{0.05} \times 0.8$, where $t_{0.05}$ is the value of $t$ at $p < 0.05$ for $(n - 1) = 7$ degrees of freedom. The value of $t$ is 2.365 (Appendix); therefore, the 95% confidence limits are $\pm 2.365 \times 0.8 = \pm 1.892$. Thus, the true mean will be expected to fall between the values 5.208 and 8.992 95% of the time. If a greater degree of confidence is desired, the 99% confidence limits can be calculated. Under these circumstances, $t_{0.01} = 3.499$. Therefore, the mean will lie between the values 4.3 and 9.899 99% of the time.

### Difference Between Two Sample Means

The statistic $t$ can be used to quantify possible differences between sample means. For example, for two samples means ($\bar{x}_1$ and $\bar{x}_2$), $t$ can be calculated as

$$t = \frac{\bar{x}_1 - \bar{x}_2}{s_p(1/n_1 + 1/n_2)} \qquad [6.2]$$

where $s_p$ is the square root of the pooled variance calculated as

$$s_p^{2} = \frac{\sum x_1^2 + \sum x_2^2 - \dfrac{\left(\sum x_1\right)^2}{n_1} - \dfrac{\left(\sum x_2\right)^2}{n_2}}{n_1 + n_2 - 2} \qquad [6.3]$$

Therefore, if a calculated value of $t$ is greater than the expected probability for a given level of confidence (for $n_1 + n_2 - 2$ degrees of freedom), then that level of confidence can be applied to the conclusion that the two sample means are different and come from two separate populations. An example of this calculation is shown in Table 6.1. The potency of nifedipine as a calcium channel blocker has been measured in two tissues, guinea pig ileum and canine coronary artery. A $t$-test can be used to determine the degree of confidence that the two mean estimates of potency are different; in this example, the potency of nifedipine is significantly greater in guinea pig ileum ($p < 0.05$). The standard error of the difference between means is given by

$$\text{SE (difference)} = [s_p^{2}(1/n_1 + 1/n_2)]^{1/2} \qquad [6.4]$$

In some cases, data can be paired; that is, there is reason to associate values. For example, if the effect of a drug that increases heart rate is to be tested, the rates for each individual heart before and after exposure to the drug can be measured; in this case, the difference in rates for each given heart before ($x$) and after ($x'$) the drug is relevant [$d$, where $d = (x - x')^2$]. Under these circumstances, the possible significance of the intervention can be calculated as

$$t = \frac{\left(\sum d\right)\left(n^{1/2}\right)}{n \cdot s_d}, \qquad \text{d.f.} = n - 1 \qquad [6.5]$$

**TABLE 6.1.** Potency[a] of nifedipine as a calcium blocker in guinea pig ileum and canine coronary artery

| Guinea pig ileum | Canine coronary artery |
|---|---|
| 8.5 | 8.35 |
| 8.3 | 8.2 |
| 8.7 | 7.95 |
| 8.4 | 8.1 |
| 8.6 | 8.3 |
| $\bar{x}_1 = 8.5$ | $\bar{x}_2 = 8.2$ |
| $SE(x_1) = 0.16$ | $SE(x_2) = 0.16$ |
| $\sum x_1 = 42.5$ | $\sum x_2 = 40.9$ |
| $\sum x_1^2 = 361.35$ | $\sum x_2^2 = 334.66$ |

$$s_p^2 = 0.02475$$
$$\text{difference} = \bar{x}_1 - \bar{x}_2 = 8.5 - 8.2 = 0.3$$
$$SE\ (\text{difference}) = [s_p^2\ (1/n_1 + 1/n_2)]^{1/2} = 0.10$$
$$\text{difference} = 0.3 \pm 0.1$$
$$t = 3.02, \qquad p < 0.0025$$

[a] Log molar concentration of nifedipine producing half-maximal response.
Data from ref. 12.

**TABLE 6.2.** Electrically stimulated force of contraction of guinea pig atria before and after lorazepam

| Control | Lorazepam (100 μM) | $d$ |
|---|---|---|
| 0.8 | 0.68 | 0.12 |
| 0.6 | 0.50 | 0.1 |
| 0.7 | 0.45 | 0.25 |
| 0.9 | 0.80 | 0.1 |
| 0.8 | 0.6 | 0.2 |
| $\bar{x} = 0.76 \pm 0.1$ g | $0.6 \pm 0.12$ g | |
| | | $\sum d = 0.77$ |
| | | $\sum d^2 = 0.1369$ |
| | | $n = 5$ |

$s_d = 0.0677$

$t = 5.09, \qquad p < 0.01$

Data from ref. 11.

where

$$s_d = \left[ \frac{n\sum d^2 - \left(\sum d\right)^2}{n(n-1)} \right]^{1/2}$$ [6.6]

An example of this calculation is shown in Table 6.2. These data describe the effects of the benzodiazepine lorazepam on the basal electrically stimulated force of contraction in guinea pig left atria. In general, a depression of inotropy of $0.16 \pm 0.08$ g was observed; a nonpaired $t$ test shows this not to be significant at the $p < 0.05$ level. However, there is an additional consideration in the fact that inotropy values for each atrium before and after lorazepam are known, and each atrium treated with the drug showed a decrease in inotropy. Under these circumstances, a paired $t$ test with each atrium serving as its own control should be done. This analysis shows the effect of lorazepam to be highly significant (Table 6.2).

## Differences Between More Than Two Means: One-Way Analysis of Variance

To estimate possible differences between a series of means, an analysis of variance can be done. This procedure considers the problem of whether, in a set of three or more samples, there are means that differ. For example, Table 6.3 shows the resting heart rates for three samples, three anesthetized

**TABLE 6.3.** *Basal heart rates in anesthetized cats*

| | Control | Phentolamine | Propranolol |
|---|---|---|---|
| | 203 | 180 | 160 |
| | 178 | 155 | 142 |
| | 147 | 139 | 148 |
| | 162 | 135 | 156 |
| | 190 | 165 | 172 |
| $\sum x$ | 880 | 674 | 778 |
| $n$ | 5 | 5 | 5 |
| $\sum x^2$ | 156,846 | 103,396 | 121,588 |

$$\sum\left(\sum x\right) = 880 + 674 + 778 = 2{,}332$$

$$\sum\left[\left(\sum x\right)^2 \Big/ n\right] = (880)^2/5 + (674)^2/5 + (778)^2/5 = 366{,}792$$

$$\sum\left(\sum x^2\right) = 156{,}846 + 103{,}396 + 121{,}588 = 381{,}830$$

Data from ref. 13.

**TABLE 6.4.**

| | Sum of squares | d.f.[a] | Mean of squares | Variance ratio |
|---|---|---|---|---|
| A. Calculations for one-way analysis of variance | | | | |
| Between groups | $\Sigma \dfrac{\left(\Sigma x_a\right)^2}{n_a} - \dfrac{\left[\Sigma\left(\Sigma x\right)\right]^2}{\Sigma n}$ | $a - 1$ | $s_c^2$ | |
| | | | | $s_c^2/s^2$ |
| Within groups | Subtraction | $N - a$ | $s^2$ | |
| Total | $\Sigma\left(\Sigma x^2\right) - \dfrac{\left[\Sigma\left(\Sigma x\right)\right]^2}{\Sigma n}$ | $N - 1$ | | |
| B. Calculations for data in Table 6.3 | | | | |
| Between groups | 4,243.7 | 2 | 2,121.8 | 1.69 |
| Within groups | 15,038 | 12 | 1,253.17 | |
| Total | 19,281.7 | 14 | | |

[a] $a$ = number of groups; $N$ = total number of values; $F$ = 1.69 (n.s.).

cats, each pretreated with a different drug. The aim of the experiment is to test the potencies of certain drugs on each of the samples and assess the significance of the pretreatments; it is important that the pretreatments produce no significant differences in the resting basal heart rates of the cats, as this could affect the subsequent measurements. Therefore, the question is asked: Do the mean basal heart rates for the three groups of cats differ? An analysis of variance can be used in this situation. The calculations for a one-way analysis of variance are shown in Table 6.4A. The relevant statistic is the variance ratio, denoted $F$, which can be calculated and compared to values in tables for various levels of significance. The calculations for the data in Table 6.3 are shown in Table 6.4B. In this instance, the variance ratio is 1.69; a comparison with tables of values for $F$ indicates that for the prescribed degrees of freedom (2, 12), this value is less than that for $p < 0.05$. Therefore, there is less than a 5% probability that this value of $F$ could arise by chance. This can be interpreted to mean that there is a 95% probability that the sample means in Table 6.3 are from the same population (they are not different).

A valuable calculation is the standard error for the difference between two of the groups; the mean square for each mean is calculated for this purpose:

$$s_i^2 = \frac{n\left(\sum x^2\right) - \left(\sum x\right)^2}{n(n-1)} \qquad [6.7]$$

Therefore, the difference between two sample means, $\bar{x}_1$ and $\bar{x}_2$, is $d = |\,x_1 - \bar{x}_2\,| \pm SE(d)$, where this standard error is

$$SE(d) = \left(\frac{s_{i1}^2}{n_1} + \frac{s_{i2}^2}{n_2}\right)^{1/2} \qquad [6.8]$$

For example, the data in Table 6.3 show the mean heart rate for untreated cats to be 176 bpm and that for propranolol-treated cats to be 155.6 bpm. The difference between these groups is $20.4 \pm 11.2$ bpm.

### Two-Way Analysis of Variance

Data may be ordered by two criteria, in which case a two-way analysis of variance can be used to determine possible differences between means. For example, assume that the sensitivities of guinea pig left atria to isoproterenol are measured in four identical organ baths on four consecutive days. Ideally, the sensitivity of the tissues should not be dependent on which organ bath is used or on which day the measurement is made; a two-way analysis of variance can be used to address this problem. Table 6.5 shows the negative logarithms of the molar concentrations of isoproterenol that produced half-maximal responses in the atria ordered by organ bath and day. Table 6.6A shows the formulas required for calculating the variance ratios required to assess whether or not the organ bath or day of measurement was a significant

**TABLE 6.5.** *Sensitivities of guinea pig isolated left atria to isoproterenol[a]*

| Organ bath | Day | | | | |
|---|---|---|---|---|---|
| | 1 | 2 | 3 | 4 | $R^b$ |
| I | 7.75 | 7.9 | 7.6 | 7.85 | 31.1 |
| II | 8.35 | 7.4 | 7.85 | 8.35 | 31.95 |
| III | 8.0 | 8.65 | 8.45 | 8.7 | 33.8 |
| IV | 7.45 | 8.25 | 8.2 | 8.55 | 32.45 |
| $C^c$ | 31.55 | 32.2 | 32.1 | 33.45 | 129.3[d] |

[a] Minus log molar concentration of isoproterenol that produces half-maximal response.
[b] R = sum of values in each row.
[c] C = sum of values in each column.
[d] T = total $\sum y$.

**TABLE 6.6.**[a]

| | Sum of squares | d.f. | Mean of squares | Variance ratio |
|---|---|---|---|---|
| A. Calculations for two-way analysis of variance | | | | |
| Between rows | $\sum R^2/c - T^2/N$ | $r - 1$ | $s_R^2$ | |
| | | | | $F_R = s_R^2/s^2$ |
| Between columns | $\sum C^2/r - T^2/N$ | $c - 1$ | $s_C^2$ | |
| | | | | $F_c = s_c^2/s^2$ |
| Residual | Subtraction | $(r - 1)(c - 1)$ | $s^2$ | |
| Total | $\sum y^2 - T^2/N$ | $N - 1$ | | |
| B. Two-way analysis of variance of data in Table 6.5 | | | | |
| Between rows (days) | 0.96 | 3 | 0.32 | |
| | | | | 2.49[b] |
| Between columns (baths) | 0.49 | 3 | 0.163 | |
| | | | | 1.27 |
| Residual | 1.155 | 9 | 0.128 | |
| Total | 2.605 | | | |

$$\left(\sum R^2\right)/c = [(31.1)^2 + (31.95)^2 + (33.8)^2 + (32.45)^2] \div 4 = 1{,}045.86$$

$$\left(\sum C^2\right)/r = [(31.55)^2 + (32.2)^2 + (32.1)^2 + (33.45)^2] \div 4 = 1{,}045.39$$

$$T^2/N = (129.3)^2 \div 16 = 1{,}044.9$$

$$\sum y^2 = 1{,}047.50$$

[a] $c$ = number of columns; $r$ = number of rows; $N$ = total number of individual $y$ values; $T = \sum R = \sum C$; $R$ = sum of each row; $C$ = sum of each column.
[b] Between rows, $F$ = 2.49 (n.s.); between columns, $F$ = 1.27 (n.s.).

factor in these studies. The calculation shown in Table 6.6B indicate no significant differences (at the 95% level of confidence) either for organ bath ($F$ between columns) or for day of measurement ($F$ between rows).

It should be noted that the $t$-test for significance and the analysis of variance rely, as do many statistical procedures, on the assumption that the values to be tested originate from normal distributions; they are referred to as parametric tests. Such normal distributions (the well-known bell-shaped curve showing the expected frequency of values over a range of standard-deviation units from the mean) are assumed in these tests, and their validity depends on this assumption. Therefore, computational metameters that clearly violate this assumption should not be used. A case in point is the distribution of concentrations of an agonist that produce half-maximal re-

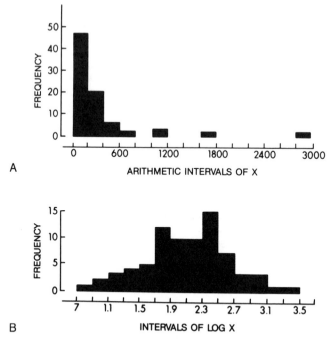

**FIG. 6.2.** Histograms of arithmetic **(A)** and logarithmic (geometric) **(B)** distributions of concentrations of norepinephrine that produce half-maximal responses in rat vasa deferentia: $N = 77$; $ED_{50} = \times 10^{-8}$ M. (From ref. 9.)

sponses in tissues. The distribution of the half-maximal concentrations of norepinephrine that produce half-maximal contractions of vasa deferentia are normally distributed only as logarithms, not as the converted $EC_{50}$ values (Fig. 6.2). Therefore, if comparisons of agonist potencies are to be made with parametric tests (like the *t* test), it is essential that *geometric means*, rather than arithmetic means, be used.

## RELATIONSHIPS BETWEEN DEPENDENT AND INDEPENDENT VARIABLES

Usually, pharmacologic experiments yield data in the form of independent (designated by the experimenter and assumed to have no error) and dependent (assumed to have only random error) variables, the most common being dose (independent) and response (dependent). It is useful to analyze such data assuming a relationship; the most commonly encountered ones are a linear relationship and one described on semilogarithmic axes by a sigmoidal curve. Statistical analysis of these can eliminate, or at least greatly reduce, bias and therefore add to the value of experiments. Although sigmoidal dose-response curves usually are chronologically the first expression of the data from an experiment, the analysis of straight lines will be discussed beforehand, because linear transformation often is used in the construction of unbiased sigmoidal curves.

## POPULATION ANALYSIS: SINGLE OR MULTIPLE POPULATIONS?

Frequently a collection of measurements are made and the question is asked, does the sample of data represent a single homogeneous population or is it comprised of samples from two or more populations? If it represents a sample from a homogeneous population, then the sample distribution should be normal. Since most statistical analyses require normal distributions for validity, it also may be important to test a sample for this assumption. The most straightforward approach is to construct a histogram of the data set and compare the result to a normal distribution curve. Any skewness, kurtosis, or multiple peaks could be interpreted as deviations from single population normality and thus sampling from two populations. Table 6.7 shows a set of hypothetical $pA_2$ measurements ($pA_2$ is the negative logarithm of molar concentration of an antagonist that produces a twofold displacement to the right of an agonist dose-response curve) made in a tissue type. The $pA_2$ can be an estimate of antagonist affinity (see Chapter 9), thus it is of practical interest to determine whether the measurements appear to be from one or several populations. This may occur if the agonist activates two similar receptors in the preparations and the antagonist is selective for one of them. Under these conditions, variations in the relative number of the two receptors in different preparations might be revealed as a two-sample population of measurements. The distribution of the data is shown in Fig. 6.3A and illustrates a common shortcoming in histogram representations of data sets. Specifically, if the number of data points is small, histograms become relatively insensitive to showing multiple populations. Also, the obligatory grouping of data into categories can cause inaccuracy. In general, bimodality is greatly influenced by the relative sizes of the two populations

**TABLE 6.7.** *Distribution of* $-log$ *(affinity) estimates*

| | | | |
|---|---|---|---|
| 1. 6.0 | 12. 6.5 | 23. 7.0 | 34. 7.45 |
| 2. 6.0 | 13. 6.55 | 24. 7.1 | 35. 7.46 |
| 3. 6.0 | 14. 6.56 | 25. 7.1 | 36. 7.47 |
| 4. 6.2 | 15. 6.6 | 26. 7.11 | 37. 7.47 |
| 5. 6.2 | 16. 6.6 | 27. 7.2 | 38. 7.6 |
| 6. 6.3 | 17. 6.67 | 28. 7.2 | 39. 7.6 |
| 7. 6.3 | 18. 6.67 | 29. 7.2 | 40. 7.8 |
| 8. 6.4 | 19. 6.7 | 30. 7.23 | 41. 7.9 |
| 9. 6.4 | 20. 6.8 | 31. 7.30 | 42. 7.9 |
| 10. 6.4 | 21. 6.8 | 32. 7.4 | 43. 8.1 |
| 11. 6.5 | 22. 6.9 | 33. 7.4 | 44. 8.2 |

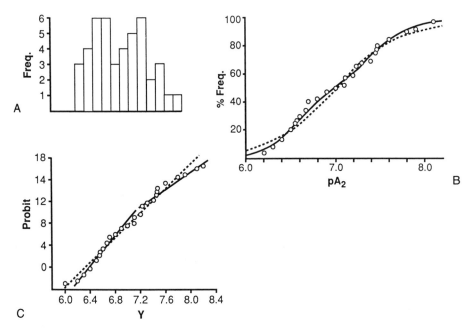

**FIG. 6.3.** Population analysis. **A:** Histogram representation of 44 estimates of $pA_2$ values in various tissue preparations. Ordinates: Number of values within a given category. Abscissae: Categories divided as increments of standard error units away from the mean. **B:** Cumulative frequency curve. Ordinates: Percentage of values below a given value. Abscissae: $pA_2$ estimates. *Broken line* indicates the best-fit curve describing a single logistic equation (Eq. 6.9). *Solid line* respresents a two-population logistic curve fit (Eq. 6.10). **C:** Probits of cumulative frequency. Ordinates: Probit calculation (Eq. 6.11) of cumulative frequencies. Abscissae: $pA_2$ estimates. *Broken line* indicates best-fit straight line to the data (single population). *Solid lines* indicate two straight-line fits with a single inflection point indicative of two populations.

and the separation between them; i.e., it is most easily detected if the two samples are of comparable size and separated by a large margin.

An alternative method of analysis of potentially bimodal distributions is by cumulative frequency analysis. By this method, the values of $Y$ are plotted as a function of the proportion of results that have values less than or equal to $Y$, i.e., the cumulative frequency (C.F.). A perfectly normal distribution would yield an S-shaped curve representing the integrated normal frequency curve. One approximation to this curve is the logistic function:

$$\text{C.F.} = \frac{M \cdot Y^p}{Y^p + K^p} \qquad [6.9]$$

where $p$ is the component of steepness of the curve, and $K$ is the value of $Y$ at the midpoint of the data set. If the data deviate from such a curve, then it is possible that a two-population equation better represents the data. Under these circumstances, the curve would resemble a two-term logistic of the form:

$$\text{C.F.} = \frac{Q \cdot Y^{p1}}{Y^{p1} + K_1{}^{p1}} + \frac{(1 - Q) \cdot Y^{p2}}{Y^{p2} + K_2{}^{p2}} \qquad [6.10]$$

where $Q$ represents the fraction of the sample coming from one population and $(1 - Q)$ the remaining fraction from the other population. A better fit of the data set to Eq. 6.10 over Eq. 6.9 might constitute evidence that the data are a mixture of two samples. Figure 6.3B shows the cumulative frequency curve for the data in Table 6.7. In this case, the two-population logistic provided a significantly better fit of the data set ($F = 29.3$, d.f. $= 3,39$, $p < 0.01$), thereby suggesting that the $pA_2$ values come from a mixture of two populations. A further representation of these data can be made with a probit plot where the probit of the cumulative frequency is plotted as a function of the data points.

$$\text{probit} = \frac{\text{C.F.} - \overline{(\text{C.F.})}}{\text{SEM (C.F.)}} + 5 \qquad [6.11]$$

where $\overline{(\text{C.F.})}$ and SEM (C.F.) are the mean and standard error of the mean of the cumulative frequencies. The probit plot for the data in Table 6.7 is shown in Fig. 6.3C. A single straight line would indicate a single normal population, whereas a single inflection point indicates bimodality.

### Analysis of Straight Lines

There are many instances, either by chance or through mathematical manipulation, in which given dependent variables are apparently linearly related to independent variables. This is convenient, because straight lines are readily amenable to analysis, and there are standard statistical methods to fit straight lines to data points. The following discussion is for the fitting of a straight line to data points on the cartesian coordinates $x$ and $y$, where $x$ can be manipulated by the experimenter, and random variability is encountered *only* in $y$. Data points are fitted to a straight line by the method of least squares, which simply minimizes the squares of the deviations of the observed $y$ values from the line. In general, the squared deviations of $y$ values from the mean value of $y$ ($\bar{y}$) are composed of the squared deviations of the least-squares line from $y$ and of the squared deviations due to random scatter of the observed points about the line. This sum of squares for residual or uncontrolled variation is minimized in the method of least squares, and data points are fitted to the equation for a straight line (*vide infra*). The analysis of data described by a straight line can be demonstrated conveniently by an example. The catecholamine isoproterenol stimulates cardiac β-adrenoceptors in cats to produce positive inotropy and increases in heart rate (tachycardia). The first question to be answered is: Are the isoproterenol-induced

increases in heart rate related to the isoproterenol-induced increases in inotropy? The independent variable will be inotropy, a designated increase being
$x$, and considered to have no error, and the dependent variable $y$ being tachycardia, which is observed for defined (i.e., chosen by the investigator) increases in inotropy. In terms of regression analysis, the first question to
answer is, Does $y$ depend on $x$? Table 6.8 shows the increases in heart rate
produced by isoproterenol in cats for designated isoproterenol-induced increases in cardiac inotropy; $x$ is a given increase in inotropy (designated and
assumed to have no error), and $y$ is the corresponding increase in heart
rate. It will be evident in the following calculations that six sums are used
repeatedly; therefore, calculation of these at the beginning of linear-regression analysis greatly expedites the procedure. These sums are shown in Table
6.8. From these sums, three useful products can be calculated to facilitate
calculation of the *regression coefficient*:

$$s_x^2 = \sum x^2 - \left(\sum x\right)2/n \qquad [6.12]$$

$$s_y^2 = \sum y^2 - \left(\sum y\right)2/n \qquad [6.13]$$

$$s_{xy} = \sum xy - \left(\sum x\right)\left(\sum y\right)/n \qquad [6.14]$$

The regression coefficient ($b$) is given by

$$b = \frac{\left(\sum x\right)\left(\sum y\right) - \left(\sum xy\right)n}{\left(\sum x\right)^2 - \left(\sum x^2\right)n} \qquad [6.15]$$

and the standard deviation of the regression coefficient ($s_b$) is given by

$$s_b = \left[\frac{(s_y^2)(s_x^2) - (s_{xy})^2}{(n-2)(s_x^2)^2}\right]^{1/2} \qquad [6.16]$$

The statistic $t$ is calculated as

$$t = \frac{b}{s_b}, \qquad \text{d.f.} = n - 2 \qquad [6.17]$$

For the data in Table 6.8, $b = 1.17$ and $s_b = 0.143$; therefore, the statistic
$t$ is 8.19 for $(n - 2) = 16$ degrees of freedom. In this case, there is a highly
significant ($p < 0.001$) regression coefficient demonstrating a dependence of
$y$ (heart rate) on $x$ (inotropy) with isoproterenol.

The equation for a straight line is

$$y = m \cdot x + c \qquad [6.18]$$

where $m$ is the slope and $c$ is the $y$ intercept (when $x = 0$). The method of
least squares can now be used to calculate the best-fit straight line through

**TABLE 6.8.** *Increases in heart rate in anesthetized cats with isoproterenol as a function of positive inotropy*

| (+)Inotropy $x$ (sec$^{-1}$) | Tachycardia $y$ (beats min$^{-1}$) | $\hat{y}$ | $(y - \hat{y})^2$ |
|---|---|---|---|
| 5 | 12 | 13.85 | 3.422 |
| 5 | 18 | | 17.22 |
| 5 | 9 | | 23.52 |
| 10 | 20 | 19.71 | 0.0841 |
| 10 | 22 | | 5.244 |
| 10 | 17 | | 7.344 |
| 15 | 26 | 25.56 | 0.1936 |
| 15 | 31 | | 29.594 |
| 15 | 24 | | 2.434 |
| 20 | 31 | 31.42 | 0.176 |
| 20 | 38 | | 43.296 |
| 20 | 25 | | 41.216 |
| 25 | 37 | 37.275 | 0.076 |
| 25 | 44 | | 45.225 |
| 25 | 32 | | 27.83 |
| 30 | 42 | 43.13 | 1.277 |
| 30 | 52 | | 78.68 |
| 30 | 33 | | 102.62 |

Note:  $\sum x = 315,$  $\sum y = 513$

$\sum x^2 = 6{,}825,$  $\sum y^2 = 16{,}851$

$n = 18,$  $\sum xy = 10{,}515$

$SS = \sum (y - \hat{y})^2 = 429.512$

Data from ref. 13.

the data points. The slope $m$ is the regression coefficient ($m = b$), and the intercept ($c$) is

$$c = \frac{\left(\sum y\right) - m\left(\sum x\right)}{n} \qquad [6.19]$$

Thus, $m$ and $c$ can be calculated and used in Eq. 6.18 to define the best-fit straight line through the data points. In the case of the data given in Table 6.8, the best-fit straight line is $y = 1.17 x + 8.0$; the data points and best-fit straight line are shown in Fig. 6.4B.

The confidence with which this line can be used to describe the data is quantified by estimation of the standard error of the slope, $y$ intercept, and $x$ intercept. To do this, the sum of squares about the regression (SS) must be calculated. This is done by subtracting the observed $y$ values ($y$) from the $y$ values calculated by the regression line (denoted $\hat{y}$); SS is calculated as

$$SS = \sum (y - \hat{y})^2 \qquad [6.20]$$

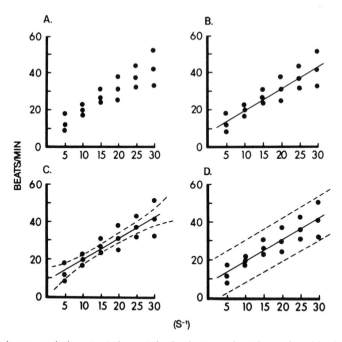

**FIG. 6.4.** Increases in heart rate in anesthetized cats as functions of positive inotropy to intravenously administered isoproterenol. Ordinates: Increases in heart rate in beats per minute. Abscissae: Increases in rate of rise of left ventricular pressure at a developed pressure of 40 mm Hg divided by 40 mm Hg (in sec$^{-1}$). **A:** Data points. **B:** Data points with best-fit straight line by linear regression; $y = 1.171x + 8.0$. **C:** Data points, best-fit straight line, and 95% confidence limits of the regression line. **D:** Data points, best-fit straight line, and 95% confidence limits of calculated values of $y$ from the regression line. (Data, in Table 6.8, from ref. 13.)

The standard error of the slope is given by

$$\text{SE}(m) = \left( \frac{n \cdot \text{SS}}{(n-2)\left[ n \cdot \left(\sum x^2\right) - \left(\sum x\right)^2 \right]} \right)^{1/2} \qquad [6.21]$$

The standard error of the $y$ intercept is given by

$$\text{SE}(c) = \left( \frac{\text{SS} \cdot \left(\sum x^2\right)}{(n-2)\left[ n \cdot \sum x^2 - \left(\sum x\right)^2 \right]} \right)^{1/2} \qquad [6.22]$$

For the data in Table 6.8, the slope is $1.17 \pm 0.143$ and the intercept is $8.0 \pm 2.78$.

It may be useful to predict the regression line for the population (i.e., for a given level of confidence, the confidence limits of the regression line). To do this, the estimate of the standard error of $y$ must be calculated:

$$SE(y) = \left[ \frac{SS}{n-2} \left( \frac{1}{n} + \frac{(x - \bar{x})^2}{\sum x^2} \right) \right]^{1/2} \qquad [6.23]$$

The confidence limits of $\hat{y}$ for each $x$ then can be estimated by calculating $SE(\hat{y})$ and multiplying by $t$ [confidence limits $= \pm t \cdot SE(\hat{y})$]. It can be seen that the confidence limits for the calculated population of regression lines greatly increase as $x$ gets larger or smaller than the mean value ($\bar{x}$). For the data in Table 6.8, the calculated 95% confidence limits for the regression line ($t_{0.05}$ used) are shown in Table 6.9 and Fig. 6.4C. The 95% confidence limits for the regression consist of a curved envelope on either side of the calculated regression line.

It may be desirable to calculate the confidence limits of $y$ for any given value of $x$ according to the regression line: these will be wider than the confidence limits for the regression line. Thus, the 95% confidence limits for $y$ will define the region around the regression line that will contain all values of $y$ for a given $x$ according to the calculated regression 95% of the time. The standard error for the predicted $y$ for a new value of $x$ under these circumstances is

$$SE(\hat{y}') = \left[ \frac{SS}{n-2} \left( 1 + \frac{1}{n} + \frac{(x - \bar{x})^2}{\sum x^2} \right) \right]^{1/2} \qquad [6.24]$$

The confidence limits are calculated as C.L. $= \pm t \cdot SE(\hat{y}')$. The 95% confidence limits on $y$ for the data in Table 6.8 are shown in Table 6.9.

It may be desirable to make a best estimate of $x$ for a given $y$ according to the regression line (linear calibration). Whereas $y$ can readily be calculated from the equation for the straight line, the confidence limits on $x$ require

**TABLE 6.9.** *Confidence limits for data in Table 6.6.*

| $x$ | $\bar{y}$ | 95% confidence for regression | 95% confidence for $y$ |
|---|---|---|---|
| 5 | 13.85 | ±3.08 | ±11.4 |
| 10 | 19.71 | ±2.77 | ±11.3 |
| 15 | 25.56 | ±2.61 | ±11.2 |
| 20 | 31.42 | ±2.61 | ±11.2 |
| 25 | 37.275 | ±2.77 | ±11.3 |
| 30 | 43.13 | ±3.08 | ±11.4 |

specialized calculation. The confidence limits on a calculated $x$ (denoted $\hat{x}$) are

$$x = \frac{\hat{x} \pm \dfrac{t}{b}\left\{\dfrac{SS}{n-2}\left[\dfrac{n+1}{n}(1-c)^2 + \dfrac{\hat{x}^2}{\sum x^2}\right]\right\}^{1/2}}{1-c^2} \qquad [6.25]$$

where

$$c^2 = \frac{t^2 \cdot SS \cdot \sum x^2}{(n-2)\left(\sum xy\right)^2} \qquad [6.26]$$

For the value of $\bar{x}$ at $\bar{y} = 20$ on the regression line shown in Fig. 6.4D, the 95% confidence limits are 7.0 (C.L. $= -0.38$ to 14.38).

### Straight Lines Through the Origin

In some cases there may be reason to believe that a straight line goes through the origin ($x = y = 0$). For example, Table 6.10 shows data describing a calibration curve for pen displacement on a chart recorder as a function of the maximal rate of rise of left ventricular pressure in anesthetized rats.

**TABLE 6.10.** *Calibration curve for dP/dt$_{max}$ of left ventricular pressure*

| Chart displacement (mm) | dP/dt$_{max}$ (mm sec$^{-1}$) | $(y - \hat{y})^2$ |
|:---:|:---:|:---:|
| 2 | 1,000 | 50,176 |
| 4 | 2,500 | 288,369 |
| 6 | 3,200 | 249,001 |
| 8 | 2,900 | 290,521 |
| 10 | 3,800 | 142,884 |
| 12 | 5,000 | 7,056 |
| 14 | 5,300 | 125,316 |
| 16 | 6,100 | 85,849 |
| 18 | 7,800 | 447,561 |

Note: $\sum x = 90$, $\sum y = 37{,}600$

$\sum x^2 = 1{,}140$, $\sum y^2 = 1.9148 \times 10^8$

$n = 9$, $\sum xy = 464{,}600$

$m = 369.2$, $SS = 1{,}686{,}733$

$c = 486.1$

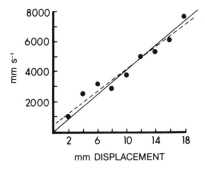

**FIG. 6.5.** Calibration curve for displacement of chart-recorder pen for given increases in rate of rise of left ventricular pressure in anesthetized rats. Ordinate: Rate of rise of left ventricular pressure in mm Hg sec$^{-1}$. Abscissa: Millimeters displacement on chart recorder. *Broken line* is the best-fit line by linear regression; $m = 369.2$, $c = 486.1$. *Solid line* is the best-fit straight line through the origin; $m = 407.5$. Data from Table 6.10.

The data describe a straight line with a slope of 369.2 and intercept of 486.1; this is the broken line in Fig. 6.5. What this implies is that when there is no pen displacement on the chart recorder, the pressure transducer records a response of 486.1 mm sec$^{-1}$. Although this may reflect inertia in the recording system, it can also be artificial. It would be expected that zero pen deflection would represent zero response; that is, the calibration curve would go through the origin. The statistic $t$ can be calculated to test the significance of an intercept different from zero with the following equation:

$$t = \frac{\bar{y} - m\bar{x}}{\left[\dfrac{SS}{n-2}\left(\dfrac{1}{n} + \dfrac{(\bar{x})^2}{\sum x^2}\right)\right]^{1/2}}, \qquad \text{d.f.} = n - 2 \qquad [6.27]$$

where $\bar{y}$ and $\bar{x}$ represent mean values. For the data in Table 6.10 the calculated value of $t$ is 2.22, which is insignificant at the $p = 0.05$ level. Therefore, the data points could just as well be described by a straight line through the origin with a slope calculated as

$$m = \sum xy / \sum x^2 \qquad [6.28]$$

This is shown in Fig. 6.5 ($m = 407.5$) as the solid line.

### Test for Linearity

Often it is important to know whether there is reason to doubt the assumption of linearity of a regression. This can be tested easily if there are replicate readings of $y$ for each $x$. Table 6.11 shows values for changes in heart rates of anesthetized cats with given increases in inotropic state to the catecholamine dobutamine. The data points are shown in Fig. 6.6A with the best-fit straight line. However, when a simple line is drawn through the means of each array, a definite curve in the mean points is evident (Fig. 6.6B). A test for linearity analyzing the deviations of the array means from the regression can quantify

**TABLE 6.11.** *Increases in heart rate in anesthetized cats with dobutamine as a function of positive inotropy*

| x | y | $T^a$ |
|---|---|---|
| 25 | 13 | |
| | 4 | 25 |
| | 10 | |
| | −2 | |
| 30 | 6 | |
| | 4 | 22 |
| | 12 | |
| | 0 | |
| 35 | 8 | |
| | 13 | 61 |
| | 18 | |
| | 22 | |
| 40 | 30 | |
| | 28 | 117 |
| | 33 | |
| | 26 | |
| 45 | 44 | |
| | 48 | 170 |
| | 36 | |
| | 42 | |

*Note:* $\sum x = 700,$  $\sum y = 395$

$\sum x^2 = 25{,}500,$  $\sum y^2 = 12{,}275$

$n = 20,$  $\sum xy = 15{,}750$

$\sum (T_i^2/n_i) = (25)^2/4 + (22)^2/4 + (61)^2/4 + (117)^2/4 + (170)^2/4$

$k = 5,$

$^a T = \sum y$ for each common $x$.
Data from ref. 13.

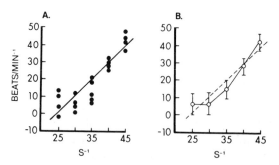

**FIG. 6.6.** Increases in heart rate in anesthetized cats as functions of increased inotropy to intravenously administered dobutamine. Ordinates: Increases in heart rate in beats per minute. Abscissae: Rate of rise of left ventricular pressure at a developed pressure of 40 mm Hg divided by 40 mm Hg. **A:** Data points with best-fit straight line by linear regression. **B:** Mean data points for each array (with SEM) joined by straight lines. *Broken line* is the best-fit straight line through the data points. (Data, in Table 6.11, from ref. 13.)

the significance of the deviation from linearity; the calculations are shown in Table 6.12A and carried out for the data (shown in Table 6.11) in Table 6.12B. The fact that $F_2$ is significant at the $p < 0.05$ level indicates a significant deviation from linearity in these data.

### Comparison of Straight Lines

Frequently it is desirable to compare straight lines to determine if they are statistically the same or different. That is, given two (or more) samples of data points, do they describe two (or more) lines or scatter about one single

**TABLE 6.12.**

| | Sum of squares | d.f.[a] | Mean of squares | Variance ratio |
|---|---|---|---|---|
| **A. Analysis of variance with test for linearity** | | | | |
| Due to regression | $\sum xy - \left[\dfrac{\left(\sum x\right)\left(\sum y\right)}{n}\right]^2$ $\sum x^2 - \left(\dfrac{\sum x}{n}\right)^2$ | 1 | $s_1^2$ | |
| | | | | $F_1 = s_1^2/s_3^2$ |
| Deviation of assay means | By subtraction | $k - 2$ | $s_2^2$ | |
| | | | | $F_2 = s_2^2/s_3^2$ |
| Within-assay residual | $\sum y^2 - \sum_i (T_i^2/n_i)$ | $n - k$ | $s_3^2$ | |
| Total | $\sum y^2 - \left(\sum y/n\right)^2$ | $n - 1$ | | |
| **B. Calculations for data in Table 6.11** | | | | |
| Due to regression | 3,705.62 | 1 | 3,705.62 | |
| | | | | 132.24 |
| Deviation of assay means | 347.88 | 3 | 115.96 | |
| | | | | 4.14 |
| Within-assay residual | 420.25 | 15 | 28.02 | |
| Total | 4,473.75 | | | |

[a] $k$ = number of arrays.

line? There are two criteria for difference: slope and position (also referred to as elevation). The first to be considered here is slope.

Much pharmacologic inference derives from comparisons of tissue sensitivities to drugs before and after an intervention. This approach permits the use of null methods, so vital to pharmacologic procedures, because stimulus-response mechanisms usually are unknown. Thus, the sensitivity of a tissue to a drug can be quantified by a dose-response curve, then the preparation altered in some way (e.g., addition of a receptor antagonist) and the effect of the alteration measured by a repeated quantification of tissue sensitivity. Ideally, these measures should be independent of the level of response; otherwise the null requirement is not met, and the data are much less useful. Frequently, two straight lines are generated that differ in location (along the *x* axis) and *somewhat* in slope. This latter fact greatly complicates interpretation of the data, because how much the lines differ in location then depends on the value of the ordinate (i.e., where along the line the difference is measured); this makes the analysis cumbersome. However, if the lines were parallel, there would be no dependence of location on ordinate values, and an unambiguous measurement would result. Therefore, an unbiased test of whether two straight lines truly are parallel can be useful.

The test for parallelism uses the following parameters (to be calculated for each *x*, *y* data set):

$$s = \left( \frac{\sum (y - \hat{y})^2}{n - 2} \right)^{1/2} \qquad [6.29]$$

$$s_x^2 = \sum x^2 - \left( \sum x \right)^2 / n \qquad [6.30]$$

Comparing two lines defined by data points $xy$ (line 1) and $x_2y_2$ (line 2), the statistic $t$ can be calculated and used to determine significant differences in slopes:

$$t = \frac{m_1 - m_2}{s_p (1/s_{x_1}^2 + 1/s_{x_2}^2)^{1/2}}, \qquad \text{d.f.} = n_1 + n_2 - 4 \qquad [6.31]$$

where $m_1$ and $m_2$ are the respective slopes of lines 1 and 2, and

$$s_p = \left( \frac{(n_1 - 2)(s_1)^2 + (n_2 - 2)(s_2)^2}{n_1 + n_2 - 4} \right)^{1/2} \qquad [6.32]$$

Table 6.13 shows the percentage depressions of guinea pig atrial contractions produced by adenosine in the absence and presence of an adenosine-uptake-blocking dose of diazepam. It can be seen from Table 6.13 and Fig. 6.7 that diazepam significantly shifted the dose-response curve to adenosine to the left. Figure 6.7A shows the mean least-squares straight line through

**TABLE 6.13.** *Percentage depressions of contraction caused by adenosine in the absence and presence of diazepam*

| $x_1, x_2$ | $y_1$ | $(y - \hat{y})_1^2$ | $y_2$ | $(y - \hat{y})_2^2$ |
|---|---|---|---|---|
| −6.5 | 12 | 80.1 | | |
| | 20 | 0.90 | | |
| | 27 | 36.6 | | |
| −6.0 | 38 | 26.01 | 0 | 4.93 |
| | 45 | 3.61 | 3 | 0.61 |
| | 52 | 79.21 | 8 | 33.41 |
| −5.5 | 58 | 52.56 | 12 | 65.37 |
| | 65 | 0.0625 | 16 | 16.69 |
| | 69 | 14.06 | 26 | 34.99 |
| −5.0 | | | 26 | 142.8 |
| | | | 38 | 0.0025 |
| | | | 49 | 122.1 |
| −4.5 | | | 44 | 139.6 |
| | | | 56 | 0.034 |
| | | | 70 | 201.21 |

Note: $\sum x_1 = -54$, $\sum y_1 = 386$, $\sum x_2 = -63$, $\sum y_2 = -348$

$\sum x_1^2 = 325.5$, $\sum y_1^2 = 19{,}796$, $\sum x_2^2 = 334.5$, $\sum y_2^2 = 15{,}642$

$n_1 = 9$, $\sum x_1 y_1 = -2{,}249.5$, $n_2 = 12$, $\sum x_2 y_2 = -1{,}693$

$m_1 = 44.3$, $m_2 = 35.73$

$c_1 = 308.9$, $c_2 = 216.6$

$\sum (y - \hat{y})_1^2 = 293.11$, $\sum (y - \hat{y})_2^2 = 761.75$

$\bar{x}_1 = -6$, $\bar{x}_2 = -5.25$

$\bar{y}_1 = 42.89$, $\bar{y}_2 = 29$

Data from ref. 11.

each of the data sets; the slopes of these lines appear different. In terms of quantifying the potentiation of adenosine by diazepam, the differences in slopes can be quite significant. For example, if a 20% response is chosen to calculate potentiation, a 10-fold sensitization is observed, whereas at 80% response there is a 22-fold sensitization; on a logarithmic concentration scale, this difference (120%) is substantial and raises a question: What is the most unambiguous method of quantifying sensitization? The difference results from the different slopes of the two lines, and therefore the first question to ask is, Are the slopes truly different? Although the lines shown in Fig. 6.7A are the best-fit calculated slopes, the scatter of the data points indicates that these need not be the only slopes capable of describing an adequate line through the data points. In this type of situation, a test for parallelism between the dose-response curves for the two sets of data points can be helpful.

Table 6.14 shows the calculated values in the test for parallelism for the data in Fig. 6.7. The calculated value of $t$ is not significant at the 5% level,

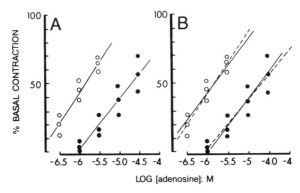

**FIG. 6.7.** Depressions of cardiac inotropy by adenosine in the presence and absence of diazepam. Ordinates: Percentage of depression of basal electrically stimulated force of contraction in guinea pig atria. Abscissae: Logarithms of molar concentrations of adenosine. Responses in the absence (•) and presence (○) of diazepam (100 μM). **A:** Best-fit straight line through each set of data points. **B:** Lines shown in **A** as *broken lines*; *solid lines* are best-fit regression lines of common slope. (Data, in Table 6.13, from ref. 11.)

indicating that there is less than a 5% chance that the lines drawn through the two sets of data points will truly differ in slope. Given this, the best-fit lines of *common* slope can be calculated. The common slope is given by

$$m_c = \frac{W_1 m_1 + W_2 m_2}{W_1 + W_2} \qquad [6.33]$$

where $W_1$ and $W_2$ are weighting factors calculated as

$$W = [SE(m)]^{-2} \qquad [6.34]$$

For the data in Fig. 6.7A, the common slope is 39.35. The best-fit straight lines through the data points can be calculated by

$$y = \bar{y} + m_c(x - \bar{x}) \qquad [6.35]$$

where $\bar{x}$ and $\bar{y}$ are the mean values of $\bar{x}$ and $\bar{y}$ for each data set. The common-slope best-fit straight lines through the two sets of data points are shown in Fig. 6.7B. This changes the interpretation of the experimental data; under these circumstances, there is no reason to assume that a nonparallel shift of

**TABLE 6.14.** *Test for parallelism: data from Table 6.13*

|  | n | S | $s_x^2$ | m |
|---|---|---|---|---|
| Line 1 (control) | 9 | 6.47 | 1.5 | 44.3 |
| Line 2 (diazepam) | 12 | 8.73 | 3.75 | 35.73 |

*Note:* $s_p = 7.88$; $t = 1.13$, d.f. $= 17$ (n.s.).

the dose-response curve is not produced by diazepam, and the potentiation is calculated to be 13.6.

A useful approach to the question of whether a data set can best be described by one or two straight lines is based on the principle of the extra sum of squares. By this method, a given data set is compared to three models of varying complexity. The first is to fit the data to two separate straight lines with individual slopes and intercepts:

$$y_1 = A_1 + B_1 \cdot x$$
$$y_2 = A_2 + B_2 \cdot x$$
[Model 1]

where the subscripts refer to data sets 1 and 2, respectively. This analysis then could be compared to another model in which a common slope B is assumed with differing intercepts:

$$y_1 = A_1 + B \cdot x$$
$$y_2 = A_2 + B \cdot x$$
[Model 2]

and then finally to a single line of common slope and intercept:

$$y_1 = y_2 = A + B \cdot x$$
[Model 3]

The statistical preference of one model over another is estimated by calculation of the sum of squares of the residuals (Eq. 6.20) and subsequent calculation of an $F$ statistic:

$$F(2,1) = \frac{(SS_1 - SS_2)/(d.f._2 - d.f._1)}{SS_1/d.f._1}$$
[6.36]

where the subscripts refer to the two models being compared and the degrees of freedom for the $F$ comparison are given by $(d.f._1 - d.f._2)$ and $d.f._1$. If the $F$ is significant, this indicates that Model 1 is preferred and if $F$ is less than the chosen significance level, then Model 2, the simpler model, is preferred.

Table 6.15 shows the increases in cardiac inotropy in anesthetized cats with dobutamine when the animals were pretreated or not pretreated with the $\alpha$-adrenoceptor blocking agent phentolamine. The question asked is: Does a component of the positive inotropic activity of dobutamine result from activation of $\alpha$-adrenoceptors? One approach is to test whether the dose-response curve for positive inotropy by dobutamine is different after phentolamine; an analysis of the regression lines describing the two dose-response curves by the extra sum of squares may be useful in this situation. The raw data are shown in Fig. 6.8A; it is not evident from this figure whether the data describe one or two regression lines. Figure 6.8B shows two separate regression lines drawn for each data set with separate slopes and intercepts (Model 1). From this figure, two lines could easily fit the data, but the standard errors on the means of the arrays do not make it clear whether it is justifiable to fit the data to two lines of common (Model 2) or differing slope

**TABLE 6.15.** *Increased inotropy[a] in anesthetized cats by dobutamine in the presence and absence of phentolamine*

| No phentolamine | | Phentolamine (2 mg kg$^{-1}$) | |
|---|---|---|---|
| $x_1$ (sec$^{-1}$) | $y_1$ (bpm) | $x_2$ (sec$^{-1}$) | $y_2$ (bpm) |
| 0 | 5 | 0 | 4.5 |
| 0 | 7 | 0 | 6 |
| 0 | 4 | 0 | 9 |
| 0.5 | 14.5 | 0.5 | 15 |
| 0.5 | 15.5 | 0.5 | 16 |
| 0.5 | 13 | 0.5 | 18 |
| 1 | 25 | 1 | 24.5 |
| 1 | 26 | 1 | 26 |
| 1 | 23 | 1 | 27.5 |

Note: $\sum x_1 = 4.5$,   $\sum y_1 = 133$,   $\sum x_2 = 4.5$,   $\sum y_2 = 146.5$

$\sum x_1^2 = 3.75$,   $\sum y_1^2 = 2{,}539.5$,   $\sum x_2^2 = 3.75$,   $\sum y_2^2 = 2{,}974.75$

$n_1 = 9$,   $\sum x_1 y_1 = 95.5$,   $n_2 = 9$,   $\sum x_2 y_2 = 102.5$

Data taken as one total set:

$\sum x_T = 9$,   $\sum y_T = 279.5$

$\sum x_T^2 = 7.5$,   $\sum y_T^2 = 5{,}514.25$

$n = 18$,   $\sum xy_T = 198$

[a] Increases in $dP/dt$ (sec$^{-1}$) at a left ventricular pressure of 40 mm Hg. Data from ref. 13.

(see Fig. 6.8C). A comparison of the sum of squares between these two models $[F(2,1)]$ yields $F = 0.007$ (d.f. $= 1{,}14$), thus indicating that Model 2 is preferable to Model 1; i.e., the data are better fit by the simpler model of two lines with common slope. The descriptive data for these calculations are given in Table 6.16. A similar analysis then can be done for comparisons of

**TABLE 6.16.** *Extra sum of squares for regression lines*

Model 1 (two lines with different slope and intercept)
  Data set I (no phentolamine)     $Y = 19.33 \cdot x + 5.11$
    SS $= 13.39$
  Data set II ($+$ phentolamine)     $Y = 19.5 \cdot x + 6.53$
    SS $= 19.68$
  SS$_1$ for Model 1 $= 33.07$, d.f.$_1 = 14$
Model 2 (two lines with common slope, different intercept)
  Data set I     $Y = 19.41 \cdot X + 5.07$
    SS $= 13.4$
  Data set II     $Y = 19.41 \cdot X + 6.57$
    SS $= 19.69$
  SS$_2$ for Model 2 $= 33.087$, d.f.$_2 = 15$
Model 3 (one common line)
  $Y = 19.41 \cdot x + 5.82$
  SS for Model 3 $= 43.22$, d.f. $= 16$

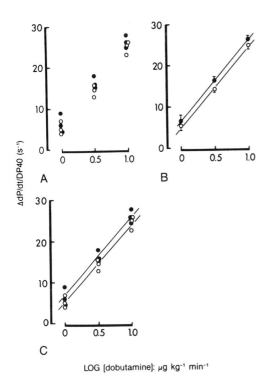

**FIG. 6.8.** Increases in inotropy in anesthetized cats to intravenous dobutamine in the absence (•) and presence (○) of phentolamine. Ordinates: Rate of rise of left ventricular pressure at a left ventricular pressure of 40 mm Hg divided by 40 mm Hg. Abscissae: Logarithms of intravenous concentrations of dobutamine in $\mu g\ kg^{-1}\ min^{-1}$. **A:** Data points. **B:** Best-fit straight line through mean of each array; bars represent SEM. **C:** Best-fit straight line for each data set (presence and absence of phentolamine). (Data, in Table 6.15, from ref. 13.)

Models 2 and 3. In this case, the $F$ statistic $[F(3,2)]$ is 4.6, d.f. = 1,15, a value indicating $p < 0.05$. Therefore, Model 2 is preferred over Model 3 (see Table 6.16). This analysis indicates that two straight lines of common slope but differing intercepts best describe these data.

Cumulative frequency analysis also can be utilized in the analysis of straight lines. In this case, the cumulative frequency of the distance of each data point from the best-fit single straight line may be used to detect whether the data are best fit by one or two straight lines. The data shown in Table 6.15 were subjected to this analysis and the cumulative frequencies of the residuals ($Y_{observed} - Y_{calculated}$) shown as a function of $Y$ in Fig. 6.9. From this figure it can be seen that a two-population logistic fit (Eq. 6.10) is better for the residuals than a single logistic fit (Eq. 6.9). This indicates that the distances of the data points from a single calculated line can be separated into two samples; i.e., there is no one single normal distribution of residuals about one line that would indicate that a single line best describes the data. The $F$ statistic for the improvement of fit of Eq. 6.10 over Eq. 6.9 ($F = 29.3$, d.f. = 3,39) indicates a highly significant possibility that the data are best described by more than one straight line.

Comparison of regression lines also can be conveniently carried out with an analysis of covariance. Two variance ratios are calculated: $F_{slope}$ for dif-

**TABLE 6.17.** *Calculation of analysis of covariance of regression lines*

|          | d.f.            | $s_x^2$ | $s_{xy}$ | $s_y^2$ | d.f.              | Sum of squares | Mean of squares |
|----------|-----------------|---------|----------|---------|-------------------|----------------|-----------------|
| 1. Within |                |         |          |         |                   |                |                 |
| 1.       | $n_1 - 1$       | A       | B        | C       | $n_1 - 2$         | D              |                 |
| 2.       | $n_2 - 1$       | E       | F        | G       | $n_2 - 2$         | H              |                 |
|          |                 |         |          |         | Sum               | Sum            |                 |
|          |                 |         |          |         | I                 | J              | K               |
|          |                 | Sum     | Sum      | Sum     |                   |                |                 |
| 2. Pooled | $n_1 + n_2 - 2$ | L       | M        | N       | $n_1 + n_2 - 3$   | O              | P               |
|          |                 |         |          |         |                   | Subt.          |                 |
|          |                 |         |          |         | 1                 | Q              | Q               |
| 3. Overall | $n_1 + n_2 - 1$ | R      | S        | T       | $n_1 + n_2 - 2$   | U              |                 |
|          |                 |         |          |         |                   | Subt.          |                 |
|          |                 |         |          |         | 1                 | V              | V               |

*Note:* Difference in slopes $F_{slope} = Q/K$; d.f. $= 1, I$; difference in elevations $F_{elevation} = V/P$; d.f. $= 1, n_1 + n_2 - 3$.

$$A = s_x^2 = \sum x_1^2 - \frac{\left(\sum x\right)_1^2}{n_1}, \qquad B = s_{xy} = \sum xy_1 - \frac{\left(\sum x\right)_1 \left(\sum y\right)_1}{n_1},$$

$$C = s_y^2 = \sum y_1^2 - \frac{\left(\sum y\right)_1^2}{n_1}, \qquad D = C - (B)^2/A$$

$E$, $F$, and $G$ as for $A$, $B$, and $C$, respectively, but substitute 2 for 1:

$H = G - (F)^2/E,$     $I = n_I + n_{II} - 4,$     $J = D + H,$     $K = J \div I$

$L = A + E,$     $M = B + F,$     $N = C + G,$     $O = N - (M)^2/L$

$$P = O \div (n_I + n_2 - 3) \qquad Q = O - J, \qquad R = \left(\sum x_1^2 + \sum x_2^2\right) - \frac{\left(\sum x_1 + \sum x_2\right)^2}{n_1 + n_2}$$

$$S = \left(\sum xy_1 + \sum xy_2\right) - \frac{\left(\sum x_1 + \sum x_2\right)\left(\sum y_1 + \sum y_2\right)}{n_1 + n_2}$$

$$T = \left(\sum y_1^2 + \sum y_2^2\right) - \frac{\left(\sum y_1 + \sum y_2\right)^2}{n_1 + n_2}, \qquad U = T - \frac{(S)^2}{R}, \qquad V = U - O$$

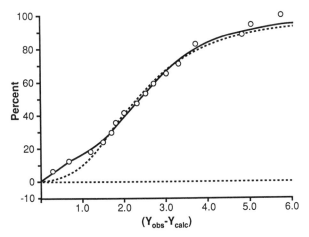

**FIG. 6.9.** Cumulative frequency analysis for two populations. Ordinate: Percentages of a given value below the maximal value. Abscissa: Differences between a value and the calculated value from the best-fit single straight line. *Broken line* represents the best-fit single logistic equation (single population) to the data set, the *solid line* the fit to two populations. Data from Table 6.15.

ferences in slope and $F_{elevation}$ for differences in elevation (position) of the two lines. The calculation for the analysis of covariance of regression lines is shown in Table 6.17 and carried out in Table 6.18. Again, as can be seen from the nonsignificance of $F_{slope}$ and the significance at $p < 0.05$ of $F_{elevation}$, the data are best fit by two lines that differ in position, but not in slope (Fig. 6.8C).

**TABLE 6.18.** *Analysis of covariance of regression lines for data in Table 6.15*

| | | d.f. | $s_x^2$ | $s_{xy}$ | $s_y^2$ | d.f. | Sum of squares | Mean of squares |
|---|---|---|---|---|---|---|---|---|
| 1. | Within | | | | | | | |
| | I | 8 | 1.5 | 29 | 574.05 | 7 | 13.38 | |
| | II | 8 | 1.5 | 29.25 | 590.05 | 7 | 19.675 | |
| | | | | | | 14 | 33.05 | 2.36 |
| 2. | Pooled | 16 | 3.0 | 58.25 | 1,164.0 | 15 | 32.98 | 2.20 |
| | | | | | | 1 | 0.07 | 0.07 |
| 3. | Overall | 17 | 3.0 | 58.25 | 1,174.2 | 16 | 43.18 | |
| | | | | | | 1 | 10.20 | 10.20 |

*Note:* $F_{slope} = 0.07/2.36 = 0.030$, d.f. $= 1, 14$ (n.s.); $F_{elevation} = 10.20/2.2 = 4.64$, d.f. $= 1, 15; p < 0.05$.

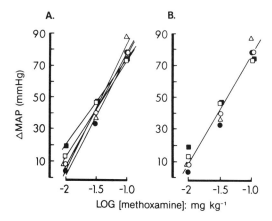

**FIG. 6.10.** Pressure responses to intravenous methoxamine in anesthetized cats. Ordinates: Increases in mean arterial pressure in mm Hg. Abscissae: Logarithms of intravenous doses of methoxamine in mg kg$^{-1}$. **A:** Best-fit straight line for data set from each cat. **B:** Best-fit straight line for all data points. (Data, in Table 6.19, from ref. 13.)

## COVARIANCE OF REGRESSION LINES: MULTIPLE LINE COMPARISONS

Analysis of covariance of regression lines can be carried out in which more than two regressions can be compared with one another. Table 6.19 shows increases in mean arterial blood pressure in five cats caused by methoxamine; the sensitivity of each cat to methoxamine is characterized by a straight-line dose-response curve. A relevant question to ask is, Do the five cats differ in their sensitivities to the methoxamine? Five separate dose-response curves can be drawn through the data points, as shown in Fig. 6.10A; an analysis of covariance of multiple regression lines can be used to

**TABLE 6.19.** *Increases in mean blood pressure for five cats given methoxamine i.v.*

| | Pressure (mm Hg) | | | | |
|---|---|---|---|---|---|
| log[methoxamine] | 1 | 2 | 3 | 4 | 5 |
| $-2$ | 4 | 8 | 8 | 12 | 20 |
| $-1.5$ | 33 | 40 | 36 | 46 | 48 |
| $-1.0$ | 78 | 78 | 88 | 72 | 74 |

*Note:* $\sum x_i = -4.5$    $\sum y_i = 115$

| | | | | | | |
|---|---|---|---|---|---|---|
| $\sum x_i^2 = 7.25$ | $\sum y_i =$ | 115 | 126 | 132 | 130 | 142 |
| | $\sum y_i^2 =$ | 7,189 | 7,748 | 9,104 | 7,444 | 8,180 |
| | $\sum xy_i =$ | $-135.5$ | $-154$ | $-158$ | $-165$ | $-186$ |
| | $s_y^2 =$ | 2,780.7 | 2,456 | 3,296 | 1,810.7 | 1,458.7 |
| | $s_{xy} =$ | 37 | 35 | 40 | 30 | 27 |
| | $s_x^2 =$ | 0.5 | 0.5 | 0.5 | 0.5 | 0.5 |

Data from ref. 13.

**TABLE 6.20.** *Analysis of covariance of multiple regression lines: calculations of differences in slopes*

| | Sum of squares | d.f. | Mean of squares |
|---|---|---|---|
| Due to common slope | A | 1 | |
| Differences between slopes | B | $k - 1$ | C |
| Residual | D | $n - 2k$ | E |

*Note:* $F_{slope} = C \div E$, d.f. $= k - 1, n - 2k$; total number of $x, y$ values $= n$; number of groups (regressions) $= k$.

$$s_{x_i}^2 = \sum x_i^2 - \frac{\left(\sum x_i\right)^2}{n_i}, \quad s_y^2 = \sum y_i^2 - \frac{\left(\sum y_i\right)^2}{n_i}, \quad s_{xy} = \sum xy_i - \frac{\left(\sum y_i\right)\left(\sum x_i\right)}{n_i}$$

$$A = \frac{\left[\sum_{i=1}^{k}\left(s_{xy}\right)_i\right]^2}{\sum_{i=1}^{k}\left(s_x^2\right)_i}, \quad B = \sum_{i=1}^{k}\frac{\left(s_{xy}\right)_i^2}{\left(s_x^2\right)_i} - A, \quad C = B \div (k - 1)$$

$$D = \sum_{i=1}^{k}\left(s_y^2\right)_i - \sum_{s_x^2}^{k}\frac{\left(s_{xy}\right)_i^2}{\left(s_x^2\right)_i}, \quad E = D \div (n - 2k)$$

determine whether the dose-response curves are significantly different. First, a test for differences in slope can be carried out; the calculation is shown in Table 6.20 and carried out for the data in Table 6.21. In this case, $F_{slope}$ is not significant at the $p < 0.05$ level; thus, the individual regression lines through the data points are not significantly different with respect to slope. The calculation for differences in position is shown in Table 6.22 and carried

**TABLE 6.21.** *Analysis of covariance of multiple regression lines: differences in slope—calculations for data in Table 6.19*

| | Sum of squares | d.f. | Mean of squares |
|---|---|---|---|
| Due to common slope | 11,424.4 | 1 | |
| Differences between slopes | 221.6 | 4 | 55.4 |
| Residual | 156.1 | 5 | 31.22 |

*Note:* $F = 55.4 \div 31.22 = 1.77$, d.f. $= 4, 5$ (n.s.).

**TABLE 6.22.** *Analysis of covariance of multiple regression lines: calculations of differences in position*

| | $s_x^2$ | $s_{xy}$ | $s_y^2$ | Sum of squares | d.f. | Mean of squares |
|---|---|---|---|---|---|---|
| Within groups | A | B | C | D | $n - k - 1$ | E |
| Total | F | G | H | I | | |
| Between groups | | | | J | $k - 1$ | K |

*Note:* $F_{elevation} = K \div E$, d.f. $= (k - 1), (n - k - 1)$.

$$A = \left( \sum x^2 \right)_T - \frac{\sum \left( x \right)_1^2}{n_1} + \cdots + \frac{\left( \sum x \right)_k^2}{n_k} = \left( \sum x^2 \right)_T - \sum_{i=1}^{k} \frac{\left( \sum x \right)_i^2}{n_i}$$

$$B = \left( \sum xy \right)_T - \frac{\sum \left( x \right)_1 \left( y \right)_1}{n_1} + \cdots + \frac{\sum \left( x \right)_k \left( y \right)_k}{n_k} = \left( \sum xy \right)_T - \sum_{i=1}^{k} \frac{\left( \sum x \right)_i \left( \sum y \right)_i}{n_i}$$

*C* as for *A*, but substitute *y* for *x*

$$D = C - (B)^2/A, \qquad E = D \div (n - k - 1)$$

$$F = \left( \sum x^2 \right)_T - \frac{\left( \sum x \right)_T^2}{n_T}, \qquad G = \left( \sum xy \right)_T - \frac{\left( \sum x \right)_T \left( \sum y \right)_T}{n_T}$$

*H* as for *F*, but substitute *y* for *x*

$$I = H - (G)^2/F \qquad J = |D - I| \qquad K = J \div (k - 1)$$

out for the data in Table 6.23. Again, $F_{elevation}$ is not significant at the $p < 0.05$ level, and it can be seen that the regression lines are not significantly different from each other. Thus, it was found that there was no evidence to conclude that the agonists activated different $\alpha$-adrenoceptors in this tissue. The common regression line is shown in Fig. 6.10B.

**TABLE 6.23.** *Analysis of covariance of multiple regression lines: differences in position—calculations for data in Table 6.19*

| | $s_x^2$ | $s_{xy}$ | $s_y^2$ | Sum of squares | d.f. | Mean of squares |
|---|---|---|---|---|---|---|
| Within groups | 2.5 | 169 | 11,802 | 377.6 | 9 | 41.95 |
| Total | 2.5 | 169 | 11,930 | 505.6 | | |
| Between groups | | | | 161 | 4 | 40.25 |

*Note:* $F = 40.25 \div 41.95 = 0.96$, d.f. $= 4, 9$ (n.s.).

**Regression and Correlation**

One method of measuring the possible relationship between two variables is by calculating the correlation coefficient ($r$):

$$r = \frac{\sum xy}{\left(\sum x^2 \cdot \sum y^2\right)^{1/2}}$$

[6.36]

A perfect correlation corresponds to $r = +1$ or $-1$, and no correlation (interrelationship) to $r = 0$. The magnitude of $r$ always lies between $+1$ and $-1$. The null hypothesis that no relationship exists between two variables can be tested by calculation of the statistic $t$ by the following equation:

$$t = r \cdot [(n - 2)/(1 - r^2)]^{1/2}, \qquad \text{d.f.} = n - 2$$

[6.37]

It should be noted that the correlation coefficient $r$ estimates only a degree of closeness of a linear relationship between $x$ and $y$. It cannot be used to approach questions much more relevant to the researcher, for example, How much does $y$ change for a given change in $x$? How well can we predict $y$ from $x$? Insight into these questions can be gained from regression analysis, a fact that probably accounts for the increasing use of regression over correlation in pharmacologic research.

## NONLINEAR REGRESSION

Although straight lines are simple to analyze, the transformation of data to this form may be statistically incorrect; i.e., experimental uncertainty of $y$ values should not be related to values of $x$ or $y$. This often is not the case after linear transformation. For example, an exponential decay curve with random ordinate error can be linearized on a logarithmic scale, but then the errors become heteroscedastic (i.e., dependent on $x$, being relatively larger at higher values of $x$). This makes statistical comparison, which assumes a normally distributed error, suspect. The availability of computers has made analysis of untransformed data accessible.

In practical terms, a complex pattern of dependent variables obtained as a function of a set of independent variables (i.e., responses from drug concentrations) can be difficult to quantify. Nonlinear curve-fitting procedures allow for a general mathematical relationship to be derived that can depict the response pattern or analyze changes in the response pattern due to other factors. Also, these mathematical relationships can be used to compare data to pharmacologic models of drug-receptor interaction. In general, as with linear regression, a procedure is utilized that determines parameters and minimizes the sum of the squares of the distances between the data points

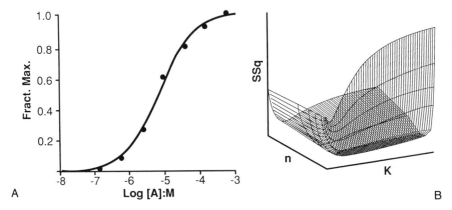

**FIG. 6.11.** Nonlinear regression. **A:** Best-fit line according to Eq. 6.38 for the data points. **B:** Surface topology for sum of squares as n and *K* are varied in Eq. 6.38 for the fit shown in A.

and the calculated curve. This is done iteratively and the process stops after subsequent modification of the parameters fails to reduce the sum of squares by a predetermined amount. For example, Fig. 6.11A shows a data set ($y$ as a function of $x$) fit to a form of the general logistic function given as:

$$y = \frac{x^n}{x^n + K}$$ [6.38]

Initial values for $n$ and $K$ are chosen and the function evaluated. The calculated values of $y$ then are compared to the real data and the individual differences between each calculated and experimental $y$ value for each $x$ is squared (see Eq. 6.20). The sum of these values, called the sum of squares, is an indication of how well the parameters in the function fit the data. These parameters then are altered, the procedure repeated, and the resulting sum of squares compared to the previous one. For a two-parameter equation such as Eq. 6.38, the influence of changes in the parameters $n$ and $K$ on the sum of squares can be depicted as a three-dimensional surface. Figure 6.11B shows the sum of squares surface for various values of $n$ and $K$ for the fit shown in Fig. 6.11A. The aim of nonlinear regression techniques is to find the minimum on this surface and thus achieve the best fit. With equations of greater than two parameters, the topography of the sum of squares versus the parameters cannot be visualized in three-dimensional space but the principles are the same. There are numerous algorithms available to iteratively reduce the sum of squares, and generally there is a balance between the time required for finding the minimum sum of squares and the potential hazards of missing the true minimum and ending at a local minimum removed from the true one.

In fitting data points to models described by equations, the number of parameters can vary. Thus, a model can be made variably flexible to accom-

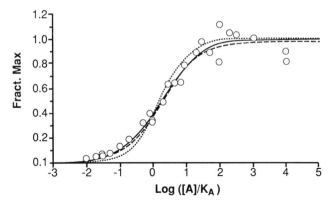

**FIG. 6.12.** Fitting of three equations to dose-response data. *Dotted line* represents the best fit to a single-parameter model (Eq. 6.39), *solid line* to a two-parameter model (Eq. 6.40), and *dashed line* to a three-parameter model (Eq. 6.42). Note the small difference between the last two curves at the expense of the loss of a degree of freedom.

modate nuances in data. For example, Fig. 6.12 shows a set of dependent variables obtained for a given set of independent variables (i.e., a set of responses observed in the presence of a set of drug dosages). These data appear by eye to fit a common sigmoidal curve described by a logistic function. The most simple function would be:

$$Y = \frac{X}{X + K} \qquad [6.39]$$

where $K$ is a location parameter on the $x$ axis. The data set was fit to Eq. 6.39 and the resulting statistical data describing this fit are given in Table 6.24A. A more flexible fit can be achieved by allowing the slope of the logistic

**TABLE 6.24.** *Fitting of different models to a data set*

| Parameter | Standard Error | 95% Confidence limits | d.f. | F |
|---|---|---|---|---|
| *One-parameter logistic* (SS = 0.195) | | | | |
| K = 1.79 | ±0.23 | 1.33–2.26 | 27 | |
| *Two-parameter logistic* (SS = 0.134) | | | | |
| K = 1.84 | ±0.24 | 1.35–2.32 | 26 | Model A to B |
| n = 0.726 | ±0.065 | 0.59–0.86 | | F = 11.12 |
| | | | | d.f. = 1,26 |
| *Three-parameter logistic* (SS = 0.132) | | | | |
| K = 1.71 | ±0.31 | 1.07–2.34 | 25 | Model B to C |
| n = 0.76 | ±0.09 | 0.57–0.94 | | F = 0.45 |
| M = 0.98 | ±0.03 | 0.91–1.05 | | d.f. = 1,25 |

function to vary. Thus, the same data set can be fit to the more flexible equation:

$$Y = \frac{X^n}{X^n + K^n} \qquad [6.40]$$

The fit of the data set to Eq. 6.40 also is shown in Fig. 6.12. The statistical data describing how well Eq. 6.40 fit the data are given in Table 6.24B. These results raise a common question in data analysis, i.e., how flexible should a model be to adequately describe the data and yet be precise enough to allow discernment of difference? One approach to this problem is to calculate an $F$ statistic for the improvement of fit to a model. If two models have the same number of degrees of freedom, then the $F$ statistic is given by $F = SS_1/SS_2$, where $SS_1$ is the sum of squares for Model 1 and $SS_2$ the same for Model 2. Usually, the number of parameters varies between successive models, thus the degrees of freedom are not constant. Under these circumstances, an assessment of the improvement of fit with two models is given by:

$$F = \frac{(SS_1 - SS_2)/(d.f._1 - d.f._2)}{SS_2/d.f._2} \qquad [6.41]$$

where the subscript 1 refers to the simplest model (i.e., larger number of degrees of freedom). Considering the example in Fig. 6.12, the $F$ value for increasing the flexibility of the model by allowing the slope of the logistic function to vary ($n = 1$) is 11.12 (d.f. $= 1,26$). This value is highly significant, indicating that the more complex model fits the data better. A *further* refinement of the model used to describe the data set would be to let the maximum value for the function to vary. Thus, the data could be fit to a three-parameter logistic function of the form:

$$Y = \frac{M \cdot X^n}{X^n + K^n} \qquad [6.42]$$

The fit of the data to Eq. 6.42 is shown in Fig. 6.12 where it can be seen that only a slight reduction in the maximal response is discernible over the fit with Eq. 6.40; the statistical data describing this fit are given in Table 6.24C. The $F$ value for this third model over the second is 0.45 (d.f. $= 1,25$), not statistically significant at the $p < 0.05$ level, thereby indicating that the added flexibility (i.e., loss in degree of freedom) of another parameter did not significantly improve the fit. In general, the larger the number of parameters is, the closer the fit will be to the data. However, the corollary to this is the fact that the larger the number of parameters, the more difficult it will be to discern the determining factors in changes in data and their relationship to pharmacologic models. In general, the simplest model with the fewest parameters is the most useful one for assessing drug-receptor interactions.

Figure 6.12 shows the fit of a single set of data to a model. Another frequently encountered situation is the fit of multiple data sets to a single model.

For example, a simple competitive antagonist of an agonist produces parallel displacement of agonist dose-response curves (see Chapter 9). The responses to any number of agonist ($[A]$) concentrations in the absence and presence of various concentrations of a competitive antagonist ($[B]$) can be modeled with the Gaddum equation:

$$R = \frac{([A]/K_A)^n}{([A]/K)^n + ([B]/K_B)^m + 1}$$ [6.43]

where $K_A$ and $K_B$ are the equilibrium dissociation constants of the agonist-receptor and antagonist-receptor complexes, respectively, and n and m are fitting parameters. The constant m is particularly pharmacologically significant in that a value different from unity implies deviation from simple competitive kinetics (see Chapter 9). Figure 6.13A shows a set of responses to an agonist obtained in the absence (filled circles) and presence of various

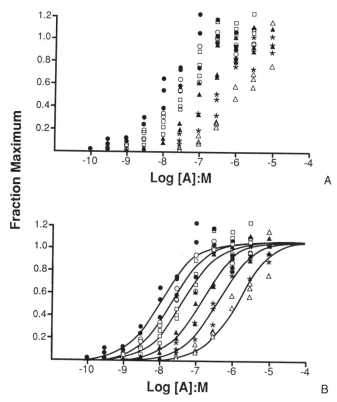

**FIG. 6.13.** Fit of multiple data sets to a single equation. **A:** Responses (ordinates) as a function of various concentrations of an agonist (abscissae, logarithmic scale) obtained in the absence (•) and presence of various concentrations of a competitive antagonist added from 10 nM in threefold increased increments. •, control. **B:** Data fit simultaneously to Eq. 6.43 (see Table 6.26 for parameter values).

**TABLE 6.25.** *Iterative sum of squares*

| Iteration | SS |
|-----------|--------|
| 1 | 1.1273 |
| 2 | 1.117 |
| 3 | 1.093 |
| 4 | 1.086 |
| 5 | 1.085 |
| 6 | 1.084 |
| 7 | 1.084 |

concentrations of antagonist. This data set was fit to Eq. 6.43 utilizing the term $[A]/K_A$ as an operational multiple of agonist concentration and n, m as fitting constants ($[B]$ is known as an added concentration). The reduction in the total sum of squares for this fitting procedure is shown in Table 6.25. The parameters for the best-fit curve are given in Table 6.26. The resulting dose-response curves, shown in Fig. 6.13B, indicate that $[B]$ behaves as a simple competitive antagonist in this system (m is not significantly different from unity) with an equilibrium dissociation constant of 10 nM.

A further advantage can be gained from the fitting of data to simultaneous equations. For example, in biochemical binding studies, the quantity of radioactive ligand that is bound to protein is measured (see Chapter 12). It is assumed in these types of experiments that the ligand binds to a specific population of receptors *and* a number of other nonreceptor sites collectively referred to as "nonspecific" binding. Pharmacologically, the aim is to accurately estimate the relative quantity of ligand bound to the receptors versus the nonspecific binding. The receptor binding, by definition, is assumed to be saturable; thus, a simple Langmuir binding isotherm can be used to model this reaction. The nonspecific binding is nonsaturable and is linear with respect to ligand concentration. Experimentally, a measure of total binding is obtained (i.e., bound radioactivity as a function of radioactive ligand concentration) and also the binding in the presence of a receptor-protecting concentration of nonradioactive ligand that protects receptor, but not nonspecific, binding. This latter measurement defines nonspecific binding. Ostensibly, the difference between the levels of bound radioactivity represents specific receptor binding. Figure 6.14A shows the total binding of radioactive calcito-

**TABLE 6.26.** *Parameters for best-fit curve*

| Parameter | Value | 95% Confidence limits |
|-----------|-------|------------------------|
| n | 0.94 | 0.83–1.05 |
| Max | 1.03 | 0.98–1.07 |
| $K_A$ | $3 \times 10^{-8}$ | $3 \times 10^{-9}$–$1.04 \times 10^{-7}$ |
| m | 1.0 | 0.87–1.14 |
| $K_B$ | $1 \times 10^{-8}$ | $1 \times 10^{-9}$–$3.6 \times 10^{-8}$ |

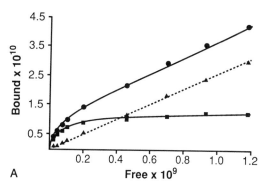

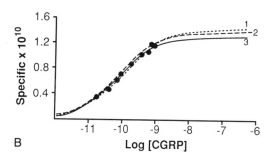

**FIG. 6.14.** Saturation binding experiment for [$^{125}$I]CGRP in membranes from rat cerebellum. **A:** Ordinates; bound radioactivity (i.e., [$A^* \cdot R$]). Abscissae; free radioactive ligand (i.e., [$A^*_f$]). Total bound radioactivity (specific + nonspecific [●]). Nonspecific binding (▲) defined as total binding not displaced by 1 μM unlabeled CGRP. Saturable binding (■) calculated as a rectangular hyperbolic function obtained from a simultaneous curve-fitting procedure on total binding curves and curve for nonspecific binding according to Eqs. 6.45 and 6.46, respectively. The data points on the specific binding curve are experimentally obtained values for specific binding. **B:** The specific binding of [$^{125}$I]CGRP on a logarithmic scale. Curve 1 represents the best fit of the specific binding to Eq. 6.44. Curve 2 is the saturation curve obtained by a fit of the total binding (curve 1 in A.) to Eq. 6.45. Curve 3 obtained from the simultaneous fitting of the total binding (curve 1 in A) and nonspecific binding (curve 2 in A) to Eqs. 6.45 and 6.46. (Data from ref. 3.)

nin gene-related peptide (CGRP) to membranes from rat cerebellum in the absence (total binding) and presence (nonspecific) binding of a receptor-protecting concentration of nonradioactive CGRP. The difference between these values is assumed to be receptor-specific binding. One approach to the quantification of specific receptor binding is to fit the experimentally derived (by subtraction), specific binding values to the model of the Langmuir adsorption isotherm:

$$[A^* \cdot R] = \frac{[A^*]^n \cdot [R_t]}{[A^*]^n + K_A} \qquad [6.44]$$

where $K_A$ is the equilibrium dissociation constant of the ligand-receptor complex. Figure 6.14B shows the experimentally derived values for specific binding fit to Eq. 6.44. A frequent practical problem in these types of experiments is the accurate determination of maximal binding (i.e., [$R_t$]) since this can only be obtained when [$A$] → ∞). This quantity, however, is experimentally important because it scales quantitative measures of ligand activity such as $K_A$. As can be seen from Fig. 6.14, Eq. 6.44 can be used to fit the existing data points and estimate the maximum for the curve. However, the paucity of data points at the higher end of the curve can cause overestimation of the maximum. A refinement of this estimate can be made with the added term for nonspecific binding to the total bound radioactivity curve. Since total binding ([TB]) is the sum of the saturable binding to the receptors and the linear unsaturable binding to nonreceptor sites, it can be described by the sum of a hyperbolic and linear function:

$$[TB] = \frac{[A^*]^n \cdot [R_t]}{[A^*]^n + K_A} + d \cdot [A^*] \qquad [6.45]$$

where $d$ reflects the slope of the linear relationship between ligand concentration and binding to nonreceptor sites and nonspecific binding ([NSB]) is described by the straight-line relationship:

$$[NSB] = d \cdot [A^*] \qquad [6.46]$$

A fit of the total binding curve (shown in Fig. 6.14A) to Eq. 6.45 yields estimates for n and $K_A$ to define curve 2 for the specific receptor binding shown in Fig. 6.14B. However, a more accurate estimate of the binding parameters can be made by utilizing all of the total and nonspecific binding data simultaneously. Thus, the total binding curve can be fit to Eq. 6.45 and the nonspecific binding to the linear Eq. 6.46 simultaneously. Under these circumstances the maximal value $[R_t]$ is the difference between the total binding and nonspecific binding at high ligand concentrations and can be estimated from the parallel regions of the nonspecific and total binding curves. A simultaneous fit of the total and nonspecific binding curves to estimate specific receptor binding yields values of n and $K_A$ to define curve 3 shown in Fig. 6.14B. As can be seen from this figure, the maximal value for receptor saturation ($[R_t]$) is significantly lower when this method is used but also more accurate because more of the available experimental data are used. This is an example of where simultaneous curve fitting methods can provide an added advantage in the utilization of obtainable experimental data.

Once a model has been chosen to fit the data, an assessment must be made of the goodness of fit. If a minimal sum of squares converges but the calculated curve does not fit the data particularly well, it is possible that an inappropriate model has been chosen. One way to assess the appropriateness of a model is to examine residuals, which are the distance of each y value from the calculated curve. If the model is appropriate, then the residuals should represent only experimental error and be randomly distributed, i.e., not be systematically related to $x$ values. An inappropriate model would tend to cluster in parts of the residual graph when plotted as a function of $y$; i.e., the data points differ systematically from the curve. Figure 6.15 shows a data set fit to a hyperbola and an exponential function. Both calculated lines appear by eye to fit the data aduately, but it can be seen from the residual plots that, whereas the residuals from the hyperbolic fit vary in a random fashion above and below zero, the residuals from the exponential plot are

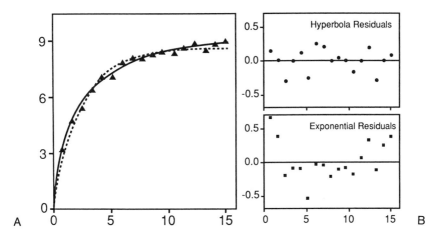

**FIG. 6.15.** Residual plots. **A:** Data set fit to two different models, namely, a hyperbola ($y = Ax/(B + x)$ [*solid line*]) and exponential function ($y = A[1 - e^{-Bx}]$ [*dotted line*]). *Insets* show the resulting residuals for each model and indicate that the residuals from the hyperbolic fit are more randomly distributed about 0. (From ref. 14.)

systematic; i.e., they are repeatedly below zero in the middle of the curve. These data indicate that a hyperbolic function best fits the data.

## REFERENCES

1. Armitage, P. (1971): *Statistical Methods in Medical Research.* Blackwell, Oxford.
2. Barlow, R. (1990): Cumulative frequency curves in population analysis. *Trends Pharmacol. Sci.,* 11:404–406.
3. Chatterjee, T. K., and Fisher, R. (1991): Multiple affinity forms of the calcitonin gene-related peptide receptor in rat cerebellum. *Mol. Pharmacol.,* 39:798–804.
4. Colquhoun, D. (1971): *Lectures in Biostatistics.* Clarendon Press, Oxford.
5. Cook, D. A., and Bielkiewicz, B. (1984): A computer assisted technique for analysis and comparison of dose-response curves. *J. Pharmacol. Meth.,* 11:77–89.
6. Dowd, J. E., and Riggs, D. S. (1965): A comparison of estimates of Michaelis-Menten kinetic constants form various linear transformations. *J. Biol. Chem.,* 240:863–869.
7. Endrenyi, L., and Patel, M. (1991): Evaluation of two assumptions: Single line, and single normal distribution. *Trends Pharmacol. Sci.,* 12:293–296.
8. Finney, D. J. (1955): *Experimental Design and Its Statistical Basis.* University of Chicago Press, Chicago.
9. Fleming, W. W., Westfall, D. P., De La Lande, I. S., and Jellet, L. B. (1972): Log-normal distribution of equieffective doses of norepinephrine and acetylcholine in several tissues. *J. Pharmacol. Exp. Ther.,* 181:339–345.
10. Gaddum, J. H. (1953): Bioassays and mathematics. *Pharmacol. Rev.,* 5:87–134.
11. Kenakin, T. P. (1982): The potentiation of cardiac responses to adenosine by benzodiazepines. *J. Pharmacol. Exp. Ther.,* 222:752–758.
12. Kenakin, T. P., and Beek, D. (1985): The activity of nifedipine, diltiazem, verapamil and lidoflazine in isolated tissues: An approach to the determination of calcium channel blocking activity. *Drug Dev. Res.,* 5:347–358.
13. Kenakin, T. P., and Johnson, S. F. (1985): The importance of the α-adrenoceptor agonist activity of dobutamine to inotropic selectivity in the anaesthetized cat. *Eur. J. Pharmacol.,* 111:347–354.

14. Motulsky, H. J., and Ransnas, L. A. (1987): Fitting curves to data using nonlinear regression: A practical and nonmathematical view. *FASEB J.*, 1:365–374.
15. Plumbridge, T. W., Aarons, L. J., and Brown, J. R. (1978): Problems associated with analysis and interpretation of small molecule/macromolecule binding data. *J. Pharm. Pharmacol.*, 30:69–74.
16. Riggs, D. S. (1963): *The Mathematical Approach to Physiological Problems.* Williams & Wilkins, Baltimore.
17. Snedecor, G. W., and Cochran, W. G. (1979): *Statistical Methods.* Iowa State University Press, Ames.
18. Tallarida, R. J., and Murray, R. G. (1979): *Manual of Pharmacologic Calculations with Computer Programs.* Springer-Verlag, Berlin.
19. Waud, D. R. (1976): Analysis of dose-response relationships. In: *Advances in General and Cellular Pharmacology,* edited by T. L. Narahashi and C. P. Bianchi, pp. 145–178. Plenum Press, New York.
20. Waud, D. R., and Parker, R. B. (1971): Pharmacological estimation of drug-receptor dissociation constants. Statistical evaluation. II. Competitive antagonists. *J. Pharmacol. Exp. Ther.*, 177:13–24.
21. Waud, D. R., Son, S. L., and Waud, B. E. (1978): Kinetic and empirical analysis of dose-response curves illustrated with a cardiac example. *Life Sci.*, 22:1275–1286.
22. Wilkinson, G. N. (1961): Statistical estimations in enzyme kinetics. *Biochem. J.*, 80: 324–332.

# 7

## Agonist Affinity

*[The equilibrium dissociation constant] defines the signal-to-noise ratio in the
chemical cacophony which surrounds every cell.*

—SIR JAMES BLACK, 1982

It is presumed that an agonist must intimately associate with a receptor to
produce a response. The property of attraction of a drug for a receptor is
termed the *affinity*. The numerical representation of affinity is the reciprocal
of the equilibrium dissociation constant of the agonist-receptor complex denoted $K_A$ (see Chapter 1). This term is used to quantify the affinity of a drug
because it is chemical in nature, with thermodynamic theoretical rationale;
specifically, it is the rate constant for offset ($k_2$) divided by the rate constant
for onset ($k_1$). The binding of a drug to a receptor is stochastic and should
be viewed not as a static process of binding and occupation but rather as a
kinetic process of drug molecules moving toward and away from drug receptors at various rates. The fraction of drug receptors occupied at any one
instant depends on the relative rates of onset and offset of the drug for the
receptor. As noted in Chapter 2, because of cellular amplification systems for
receptor stimuli, the concentration of agonist that produces half the maximal
response, especially for full agonists, most often does not correspond to the
agonist concentration that occupies half of the receptor population. For this
reason, null methods must be used to measure $K_A$ for agonists. Before discussion of these methods, some background on the molecular nature of affinity
will be useful.

### THE MOLECULAR NATURE OF AFFINITY

The affinity of a drug for a receptor can be thought of as the frequency
with which the drug, when brought into the proximity of a receptor by diffusion, will reside at a position of minimum free energy (the equilibrium position) within the force field of that receptor. The first step to drug binding is

*221*

diffusion to the receptor ($k_{D1}$, $k_{D2}$); the second is formation of the drug-receptor complex when the drug enters the force field of the receptor [i.e., when intermolecular forces modify diffusion rate constants ($k'_{D1}$, $k'_{D2}$)].

$$D + R \underset{k_{D2}}{\overset{k_{D1}}{\rightleftharpoons}} D{\cdot}R \underset{k'_{D2}}{\overset{k'_{D1}}{\rightleftharpoons}} D{\cdot}R \qquad [7.1]$$

The association rate constant for diffusion to the receptor ($k_{D1}$) can be calculated with Smoluchowski's equation:

$$k_{D1} = \frac{4\pi NDr}{1,000} \qquad [7.2]$$

where $N$ is Avogadro's number, $D$ is the coefficient of diffusion, and $r$ is the radius of the target on the receptor. When combined with the Stokes-Einstein equation (Eq. 4.8), the diffusion rate constant becomes

$$k_{D1} = \frac{2RT}{3,000\eta} \qquad [7.3]$$

where $R$ is the universal gas constant, $T$ is absolute temperature, and $\eta$ is the viscosity of the medium. This equation assumes a close spatial correspondence between the target on the receptor and the drug molecule; in certain cases of polymeric drugs or large peptides, this may not be a valid assumption (i.e., the site corresponding to the target may be considerably smaller than the effective radius of the molecule). Assuming that the effective radii correspond, $k_{D1}$ in water at 37°C was calculated by Burgen (5) to be $2.5 \times 10^9$ sec mol$^{-1}$. It should be noted that there can be factors present in drug-receptor interactions that can seriously affect $k_{D1}$. For example, the arrangement of water molecules into an icelike structure around hydrophobic regions of drug molecules can increase the effective radius of the molecule; in this event, the Stokes-Einstein equation (Eq. 4.8) predicts a decrease in diffusion rate. Hydration of proteins and other structures near the receptor may produce an anisotropic medium (nonhomogeneous), the result being a decrease in the diffusion coefficient. Another major factor in the modification of $k_{D1}$ is possible steric hindrance to the drug on its path to the receptor (i.e., the receptor may reside at the end of an effective tunnel of structures with respect to forces of diffusion). In this case, diffusive displacements are no longer random.

Once the drug closely approaches the receptor, a series of intermolecular forces can modify $k_{D1}$, and the effective rate constant for association within the force field of the receptor becomes $k_{D1}$, multiplied by Debye's function:

$$k'_{D1} = k_{D1}{\cdot}Y \qquad [7.4]$$

Debye's function is

$$Y = \left( a \int_a^\infty e^{(u/\kappa T)} \frac{dr}{r^2} \right)^{-1} \qquad [7.5]$$

where $a$ is the distance of closest approach, $u$ is the potential energy of interaction, $r$ is the distance between reactants, and $\kappa$ is Boltzmann's constant.

The force field normal to the receptor surface experienced by a drug molecule consists of electrostatic, dispersion, and hydrophobic forces. Electrostatic interactions probably are important in the first orientation of the drug to the receptor. The attractive forces between oppositely charged groups vary with the reciprocal of the distance between the drug and receptor and thus form the long-range intermolecular forces (although shielding effects shorten the effective distance at which these forces are operative). Other forces that become important at different distances between the drug and receptor are dipole-dipole or ion-dipole bonds (created by unequal distribution of electrons), hydrogen bonds (between hydrogen atoms), and induced dipole bonds (due to distortion of outer electron orbits). A major contribution results from the interaction of hydrophobic groups and water. The icelike structures of water around hydrophobic groups on the drug molecule and the receptor rearrange when these groups approach one another to form an all-inclusive structure around both, leading to a transfer of free energy, possibly by a gain in entropy. Hydration can also affect coulombic interactions by affecting the dielectric constant near the receptor.

Burgen (5) showed that most intermolecular forces depend on distance by a general function:

$$u = cr^{-p} \qquad [7.6]$$

where $c$ is a constant and $p$ is a power of inverse relationship. The effects of distance on various intermolecular forces are shown in Table 7.1, it can be seen that different forces take on different orders of importance as the drug approaches the target site.

**TABLE 7.1.** *Strengths of electrostatic bonds*

| Type | Energy of bond[a] (kJ mol$^{-1}$ per bond) | Strength-vs.-distance relationship |
|---|---|---|
| Ion-ion | 20–40 | $1/d$ |
| Ion-dipole | 8–20 | $1/d^2$ |
| Dipole-dipole | 3–15 | $1/d^3$ |
| Hydrogen | 5–25 | $1/d^4$ |
| Induced dipoles | 0.5–5 | $1/d^5$–$1/d^8$ |

[a] At typical bond length.
From ref. 4.

Thus, the rate constant for association is given by the $k_{D1}$ from Smoluchowski's equation modified by $Y$, the magnitude of this latter function being dependent on the nature of the intermolecular forces and the distances between the drug and the receptor. In general, as the drug closely approaches the receptor, repulsive forces have a strong reducing effect on $k_{D1}$, and attractive forces do not raise $k_{D1}$ substantially.

The universal repulsive force results from invasion of the van der Waals envelope of atoms, for which $p = 9$ to $12$. Because attractive forces predominate in drug-receptor interactions, the rate constant for dissociation in the force field ($k'_{D2}$) will be decreased below the limit for diffusion-controlled dissociation ($k_{D2}$). This decrease can be quantified by a multiplicative factor $Y'$ for $k_{D2}$ that depends on the nature of the forces and distance. For example, for predominant coulombic forces,

$$k'_{D2} = k_{D2} \cdot Y' \qquad [7.7]$$

where

$$Y' = \omega/(1 - e^{-\omega}) \qquad [7.8]$$

The magnitude of the factor $\omega$ depends on the respective valencies of the drug and receptor sites, the electronic charge, temperature, and the dielectric constant of the medium.

The combination of these effects creates a distance of minimum free energy at which the drug will reside in the influence of the receptor. The changes in energy when this distance is increased or decreased are shown in Fig. 7.1A. The drug will escape the force field of the receptor only when it gains enough kinetic energy (by thermal agitation) to do so. The proportion of molecules that attain this energy is given by the Boltzmann equation:

$$f = e^{-u/RT} \qquad [7.9]$$

Therefore, if a drug is bound to a receptor with an electrostatic-bond energy of 5 kJ mol$^{-1}$, the probability that it will attain sufficient kinetic energy from random thermal collision between molecules to escape the force field of the receptor can be calculated with Eq. 7.9 to be 0.14 (i.e., at any given instant, seven of every 50 drug molecules will attain escape energy and diffuse away from the receptor). A drug with a higher bond energy (e.g., 35 kJ mol$^{-1}$) will have a much lower probability of attaining escape energy ($f = 1.2 \times 10^{-6}$, or six in every 5 million drug molecules). Because molecular collisions supply thermal kinetic energy, drug molecules are constantly moving toward and away from the receptor; they do not reside motionless in the receptor target site. Thus, a drug with newly acquired kinetic energy will move away from the receptor and stop when its kinetic energy is balanced by the increased potential energy of its new position; then the potential-energy gradient will return the molecule to the equilibrium distance. The same occurs when the drug moves toward the receptor, only it will not go

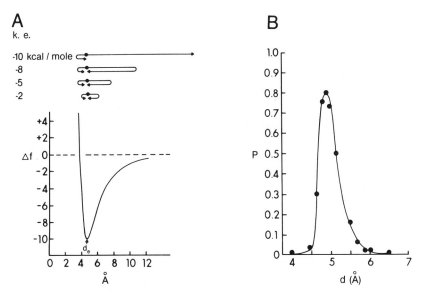

**FIG. 7.1.** Position of a drug in the force field of a receptor. **A:** Potential-energy diagram for a drug residing at the equilibrium distance ($d_e$ = 5Å at the energy minimum assuming a free energy of interaction of $-10$ kcal mol$^{-1}$). Attractive forces assumed to be $p$ = 3–6, and repulsive force $p$ = 9; energy $\Delta f$ in kcal mol$^{-1}$. Upper part of diagram shows behavior of molecules initially at $d_e$ and acquiring various levels of kinetic energy. **B:** Probability (ordinate) of finding a drug at a given distance at any instant in the lifetime of the drug-receptor complex for model given in A. (From ref. 5.)

as far because of the much larger increases in the field produced (i.e., $p$ = 9–12). The probability of finding the drug at a distance of greater or lesser magnitude than the equilibrium distance at any instant can be calculated with Boltzmann's equation and is shown in Fig. 7.1B.

## AFFINITY OF FULL AGONISTS: PARTIAL ALKYLATION METHOD

Measurements of full-agonist affinity can be made by a procedure developed by Furchgott (9) that compares dose-response curves for the agonist before and after irreversible elimination (usually by chemical alkylation) of some portion of the receptor population. The receptor stimulation by the agonist in the control situation (no receptors alkylated) is given by

$$S_A = \frac{\epsilon_A[A][R_t]}{[A] + K_A} \qquad [7.10]$$

After controlled alkylation of a certain proportion of receptors, a fraction $q$ remains operative for production of a stimulus. The receptor stimulation to a dose of agonist $[A']$ becomes

$$S_A = \frac{\epsilon_A[A'][R_t \cdot q]}{[A'] + K_A} \quad\quad [7.11]$$

If this procedure is carried out in a given tissue, then comparison of equal responses should compare conditions of equal receptor occupancies for the agonist (assuming no change has occurred with respect to stimulus-response coupling). Therefore, equating 7.10 and 7.11,

$$\frac{[A]}{[A] + K_A} = \frac{[A']}{[A'] + K_A} \cdot q \quad\quad [7.12]$$

which rearranges to the double-reciprocal equation

$$\frac{1}{[A]} = \frac{1}{[A']} \cdot \frac{1}{q} + \frac{1}{K_A} \cdot \frac{1 - q}{q} \quad\quad [7.13]$$

where $[A]$ and $[A']$ are equiactive agonist concentrations before and after receptor alkylation, respectively. According to this equation, a double-reciprocal plot of $1/[A]$ versus $1/[A']$ should yield a straight line with a slope of $1/q$ and intercept of $(1 - q)/q \cdot K_A$. Therefore, $K_A$ can be calculated as

$$K_A = \frac{\text{slope} - 1}{\text{intercept}} \quad\quad [7.14]$$

Noting the caveats associated with double-reciprocal plots given in an earlier section, Eq. 7.13 can be rewritten

$$\frac{[A']}{[A]} = \frac{1 - q}{q \cdot K_A} \cdot [A'] + \frac{1}{q} \qu\quad [7.15]$$

where

$$K_A = \frac{\text{intercept} - 1}{\text{slope}} \quad\quad [7.16]$$

and

$$[A] = \frac{q \cdot K_A}{1 - q} - \frac{K_A}{1 - q} \cdot \frac{[A]}{[A']} \quad\quad [7.17]$$

where

$$K_A = -(S + I) \quad\quad [7.18]$$

In practical terms, this technique requires that a sufficient fraction of the receptor population be irreversibly inactivated such that the maximal response to the full agonist is depressed.

As discussed in Chapter 1, another major theoretical framework for drug-receptor kinetics is the operational model. It is useful to discuss the various methods of estimating agonist affinity with both occupation theory and the operational model. As shown in Chapter 1, the equation for agonist response in the operational model is:

$$\frac{E_a}{E_m} = \frac{[A]\cdot\tau}{K_A + (\tau + 1)\cdot[A]} \qquad [7.19]$$

where $\tau$ is defined as the receptor density $[R_t]$ divided by $K_E$, the quantity of ternary complex required for half-maximal response, and $E_m$ the maximal response of the receptor system in the tissue. Therefore, receptor alkylation to depress the maximal response to a factor $q$ (multiple of $[R_t]$) would correspond to a new value for $\tau$ (denoted $\tau'$ where $\tau' = \tau\cdot q$). Under these circum-

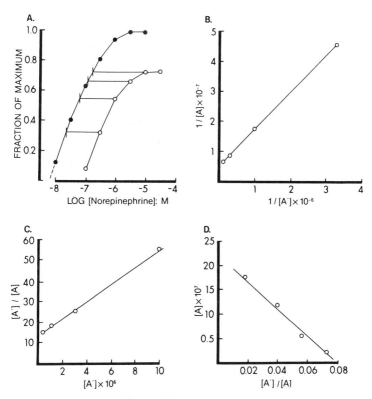

**FIG. 7.2.** Estimation of $K_A$ for norepinephrine in rat anococcygeus muscle. **A:** Dose-response curves to norepinephrine. Ordinate: Contractions as fractions of the maximal contraction to norepinephrine before receptor alkylation. Abscissa: Logarithms of molar concentrations of norepinephrine. Responses before (●) and after (○) treatment with phenoxybenzamine (0.3 μM, 10 min). **B:** Double-reciprocal plot for equiactive concentrations of norepinephrine according to Eq. 7.13. Intercept = $4.56 \times 10^6$; slope = 12.4; $K_A = 2.49$ μM. **C:** Regression from same data according to Eq. 7.22. Intercept = 12.7; slope = $4.32 \times 10^6$; $K_A = 2.7$ μM. **D:** Regression according to Eq. 7.24. Intercept = 0.23 μM; slope = $-2.92$ μM; $K_A = 2.69$ μM.

stances, the double-reciprocal equation for the partial alkylation method would be:

$$\frac{1}{[A]} = \frac{1}{[A']} \cdot \frac{\tau}{\tau'} + \left[\frac{\tau - \tau'}{\tau'}\right] \cdot \frac{1}{K_A} \qquad [7.20]$$

It can be seen from Eq. 7.20 that a double-reciprocal plot within this framework would still be linear and that Eq. 7.14 would still yield an estimate of the $K_A$. Figure 7.2 shows the use of the partial alkylation method for the estimation of $K_A$ for norepinephrine in the rat anococcygeus muscle.

As discussed in Chapter 6, with the availability of computer modeling and data-fitting packages, there is less need to rely on transformed data (i.e., linearized versions of data sets). With these techniques the dose-response curves to an agonist from a control and partially alkylated state could be compared directly with equations describing classical occupation theory (Eq. 7.12 where $[A]$ and $[A']$ are fit with a given value for $q$ and common $K_A$) or the operational model. For example, a series of serially alkylated, and thus depressed, dose-response curves could be fit with a set of common values for $K_A$ and $E_m$ and a curve fit for varying values of $\tau'$. Figure 7.3 shows an example of this procedure for serotonin on rabbit aorta. The data set was simultaneously fit to the nonconstrained (not necessarily hyperbolic) form of Eq. 7.19 with constant $E_m$, $K_A$, n, and varying values for $\tau$. It can be seen from this figure that a common $K_A$ value of 0.16 μM adequately fits the complete data set.

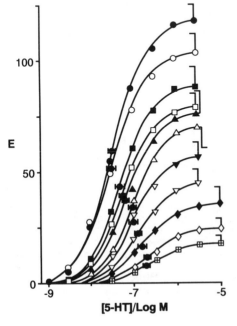

FIG. 7.3. Concentration-response curves for serotonin (5-HT) contraction of rabbit aorta. Ordinate: Response as a percentage of the value observed at 5-HT = 10 μM. Abscissa: Logarithms of molar concentrations of 5-HT. Curves obtained after treatment with phenoxybenzamine (10 min exposure) at the following concentrations (in nM): 0 (●), 12.5 (○), 30 (■), 80 (□), 125 (▲), 200 (△), 300 (▼), 500 (▽), 800 (◆), 1250 (◇), and 3000 (⊞). Bars represent SEM. (From ref. 3.)

E

[5-HT]/Log M

## TWO-STAGE AGONIST BINDING AND RECEPTOR DISTRIBUTION

By their very nature agonists change receptors to impart a message to the physiological system. This process can be viewed as an isomerization of the receptor from a state $R$ to $R^*$, the latter form being the transformed receptor (i.e., message received) altered by binding of agonist.

$$A + R \xrightarrow{K_A} A \cdot R \underset{\alpha}{\overset{\beta}{\longrightarrow}} A \cdot R^* \qquad \overset{K_{obs}}{\longrightarrow}$$

[7.21]

It should be noted that no mechanism is implied by this scheme and that the change could come about either by conformational induction (the agonist imposes a conformational change in the tertiary structure of the receptor) or conformational selection (the agonist preferentially binds to one or more of preexisting conformations of the receptor). These mechanisms are discussed more fully in Chapter 8. The difference between $R$ and $R^*$ could take on many forms including the change from a shut to an open ion channel, or the formation of a ternary complex with other membrane-bound coupling proteins. The essential part of the scheme is that $R$ is not identical to $R^*$, and thus the equilibrium between the agonist $A$ and $R$ cannot only be described by $K_A$. This is because the isomerization process removes $A \cdot R$ from the equilibrium by driving the reaction toward $A \cdot R^*$, thus allowing the formation of more $A \cdot R$ than would normally be allowed by $K_A$. The extent to which this secondary reaction perturbs the equilibrium between $A$ and $R$ depends on the relative magnitudes of $\alpha$ and $\beta$. Therefore, the observed equilibrium dissociation constant ($K_{obs}$) for $A \cdot R^*$ is comprised of $K_A$ *and* $K_{obs}$ defined by $\alpha$ and $\beta$:

$$K_{obs} = \frac{K_A}{1 + \beta/\alpha}$$

[7.22]

It can be seen from Eq. 7.22 that the isomerization process causes the observed affinity of the agonist to appear to be higher than the true affinity of the agonist for the receptor ($K_{obs} < K_A$).

One of the most well-defined systems for such receptor isomerization is the two-stage binding of agonists to G protein–linked receptors to form ternary complexes. Thus, the agonist $[A]$ binds to the receptor $[R]$ and promotes the further binding of the receptor to a membrane-bound protein coupler $[T]$ for the production of response

$$A + R \xrightarrow{K_1} A \cdot R + T \xrightarrow{K_2} A \cdot R \cdot T \qquad \overset{K_{obs}}{\longrightarrow}$$

[7.23]

As with the general isomerization model, the observed equilibrium dissociation constant is given by:

$$K_{obs} = \frac{K_1}{1 + ([T] - [A \cdot R \cdot T])/K_2} \qquad [7.24]$$

For functional systems it might be assumed that, due to receptor-stimulus cellular amplification systems, the amount of ternary complex required for the production of measurable response is low and that $[A \cdot R \cdot T] \ll [T]$. Under these circumstances:

$$K_{obs} = \frac{K_1}{1 + [T]/K_2} \qquad [7.25]$$

From Eq. 7.25 it can be seen that the difference between the observed affinity of the agonist for the receptor system and $K_1$, the equilibrium dissociation constant of the $A \cdot R$ complex, is dependent on the magnitude of $K_2$ and the quantity of receptor coupler $[T]$. Table 7.2 shows the effects of increasing amounts of coupling protein $[T]$ (in this case $G_o$) on the $K_{obs}$ for oxotremorine in a reconstituted system for muscarinic receptors. It can be seen from this table that increasing amounts of $[G_o]$ produce increasing affinity of the system for the agonist. Figure 7.4 shows the relationship between these parameters. The greater the propensity of the agonist to produce secondary coupling (i.e., the smaller $K_2$ is), the smaller the $K_{obs}$ will be relative to the true $K_A$. Mechanistically, the magnitude of $K_2$ can be linked to intrinsic efficacy (see Chapter 8) if the resulting ternary complex ($[A \cdot R \cdot T]$) leads to activation of a response pathway in the cell. Therefore, Eq. 7.25 predicts that $K_{obs}$ can be lower than $K_1$ for agonists of high efficacy.

Two-stage binding can produce differences between the estimation of the true $K_A$ ($K_1$ in terms of the initial binding of agonist to receptor) and the observed $K_A$ by the partial alkylation method. If a two-stage binding process

**TABLE 7.2.** Effect of coupling protein $(G_0)$ on oxotremorine potency

| $[R_t]^a$ (pmol) | $[T]^b$ (pmol) | IC$_{50}$ ($-$GTP)$^c$ ($\mu$M) | IC$_{50}$ ($+$GTP)$^d$ ($\mu$M) | Ratio |
|---|---|---|---|---|
| 5.7 | 36 | 4.0 | 9 | 2 |
| 5.7 | 180 | 1.5 | 7 | 5 |
| 5.7 | 920 | 0.25 | 8 | 30 |
| 5.7 | 4,600 | 0.02 | 15 | 800 |

[a] Purified muscarinic receptor.
[b] $G_0$.
[c] Concentration of oxotremorine required for half-maximal displacement of [$^3$H]L-quinuclidinyl benzilate from muscarinic receptors. This value measured in system favoring ternary complex formation (no GTP present).
[d] As for note c but in the presence of an excess of GTP where ternary complex formation does not occur (i.e., production of $[A \cdot R]$ only).
From ref. 8.

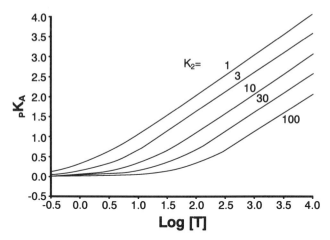

**FIG. 7.4.** Observed agonist affinity as a function of coupler protein [T] availability. Ordinate: $-\text{Log } K_{\text{obs}}$. Abscissa: Logarithms of molar concentration of coupling protein [T]. Curves shown for agonists with $K_2 = 1,3,10,30,100$.

is operable, then the double-reciprocal relationship for Eq. 7.13 represents:

$$\frac{1}{[A]} = \frac{1}{[A]} \cdot \frac{1}{q} + 1 + \left(\frac{([T] - [A \cdot R \cdot T])}{K_2}\right)\left(\frac{1-q}{q}\right) \cdot \frac{1}{K_1} \qquad [7.26]$$

If $[A \cdot R \cdot T]$ is negligible, Eq. 7.26 reduces to:

$$\frac{1}{[A]} = \frac{1}{[A']} \cdot \frac{1}{q} + \frac{1}{K_1} \cdot \left(\frac{(1-q)}{q}\right)\left(1 + \frac{[T]}{K_2}\right) \qquad [7.27]$$

Therefore, using Eq. 7.14 to estimate $K_A$ still yields an estimate of an apparent $K_A$ given by Eq. 7.25; i.e., the partial alkylation method will yield $K_{\text{obs}}$ and not necessarily $K_1$.

In terms of the methods of measuring the initial binding of agonists to receptors (i.e., of accurately determining $K_1$), two-stage binding such as that shown in Eq. 7.23 can be a serious obfuscation. Black and Shankley (3) have termed the effective removal of free receptor from the equilibrium between agonist and receptor by isomerization *receptor distribution* since the receptors are distributed among the states $[R]$, $[A \cdot R]$, and $[A \cdot R \cdot T]$. It is worth considering possible methods to determine whether receptor distribution is a tangible problem in $K_A$ measurements. A straightforward approach to the study of receptor distribution is to use the operational model. It should be noted that the equations describing classical occupation theory are consistent with this analysis as well, but that the operational model offers an explicit and convenient theoretical framework for the effect. In terms of the operational model (see Chapter 1 for details), the response $E_a$ to an agonist $[A]$

is given by Eq. 7.19. The experimentally measurable maximal response to an agonist (not necessarily the maximal tissue response) can be defined by a term $\alpha$:

$$\text{asymptote} \atop {\scriptstyle (E_a \text{ as } [A] \to \infty)} = \alpha = \frac{E_m \tau}{\tau + 1} \tag{7.28}$$

Similarly, the concentration of agonist producing half-maximal response (denoted as $A_{50}$) can be obtained by calculating $[A]$ when $E_a/\alpha = 0.5$. With this quantity and combining Eqs. 7.19 and 7.28:

$$\frac{E_a}{\alpha} = 0.5 = \frac{A_{50}(1 + \tau)}{K_A + A_{50}(1 + \tau)} \tag{7.29}$$

which reduces to:

$$[A_{50}] = \frac{K_A}{1 + \tau} \tag{7.30}$$

Equating $\tau$ from Eqs. 7.28 and 7.30, it can be shown that:

$$-\log(1 - \alpha/E_m) = -\log[A_{50}] + \log K_A \tag{7.31}$$

This equation can be useful as a means to compare experimentally observed parameters in systems that do and do not demonstrate receptor distribution. As discussed earlier, a common method to experimentally estimate the equilibrium dissociation constant of an agonist-receptor complex is to serially decrease the receptor density and compare equiactive responses to the agonist. Equation 7.31 can be used to predict the relationship between the maximal response to the agonist before and after receptor alkylation and the $A_{50}$ concentrations. Figure 7.5A shows the effect of decreasing receptor density on dose-response curves to an agonist in a measuring system where receptor distribution is not obtained. The ordinate axis for response is the quantity of $[A \cdot R \cdot T]$ complex formed by the agonist. It should be stressed that this restricts the conclusions of these simulations to the simplest, but not necessarily most common, model of receptor coupling, namely, a linear relationship between receptor occupancy and tissue response. Also, it is assumed that receptor occupancy and the subsequent production of $[A \cdot R \cdot T]$ follows a hyperbolic relationship. The analysis will be extended beyond these confining conditions further on. As can be seen from this simulation, receptor diminution produces dextral displacement of the dose-response curve followed by depression of the maximal response. As predicted for this system, location parameters of the dose-response curves ($A_{50}$ values) converge to the true $K_A$. Figure 7.5B shows the relationship between the metameter for maximal response ($1 - \alpha/E_m$) and $A_{50}$. As with the $A_{50}$ values of the depressed dose-response curves, the $A_{50}$ at zero response equals the true $K_A$. In contrast, Fig. 7.5C shows the effect of decreases in receptor density in a

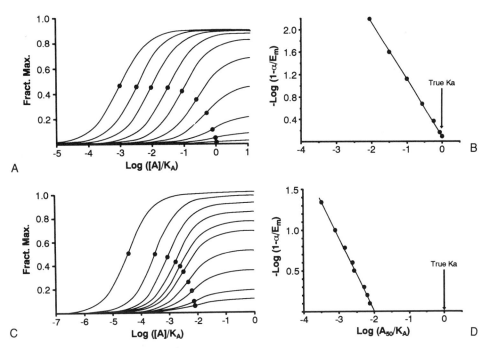

**FIG. 7.5.** Effects of decreases in receptor density on dose-response curves to agonists. **A:** Theoretical dose-response curves to an agonist where receptor distribution does not occur. $K_2 = 10^{-2}$, $[T] = 0.0001$, $[R]$ for curves left to right in threefold decreasing increments from 10 to 0.0003. **B:** Plot of maximal effect (as $-\log(1 - \alpha/E_m)$ versus $-\log$ of the molar concentration of agonist producing 50% maximal effect. Data points from curves shown in A. Abscissal intercept equals the true $K_A(K_1)$ for agonist-receptor binding. **C:** Theoretical dose-response curves for the agonists in a system in which receptor distribution occurs. $[T] = 1$, $[R]$ for curves from left to right 3, 1, 0.3, 0.2, 0.1, 0.05, 0.03, 0.01, 0.005, 0.003, and 0.0003. **D:** Plot as for B, where data points taken from curves shown in C. Although the plot is linear, the abscissal intercept is far short of the true $K_A(K_1)$.

system in which the receptor is significantly distributed between the states $[R]$, $[A \cdot R]$, and $[A \cdot R \cdot T]$. In this system, the secondary coupling of receptor to $[T]$ effectively consumes $[R]$, making the total binding reaction subject to $K_1$, $K_2$, and $[T]$. Under these circumstances, the observed $K_A$ is abstracted from the true one by the secondary binding process and $K_{obs}$ is less than $K_A$. This is shown by the fact that the dose-response curves collapse to a point of lower magnitude than the true $K_A$. The relationship between $(1 - \alpha/E_m)$ and $A_{50}$ is shown in Fig. 7.5D. In this case the relationship between the $(1 - \alpha/E_m)$ and $A_{50}$ again is linear with an intercept far short of the true $K_A$.

One hallmark of receptor distribution is the considerably steeper parabolic relationship between the $A_{50}$ values of the depressed dose-response curves and the maximal response. A comparison of Fig. 7.5A and C shows how receptor alkylation in the receptor-distributed system (Fig. 7.5C) produces a steeper decline in the response than in systems with no receptor distribution. Unfortunately, this experimentally observable feature of receptor distribution can be masked by nonlinear stimulus-response mechanisms. The simulations shown in Fig. 7.5 are for systems in which the tissue response is linearly related to the production of $[A \cdot R \cdot T]$. If this is not the case and if a nonlinear function intervenes between receptor occupancy and tissue response, then the relationship between $A_{50}$ and the maximal response is similarly buffered and need not necessarily be steep in receptor-distributed systems. This is shown in Fig. 7.6, where a clearly receptor-distributed system that produces response via a hyperbolic relationship between $[A \cdot R \cdot T]$ and the response also demonstrates a more gradual decline in $A_{50}$ values with receptor alkylation in

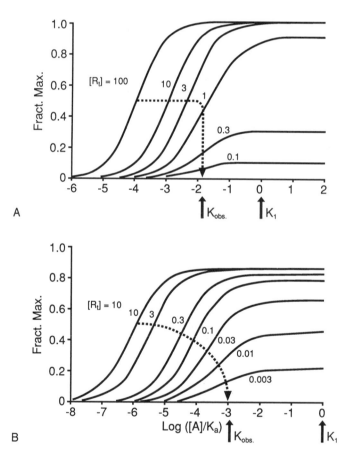

**FIG. 7.6.** Decline of $A_{50}$ values in a system in which receptor occupancy and response are linearly related **(A)** and linked via a hyperbolic function with $\beta = 0.01$ **(B)** (see Eq. 2.7). For this simulation, $K_2 = 0.01$, $[T] = 1$.

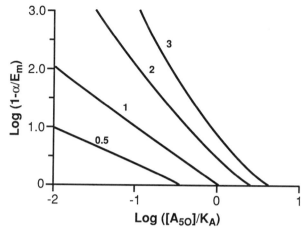

**FIG. 7.7.** Plots for $-\log(1 - \alpha/E_m)$ versus $-\log[A_{50}]$ in hyperbolic systems (Hill coefficient for dose-response curve = 1) and nonhyperbolic systems ($n \neq 1$).

a system in which there is a nonlinear relationship between receptor occupancy and response.

Another potential hazard in the experimental detection of receptor distribution is the fact that nonhyperbolic curves often are encountered. Under these circumstances, the simple relationships between $A_{50}$, maximal response, and $K_A$ described above become distorted. If the hyperbolic form of the operational equation (Eq. 7.19) cannot be used to fit data, then the relationship between $A_{50}$ and $K_A$ is given by:

$$[A_{50}] = \frac{K_A}{((2 + \tau^n)^{1/n} - 1)} \qquad [7.32]$$

Thus, although $A_{50}$ approaches the true $K_A$ after receptor alkylation with hyperbolic dose-response curves (i.e., when $n = 1$), it approaches a value of $K_A/(2^{1/n} - 1)$ when $n \neq 1$. This effectively distorts plots of $-\log(1 - \alpha/E_m)$ versus $A_{50}$ to where they cannot reliably be used to define $K_A$ values. Figure 7.7 shows plots according to Eq. 7.31 for systems of varying values for $n$.

In general there is as yet no simple experimental method to demonstrate effective receptor distribution in a functional system to where estimates of $K_A$ are affected. It is also unclear to what extent receptor distribution occurs in living systems, at least where G proteins are involved. This is because the couplers $[T]$ for G protein–linked receptors are GTPase proteins that substitute a bound molecule of GDP with GTP upon binding of activated receptor to subsequently hydrolyze the GTP. The rate of this reaction can be controlled by availability of GTP and in cases where GTP is plentiful, the binding and recycling of receptor/G-protein complexes may be so fast that no appreciable ternary complex ($[A \cdot R \cdot T]$) accumulates. Under these circumstances, no $[A \cdot R]$ is abstracted to $[A \cdot R \cdot T]$ under steady-state conditions and the equilibrium among $[A]$, $[R]$ and $[A \cdot R]$ can be adequately described by $K_1$. Therefore, in the presence of GTP, the effective recycling to $[A \cdot R \cdot T]$ to regenerate $[T]$ is so rapid that the magnitude of $K_2$ increases to the point where $[T]/K_2 \to 0$. Under these circumstances $K_{obs} = K_1$ (see Eq. 7.25). Table 7.2 shows the effect of GTP on the two-stage binding of oxotremorine to muscarinic receptors and $G_o$ proteins. As can be seen from this table, a

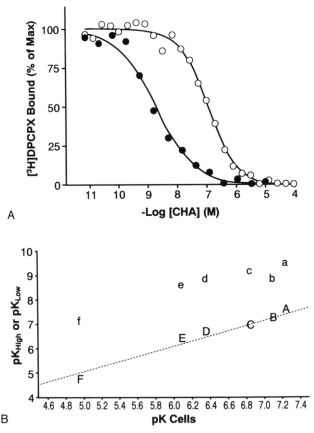

**FIG. 7.8.** Binding of agonists in membranes and intact cellular systems. **A:** Displacement of [³H]8-cyclopentyl-1,3-dipropylxanthine ([³H]DPCPX) by the adenosine receptor agonist $N^6$-cyclohexyladenosine (CHA). Binding in intact $DDT_1$ MF-2 cells (o) or membranes from the same cells (•). **B:** Correlation of displacement -$pK_i$ estimates measured in intact cells (abscissae) with apparent high- ($pK_H$, denoted by lower case letters) and low- ($pK_L$, denoted by upper case letters) affinity binding (two-site model) for displacement by the same agonists in membranes. a,A = $N^6$-cyclopentyladenosine, b,B = (−)-(R)-$N^6$-phenylisopropyladenosine, c,C = CHA, d,D = 5′-N-ethylcarboxamidoadenosine, e,E = 2-chloroadenosine, f,F = 2-phenylminoadenosine. (Data from ref. 10.)

striking 800-fold increase in apparent potency is produced by the presence of coupling protein $G_o$. The 800-fold discrepancy is canceled by GTP, and a constant value for the affinity (equal to $K_1$) is obtained. This phenomenon is described further in Chapters 8 and 12.

It has been demonstrated that coupler-induced diminutions in the magnitude of $K_{obs}$ observed in membrane preparations devoid of GTP are *not* seen in some intact physiological systems in which GTP may be abundant. For example, Fig. 7.8A shows displacement binding curves for the adenosine receptor agonist $N^6$-cyclohexyladenosine (CHA) on intact cells and membrane preparations from $DDT_1$ MF-2 cells. These data are consistent with a higher affinity two-stage binding for the agonist in the membrane preparations and a single-state (i.e., presumably high GTP state) binding in intact cells. Figure 7.8B shows $K_i$ values for the two affinity states for a collection of adenosine receptor agonists in membranes plotted against the single $K_i$ obtained in intact cells. The line of identity closely corresponds to the low-affinity state in membranes and that in whole cells, indicating that $K_1$ adequately describes the binding of the agonists in the intact system. These data indicate that two-stage binding may, in some cases, be an artifact of membrane systems devoid of GTP and may have less relevance to physiological systems. However, in contrast, there are whole cell systems in which complex-binding curves for agonists are obtained, thereby indicating possible two-stage binding. For example, Table 7.3 shows binding parameters for muscarinic receptor ligands in dissociated rat brain cell aggregates. As can be seen from this table, antagonist binding can be described by a single-site receptor model (Hill coefficient not different from unity), whereas the binding of agonists fits a two-site binding scheme. These data indicate that agonist

**TABLE 7.3.** *Binding parameters for [³H]NMS in intact rat brain aggregates*

| Displacer | $n^a$ | $K_H{}^b$ | $\%R_H{}^c$ | $K_L{}^d(\mu M)$ | $\%R_L{}^e$ |
|---|---|---|---|---|---|
| Antagonists | | | | | |
| Atropine | 0.96 | 0.42 nM | | | |
| Scopolamine | 0.94 | 1.27 nM | | | |
| (−)-QNB$^f$ | 0.81 | 0.25 nM | | | |
| Agonists | | | | | |
| Carbamylcholine | 0.64 | 4.3 $\mu$M | 18.5 | 89 | 81.5 |
| Oxotremorine | 0.65 | 89.8 nM | 18.9 | 1.8 | 81.1 |
| Pilocarpine | 0.78 | 1.6 $\mu$M | 34.5 | 18.1 | 65.5 |

[a] Hill coefficient for displacement curve
[b] Apparent equilibrium dissociation constant for 'high' affinity site
[c] Percentage 'high' affinity sites
[d] Apparent equilibrium dissociation constant for 'low' affinity sites
[e] Percentage 'low' affinity sites
[f] (±)-quinuclidinyl benzilate
[³H]NMS, [³H]N-Methylscopolamine.
From ref. 17.

binding induces significant steady-state formation of ternary complex in the intact system. In general, the potential for dissimilation in the measurement of $K_A$ for agonist and receptor classification should be considered, especially when binding studies are used to quantify affinity (see Chapter 12).

## ESTIMATION OF AGONIST AFFINITY WITH FUNCTIONAL ANTAGONISM

The partial alkylation method described previously requires that a dose-response curve to agonist be obtained under two conditions of differing receptor density, the lower one demonstrating a depressed maximal response to the agonist. Other interventions to effect the same qualitative changes in dose-response curves that do not stem from diminution of receptor density have been used to furnish equiactive agonist concentrations for Eq. 7.13. These interventions can be generally described as physiological antagonism, whereby the response to an agonist is pharmacologically impaired by antagonism of the stimulus-response machinery of the tissue or by the generation of an opposing stimulus. For example, the contraction of an agonist may be countered by the addition of a relaxant agent. In many cases, the data generated by these techniques appear to fit very well with the Furchgott method of estimating $K_A$. The use of functional antagonism for the estimation of $K_A$ has a major practical advantage in that receptor-alkylating drugs for many receptor types are still not available. Therefore, any physiological intervention that opposes the production of a response to an agonist can be used for this technique. The major *disadvantage* to the use of this technique is the lack of theoretical rationale within the framework of receptor theory for the calculation of $K_A$ with functional antagonism. Therefore, it is often impossible to identify the calculated parameter as the true $K_A$.

This problem has been analyzed theoretically by Leff and colleagues (18). Figure 7.9 shows a schematic of the binding of an agonist $[A]$ to a receptor $[R]$ to produce a complex $[A \cdot R]$, which goes on, through a hyperbolic function, to produce an initial product $P_1$, which in turn goes on to produce other products $P_2, P_3, \ldots$ Pn and finally an effect $E_a$. It is assumed that the functions linking these intermediate products are hyperbolic in nature (see Fig. 2.13 for an example). Under these circumstances, the production of $P_1$ is given by:

$$P_1 = \frac{\Phi[A \cdot R]}{\gamma + [A \cdot R]} \qquad [7.33]$$

The subsequent production of response from $P_1$ can be described by a second hyperbolic function defined:

$$E_a = \frac{\Omega P_1}{\sigma + P_1} \qquad [7.34]$$

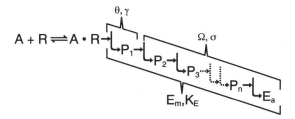

**FIG. 7.9.** Schematic diagram of the binding of an agonist [A] to a receptor [R] to form an initial complex [A·R], which then is translated via a series of hyperbolic functions into an effect (E). The complete process from [A·R] to E can be described by a hyperbolic function with maximal asymptote $E_m$ and location parameter $K_E$ or a pair of hyperbolic functions with asymptotes $\Phi$ and $\Omega$ and location parameters $\gamma$ and $\sigma$ (see Eqs. 7.33 to 7.36).

substituting for $P_1$:

$$E_a = \frac{\Phi\Omega[A·R]}{\gamma\sigma + (\Phi + \sigma)[A·R]} \qquad [7.35]$$

This equation resembles the one for the description of response with [A·R]:

$$E_a = \frac{E_m[A·R]}{K_E + [A·R]} \qquad [7.36]$$

where $E_m$ is the maximal response and $K_E$ is the concentration of [A·R], which produces half-maximal response. Comparing Eqs. 7.35 and 7.36, the maximal response $E_m$ and location parameter $K_E$ are given by:

$$E_m = \frac{\Phi\Omega}{\Phi + \sigma} \qquad [7.37]$$

and

$$K_E = \frac{\gamma\sigma}{\Phi + \sigma} \qquad [7.38]$$

Functional antagonism could change all parameters $\Phi$, $\Omega$, $\gamma$, and $\sigma$ to effect changes in dose-response curves to agonists. However, to be consistent with the theoretical rationale for the partial alkylation method (i.e., the change in the dose-response curve occurs only with a change in $[R_t]$), *only* a change in $K_E$ is permissible since that would change $\tau([R_t]/K_E$ in terms of the operational model [see Fig. 7.3]). The only way to ensure this would be to show that the functional antagonist produces an increase only in $\gamma$, the location parameter for the first saturable function relating [A·R] and the remaining stimulus-response apparatus. Therefore, it can be seen that a functional intervention cannot be guaranteed to bring about the theoretically required impairment of agonist function for the correct application of the partial alkylation method for the estimation of $K_A$. Under these circumstances, estimates of $K_A$ with this approach must be considered with caution.

## AFFINITY OF PARTIAL AGONISTS

Classic receptor theory predicts the following relationship between equiactive concentrations of two agonists, $A$ and $P$. The stimulus to $A$ is given by

$$S_A = \frac{\epsilon_A \cdot [A] \cdot [R_t]}{[A] + K_A} \qquad [7.39]$$

where $\epsilon_A$ is the intrinsic efficacy of $A$ and $[R_t]$ is the total receptor density. An analogous equation can be given for the stimulus to agonist $P$:

$$S_P = \frac{\epsilon_P \cdot [P] \cdot [R_t]}{[P] + K_P} \qquad [7.40]$$

Comparing equiactive ($S_P = S_A$) concentrations of $A$ and $P$ in the same tissue ($[R_t]$ is constant and cancels), the following relationship results:

$$\frac{1}{[A]} = \frac{\epsilon_A}{\epsilon_P} \cdot \frac{K_P}{K_A} \cdot \frac{1}{[P]} + \frac{1}{K_A}\left(\frac{\epsilon_A}{\epsilon_P} - 1\right) \qquad [7.41]$$

Here it can be seen that

$$K_P = \frac{\text{slope}}{\text{intercept}}\left(1 - \frac{\epsilon_P}{\epsilon_A}\right) \qquad [7.42]$$

Forms of Eq. 7.41 that do not have some of the disadvantages of double-reciprocal plots are

$$\frac{[P]}{[A]} = \frac{1}{K_A}\left(\frac{\epsilon_A}{\epsilon_P} - 1\right) \cdot [P] + \frac{\epsilon_A}{\epsilon_P} \cdot \frac{K_P}{K_A} \qquad [7.43]$$

where

$$K_P = \frac{\text{intercept}}{\text{slope}}\left(1 - \frac{\epsilon_P}{\epsilon_A}\right) \qquad [7.44]$$

and

$$[A] = \frac{K_A}{(\epsilon_A/\epsilon_P) - 1} + \frac{K_P}{(\epsilon_P/\epsilon_A) - 1} \cdot \frac{[A]}{[P]} \qquad [7.45]$$

where

$$K_P = \text{slope}\left(\frac{\epsilon_P}{\epsilon_A} - 1\right) \qquad [7.46]$$

Equation 7.45 has the added advantage of yielding an estimate of the error on the measurement of $K_P$. Because $K_P$ is given only by the slope of the

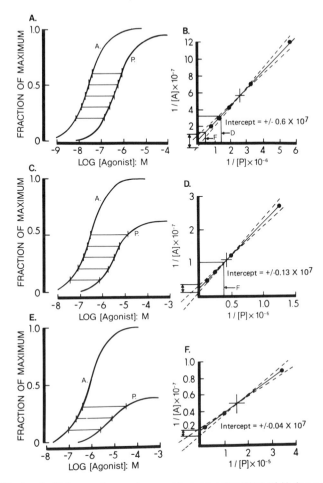

**FIG. 7.10.** Effects of efficiency of receptor coupling on estimation of $K_P$ for a partial agonist. **A, C,** and **E:** Dose-response curves for a full agonist ($A$) (intrinsic efficacy = 3, $K_A$ = $10^{-5}$ M) and a partial agonist ($P$) (intrinsic efficacy = 0.15, $K_A$ = $10^{-5}$ M) in three tissues with different efficiencies of receptor coupling. Response given by the function stimulus ÷ (stimulus + β), where the β constant reflects the efficiency of coupling. For A, β = 0.01 (well coupled); $P$ produces 94% of the maximal response to $A$. For C, β = 0.1; $P$ produces 62% of the maximal response to $A$. For E, β = 0.5 (poorly coupled); $P$ produces 36% of the maximal response to $A$. **B, D,** and **F:** Double-reciprocal plots of equiactive concentrations of $A$ and $P$ corresponding to adjacent sets of dose-response curves. In the tissue in which $P$ produces near-maximal response, errors in the regression line (rotations of line about mean $x$ and $y$) produce large variation in intercept values. The inset boxes show scales of plots in parts D and F. D shows less effect of variation in the regression line on the intercept, and F (poorly coupled tissue) allows the most accurate estimate of the intercept.

regression, Eq. 6.21, which calculates the standard error on the slope of the regression line, can be used to estimate an error on the estimate of $K_P$.

It should be noted that Eq. 7.41 also is compatible with the operational model. The derivation for the double-reciprocal equation results in:

$$\frac{1}{[A]} = \frac{1}{[P]}\frac{K_P \tau_A}{K_A \tau_P} + \frac{\tau_A - \tau_P}{K_A \tau_P} \qquad [7.47]$$

And $K_P$ then can be calculated:

$$K_P = \frac{\text{slope}}{\text{intercept}}\left(1 - \frac{\tau_P}{\tau_A}\right) \qquad [7.48]$$

There are two important features of these equations that dictate their applicability for measurement of agonist affinity. The first relates to the nature of $A$ and $P$. In each case, the mathematical manipulations lead to a calculation of $K_P$ that is multiplied by a term involving the intrinsic efficacies of $A$ and $P$. Therefore, unless the relative efficacies of the drugs are known, the estimate of $K_P$ will be in error. However, the magnitude of this error will diminish to insignificance as $\epsilon_A \gg \epsilon_P$. Therefore, this method does become practical for comparison of high- and low-efficacy agonists to calculate the affinity of the low-efficacy agonist. The second practical aspect of this method concerns the type of response system chosen to make the measurement. Figure 7.10A, C, and E shows theoretical dose-response curves for two agonists, $A$ and $P$; the efficacy of $P$ is only 0.05 that of $A$, making the efficacy correction term relatively insignificant. The differences in dose-response curves in Fig. 7.10A, C, and E result from differences in receptor coupling; Fig. 7.10A shows the effects of $A$ and $P$ in a well-coupled tissue, Fig. 7.10C is for a less efficiently coupled tissue, and Fig. 7.10E is for an even less efficiently coupled tissue. The effect of decreased efficiency in receptor coupling is to shift the curve for the high-efficacy agonist to the right and depress the curve for the low-efficacy agonist. Regressions, according to Eq. 7.41, for reciprocals of equiactive doses of $A$ and $P$ from the respective dose-response curves illustrate the effects of errors in the regression lines (rotations about mean $x$ and $y$) on the ordinate intercepts. It can be seen that measurement errors are much less devastating to estimates of $K_P$ if data are obtained from tissues in which the partial agonist produces a relatively low maximal response (i.e., poor receptor coupling). In practice, this method works best for comparison of a full agonist and a partial agonist in tissues in which the partial agonist produces less than 50% of maximal response.

Figure 7.11A shows estimation of $K_P$ for the β-adrenoceptor partial agonist prenalterol. The efficacy of the full agonist (isoproterenol) is 220 times that of prenalterol, making the efficacy correction term insignificant. The estimate of $K_P$ using a plot of $1/[A]$ versus $1/[P]$ is 53.7 nM (Fig. 7.11B), that using $[P]/[A]$ versus $[P]$ is 58.9 nM (Fig. 7.11C), and that using $[A]$ versus

$[A]/[P]$ is 55 nM (Fig. 7.11D). The estimate of the standard error in $K_P$ from the slope in the regression of $[A]$ versus $[A]/[P]$ is $\pm 4.3$ nM, giving the 95% confidence limits on the estimate of $K_P = 55$ nM, 43 to 67 nM.

In some cases the efficacy correction term may produce a significant difference in the estimate of $K_P$. Oxymetazoline is an $\alpha$-adrenoceptor agonist with 0.3 of the intrinsic efficacy of norepinephrine. Estimation of the $K_P$ for oxymetazoline by the method of equiactive concentrations yields $K_P$ values smaller than that given by an independent method not affected by efficacy (Schild analysis, see Chapter 9). The dose-response curves and regressions are shown in Fig. 7.12, and the resulting estimates of $K_P$ in Table 7.4. In general, the estimates are 20% to 30% higher than that given by Schild analy-

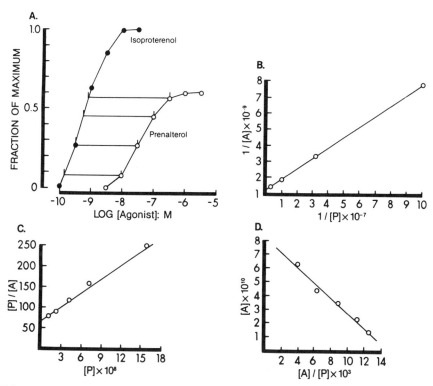

**FIG. 7.11.** Calculation of $K_P$ for prenalterol by comparison of equiactive concentrations. **A:** Dose-response curves for isoproterenol ($[A]$) and prenalterol ($[P]$) in rat left atria. Ordinate: Increases in twitch contraction as fractions of the maximal response to isoproterenol. Abscissa: Logarithms of molar concentrations of agonist. Horizontal lines connect equiactive concentrations used for estimation of $K_P$. **B:** Double-reciprocal plot according to Eq. 7.41 for data in A. Intercept $= 1.24 \times 10^9$; slope $= 65.77$; $K_P = 53$ nM. **C:** Regression according to Eq. 7.43. Intercept $= 68.24$; slope $= 1.17 \times 10^9$; $K_P = 58$ nM. **D:** Regression according to Eq. 7.45. Intercept $= 8.27 \times 10^{-10}$; slope $= -5.48 \times 10^{-8}$; $K_P = 55$ nM. (Data from ref. 15.)

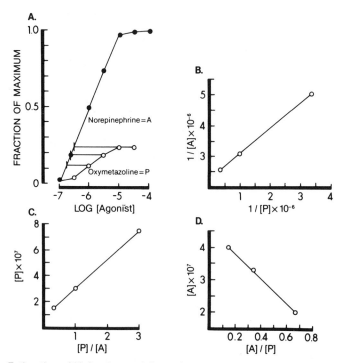

**FIG. 7.12.** Estimation of $K_P$ for the partial agonist oxymetazoline by comparison of equiactive concentrations. **A:** Dose-response curves for norepinephrine (●) and oxymetazoline (○) in rat vas deferens. Ordinate: Contractions as fractions of the maximal response to norepinephrine. Abscissa: Logarithms of molar concentrations of agonist. Horizontal lines indicate levels of response used for calculation of $K_P$. **B:** Double-reciprocal plot of equiactive concentrations of norepinephrine (ordinate) and oxymetazoline (abscissa) from A. Slope = 0.663; intercept = $3.79 \times 10^6$; uncorrected $K_P = 0.174$ μM; corrected for efficacy of oxymetazoline, $K_P = 0.24$ μM. **C:** Data plotted according to Eq. 7.43. **D:** Data plotted according to Eq. 7.45. (Data for A, C, and D from ref. 14.)

sis. The correction term for efficacy is a multiplicative factor of 0.71; when this is applied, the estimates of $K_P$ agree more closely with the independent estimate (Table 7.4).

Another method of estimating $K_P$ for a partial agonist, derived by Stephenson (24), is to compare equiactive concentrations of a full agonist in the absence and presence of a partial agonist. In the absence of a partial agonist, the stimulus to a concentration $[A]$ of a full agonist of intrinsic efficacy $\epsilon_A$ is given by Eq. 7.39. In the presence of a concentration of partial agonist (of intrinsic efficacy $\epsilon_P$) $[P]$, and assuming that receptor stimuli are additive, the total stimulus to a concentration of full agonist $[A']$ and partial agonist $[P]$ is

$$S_T = \frac{\epsilon_A \cdot [A']}{[A'] + K_A(1 + [P]/K_P)} + \frac{\epsilon_P \cdot [P]}{[P] + K_P(1 + [A']/K_A)} \quad [7.49]$$

**TABLE 7.4.** *Estimates of $K_p$ for oxymetazoline*

| Method | Uncorrected[a] $K_P$ (μM) | Δ%[b] | Corrected[c] $K_P$ (μM) | Δ% |
|---|---|---|---|---|
| 1/[A] vs. 1/[P] | 0.383 | +28% | 0.272 | −12% |
| [P]/[A] vs. [P] | 0.363 | +21% | 0.260 | −14% |
| [A] vs. [A]/[P] | 0.376 | +25% | 0.270 | −11% |
| Schild analysis[d] | $K_P$ = 0.30 | | | |

[a] Correction for $\epsilon_P/\epsilon_A$ not applied.
[b] Percentage difference from estimate given by Schild analysis.
[c] Correction for $\epsilon_P/\epsilon_A$ applied.
[d] Method of estimating $K_p$ not affected by the efficacy of the partial agonist; in this case, the receptor population was alkylated to a point at which oxymetazoline produced no agonist response and functioned as a competitive antagonist of norepinephrine.
Data from ref. 14.

Assuming that equal responses emanate from equal stimuli. Eqs. 7.39 and 7.49 can be equated and rearranged to the following relationship:

$$[A] = \frac{[A']}{1 + \{1 - (\epsilon_P/\epsilon_A)\}\cdot([P]/K_P)} + \frac{(\epsilon_P/\epsilon_A)\cdot([P]/K_P)\cdot K_A}{1 + \{1 - (\epsilon_P/\epsilon_A)\}\cdot([P]/K_P)} \quad [7.50]$$

Therefore, a regression of [A] on [A'] should yield a straight line with

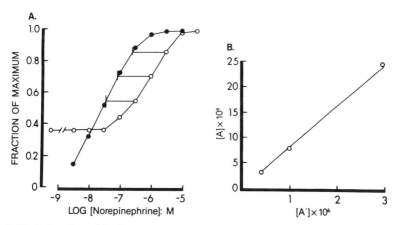

**FIG. 7.13.** Estimation of $K_P$ for dobutamine by the method of Stephenson. **A:** Response of rat anococcygeus muscle to norepinephrine in the absence (•) and presence (o) of dobutamine (1 μM). Ordinate: Contraction as a fraction of the maximal contraction to norepinephrine. Abscissa: Logarithms of molar concentrations of norepinephrine. Horizontal lines join equiactive concentrations. **B:** Regression of equiactive concentrations of norepinephrine according to Eq. 7.50. Concentrations of norepinephrine in the absence (ordinate) and presence (abscissa) of dobutamine. Slope = 0.081; $K_P$ = 89 nM. (Data from ref. 14.)

slope = $[1 + \{1 - (\epsilon_P/\epsilon_A)\}([P]/K_P)]^{-1}$, and $K_P$ can be calculated as

$$K_P = \frac{[P]\cdot\text{slope}}{1 - \text{slope}}\left(1 - \frac{\epsilon_P}{\epsilon_A}\right) \qquad [7.51]$$

Again, it can be seen that the estimate of $K_P$ is affected by the relative efficacies of the agonists; for this to be insignificant, $\epsilon_A$ should be considerably larger than $\epsilon_P$. Also, because concentrations of full agonist need to be determined accurately in the presence of the partial agonist, the partial agonist should not produce a sizable response. For example, if the partial agonist produces 80% of maximal response, then doses of full agonist producing 81% to 100% response in the presence of partial agonist will have to be used; estimates of responses in this region of the curve are much more susceptible to error than in a response range of 25% to 75%. Therefore, as with the previous method of comparison of equiactive doses, this method works best when measuring the affinity of low-efficacy partial agonists in tissues in which the partial agonist produces less than 50% of maximal response. Figure 7.13 shows estimation of $K_P$ for the $\alpha$-adrenoceptor partial agonist dobutamine by this method.

Equations 7.50 and 7.51 yield estimates of $K_P$ from one concentration of $P$, but this method can be extended to the use of a range of partial-agonist concentrations. Thus, an estimate of $K_P$ can be derived from a number of tissues. Repeated analysis by Eq. 7.50 for a range of partial-agonist concen-

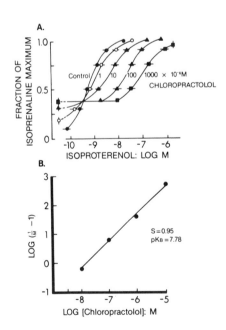

FIG. 7.14. Estimation of $K_P$ for chloropractolol by the method of Stephenson with data from more than one tissue. **A:** Concentration-response curves in rat isolated right atria in the absence and presence of various concentrations of chloropractolol. Ordinate: Increases in atrial rate as fractions of the maximal increase in rate to isoproterenol. Abscissa: Logarithms of molar concentrations of isoproterenol. Responses in the absence (•) and presence of chloropractolol, 10 nM (▲), 100 nM (▲), 1 μM (o), and 10 μM (■). (From ref. 16.) **B:** Regression of slopes of regressions according to Eq. 7.52 [metameter log(1/$m$ − 1)] on logarithms of molar concentrations of chloropractolol. Slope = 0.95; intercept = 7.78; $K_P$ = 16.5 nM.

trations yields a data set of pairs of slopes and concentrations $[P]$. These data yield $K_P$ by (12),

$$\log \left( \frac{1}{\text{slope}} - 1 \right) = \log [P] - \log K_P \qquad [7.52]$$

An estimate of $K_P$ for the $\beta$-adrenoceptor partial agonist chloropractolol was made by this method and is shown in Fig. 7.14.

## REFERENCES

1. Black, J. W. (1982): Receptor function and control. In: *Catecholamines in the Non-Ischaemic and Ischaemic Myocardium*, edited by R. Riemersma and W. Oliver, pp. 3–12. Elsevier/North Holland, Amsterdam.
2. Black, J. W., Leff, P., Shankley, N. P., and Wood, J. (1985): An operational model of pharmacological agonism: The effect of E/[A] curve shape on agonist dissociation constant estimation. *Br. J. Pharmacol.*, 84:561–571.
3. Black, J. W., and Shankley, N. P. (1990): Interpretation of agonist affinity estimations: The question of distributed receptor states. *Proc. R. Soc. Lond. [Biol]*, 240:503–518.
4. Bowman, W. C., and Rand, M. J. (1980): Principles of drug action. In: *Textbook of Pharmacology*, ed. 2. Blackwell, Oxford.
5. Burgen, A. S. V. (1966): The drug-receptor complex. *J. Pharm. Pharmacol.*, 18:137–149.
6. Chang, K.-J., Jacobs, S., and Cuatrecasas, P. (1975): Quantitative aspects of hormone-receptor interactions of high affinity. Effect of receptor concentration and measurement of dissociation constants of labeled and unlabeled hormones. *Biochim. Biophys. Acta*, 406:294–303.
7. Clark, A. J. (1937): General pharmacology. In: *Heffter's Handbuch d-exp. Pharmacol. Erg. band 4*, Springer Verlag, Berlin.
8. Florio, V. A., and Sternweis, P. C. (1989): Mechanism of muscarinic receptor action on $G_o$ in reconstituted phospholipid vescicles. *J. Biol. Chem.*, 264:3909–3915.
9. Furchgott, R. F. (1966): The use of $\beta$-haloalkylamines in the differentiation of receptors and in the determination of dissociation constants of receptor-agonist complexes. In: *Advances in Drug Research, Vol. 3*, edited by N. J. Harper and A. B. Simmonds, pp. 21–55. Academic Press, New York.
10. Gerwins, P., Nordstedt, C., and Fredholm, B. B. (1990): Characterization of adenosine $A_1$ receptors in intact $DDT_1$ MF-2 smooth muscle cells. *Mol. Pharmacol.*, 38:660–666.
11. Jenkinson, D. H. (1979): Partial agonists in receptor classification. In: *Proceedings of the VI International Symposium on Medicinal Chemistry*, edited by M. A. Simpkins, pp. 373–383. Cotswold Press, Oxford.
12. Kaumann, A. J., and Marano, M. (1982): On equilibrium dissociation constants for complexes of drug-receptor subtypes. Selective and nonselective interactions of partial agonists with two plausible $\beta$-adrenoceptor subtypes mediating positive chronotropic effects of $(-)$-isoprenaline in kitten atria. *Naunyn Schmeidebergs Arch. Pharmacol.*, 318:192–201.
13. Kenakin, T. P. (1981): An in vitro quantitative analysis of the alpha adrenoceptor partial agonist activity of dobutamine and its relevance to inotropic selectivity. *J. Pharmacol. Exp. Ther.*, 216:210–219.
14. Kenakin, T. P. (1984): The relative contribution of affinity and efficacy to agonist activity: Organ selectivity of noradrenaline and oxymetazoline with reference to the classification of drug receptors. *Br. J. Pharmacol.*, 81:131–141.
15. Kenakin, T. P., and Beek, D. (1984): Relative efficacy of prenalterol and pirbuterol for $\beta_1$-adrenoceptors: Measurement of agonist affinity by alteration of receptor number. *J. Pharmacol. Exp. Ther.*, 229:340–345.
16. Kenakin, T. P., and Black, J. W. (1978): The pharmacological classification of practolol and chloropractolol. *Mol. Pharmacol.*, 14:607–623.

17. Lee, J-L., and El-Fakahany, E. E. (1985): [$^3$H]$N$-Methylscopolamine binding to muscarinic receptors in intact adult rat brain cell aggregates. *Biochem. Pharmacol.*, 34:4299–4303.
18. Leff, P., Martin, G. R., and Morse, J. M. (1985): Application of the operational model of agonism to establish conditions when functional antagonism may be used to estimate agonist dissociation constants. *Br. J. Pharmacol.*, 85:655–663.
19. Mackay, D. (1966): A general analysis of the receptor-drug interaction. *Br. J. Pharmacol.*, 26:9–16.
20. Mackay, D. (1966): A new method for the analysis of drug-receptor interactions. In: *Advances in Drug Research, Vol. 3*, edited by N. J. Harper and A. B. Simmonds, pp. 1–19. Academic Press, New York.
21. Mackay, D. (1988): Continuous variation of agonist affinity constants. *Trends Pharmacol. Sci.*, 9:156–157.
22. Parker, R. B., and Waud, D. R. (1971): Pharmacological estimation of drug-receptor dissociation constants. Statistical evaluation. I. Agonists. *J. Pharmacol. Exp. Ther.*, 177:1–12.
23. Plumbridge, T. W., Arrons, L. J., and Brown, J. R. (1978): Problems associated with the analysis and interpretation of small molecule/macromolecule binding data. *J. Pharm. Pharmacol.*, 30:69–74.
24. Stephenson, R. P. (1956): A modification of receptor theory. *Br. J. Pharmacol.*, 11:379–393.
25. Thron, D. C. (1970): Graphical and weighted regression analyses for the determination of agonist dissociation constants. *J. Pharmacol. Exp. Ther.*, 175:541–553.
26. Van Ginneken, C. A. M. (1977): Kinetics of drug-receptor interaction. In: *Kinetics of Drug Action*, edited by J. M. Van Rossum, pp. 357–396. Springer-Verlag, Berlin.

# 8

## Efficacy

*The distinction between affinity and intrinsic activity therefore seems of general importance.*

—E. J. ARIËNS, 1954

Perhaps no other interaction between a small molecule and a receptor is as shrouded in mystery as the interaction that results in a physiological response. The property that enables drugs to produce responses is given the name *intrinsic efficacy*, and it can be studied in terms of molecular processes or as an empirical proportionality factor. Conceptually, it is convenient to differentiate the properties of drugs that cause them to associate with the receptor (affinity) and those that produce a change in the receptor (efficacy to produce stimulus), as put by Clark (5), "[to differentiate] the capacity to bind and the capacity to excite." Molecular mechanisms of agonism are varied and, for many receptor systems, are not yet completely understood, but quantification of the *relative* efficacies of agonists on an operational level has great value in terms of the classification of drugs and drug receptors. Experiments with agonists on a biochemical level probably will define the nature of efficacy.

### THE MOLECULAR NATURE OF EFFICACY

For a tissue to respond to a drug, a message must be transmitted via the receptor to the organ response mechanisms. In general, there are two possible molecular mechanisms by which this can occur. One involves a conformational change in the tertiary structure of the receptor protein brought about by the binding of the agonist. Many proteins have more than one conformation of minimal free energy, and the energy barriers between these can be overcome by drug binding; this process is referred to as *conformational induction*. A second mechanism for an agonist-induced receptor stimulus can be by selective binding of the agonist to two or more coexisting

249

conformations of the receptor (in thermodynamic equilibrium). When an agonist binds selectively to one of these, the equilibrium shifts, and a bias, in terms of which conformation prevails, is introduced by the presence of the agonist; this is referred to as *conformational selection*.

Not all agonists are capable of inducing identical levels of maximal responses. This raises a fundamental question: What is the nature of such a graded scale of maximal stimulation? One possibility is that the intensity of a stimulus may be related to the extent of the conformational induction (allosteric aberration of the receptor protein) or conformational selection (relative affinities of the agonist for the various conformers), or the stimulus may depend on how often the agonist-induced change occurs (i.e., rate theory, see Chapter 1) and thus will be related to the kinetics of drug-receptor interactions. Another scenario relates the intensity of the stimulus to the time period that the receptor is affected by the agonist; i.e., various activated receptor-transducer complexes may retain activity for various periods after agonist dissociation. It is probable that in the spectrum of neurotransmitter, hormone, and drug interactions with mammalian organs, all of these mechanisms are relevant; so to a certain extent the molecular mechanism of agonism depends on the particular drug, organ, and receptor type, as well as the pharmacologic model one chooses to depict responses.

As with allotopic drug effects (see Chapter 10), conformational induction is difficult to quantify. In contrast, efficacy by conformational selection offers a model whereby molecular quantities (affinities) can be used to describe the degree of drug effect produced by an agonist. For example, studies of single-ion channels opened by nicotinic agonists suggest that these drugs produce effects by a common mechanism. When single ion–channel currents produced by a range of nicotinic agonists are recorded, the single ion–channel conductance is found to remain the same (Table 8.1). This suggests that the conductance of an ion channel does not depend on the nature of the agonist

TABLE 8.1. *Single-channel slope conductance ratios for agonists relative to acetylcholine (on rat myotubules)*

| Agonist | N | Slope |
|---|---|---|
| Carbachol | 3 | $1.00 \pm 0.03$ |
| Suberyldicholine | 3 | $1.02 \pm 0.05$ |
| Nicotine | 2 | $0.98 \pm 0.02$ |
| 1,1-Dimethyl-4-phenylpiperazinium | 2 | $1.00 \pm 0.02$ |
| Decamethonium | 3 | $1.03 \pm 0.05$ |
| Succinylcholine | 2 | $1.01 \pm 0.04$ |
| 3-(*m*-Hydroxyphenyl)propyltrimethylammonium | 3 | $1.00 \pm 0.03$ |
| 3-Phenylpropyltrimethylammonium | 3 | $1.01 \pm 0.05$ |
| 3-Phenylethyltriethylammonium | 2 | $0.98 \pm 0.10$ |

From ref. 13.

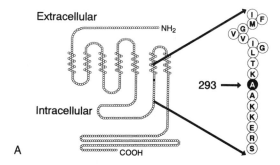

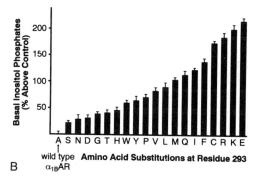

FIG. 8.1. Schematic diagram of the $\alpha_{1B}$-adrenoceptor and the activation by substitution of amino acids at position 293. **A:** Topography of the $\alpha_{1B}$-adrenoceptor and position of residue 293. **B:** Basal levels of inositol phosphate in COS-7 cells expressing the wild type $\alpha_{1B}$-adrenoceptor and mutant receptors with the designated substitutions at position 293. (From ref. 27.)

that opens it, but rather on the effect of the agonist on the equilibrium between the open and shut states of the agonist-channel complexes (see Chapter 1).

Sophisticated biochemical techniques have yielded models to describe events beyond agonist-receptor interaction. A common theme is the interaction of an agonist-activated receptor with other membrane-bound proteins (variously called collision-coupling, ternary complex, fluid mosaic, and floating receptor models). In general, the binding of an agonist to a receptor either facilitates or stabilizes receptor coupling to a transducer protein to produce activation of the transducer protein and subsequent production of response. There is evidence to suggest that, for at least some receptors, efficacy by conformational selection may be operative. By this mechanism the relative affinity of the agonist for the two receptor states (active and inactive) would determine efficacy (see Eq. 1.38). A possible example for such a scheme is the $\alpha_{1B}$-adrenoceptor. It has been demonstrated that substitution of virtually any other amino acid at position 293 (Fig. 8.1A) produces a mutant receptor capable of spontaneously interacting with membrane-coupling components and thus producing cellular responses (Fig. 8.1B). The intriguing aspect of this phenomenon from the point of view of conformational selectional efficacy is the fact the affinity of the agonist epinephrine for these mutants is *selectively* enhanced (over that of the antagonist HEAT). This implies that the mutations mimic the "active" state of the receptor and that this active state has a different affinity for agonists than the inactive state.

A large class of receptors utilize membrane-bound proteins (called G proteins for their involvement with GTP) to elicit response. In general, the activated receptor (agonist bound or otherwise) binds to the G protein, which has a bound GDP molecule. Graphic evidence for the association between proteins after agonist binding has been obtained in biochemical studies on β-adrenoceptors. For example, Fig. 8.2 shows results from gel exclusion chromatography of β-adrenoceptors after binding with the agonist [³H]hydroxybenzylisoproterenol and the antagonist [³H]dihydroalprenolol; the slower elution of that agonist-receptor complex indicates a larger apparent size. As can be seen from this figure, association of the receptor with the agonist, as opposed to the antagonist, produced a larger protein complex (i.e., associated proteins).

As discussed in Chapter 7, the formation of the ternary complex [$A \cdot R \cdot G$] distorts the equilibrium among [$A$], [$R$], and [$A \cdot R$], thus creating an apparently high-affinity state (compared to the affinity of [$A$] for [$R$]). This process can be shown schematically as:

$$A + R \xrightleftharpoons{K_1} A \cdot R + G \xrightleftharpoons{K_2} A \cdot R \cdot G \qquad \overset{\xrightarrow{\hspace{3cm}}}{K_{obs}}$$

$$[8.1]$$

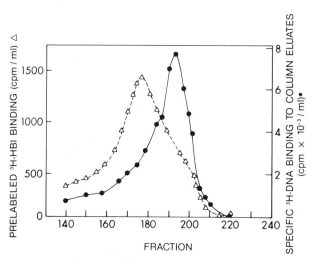

**FIG. 8.2.** Gel exclusion chromatography for β-adrenergic receptors solubilized from rat reticulocyte membranes with digitonin. Receptors were prelabeled with either the agonist [³H]hydroxybenzylisoproterenol (³H-HBI, △) or the antagonist [³H]dihydroalprenolol (³H-DNA, ●). The staggered elution pattern shows a difference in molecular sizes of the receptors. (From ref. 29.)

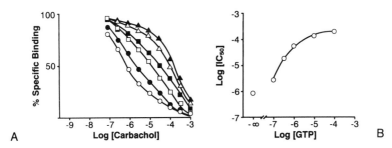

**FIG. 8.3.** Effect of GTP on the displacement of [³H]N-methylscopolamine binding by carbachol in membranes from rat myocardium. **A:** Displacement measured in the absence (o) and presence of GTP at concentrations of 0.1 μM (•), 0.3 μM (□), 1.0 μM (■), 10 μM (▵), and 100 μM (▴). **B:** Log IC₅₀ of the displacement curves shown in A expressed as a function of GTP concentrations. (From ref. 10.)

Therefore, under conditions where the receptor coupler can abstract $[A \cdot R]$, the affinity of the agonist for the receptor can be described by an experimentally determined high-affinity dissociation constant denoted $K_H$. If an excess of GTP is introduced into this system, then the $[A \cdot R \cdot G]$ complex rapidly dissolves (GDP replaced by GTP and dissociation of the G protein results) and the receptor is quickly recycled to the $[R]$ state again. The time scale for this reaction often is sufficient to effectively cancel any steady-state formation of $[A \cdot R \cdot G]$. This results in the formation of a system in which the binding of $[A]$ to $[R]$ is not distorted. Under these circumstances, the experimentally observed affinity of the agonist for the receptor is described by the dissociation constant of the $[A \cdot R]$ complex. This will be of a lower magnitude than that of the dissociation constant describing the two-stage binding (to $[A \cdot R \cdot G]$) and thus is labeled $K_L$. Figure 8.3A shows the progressive GTP-dependent loss of apparent affinity of carbachol for the muscarinic receptor in membranes from rat myocardium. As seen in Fig. 8.3B, the GTP effect is concentration related. Therefore, if the resulting affinity is to be considered an estimate of $K_L$, it must be confirmed that the maximal dextral displacement of the binding curve has been obtained.

The ratio of $K_L/K_H$ quantifies the magnitude of the G protein–coupling effect linked to efficacy. As discussed in Chapter 7, the observed affinity for an agonist that binds to a receptor to subsequently form a ternary complex with a coupler protein $[T]$ is given by:

$$K_{obs} = K_H = \frac{K_1}{1 - \left( \dfrac{([G] - [A \cdot R \cdot G])}{K_2} \right)} \qquad [8.2]$$

In the presence of a large concentration of GTP, $K_2$ increases to the point where $((([G] - [A \cdot R \cdot G])/K_2 \rightarrow 0)$ and $K_{obs} \rightarrow K_1$. This would be the low-affinity state of the receptor, thus $K_{obs} = K_L$. From Eq. 8.2, the ratio of $K_L/K_H$ is:

$$K_L/K_H = 1 + [G]/K_2 - [A \cdot R \cdot G]/K_2 \qquad [8.3]$$

Thus, for two agonists, A1 and A2, the relative GTP shift ($K_L/K_H$ designated SHIFT$_{A1}$ and SHIFT$_{A2}$) is given by:

$$\frac{\text{SHIFT}_{A1}}{\text{SHIFT}_{A2}} = \frac{1 + [G]/K_{2(A1)} - [A1 \cdot R \cdot G]/K_{2(A1)}}{1 + [G]/K_{2(A2)} - [A2 \cdot R \cdot G]/K_{2(A2)}} \qquad [8.4]$$

Under circumstances where little ternary complex $[A \cdot R \cdot G]$ is required for response production (i.e., functional studies), then $[A \cdot R \cdot G] \ll [G]$ and Eq. 8.4 reduces to:

$$\frac{\text{SHIFT}_{A1}}{\text{SHIFT}_{A2}} = \frac{K_{2(A2)}(K_{2(A1)} + [G])}{K_{2(A1)}(K_{2(A2)} + [G])} \qquad [8.5]$$

If the magnitude of the equilibrium dissociation constant of the ternary complex is considerably lower than the concentration of coupling protein (i.e., if $[G] \gg K_{2(A1)}, K_{2(A2)}$, it can be seen from Eq. 8.5 that the relative magnitudes of the GTP shift approximate $K_2$ ratios. Since $K_2$ is the dissociation constant of the agonist-ternary complex unique for agonist and receptor pairs, it can be defined as a measure of the intrinsic efficacy of an agonist. Under these circumstances the relative GTP shifts of two agonists would reflect their relative intrinsic efficacy. Note that if $[T] \ll K_{2(A1)}, K_{2(A2)}$, then little abstraction of binding by $[G]$ will occur (no shift will be observed).

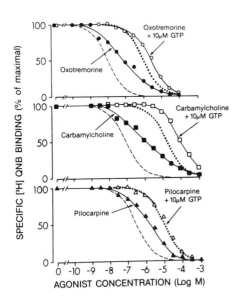

FIG. 8.4. Displacement of [³H]-L-[benzilic-4,4'-³H]quinuclidinyl benzilate (QNB) from muscarinic receptors of rat heart membranes by cholinergic agonists. *Closed symbols* represent binding in the absence, and *open symbols* in the presence, of GTP. *Dashed lines* represent binding to a high-affinity site, dots to a low-affinity site. The magnitudes of the effects of GTP on the binding curve [carbamylcholine (■, □) > oxotremorine (●, ○) > pilocarpine (▲, △)] are of the same rank order as their respective relative efficacies in physiological systems (carb > oxo > pilo). (Binding curves from ref. 37.)

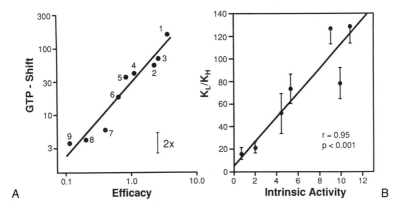

FIG. 8.5. Correlations of the GTP shift for agonists observed in binding studies and tissue-based estimates of relative efficacy. **A:** Data for muscarinic agonists in rat myocardium. (From ref. 9.) **B:** Data for β-adrenoceptor agonists in turkey erythrocytes. (From ref. 28.)

The propensity of an agonist to predispose ternary complex formation can be considered a measure of efficacy. This agonist property can be related to the degree of abstraction of binding produced by a coupler, i.e., the greater the efficacy, the greater the tendency to produce $[A \cdot R \cdot G]$ and thus to enhance agonist binding. Under these circumstances, it would be expected that there would a greater difference between $K_H$ and $K_L$ in experimental systems. This ratio has been correlated with observed tissue efficacy of agonists. For example, the changes in the affinities of three muscarinic agonists carbamylcholine, oxotremorine, and pilocarpine (relative intrinsic efficacies $1:0.14:0.05$) are shown in Fig. 8.4. From Eq. 8.5 it can be seen that, under certain conditions, the magnitude of the GTP shift ($K_L/K_H$) should be directly related to the $K_2$ values of the agonists, i.e., be agonist-specific estimates of intrinsic efficacy. In fact, close correlations between this experimentally measurable quantity and relative efficacy in functional studies have been shown. For example, Fig. 8.5A shows the correlation between the experimentally observed GTP shift and relative efficacy of a series of muscarinic receptor agonists for the inhibition of adenylate cyclase in rabbit myocardial membranes. Similarly, the relative efficacy of β-adrenoceptor agonists can be correlated with $K_L/K_H$ in turkey erythrocytes (Fig. 8.5B).

## INTRINSIC ACTIVITY

A term introduced by Ariëns (1) that is widely used to describe the property of agonism is *intrinsic activity*. We must distinguish between the meaning of this term that has evolved with common usage and the definition originally given by Ariëns. Ariëns introduced the concept of intrinsic activity as a proportionality factor between tissue response and receptor occupancy to represent the "effect per unit of pharmacon-receptor complex." By this definition, intrinsic activity was intended to describe a molecular quantity. The numerical value of intrinsic activity ($\alpha$) could range from unity (for full agonists) to zero (for antagonists), the fractional values within this range denoting partial agonists. Because Ariëns's modeling assumed a linear relationship between receptor occupancy and tissue response, the magnitude of the intrinsic activity was equal to the magnitude of the maximal response to the agonist (i.e., a partial agonist that produced a maximal response that was 40% of that of the tissue maximal response had $\alpha = 0.4$). Since its introduction in 1954, the measurement of intrinsic activity (tissue maximal response) has become a standard method for quantifying the ability of a drug to produce a response. However, if the measure of agonism is meant to be drug related, this scale is inappropriate, because in this scheme the magnitude of the maximal response is both drug and tissue related. Therefore, the efficiency of receptor coupling, a factor that changes from tissue to tissue, greatly affects the magnitude of the maximal response to an agonist. For example, as seen in Fig. 1.3, the $\beta$-adrenoceptor agonist prenalterol has $\alpha = 0.85$ in guinea pig right atria treated with thyroxine, $\alpha = 0.4$ in cat papillary muscle, and $\alpha = 0$ in canine coronary artery and thus will be classified as a nearly full agonist, a partial agonist, or an antagonist in these different tissues; the classification will depend on the tissue in which the measurement is made. The use of intrinsic activity as a parameter to classify drugs ignores Ariëns's original careful definition, which equates the molecular nature of $\alpha$ to maximal response only when response is a linear function of receptor occupancy. Failure to comply with this prerequisite renders the use of tissue maximal re-

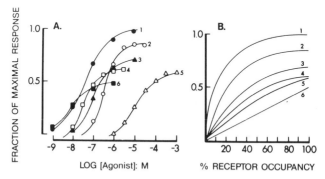

**FIG. 8.6.** Dose-response **(A)** and occupancy-response **(B)** curves for partial agonists. A: Ordinate: Responses as fractions of the tissue maximal response. Abscissa: Logarithms of molar concentrations of agonists. Responses to 1, phenylephrine (•) (data from ref. 32); 2, pirbuterol (○) (data from ref. 23); 3, oxymetazoline (▲) (data from ref. 19); 4, prenalterol (□) (data from ref. 23); 5, ethyl-2-pyretamine (△) (data from ref. 25); and 6, naphthazoline (■) (data from ref. 32). B: Ordinate: Responses as for A. Abscissa: Percentage of receptor occupancy calculated by the adsorption isotherm and $K_A$ values from sources of data. (From ref. 21.)

**TABLE 8.2.** *Effects of receptor alkylation on muscarinic responses to furtrethonium analogues*

| Drug | Exposure time (min) to dibenamine (20 μM) | | | | | |
|---|---|---|---|---|---|---|
| | 0 | 10 | 20 | 30 | 40 | 50 |
| A. Effect of dibenamine on maximal responses | | | | | | |
| HFMe$_3$ | 1.0 | 1.0 | 0.94 | 0.6 | 0.21 | 0.03 |
| MeFMe$_3$ | 1.0 | 1.0 | 0.86 | 0.59 | 0.20 | 0.02 |
| HFur | 1.0 | 0.9 | 0.6 | 0.32 | 0.07 | 0 |
| EtFMe$_3$ | 1.0 | 0.7 | 0.13 | 0.02 | 0 | 0 |
| B. Effect of dibenamine on relative intrinsic activity | | | | | | |
| HFMe$_3$ | 1.0 | 1.0 | 1.0 | 1.0 | 1.0 | 1.0 |
| MeFMe$_3$ | 1.0 | 1.0 | 0.91 | 0.98 | 0.95 | 0.67 |
| HFur | 1.0 | 0.91 | 0.65 | 0.53 | 0.33 | 0 |
| EtFMe$_3$ | 1.0 | 0.73 | 0.14 | 0.03 | 0 | 0 |

Data calculated from ref. 36.

sponses in an absolute scale of agonism incorrect. As detailed in Chapter 2, there is a predominance of evidence to suggest that stimulus-response coupling is not linear, even for partial agonists. Figure 8.6 shows dose-response curves for a number of partial agonists and the relationship between the receptor occupancy and tissue response. It can be seen from this figure that even for drugs that require 100% receptor occupancy for production of maximal response, the functions relating occupancy and response are not linear. In practical terms, this means that even the relative maximal responses of partial agonists cannot be directly equated to the molecular properties of agonism except in a sense of rank order (i.e., the agonist that produces the larger maximal response possesses the greater efficacy). This can be illustrated by the capricious behavior of the values of maximal responses to a series of cholinomimetics with changes in receptor number. Table 8.2A shows the maximal responses to four furtrethonium analogues after serial decreases in receptor density by treatment with the receptor-alkylating agent dibenamine. Normalization of these data in Table 8.2B, such that the maximal response to the most powerful agonist is taken to be $\alpha = 1$, shows that the relative values of $\alpha$ for the four analogues differ considerably as receptor number decreases. This dependence of maximal responses to partial agonists on receptor density makes calculation of a drug-specific parameter of efficacy from such data futile.

Quantification of agonism by relative maximal responses (intrinsic activity) is convenient and can be useful as long as the dependence of this measurement on the efficiency of stimulus-response coupling is recognized.

However, intrinsic activity cannot be used as a characteristic drug parameter for classification of drugs or drug receptors. For this purpose, a proportionality factor derived by null methods, namely, relative efficacy, can be useful.

## INTRINSIC EFFICACY

Theoretical considerations (see Chapter 1) suggest that a dimensionless proportionality factor can relate receptor occupancy and receptor stimulus; i.e., one drug may produce a given stimulus by occupying 5% of the available receptors, whereas another may require 40%. The proportionality factor is given the name *intrinsic efficacy*, and it represents the stimulus per receptor molecule produced by an agonist. It is strictly a drug-related term, and thus relative intrinsic efficacy can be measured by null methods and used to classify drugs and drug receptors.

One method to do this that does not require prior knowledge of agonist parameters, only two dose-response curves, uses a double-reciprocal equation to relate equiactive concentrations of two agonists, $[A_1]$ and $[A_2]$ (see Chapter 7 for derivation):

$$\frac{1}{[A_1]} = \frac{1}{[A_2]} \cdot \left( \frac{K_{A2}}{K_{A1}} \cdot \frac{\epsilon_1}{\epsilon_2} \right) + \frac{\epsilon_1}{\epsilon_2 \cdot K_{A1}} \left( 1 - \frac{\epsilon_2}{\epsilon_1} \right) \qquad [8.6]$$

where $K_A$ and $\epsilon$ are, respectively, agonist-receptor dissociation constants and intrinsic efficacies of the agonists. It can be seen from Eq. 8.6 that a double-reciprocal plot of $1/[A_1]$ on $1/[A_2]$ should yield a straight line, with intercept determined as

$$\text{intercept} = \frac{\epsilon_1}{\epsilon_2 \cdot K_{A1}} \left( 1 - \frac{\epsilon_2}{\epsilon_1} \right) \qquad [8.7]$$

Although a numerical estimate of $\epsilon_2/\epsilon_1$ cannot be made without a value for $K_{A1}$, the rank order of efficacy can be obtained from the arithmetic sign of the intercept; i.e., if $\epsilon_2 > \epsilon_1$, then the intercept will be negative, and if $\epsilon_2 < \epsilon_1$, it will be positive. In practice, dose-response curves for full agonists usually are parallel, causing the intercept of such a regression to approach zero and thereby making this procedure difficult to use. Also, the double-reciprocal regressions for two dose-response curves giving maximal responses do not yield accurate estimates of intercepts because of the variance in the regression line (see Chapter 7).

A numerical estimate of relative efficacy can be made by a method devised by Furchgott (11). The stimulus produced by an agonist is the product of the fractional receptor occupancy ($\rho$), the intrinsic efficacy ($\epsilon$), and the receptor density $[R_t]$; the respective stimuli to two agonists are given as

$$S_1 = \epsilon_1 \cdot \rho_1 \cdot [R_{t1}] \quad \text{and} \quad S_2 = \epsilon_2 \cdot \rho_2 \cdot [R_{t2}] \qquad [8.8]$$

If equal responses to the two agonists are compared, it will be assumed that these emanate from equal stimuli; therefore, $S_1 = S_2$, and

$$\frac{\epsilon_1}{\epsilon_2} = \frac{\rho_2 \cdot [R_{t2}]}{\rho_1 \cdot [R_{t1}]} \qquad [8.9]$$

If the comparison is made in the same tissue and if the agonists activate the same receptors, $[R_{t1}] = [R_{t2}]$, and Eq. 8.9 becomes

$$\epsilon_1/\epsilon_2 = \rho_2/\rho_1 \qquad [8.10]$$

Thus, the relative receptor occupancies required for the agonists to produce a common response are inversely proportional to the relative intrinsic efficacies of the agonists. This is logical if one assumes that the more efficacious is an agonist, the fewer receptors (lower $\rho$) it will need to activate to produce a given response.

Equation 8.10 leads to a practical method of estimating relative efficacy as long as the receptor occupancy can be calculated; to do this, the $K_A$ for each agonist is required. Therefore, a prerequisite for measurement of relative efficacy is measurement of relative affinity. In practice, measurement of relative $\epsilon$ is made with an occupancy-response curve; i.e., the responses to the agonist are plotted as functions of the logarithms of receptor occupancies (response versus log $\rho$). The lateral displacement between the curves on the $x$ axis is a measure of the logarithm of the relative efficacy. An example of measurement of the relative efficacies of the muscarinic agonists acetylcholine and methacholine is shown in Fig. 8.7A; the occupancy-response curves from rabbit aorta indicate that acetylcholine has 1.33 times the intrinsic efficacy of methacholine. Figure 8.7B shows a similar analysis for the β-adrenoceptor agonists pirbuterol and prenalterol. In both of these examples, the occupancy-response curves are reasonably parallel, and an unambiguous estimate of the lateral displacement between them can be made. If the occupancy-response curves are not parallel, then a practical problem arises as to where along the curves the displacement should be measured. Figure 8.7C shows occupancy-response curves for the α-adrenoceptor agonists norepinephrine and dobutamine in rat anococcygeus muscle; although the displacement at 30% maximal response was chosen to express relative efficacy, this is an arbitrary definition, because displacement at other points on the curves would yield different estimates of relative efficacy. One approach to circumvent these difficulties is to fit lines of common slope to the linear portions of occupancy-response curves. If it can be shown that the two curves are not significantly different with respect to slope (see Chapter 6), then parallel lines can be fitted to the two sets of data points. An example in which this was done is shown in Fig. 8.7D for the β-adrenoceptor agonists isoproterenol and prenalterol.

It should be noted that the Furchgott method results in a potentially agonist-specific estimate of relative efficacy within the framework of the opera-

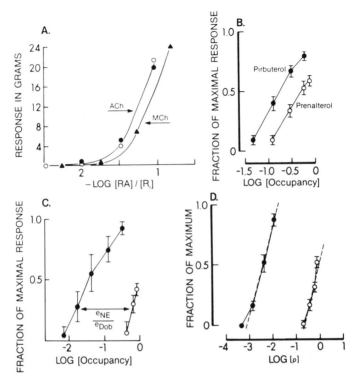

**FIG. 8.7.** Occupancy-response curves for measurement of relative efficacies of agonists. **A:** Contractions of rabbit aorta (ordinate) to acetylcholine (ACh) (●, ○) and methacholine (MCh) (▲) as functions of the logarithms of receptor occupancies (abscissa). (From ref. 12.) **B:** Positive inotropic responses (ordinate) to pirbuterol (●) and prenalterol (○) in rat left atria as functions of the logarithms of receptor occupancies. Bars represent SEM; $N$ = 6. Relative efficacy of pirbuterol/prenalterol = 2.3. (From ref. 23.) **C:** Contractions of rat anococcygeus muscle (ordinate) to norepinephrine (●) and dobutamine (○) as functions of the logarithms of receptor occupancies (abscissa). Bars represent SEM; $N$ = 8. Depending on where along the $y$ axis the displacement of the curves is measured, the relative efficacy of norepinephrine/dobutamine ranges from 57 to 25. (From ref. 17.) **D:** Positive inotropic responses (ordinate) to isoproterenol (●) and prenalterol (○) in guinea pig papillary muscles pretreated with isobutylmethylxanthine as functions of the logarithms of receptor occupancies (abscissa). *Broken lines* indicate best-fit common-slope regressions through the data points; bars represent SEM. The relative efficacy of isoproterenol/prenalterol was estimated to be $242 \pm 29$. (From ref. 22.)

tional model of drug action as well. The tissue response to two agonists, $A_1$ and $A_2$ can be described as hyperbolic functions of the ternary complexes formed between the agonist, receptor, and next-step coupling process. This need not necessarily be a coupling protein but rather any process that can be described by a hyperbolic function. Under these circumstances, the respective agonist responses are:

$$E_{A1} = \frac{[A_1{\cdot}R{\cdot}T]}{[A_1{\cdot}R{\cdot}T] + K_E} \quad E_{A2} = \frac{[A_2{\cdot}R{\cdot}T]}{[A_2{\cdot}R{\cdot}T] + K_E} \quad [8.11]$$

where $K_E$ is the concentration of ternary complex producing half the maximal response. Assuming that the stimulus-transduction steps in the same tissue are common for all agonist ternary complexes, equal responses (equating the two parts of Eq. 8.11) cancels $K_E$ and $[A_1 \cdot R \cdot T] = [A_2 \cdot R \cdot T]$. Further, the concentration of ternary complexes for each agonist is given by:

$$[A_1 \cdot R \cdot T] = \frac{[A_1 \cdot R]}{[A_1 \cdot R] + K_{AR1}} \quad [A_2 \cdot R \cdot T] = \frac{[A_2 \cdot R]}{[A_2 \cdot R] + K_{AR2}} \qquad [8.12]$$

where $K_{AR1}$ and $K_{AR2}$ are the respective equilibrium dissociation constants for the two agonist-formed ternary complexes. It is these dissociation constants that are unique to agonists and, if measurable, should furnish a system-independent measure of relative efficacy that could serve to characterize receptor and agonist pairs. Equating the two parts in Eq. 8.12 ($[A_1 \cdot R \cdot T] = [A_2 \cdot R \cdot T]$), the relative intrinsic efficacy is given as:

$$\frac{[A_2 \cdot R]}{[A_1 \cdot R]} = \frac{\rho_2}{\rho_1} = \frac{K_{AR1}}{K_{AR2}} \qquad [8.13]$$

A practical problem with this method concerns the comparison of agonists of low intrinsic efficacies. Figure 8.8A shows a series of dose-response curves for agonists with relative intrinsic efficacies of 10 to 0.01. The corresponding occupancy-response curves, shown in Fig. 8.8B, demonstrate the necessarily limited curves for low-efficacy agonists. Clearly, no values can exceed $\log \rho = 0$ (100% receptor occupancy); therefore, occupancy-response curves for low-efficacy agonists approach this limit and then are depressed. This makes unambiguous measurement of lateral distance between the curves difficult. An alternative method for measurement of relative efficacies of such low-efficacy agonists can be found in a calibration curve by interpolation. The tissue maximal responses to an agonist of given intrinsic efficacy is determined by tissue factors such as receptor number and receptor coupling to stimulus-response mechanisms. Although these largely are unknowns, they should be constant for a given receptor type in a given tissue. Under these circumstances, a linear calibration curve for efficacy can be constructed for estimation of the efficacies of partial agonists in any one tissue. Figure 8.8C shows dose-response curves for a series of α-adrenoceptor partial agonists in rat aorta. It is to be expected that a relationship will exist between efficacy and maximal response, because receptor occupancy at this point is complete, and the maximal stimulus depends only on efficacy, receptor density, and stimulus-response coupling. Figure 8.8D shows that the maximal responses to the partial agonists can adequately be described by a linear relationship between relative efficacy (logarithmic scale) and maximal response. Analysis of maximal responses in one tissue type makes the latter two tissue factors common; therefore, differences can be ascribed only to differences in efficacies. Of course, the nature of the relationships may not be linear, but empirically, if a linear relationship is obtained, then prediction

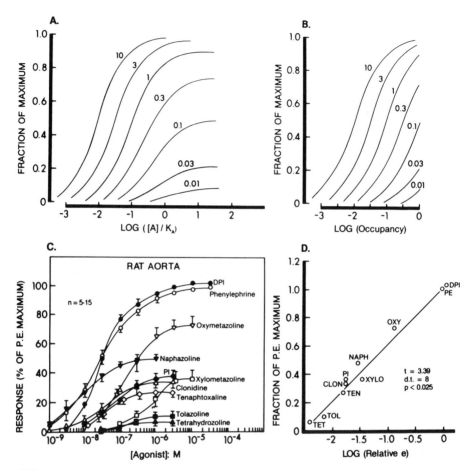

**FIG. 8.8.** Measuring relative efficacies of low-efficacy agonists. **A:** Dose-response curves for agonists of different efficacies. Ordinate: Response as a fraction of maximal tissue response. Abscissa: Logarithms of molar concentrations of agonist as fractions of $K_A$. Numbers next to the curves refer to relative efficacies (10 to 0.01). Response = $S/(S + 0.1)$, where $S = \epsilon \cdot \rho$ ($\rho$ = fractional receptor occupancy). **B:** Occupancy-response curves for data in A. Abscissa: Logarithms of receptor occupancies calculated from the adsorption isotherm. Numbers next to the curves refer to relative efficacies (10 to 0.01). **C:** Dose-response curves for $\alpha$-adrenoceptor agonists in rat aorta. Ordinate: Responses as percentages of the maximal response to phenylephrine. Abscissa: Molar concentrations of agonist on a logarithmic scale. (From ref. 33.) **D:** Calibration curve from correlation of maximal responses to $\alpha$-adrenoceptor agonists (ordinate) and logarithms of relative efficacies (abscissa). The line represents the least-squares best-fit straight line to the data points; the regression is significant, thereby allowing prediction of the maximal responses in rat aorta to $\alpha$-adrenoceptor partial agonists of low efficacies. Data from C.

is statistically simple. This suggests a practical method of estimating the relative efficacies of low-efficacy agonists. If the maximal responses to a number of agonists of known relative efficacies are determined in a given tissue, then a calibration curve will serve to predict the maximal responses to agonists of relative efficacies within that range by interpolation. This expands the scale for relative efficacies of low-efficacy agonists; i.e., rather than measurement of lateral displacements between depressed response and log-occupancy curves, as in Fig. 8.8B, the scale of efficacy for these agonists is the range of tissue maximal responses from 50% to 10%. In practical terms, accurate measurement of the maximal response to a partial agonist is considerably easier than determination of $K_A$ for the partial agonist and a complete dose-response curve that reflects the correct location parameter.

## RECEPTOR-TRANSDUCER PROMISCUITY

It is clear from studies in which receptors and transducer proteins are reconstituted in lipid membranes that some receptors are capable of associating with more than one type of G protein. For example, Fig. 8.9A shows the activation of three G proteins ($G_{i1}$, $G_{i2}$, and $G_o$) by adenosine A1 receptors

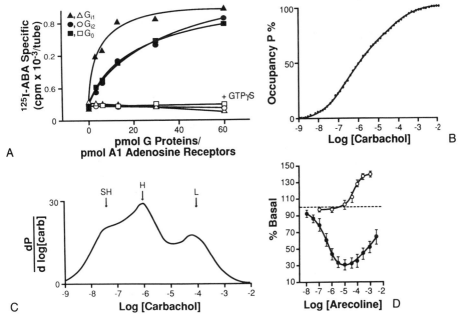

FIG. 8.9. Receptor promiscuity with respect to coupling proteins. A: Increased agonist binding of [$^{125}$I]N$^6$(3-iodo,4-amino)benzyladenosine (IABA) with reconstitution of adenosine A$_1$ receptors with either $G_{i1}$, $G_{i2}$, or $G_o$ proteins reconstituted in isolectin vesicles. (From ref. 30.) B: Muscarinic receptor occupancy in rat medulla-pons as measured by displacement of [$^3$H]propylbenzilylcholine. (From ref. 2.) C: Slope of the dose-response curve shown in B. SH, H, and L refer to potential superhigh-, high- and low-affinity states of the receptor. (From ref. 2.) D: Dose-response curves to arecoline in rat isolated left atria. Ordinates: Strength of electrically stimulated twitch contraction as a percentage of basal contraction. Abscissae: Logarithm of mole concentrations of arecoline. Response from normal (○) and atria from rats pretreated with pertussis toxin. (From ref. 24.)

reconstituted in phospholipid vesicles. When receptor activation was precluded by an excess of the stable GTP analogue GTPγS no increased agonist binding was observed. Whereas receptor promiscuity with respect to G-protein interactions can be demonstrated in reconstituted systems, it is unclear to what extent this occurs in natural physiological membranes. Figure 8.9B shows a very complex binding curve for the muscarinic agonist carbachol in rat medulla pons membranes. The extreme broadness of the curve and three different areas of slope (Fig. 8.9C) suggest a receptor with three binding affinities. A possible explanation for this type of behavior would be a single receptor interacting with three G proteins in the same membrane. There are functional studies that suggest receptor promiscuity as well. Figure 8.9D shows the biphasic inotropic response to arecoline in rat atria. The negative inotropy is thought to reflect activation of a G protein to promote potassium ion entry ($G_k$) and the positive inotropy from the activation of phosphoinositide turnover mechanisms. The involvement of two G proteins is suggested by the fact that treatment of the rats with pertussis toxin, which inactivates $G_k$ protein, converts the biphasic response to a monophasic response (Fig. 8.9D). The mediation of these two effects by a single receptor is suggested by the fact that only a single mRNA for muscarinic receptors has been detected in this tissue, and the sensitivity of both responses to a range of selective muscarinic receptor antagonists is uniform (see Table 8.3).

There also is biochemical evidence to support the notion that receptors are promiscuous in natural membranes. For example, it has been shown that adenosine A1 receptors in bovine brain copurify on an agonist affinity column with $G_{i1}$, $G_{i2}$, and $G_o$ (30). A strikingly graphic illustration of multiple ternary complexes has been shown in membranes from NG108-15 neuroblastoma X glioma cells. Figure 8.10A shows the effects of the opioid agonist D-Ala²-D-Leu⁵-enkephalin (DADLE) on [³²P] incorporation into G proteins. Incorpo-

**TABLE 8.3.** *Muscarinic receptor blockade of biphasic inotropic responses to arecoline in rat atria*

| Antagonist | Negative inotropy | | Positive inotropy | |
|---|---|---|---|---|
| | Slope[a] | pK$_B$[b] | Slope | pK$_B$ |
| Scopolamine | 0.9 | 8.8 | 0.9 | 9.0 |
| | (0.7–1.1) | (8.7–9.0) | (0.6–1.2) | (8.7–9.3) |
| AF-DX 116 | 1.05 | 6.9 | 1.0 | 7.0 |
| | (0.8–1.3) | (6.75–7.0) | (0.7–1.3) | (6.8–7.2) |
| 4-DAMP | 0.9 | 7.8 | 0.9 | 7.9 |
| | (0.8–1.0) | (7.7–7.9) | (0.8–1.1) | (7.8–8.0) |

[a] Slope of Schild regression.
[b] – Log of equilibrium dissociation constant for antagonist-receptor complex.
All values in parentheses represent 95% confidence limits of the means.
4-DAMP, 4-diphenyl-acetoxy-*N*-methylpiperidine methiodide.
From ref. 24.

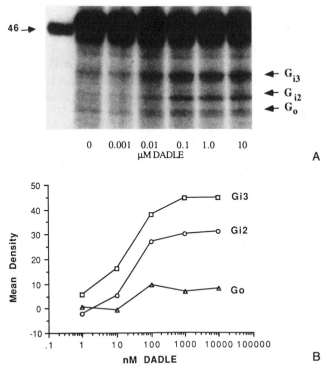

**FIG. 8.10.** Activation of three G proteins in NG108-15 neuroblastoma X glioma cells by the opioid receptor agonist DADLE. **A:** Autoradiogram of a urea gradient SDS-PAGE showing increasing incorporation of $^{32}P$ resulting from receptor activation of $G_{i1}$, $G_{i2}$, and $G_o$. *Arrows* show locations of active $\alpha$ subunits of the three G proteins. Concentrations of DADLE shown on bottom of autoradiogram. **B:** Mean density of bands shown in A by densitometry. (From ref. 31.)

ration of radioactivity indicates G-protein activation. It can be seen in Fig. 10A that increasing concentrations of DADLE produce increasingly evident bands of three activated G proteins. In Fig. 8.10B the density of the bands is quantified, thus giving the dose-response relationship for DADLE G-protein activation.

If receptors are promiscuous with respect to the type and number of coupling proteins with which they interact in cell membranes, this has broad implications for the definition of agonist efficacy. This is because it is highly unlikely that all agonists for a given receptor will produce an activated receptor with identical reactivity toward all coupling proteins. For example, although it is known that carbachol produces a biphasic dose-response effect in rat atria (Fig. 8.9D) thought to result from activation of two biochemical pathways, the muscarinic agonist oxotremorine produces a monophasic response. In the context of multiple receptor couplers, it might be supposed that oxotremorine produces an activated receptor capable of utilizing only one (not two) G protein. Alternatively, the difference could be quantitative in that a certain level of activated receptor would need to be produced to form ternary complexes with an array of G proteins. Therefore, powerful agonists might activate all possibilities, whereas a weaker agonist might only activate the most prominent. This would have the effect of shifting the curves shown in Fig. 8.10B, possibly making only the curve for $G_{i3}$ significant for a weak agonist (as opposed to three ternary complexes for DADLE).

If these types of interaction occur in natural membranes, then the uniqueness of efficacy as a drug-related term (embodied in the constants $\epsilon$ or $\tau$) is lost and the efficacy of an agonist would depend on both the receptor and the membrane-coupling proteins present in any individual system. Under these circumstances, measurements of the relative efficacy of agonists would not furnish useful data for drug and drug-receptor classification. However, the wide prevalence of promiscuous receptor-coupler reactions is thus far unproven, making this objection to the use of relative efficacy scales theoretical.


## NEGATIVE EFFICACY

In general pharmacologists have defined efficacy as the property of a drug producing a physiological response. The mechanistic implication of this definition is that the agonist has a message it imparts to the receptor, thus changing it and passing that message on to the cellular machinery via that change in the receptor. Parenthetically, the change in the receptor isomerizes it and may affect total agonist binding if the change removes the receptor from the equilibrium among agonist, free receptor, and agonist-receptor complex (see Chapter 7). Therefore a *broader* definition of efficacy would be the property that changes a receptor state or receptor equilibria between discrete states. Under this definition, a pure antagonist would be a more specialized entity in that it would bind to the receptor but in no way alter existing equilibria between receptor states or alter the receptor. This would lead to the definition of another class of drug, namely, those that alter existing receptor equilibria toward an inactive state or destabilize the formation the ternary complexes with coupling proteins (negative antagonists). These types of drugs have been described as having *negative efficacy*. In systems in which there is no way to detect inhibition of spontaneous receptor activity, negative and neutral antagonists will be indistinguishable. However, there are intriguing GTP effects that can be demonstrated with some antagonists that suggest more complex interactions than simple receptor occupancy. For example, Fig. 8.11 shows the expected decrease in specific binding of the dopamine agonist [$^3$H]$N$-propylapomorphine produced by GTP in membranes from the porcine anterior pituitary gland. However, this figure also shows an *increase*

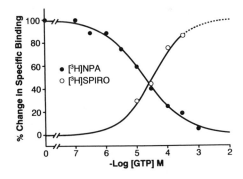

FIG. 8.11. Effect of GTP on binding of the agonist [³H]N-propylapomorphine ([³H]NPA, 155 pM) and antagonist [³H]spiroperidol ([³H]SPIRO, 160 pM) in membranes from porcine anterior pituitary gland. Specific binding expressed as a percentage of binding in the absence of GTP. (From ref. 8.)

in binding for the apparent antagonist [³H]spiroperidol produced by a similar concentration range of GTP. These data suggest that some antagonists discriminate between receptor states and that this discrimination may translate to differences in affinity under certain conditions.

A useful way to view these equilibria is with the model of drug-receptor equilibria proposed by Costa et al. (7):

$$A + R + T \overset{K}{\rightleftharpoons} A \cdot R + T$$
$$M \updownarrow \qquad \updownarrow \alpha M \qquad\qquad [8.14]$$
$$A + R \cdot T \underset{\alpha K}{\rightleftharpoons} A \cdot R \cdot T$$

Scheme 8.14 incorporates two important concepts in ligand equilibria, namely, the potential for receptors to spontaneously associate with coupling proteins (formation of $[R \cdot T]$) and the potential for ligands to destabilize ternary complex formation and predispose formation of $[R]$ from $[R \cdot T]$. The spontaneous interaction of receptors with coupling proteins is controlled by an equilibrium constant denoted $M$ and ligand-receptor interactions by the dissociation constants denoted by $K$ and $\alpha$. The dual dissociation constants for the ligand correspond to the relative affinity the ligand may have for the bare receptor $[R]$ and the precoupled receptor $[R \cdot T]$. Thus, a value of $\alpha = 1$ denotes a pure antagonist (also termed a neutral antagonist) in that the ligand has equal affinity for $[R]$ and $[R \cdot T]$ and it does not alter existing equilibria between receptor and coupling proteins. An $\alpha$ value $>1$ indicates classical agonism in that formation of the ternary complex $[A \cdot R \cdot T]$ is facilitated by the presence of $[A]$. Significantly, an $\alpha$ value $<1$ (negative antagonist) indicates an ability of the ligand to *destabilize* ternary complex formation and drive an existing tendency for the spontaneous formation of $[R \cdot T]$ back toward $[R]$ and $[T]$. In this sense, the affinity of the negative antagonist is higher for the bare receptor $[R]$ than it is for $[R \cdot T]$. Therefore, any experimental intervention that converts preexisting $[R \cdot T]$ into $[R]$ (i.e., GTP) would serve to *increase* the apparent affinity of negative antagonists. The effects of such interventions on antagonist assays such as the Schild analysis are discussed in Chapter 9. It should be noted that the precoupling of $[R]$ and $[T]$ is not essential to the differential affinity of negative antagonists, but also would occur in systems preactivated by agonists (where $[A \cdot R \cdot T]$ exists) such as binding assays displacing radiolabeled agonists. Data from these types of experiments are discussed in Chapter 12.

Figure 8.12 shows the behavior of a receptor system like that shown in scheme 8.14 toward agonists, neutral antagonists, and negative antagonists. Thus, a full agonist forms the species $[A \cdot R \cdot T]$ and depletes free $[T]$ and any existing $[R \cdot T]$. The physiological response of the system is given by the summed effects of $[A \cdot R \cdot T]$ and $[R \cdot T]$. Note how receptor precoupling increases basal activity and is additive to response produced by the ligand (curve $[A \cdot R \cdot T]$ and $[R \cdot T]$). A neutral antagonist produces no $[A \cdot R \cdot T]$ and does not deplete $[T]$. There is no change in the level of response ($[A \cdot R \cdot T]$ + $[R \cdot T]$) irrespective of whether receptor precoupling exists in the system. A negative antagonist depletes preexisting $[R \cdot T]$ and increases the level of free $[T]$. If there is a basal response emanating from a steady-state level of preformed $[R \cdot T]$, the negative antagonist, by reducing $[R \cdot T]$, will produce a reduction in basal response. If there is no basal response from receptor precoupling, a negative antagonist will appear as a neutral antagonist. However, in the presence of an agonist, differences between neutral and negative antag-

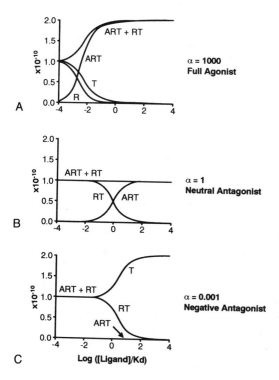

**FIG. 8.12.** Drug-receptor equilibria with transducer coupling protein $[T]$ for different ligands. Modeled according to scheme 8.14 with $[R] = [T] = 0.2$ nM, $M = 10^{10}$ M$^{-1}$, $K_d = 100$ nM. $[T]$, uncoupled transducer protein (G protein); R, uncoupled receptor; $A \cdot R$, ligand-receptor complex; $A \cdot R \cdot T$, ternary complex between ligand, receptor, and transducer protein. *Heavy line* represents $[A \cdot R \cdot T]$ + $[R \cdot T]$, which equals the physiological response of the system. (From ref. 7.)

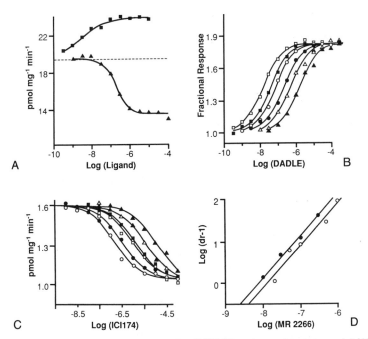

**FIG. 8.13.** Effects of opioid receptor agonist (DADLE) and negative antagonist [*N,N'*-dial-lyl-Tyr[1],Aib[2,3]]Leu[5]-enkephalin (ICI 174864) on GTPase activity in membranes from NG108-15 cells. **A:** Dose-response curves to DADLE (■) and ICI 174 (▲) in membranes assayed in 150 mM NaCl (significant spontaneous GTPase activity). **B:** Inhibition of DADLE activation by the neutral antagonist MR 2266 0 μM (□), 0.01 μM (■), 0.03 μM (○), 0.1 μM (●), 0.3 μM (△), and 1 μM (▲). **C:** Inhibition of the negative effects on basal GTPase activity by ICI 174 with MR 2266 0 μM (○), 0.02 μM (●), 0.04 μM (□), 0.1 μM (■), 0.3 μM (△), and 1 μM (▲). **D:** Schild regressions for data in B and C. The p$K_B$ estimates for the effects of MR 2266 on DADLE activation (8.2 ± 0.1) and ICI 174 negative activation (7.9 ± 0.12) are not significantly different. (From ref. 6.)

onists will appear as differences in apparent affinity because of the differential affinity of negative antagonists for [*R*], [*A·R*], and [*A·R·T*]. The magnitude of these differences will depend on the selectivity of the negative antagonist for the different receptor forms (magnitude of α), the levels of [*T*], and extent of [*A·R·T*] formation. These ideas are extended further in Chapters 7 and 9.

Figure 8.13 shows experimental data with the negative opioid receptor antagonist ICI 174 in NG108-15 cell membranes under conditions of spontaneous receptor coupling. In panel A, the functional response of the membrane system (i.e., the activity of GTPase) to an agonist DADLE and the negative antagonist ICI 174 is shown. From this figure it can be seen that, although the agonist increases response, the negative antagonist decreases basal response. The neutral antagonist MR 2266 was used to block both the positive (panel B) and negative (panel C) responses, and the resulting Schild

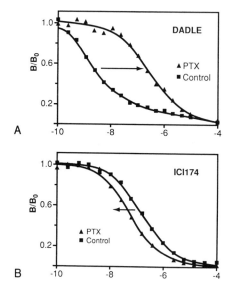

**FIG. 8.14.** Effects of inactivation of transducer coupling protein with pertussis toxin on displacement curves for DADLE **(A)** and ICI 174 **(B)**. Membranes were incubated with (▲) and without (■) pertussis toxin (PTX) 10 ng/mL. Displacement of [³H]diprenorphine (0.25 nM) measured in NG108-15 cell membranes in the presence of 100 mM NaCl. (From ref. 6.)

regressions for the blockade are shown in Fig. 8.13D. The fact that MR 2266 is equipotent as a blocker of the positive responses to DADLE and the negative responses to ICI 174 is consistent with the hypothesis that a single receptor mediates both processes. Under different ionic conditions that decrease spontaneous receptor-transducer coupling, the basal GTPase tone and the negative responses to ICI 174 decrease accordingly.

Another prediction made for spontaneously coupled receptor systems and negative antagonists is the effect of transducer protein depletion. Thus, membrane treatment with the G-protein inactivator pertussis toxin produces the well-known dextral shift in the displacement curves for agonists such as DADLE (Fig. 8.14A), but a *reverse* shift to the left in the displacement curves for the negative antagonist ICI 174 (Fig. 8.14B). This is because pertussis treatment inactivates the G protein (thus depleting $[T]$) and eliminates $[R \cdot T]$. Since the affinity of ICI 174 is greater for $[R]$ than it is for $[R \cdot T]$, this produces a net increase in the potency of this drug. In effect, the pertussis toxin is eliminating a receptor form less susceptible to blockade by ICI 174.

In general, the possibility that apparently neutral antagonists have properties that alter receptor equilibria with transducer proteins in systems in which this will not normally be detected leaves open reinterpretation of apparent receptor heterogeneity based on the premise of receptor subtypes. The impact of negative efficacy on the apparent affinity of negative antagonists would depend on the extent of receptor precoupling, which in turn is a tissue-specific phenomenon. Therefore, the apparent affinity of negative antagonists would be dependent on membrane components in addition to receptor type and thus be tissue dependent. Under these conditions receptor classification with such drugs could lead to false ascription of receptor selectivity.

## THE CONTRIBUTION OF EFFICACY TO AGONIST RESPONSE

Agonist potency depends on both affinity and efficacy, but there are instances in which knowing which of these parameters is dominant can be helpful in predicting therapeutic responses. In tissues for which given agonists have considerable reserves (i.e., maximal response is attained at low receptor occupancy), the location parameter for the dose-response curve ($EC_{50}$) depends on the quotient $\epsilon/K_A$. Parenthetically, this highlights the hazards of relying on binding data for prediction of potencies of agonists. Figure 8.15A shows theoretical curves for two agonists displacing a radioactive ligand from receptors in a binding experiment; agonist *A* has 10 times more affinity for receptors than does agonist *B*. However, if agonist *A* has 100 times the intrinsic efficacy of agonist *B*, then the dose-response curves for these drugs in physiological systems will show a striking reversal of the potency pattern from that predicted from binding data. Conceivably, two agonists could be equipotent but have different intrinsic efficacies, with compensating differences in $K_A$. An interesting differentiation of such agonists occurs on compromise of stimulus-response efficiency or decreases in receptor density in that the maximal response to the agonist of higher intrinsic efficacy is more resistant to decreases in tissue response capability. This can be illustrated by example; Fig. 8.16 (left) shows dose-response curves in rat anococcygeus muscle for the $\alpha$-adrenoceptor agonists norepinephrine and oxymetazoline. Independent experiments show that oxymetazoline has lower efficacy [$\epsilon(oxy)/\epsilon(nor) = 0.3$] but higher affinity [$K_A(oxy)/K_A(nor) = 0.2$] for $\alpha$-adrenoceptors than norepinephrine. As predicted by the $\epsilon/K_A$ ratio, oxymetazoline is a slightly more potent agonist, but its potency is more dependent on affinity than on efficacy. Figure 8.16 (center) shows the dose-response curves for the two agonists after reduction of receptor density by alkylation, with norepinephrine producing a greater maximal response than oxymetazoline. Figure 8.16 (right) shows the relative responses after further diminution of receptor number.

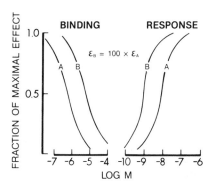

**FIG. 8.15.** Theoretical binding curves and response curves for two agonists A and B. A has 10 times the affinity of B for receptors, but B has 100 times the intrinsic efficacy. Binding: Displacements of a radioligand by various concentrations of A and B. Response: Predicted relative responses to the agonists with the specified relative $K_A$ and $\epsilon$ values in a tissue. (From ref. 18.)

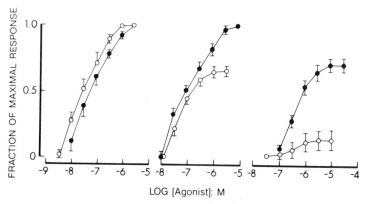

**FIG. 8.16.** Effects of receptor alkylation on responses of rat anococcygeus muscle to oxymetazoline (o) and norepinephrine (•). Ordinates: Contraction as a fraction of the control maximal response to norepinephrine. Abscissae: Logarithms of molar concentrations of agonist. **Left:** Control responses; no alkylation. **Center:** Responses after partial receptor alkylation by exposure to phenoxybenzamine (POB) (30 nM for 10 min). **Right:** Responses after 0.1 μM POB for 10 min. (From ref. 19.)

This effect has important ramifications for chronic therapy with agonists in that receptor down-regulation would be expected to reduce the responses to low-efficacy agonists to a greater extent than to those of high efficacy. For example, isoproterenol has 220 times the intrinsic efficacy of prenalterol for β-adrenoceptors. Figure 8.17A shows the effects of receptor down-regulation, produced by chronic stimulation of β-adrenoceptors, on the dose-response curves for both agonists. Whereas the dose-response curve for the agonist of high efficacy (isoproterenol) is shifted to the right, the curve for

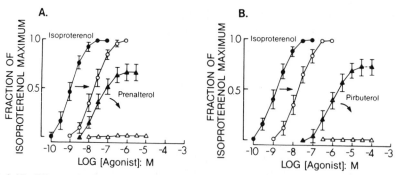

**FIG. 8.17.** Effects of receptor down-regulation on rat left atrial responses to isoproterenol (high efficacy) and prenalterol (low efficacy). Ordinates: Positive inotropy as a fraction of the maximal response to isoproterenol. Abscissae: Logarithms of molar concentrations of agonist. Responses to isoproterenol (•, o) and **(A)** prenalterol (▲, △) and **(B)** pirbuterol in normal (*filled symbols*) and desensitized (*open symbols*) atria. Receptor down-regulation (desensitization) produced by subcutaneous implantation of osmotic miniosmotic pumps delivering isoproterenol at 400 μg kg$^{-1}$ hr$^{-1}$ for 4 days. (From ref. 26.)

prenalterol (lower efficacy) is completely depressed. In down-regulated tissues, prenalterol functions as a competitive antagonist; if β-adrenoceptor agonism is a desired therapeutic event, then on chronic treatment with a low-efficacy β-adrenoceptor agonist, an opposite response could result (β-adrenoceptor antagonism). This same effect can be seen with the β-adrenoceptor agonist pirbuterol, which has 0.01 the intrinsic efficacy of isoprotere-

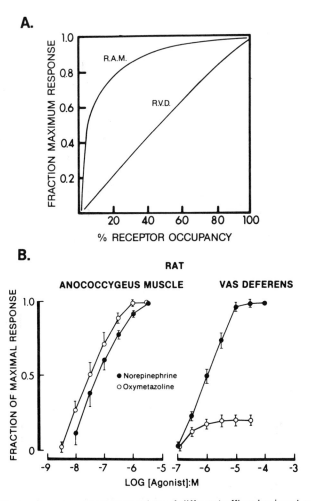

**FIG. 8.18.** Effects of α-adrenoceptor agonists of different efficacies in rat anococcygeus muscle and vas deferens. **A:** Occupancy-response curves for norepinephrine in rat anococcygeus muscle (R.A.M.) and rat vas deferens (R.V.D.). Occupancy (abscissa) calculated from an experimentally derived $K_A$ (1.26 μM). The efficiency of occupancy-response coupling is greater in the R.A.M., as shown by the steeper hyperbolic function. **B:** Dose-response curves for oxymetazoline ($N = 6$) and norepinephrine ($N = 6$) in rat anococcygeus muscle and vas deferens. Response expressed as fractions of the maximal response to norepinephrine. Bars represent SEM. (From ref. 19.)

nol (Fig. 8.17B). Therapeutically, as can be seen in Fig. 8.17, increasing the dosage of a high-efficacy agonist can overcome the effects of receptor down-regulation within limits (i.e., the curve is shifted to the right, but no depression of the maximal response occurs). Increasing the dosage of a low-efficacy agonist would not overcome receptor down-regulation (dose-response curve depressed), but rather exacerbate the loss of receptor function by producing receptor antagonism. Whereas the effects of receptor down-regulation on

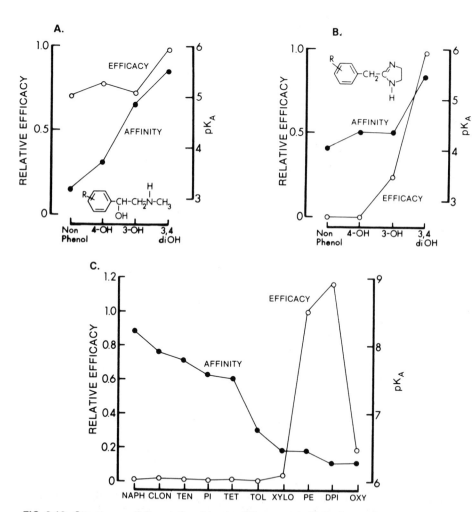

**FIG. 8.19.** Structure-activity relationships for efficacy and affinity for α-adrenoceptor agonists. p$K_A$ refers to the negative logarithm of $K_A$. Abscissa for **C**: Naphthazoline (NAPH), clonidine (CLON), tenaphtoxaline (TEN), 2-(phenylimino)imidazoline (PI), tetrahydrozoline (TET), tolazoline (TOL), xylometazoline (XYLO), phenylephrine (PE), (3,4-dihydroxyphenylamino)-2-imidazoline (DPI), and oxymetazoline (OXY). (Data for A and B [guinea pig aorta] from ref. 34 and C [rat aorta] from ref. 33.) (From ref. 20.)

low-efficacy agonists are greater, it is not clear whether low-efficacy agonists will produce receptor down-regulation to the same extent as that produced by a high-efficacy agonist.

Another aspect of the relative contributions of efficacy and affinity to agonist potency relates to drug and receptor classifications with agonists. Because the tissue response capability (receptor density and the efficiency of stimulus-response mechanisms) has a disproportionately larger effect on low- as opposed to high-efficacy agonists, such agonists may have different profiles in different tissues. For example, Fig. 8.18A shows occupancy-response curves for α-adrenoceptor activation by norepinephrine in rat anococcygeus muscle and vas deferens. The stimulus-response capability of the former tissue is greater (i.e., a lower fractional α-adrenoceptor occupancy by norepinephrine results in maximal response in rat anococcygeus muscle). Thus, whereas high- and low-efficacy agonists both produce a maximal response in this tissue (norepinephrine and oxymetazoline [Fig. 8.18B]), the low-efficacy agonist does not produce a maximal response in the tissue of lesser response capability (vas deferens [Fig. 8.18B]). This latter tissue can be compared to the tissue with a partially alkylated α-adrenoceptor pool shown in Fig. 8.16. Independent evidence shows that the strikingly different profiles of these agonists in these two tissues are not due to differences in receptor types, but rather to differences in tissue response capabilities. The relative activities of these agonists shown in Fig. 8.18B clearly are different (i.e., oxymetazoline is a more potent full agonist in rat anococcygeus muscle and a much weaker partial agonist in rat vas deferens). The fact that these differences are due to differences in efficacy rather than receptor heterogeneity should serve as a caveat against reliance on selective agonist profiles for receptor classification; this is discussed further in Chapters 11 and 13.

It is apparent that affinity and intrinsic efficacy are separate drug properties, presumably with different structure-action relationships to receptors. Figure 8.19 illustrates this for a number of α-adrenoceptor agonists. It can be seen that a change in chemical structure that produces a change in affinity may not produce a corresponding change in efficacy (i.e., 4-OH- to 3-OH-phenylethylamine [Fig. 8.19A]), and vice versa (4-OH- to 3-OH-imidazoline [Fig. 8.19B]). Therefore, quantification of efficacy is as valuable as quantification of affinity for agonists in receptor studies and drug design.

## REFERENCES

1. Ariëns, E. J. (1954): Affinity and intrinsic activity in the theory of competitive inhibition. *Arch. Int. Pharmacodyn. Ther.*, 99:32–49.
2. Birdsall, N. J. M., Hulme, E. C., Keen, M., Stockton, J. M., Pedder, E. K., and Wheatley, M. (1987): Can complex binding phenomena be resolved to provide a safe basis for receptor classification? In: *Perspectives on Receptor Classification, Receptor Biochemistry and Methodology, Vol. 6*, edited by J. W. Black, D. H. Jenkinson, and V. P. Gerskowitch, pp. 61–71. Alan R. Liss, New York.

3. Black, J. W., and Leff, P. (1983): Operational models of pharmacological agonism. *Proc. R. Soc. Lond.* [*Biol.*], 220:141–162.

4. Burgen, A. S. V. (1981): Conformational changes and drug action. *Fed. Proc.*, 40: 2723–2728.

5. Clark, A. J. (1937): General pharmacology. In: *Heffter's Handbuch d-exp. Pharmacol. Erg., band 4.* Springer, Berlin.

6. Costa, T., and Herz, A. (1989): Antagonists with negative intrinsic activity at δ-opioid receptors coupled to GTP-binding proteins. *Proc. Natl. Acad. Sci. U.S.A.*, 86:7321–7325.

7. Costa, T., Ogino, Y., Munson, P. J., Onaran, H. O., and Rodbard, D. (1992): Drug efficacy at guanine nucleotide-binding regulatory protein-linked receptors: Thermodynamic interpretation of negative antagonism and of receptor activity in the absence of ligand. *Mol. Pharmacol.*, 41:549–560.

8. De Lean, A., Kilpatrick, B. F., and Caron, M. (1982): Dopamine receptor of the porcine anterior pituitary gland: Evidence for two affinity sites discriminated by both agonists and antagonists. *Mol. Pharmacol.*, 22:290–297.

9. Ehlert, F. J. (1985): The relationship between muscarinic receptor occupancy and adenylate cyclase inhibition in the rabbit myocardium. *Mol. Pharmacol.*, 28:410–427.

10. Ehlert, F. J., and Rathbun, B. E. (1990): Signaling through the muscarinic receptor-adenylate cyclase system of the heart is buffered against GTP over a range of concentrations. *Mol. Pharmacol.*, 38:148–158.

11. Furchgott, R. F. (1966): The use of β-haloalkylamines in the differentiation of receptors and in the determination of dissociation constants of receptor-agonist complexes. In: *Advances in Drug Research, Vol. 3*, edited by N. J. Harper and A. B. Simmonds, pp. 21–55. Academic Press, New York.

12. Furchgott, R. F., and Bursztyn, P. (1967): Comparison of dissociation constants and of relative efficacies of selected agonists acting on parasympathetic receptors. *Ann. N.Y. Acad. Sci.*, 139:882–899.

13. Gardner, P., Ogden, D. C., and Colquhoun, D. (1985): Conductances of single ion channels opened by nicotinic agonists are indistinguishable. *Nature*, 309:168–172.

14. Helmreich, E. J. M., and Pfeuffer, T. (1985): Regulation of signal transduction by β-adrenergic hormone receptors. *Trends Pharmacol. Sci.*, 6:438–443.

15. Hildebrandt, J. D., Codina, J., and Birnbaumer, L. (1984): Interaction of the stimulatory and inhibitory regulatory proteins of the adenylyl cyclase system with the catalytic component of S49 cell membranes. *J. Biol. Chem.*, 259:13178–13185.

16. Katada, T., Bokoch, G. M., Smigel, M. D., Ui, M., and Gilman, A. G. (1984): The inhibitory guanine nucleotide-binding regulatory component of adenylate cyclase. *J. Biol. Chem.*, 259: 3586–3589.

17. Kenakin, T. P. (1981): An *in vitro* quantitative analysis of the alpha adrenoceptor partial agonist activity of dobutamine and its relevance to inotropic selectivity. *J. Pharmacol. Exp. Ther.*, 216:210–219.

18. Kenakin, T. P. (1983): Receptor classification by selective agonists: Coping with circularity and circumstantial evidence. *Trends Pharmacol. Sci.*, 4:291–295.

19. Kenakin, T. P. (1984): The relative contribution of affinity and efficacy to agonist activity: Organ selectivity of noradrenaline and oxymetazoline with reference to the classification of drug receptors. *Br. J. Pharmacol.*, 81:131–143.

20. Kenakin, T. P. (1984): The classification of drugs and drug receptors in isolated tissues. *Pharmacol. Rev.*, 36:165–222.

21. Kenakin, T. P. (1985): The quantification of relative efficacy of agonists. *J. Pharmacol. Meth.*, 13:281–308.

22. Kenakin, T. P., and Beek, D. (1984): The measurement of the relative efficacy of agonists by selective potentiation of tissue responses: Studies with isoprenaline and prenalterol in cardiac tissue. *J. Auton. Pharmacol.*, 4:153–159.

23. Kenakin, T. P., and Beek, D. (1984): Relative efficacy of prenalterol and pirbuterol for β₁-adrenoceptors: Measurement of agonist affinity by alteration of receptor number. *J. Pharmacol. Exp. Ther.*, 229:340–345.

24. Kenakin, T. P., and Boselli, C. (1991): Biphasic dose-response curves to arecoline in rat atria: Mediation by a single promiscuous receptor or two receptor subtypes? *Naunyn Schmiedebergs Arch. Pharmacol.*, 344:201–205.

25. Kenakin, T. P., and Cook, D. A. (1980): *N,N*-diethyl-2-(1-pyridyl)ethylamine, a partial agonist for the histamine receptor in guinea pig ileum. *Can. J. Physiol. Pharmacol.*, 58: 1307–1310.

26. Kenakin, T. P., and Ferris, R. M. (1983): Effects of in vivo β-adrenoceptor down-regulation on cardiac responses to prenalterol and pirbuterol. *J. Cardiovasc. Pharmacol.*, 5:90–97.

27. Kjelsberg, M. A., Cottechia, S., Ostrowski, J., Caron, M. G., and Lefkowitz, R. J. (1992): Constitutive activation of the $\alpha_{1B}$-adrenergic receptor by all amino acid substitutions at a single site. *J. Biol. Chem.*, 267:1430–1433.

28. Lefkowitz, R. J., Caron, M. G., Michel, T., and Stadel, J. M. (1982): Mechanisms of hormone receptor-effector coupling: The β-adrenergic receptor and adenylate cyclase. *Fed. Proc.*, 41:2664–2670.

29. Limbird, L. E., and Lefkowitz, R. J. (1978): Agonist induced increase in apparent β-adrenergic receptor size. *Proc. Natl. Acad. Sci. U.S.A.*, 75:228–232.

30. Munshi, R., Pang, I-H., Sternweis, P. C., and Linden, J. (1991): $A_1$ adenosine receptors of bovine brain couple to guanine nucleotide-binding proteins $G_{i1}$, $G_{i2}$ and $G_o$. *J. Biol. Chem.*, 266:22285–22289.

31. Roerig, S. C., Loh, H. H., and Law, P. Y. (1992): Identification of three separate guanine nucleotide-binding proteins that interact with the δ-opioid receptor in NG108-15 X glioma hybrid cells. *Mol. Pharmacol.*, 41:822–831.

32. Ruffolo, R. R., Jr. (1982): Review: Important concepts of receptor theory. *J. Auton. Pharmacol.*, 2:277–295.

33. Ruffolo, R. R., Rosing, E. L., and Waddell, J. E. (1979): Receptor interactions of imidazolines. I. Affinity and efficacy for alpha adrenergic receptors in rat aorta. *J. Pharmacol. Exp. Ther.*, 209:429–436.

34. Ruffolo, R. R., Jr., and Waddell, J. E. (1983): Aromatic and benzylic hydroxyl substitution of imidazolines and phenthylamines: Differences in activity at alpha-1 and alpha-2 adrenergic receptors. *J. Pharmacol. Exp. Ther.*, 224:559–566.

35. Stephenson, R. P. (1956): A modification of receptor theory. *Br. J. Pharmacol.*, 11:379–393.

36. Van Rossum, J. M., and Ariëns, E. J. (1962): Receptor-reserve and threshold-phenomena. II. Theories on drug-action and a quantitative approach to spare receptors and threshold values. *Arch. Int. Pharmacodyn. Ther.*, 136:385–413.

37. Waelbroeck, M., Robberecht, P., Chatelain, P., and Christophe, J. (1981): Rat cardiac muscarinic receptors. Effects of guanine nucleotides on high- and low-affinity binding sites. *Mol. Pharmacol.*, 21:581–588.

# 9

# Competitive Antagonism

*Imperfect knowledge appears to be the most probable reason for any apparent simplicity in processes of drug antagonism.*

—A. J. Clark, 1937

*If it could be verified experimentally that certain groups of agonists produce the same . . . dose ratio with antagonists, the receptor theory would be strengthened and a precise method provided of classifying agonists according to the receptors on which they act.*

—H. O. Schild, 1959

The process of inhibition or prevention of agonist-induced response is termed *antagonism*, and the chemical entities with such properties are *antagonists*. Antagonists can be classified by their kinetics of interaction with receptors. For example, an antagonist can rapidly dissociate from the receptor to produce reversible antagonism or form a chemical bond with the receptor (i.e., alkylating agents) to produce irreversible antagonism. Essentially irreversible antagonism can be produced by antagonists that do not alkylate receptors, but still dissociate very slowly from receptors (pseudo irreversible antagonism). Antagonists, depending on their sites of interference with agonist-induced responses and kinetics of interaction, may have different effects on dose-response curves. Therefore, it is best to classify antagonists on the basis of the molecular mechanisms by which they block agonist responses. First, a drug (or a surface) may block the response to an agonist chemically by preventing access to the receptor. This is dealt with in Chapter 5 under drug adsorption effects. Second, an antagonist may bind to a site on the receptor distinct from the agonist recognition site, but through allotopic or other mechanisms may prevent agonist activation of the receptor. This is termed noncompetitive and/or allotopic antagonism and is dealt with in the next chapter. Last, an antagonist may bind to the same recognition site on the receptor as the agonist and thus compete for binding with the agonist.

This is termed competitive antagonism, and it is this model that has the most formalized mathematical formulations.

## SURMOUNTABLE AND INSURMOUNTABLE ANTAGONISM

Gaddum and associates (12) termed the antagonism of an agonist response that results in a parallel displacement of the agonist dose-response curve to the right, with no concomitant depression of maximal response to the agonist, *surmountable antagonism*. Likewise, blockade of a response that results in depression of the maximal response to the agonist (whether or not it is accompanied by a shift of the dose-response curve to the right) is termed *insurmountable antagonism*. Although empirical, these categories are useful as a first means of classification. They also serve to somewhat simplify possible further classification by mechanisms, because certain molecular mechanisms of antagonism usually result in either surmountable or insurmountable blockade. The definitions of these types of antagonism in terms of effects on agonist dose-response curves and the commonly encountered molecular mechanisms giving rise to these effects are shown in Fig. 9.1. As can be seen from this figure, certain types of antagonism involve only surmountable

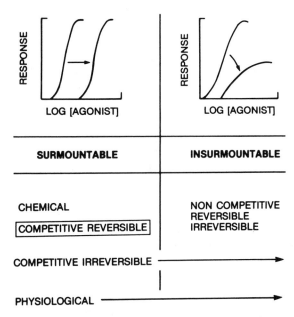

**FIG. 9.1.** Classification of molecular mechanisms of antagonism in terms of empirical effects on agonist dose-response curves. *Arrows* indicate where different concentrations of antagonist may produce both surmountable antagonism and insurmountable antagonism.

antagonism (chemical, competitive reversible); thus, experimentally observed insurmountable antagonism will tend to eliminate these mechanisms from consideration. It should be stressed, however, that a certain degree of overlap is observed that sometimes is dependent on the concentration of antagonist. For example, low concentrations of an irreversible, functional, or noncompetitive antagonist may produce surmountable antagonism in tissues efficiently receptor coupled, in which activation of only a small proportion of the receptors is sufficient to produce a maximal response to a given agonist. Therefore, the testing of a range of concentrations of antagonist, as opposed to reliance on the effects of one concentration, is essential. Also, if a range of antagonist concentrations is used, the resulting effects on agonist responses can be compared with the various theoretical quantitative models of the molecular forms of antagonism.

## MOLECULAR NATURE OF ANTAGONIST AFFINITY

The molecular forces that control the attraction and repulsion between an antagonist and a receptor are qualitatively the same as those discussed in Chapter 7 (The Molecular Nature of Affinity). However, it is possible that quantitatively the contribution of hydrophobic forces is greater for antagonists than it is for agonists. It may be assumed that for an agonist to bind to and activate a receptor, a close structural fit must be made between the agonist and target site. It would follow that the target sites for agonists on receptors would be somewhat homogeneous, because they would have to respond to the same chemicals (i.e., hormones, neurotransmitters) throughout most mammalian species. Antagonists, on the other hand, need not fit into the target site, but rather only need to occlude it; therefore, it might be expected that a range of auxiliary binding sites around the target site may be as important to antagonists as the target site itself. Antagonists in general are more lipophilic than agonists, and it would be expected that more nonspecific hydrophobic interactions would be important to such molecules. This also is in keeping with the known lower dissociation rate constants for antagonists as opposed to agonists.

Subclassification of receptor types has come about largely because of the discovery of selective antagonists. Theoretically this could be because there are numerous possible binding sites for antagonists on a receptor that could vary their orientations toward the extracellullar space with structural factors such as composition of cellular membranes; this could, in turn, vary with types of organs and/or species.

## COMPETITIVE REVERSIBLE ANTAGONISM

The condition in which the agonist and antagonist bind reversibly to the same recognition sites on the receptor, and thus when present concomitantly compete for such sites, is called competitive reversible antagonism. The original equation to predict the quantitative effects of such an antagonist on agonist dose-response curves was derived by Gaddum (10). The equilibria of the free receptors $[R]$ with an agonist $[A]$ and competitive antagonist $[B]$ can be described by the reactions

$$[A] + [R] \underset{k_{2A}}{\overset{k_{1A}}{\rightleftharpoons}} [A \cdot R], \qquad [B] + [R] \underset{k_{2B}}{\overset{k_{1B}}{\rightleftharpoons}} [B \cdot R] \qquad [9.1]$$

where $k_1$ and $k_2$ are the respective rates of onset and offset of either $A$ or $B$ for the receptor, and $[A \cdot R]$ and $[B \cdot R]$ are the complexes formed between the receptor and the agonist and antagonist, respectively. The total receptor population ($[R_t]$) is given by the sum of the free $[R]$ and complexed receptor. Therefore,

$$[R_t] = [R] + [A \cdot R] + [B \cdot R] \qquad [9.2]$$

At equilibrium, the rate of agonist-receptor formation ($k_{1A} \cdot [A] \cdot [R]$) equals the rate of agonist-receptor dissociation ($k_{2A} \cdot [A \cdot R]$); substituting for $[R]$ from Eq. 9.2, this equilibrium becomes

$$k_{1A} \cdot [A]([R_t] - [A \cdot R] - [B \cdot R]) = k_{2A} \cdot [A \cdot R] \qquad [9.3]$$

which rearranges to

$$\frac{[B \cdot R]}{[R_t]} = 1 + \frac{[A \cdot R]}{[R_t]}\left(1 + \frac{K_A}{[A]}\right) \qquad [9.4]$$

where $k_A = k_{2A}/k_{1A}$. An equation for the equilibrium between $[B]$ and $[R]$ analogous to Eq. 9.3 can be derived from which an expression for $[B \cdot R]/[R_t]$ can be obtained. Substituting for $[B \cdot R]/[R_t]$ into Eq. 9.4,

$$\frac{K_B}{[B]} = \frac{[A \cdot R]}{[R_t]}\left[\left(1 + \frac{K_A}{[A]}\right)\left(1 + \frac{K_B}{[B]}\right) - 1\right] \qquad [9.5]$$

where $K_B$ is the equilibrium dissociation constant for the antagonist-receptor complex ($k_{2B}/k_{1B}$). Rearrangement of Eq. 9.5 yields the classic equation for competitive antagonism derived by Gaddum (10):

$$\frac{[A \cdot R]}{[R_t]} = \frac{[A]}{[A] + K_A (1 + [B]/K_B)} \qquad [9.6]$$

which gives the fractional receptor occupancy by an agonist ($[A \cdot R]/[R_t]$) for any given concentrations of agonist and antagonist. This equation predicts that in the presence of a competitive antagonist, the fractional receptor occupancy by the agonist will be lower than in the absence of antagonist; this is logical in view of the defined condition that the two drugs compete for the same receptors.

To describe the effects of a competitive antagonist on the responses to a range of agonist concentrations, the concept of dose ratios is useful. If it is assumed that a given concentration of agonist [A] occupies a fraction of receptors $\rho_A$ in the absence of antagonist, then in the presence of a concentration [B] of antagonist (which also occupies a fraction of receptors), the fractional occupancy by [A] will be diminished (and therefore the response to A will be diminished as well). In order to attain the same fractional occupancy $\rho_A$, the concentration of agonist must be increased. Figure 9.2 shows fractional receptor occupancies by the agonist in the absence and presence of various concentrations of antagonist according to Eq. 9.9. It can be seen that the receptor-occupancy curve is shifted to the right in the presence of antagonist. The multiple increase in agonist concentration required to achieve a given response is termed the *dose ratio*. Because this parameter can be determined experimentally, it functions as a scale for competitive antagonist potencies.

An empirical scale for antagonist potencies based on dose ratios, termed the pA scale, was introduced by Schild (34) in 1949. The term $pA_x$ is defined as the negative logarithm of the molar concentration of antagonist that produces an equiactive dose ratio of magnitude $x$; i.e., $pA_{10}$ represents a concentration of antagonist that produces a 10-fold shift to the right in the agonist dose-response curve. It should be stressed that this is an empirical scale, with no theoretical relevance to molecular mechanisms. However, dose ratios can be used in a model that theoretically can yield a molecular parameter by the Schild equation.

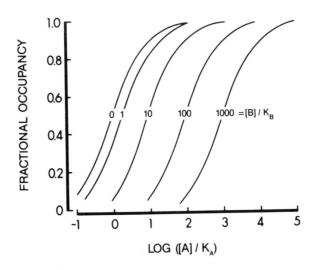

**FIG. 9.2.** Effects of a simple competitive antagonist on agonist dose-response curves. The dose ratio is [A'] ÷ [A], where these refer to equiactive concentrations of agonist in the presence and absence of antagonist, respectively.

### Measurement of Antagonist Potency: Schild Regression

The dose ratios calculated for a competitive antagonist can be compared to a quantitative model of competitive antagonism derived by Arunlakshana and Schild (2). If the criteria of simple competitive antagonism, as defined by this model, are met, then a "molecular fingerprint" for the antagonist, in the form of the equilibrium dissociation constant for the antagonist-receptor complex, can be obtained. As can be seen by Eq. 9.6, in the absence of antagonist ($[B] = 0$), the receptor occupancy by concentration $[A]$ of an agonist is given by

$$\frac{[A \cdot R]}{[R_t]} = \frac{[A]}{[A] + K_a} \qquad [9.7]$$

In the presence of an antagonist, a given concentration of agonist ($[A']$) produces an equal response and therefore presumably produces an equal receptor occupancy, given by

$$\frac{[A \cdot R]}{[R_t]} = \frac{[A']}{[A'] + K_A (1 + [B]/K_B)} \qquad [9.8]$$

Equating 9.7 and 9.8 (because equal receptor occupancies are presumed to yield equal responses), the ratio of equiactive concentrations of agonist in the presence and absence of antagonist (dose ratio, dr) is given by $[A']/[A]$:

$$\frac{[A']}{[A]} = \mathrm{dr} = \frac{[B]}{K_B} + 1 \qquad [9.9]$$

Equation 9.9 quantifies the relationship between the multiple increases in agonist concentrations required to produce equal responses in the presence of given concentrations of antagonist. It can be seen that the magnitude of the dose ratios depends on two factors: the concentration of the antagonist $[B]$ and the equilibrium dissociation constant for the antagonist-receptor complex, the constant that defines the fractional receptor occupancy attained by that concentration. Because the concentration of antagonist $[B]$ is known and the dose ratio is observed experimentally, the equilibrium dissociation constant for the antagonist-receptor complex can be calculated. This is most conveniently done by converting Eq. 9.9 into a logarithmic metameter that describes a straight-line regression of a mathematical manipulation of dr on $\log[B]$. From Eq. 9.9,

$$\log(\mathrm{dr} - 1) = \log[B] - \log K_B \qquad [9.10]$$

Regressions according to Eq. 9.10 are called Schild regressions and provide a cornerstone of pharmacologic receptor classification.

This regression is a powerful tool in the drug and receptor classification process; it has two specific applications. The first is as a determinant of simple competitive antagonism and $K_B$; the second is as an indicator of nonequilibrium states with respect to the homogeneity of receptor populations, the drug-disposition mechanisms in tissues, or multiple drug properties. These latter applications will be discussed specifically in following sections.

If a regression of $\log(dr - 1)$ on $\log[B]$ is linear and has a slope of unity, this furnishes presumptive evidence that the antagonism is competitive; i.e., the agonist and antagonist compete for the same recognition sites on the receptor. It should be noted that Eq. 9.10 as written assumes that one molecule of agonist and one molecule of antagonist bind to each receptor. There is no theoretical rationale for this constraint, but current evidence suggests this to be the general observation. Nevertheless, the more general form of the Gaddum equation describing competitive antagonism (Eq. 9.6) is

$$\frac{[A \cdot R]}{[R_t]} = \frac{[A]^{n_1}}{[A]^{n_1} + K_A (1 + [B]^{n_2}/K_B)} \qquad [9.11]$$

where $n_1$ and $n_2$ represent the numbers of agonist and antagonist molecules, respectively, that interact with the receptor. The resulting Schild equation is

$$\log(dr^{n_1} - 1) = n_2 \cdot \log[B] - \log K_B \qquad [9.12]$$

It can be seen from Eq. 9.12 that true competitive antagonism in such systems will be made manifest in regressions of slope equal to $n_2$. The following discussion will focus on the far more commonly observed condition in which $n_1 = n_2 = 1$, but it should be noted that if consistent evidence of a slope greater than unity is obtained from experiments known to have been carried out under true equilibrium conditions, this could signify multiple drugs binding to a single receptor.

It can be seen from the Schild equation that if the regression according to Eq. 9.10 is linear and has a slope of unity, then the intercept represents $-\log K_B$, and an estimate of the equilibrium dissociation constant can be obtained. Because this is a chemical term describing the molecular interaction of the antagonist and the receptor, it has obvious value in drug-receptor classification (see Chapter 11). The term $pK_B$ is the value of $-\log(dr - 1)$ when the dr $= 2$; this quantity therefore also corresponds to $pA_2$, an empirical parameter defined as the negative logarithm of the molar concentration of antagonist that produces a dr of 2. As seen from the Schild equation (Eq. 9.10), $pK_B$ always corresponds to $pA_2$, but the converse, namely, that $pA_2$ equals $pK_B$, often is not true. Only when the Schild regression is linear and has a slope of unity can $pA_2$ be equated with the molecular quantity $pK_B$. This makes the linearity and slope of experimental Schild regressions of prime importance in studies of drug and receptor classification.

The most unambiguous method to measure antagonist potency is to determine its effects on a complete-agonist dose-response curve. Thus, after determination of a dose-response curve, the agonist is removed by washing, and the tissue is equilibrated with a known concentration of the antagonist. Sufficient equilibration time must be allowed to produce a thermodynamic equilibrium between the antagonist and the receptor; after that period, a dose-response curve to the agonist is repeated in the presence of the antagonist. Ideally, the antagonist, if competitive, produces a parallel shift to the right in the agonist dose-response curve. Under these circumstances, equiactive dose ratios are independent of the level of response. There dose ratios, expressed as log(dr − 1), are used in a linear regression on log[B] to produce a Schild regression.

A practical aspect of experimental Schild regressions concerns the concentration range of antagonist used. Although it is preferable to use as wide a range as possible for greater receptor occupancy and also to define the limits of simple competitive blockade, in general, high concentrations of antagonists can produce nonspecific effects that can interfere with competitive blockade. Also, because of the nature of the ordinate axis [log(dr − 1)], small random changes in tissue sensitivities have greater effects on low as opposed to high dose ratios. This may lead to a degree of heteroscedasticity of error in the regression in that errors in the ordinate near $pK_B$ are greater.

Figure 9.3A shows the antagonism by oxymetazoline of responses of rat anococcygeus muscle to norepinephrine, and Fig. 9.3B shows the resulting

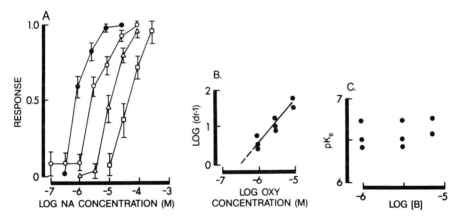

**FIG. 9.3.** Competitive antagonism of responses of rat anococcygeus muscle to norepinephrine by oxymetazoline. **A:** Ordinate: Contractions of rat anococcygeus muscle to norepinephrine as fractions of the maximal contraction. Abscissa: Logarithms of molar concentrations of norepinephrine. Responses in the absence (●, $N = 6$) and presence of oxymetazoline at 1 (○, $N = 3$), 3 (△, $N = 3$), and 100 μM (□, $N = 2$). Tissues pretreated with phenoxybenzamine (0.3 μM, 10 min) to block contractions by oxymetazoline. Bars represent SEM. **B:** Schild regression to oxymetazoline. Ordinate: Logarithms of dose ratios minus 1. Abscissa: Logarithms of molar concentrations of oxymetazoline. From data shown in A. Slope = 1.0 (95% confidence limits 0.9–1.2); $pK_B = 6.5$ (6.3–6.8). **C:** Regressions of $pK_B$ estimates calculated from individual concentrations of oxymetazoline (ordinate) on the corresponding concentrations of oxymetazoline (abscissa). From data in A and B; no significant regression is obtained. (A and B from ref. 15.)

Schild regression. In this case, the regression is linear and has a slope not significantly different from unity; thus, the intercept can be used as an estimate of the $pK_B$ for oxymetazoline for the receptors mediating norepinephrine responses in this tissue. There are statistical procedures to determine the confidence with which a regression can be considered linear and the confidence limits of the slope (see Chapter 6). Under these circumstances, Schild regressions can be analyzed quantitatively with regard to whether they furnish accurate $pK_B$ values; there is more than one method to make this estimate. If the slope of a regression of log(dr − 1) on log[B] is found to be not significantly different from unity, then a plot constrained to slope of unity can be used. Under these circumstances, it is assumed that any differences from unity in the slope obtained experimentally are due to random variation and that if a sufficient number of experiments can be done, the slope eventually will equal unity. Thus, the values log(dr − 1) and log[B] are fit to the best straight line, the intercept of which is given by

$$pK_B = \frac{\sum_{i=1}^{n} \log(dr_i - 1)}{n} - \frac{\sum_{i=1}^{n} \log[B_i]}{n} \qquad [9.13]$$

The standard error of the intercept is given as

$$SE(c) = s/n \qquad [9.14]$$

Denoting log[B] as $x$ and log(dr − 1) as $y$, $s$ is given as

$$s = \frac{\sum_{i=1}^{n} [y_i = \bar{y}) + (x_i - \bar{x})]^2}{n - 1} \qquad [9.15]$$

where $\bar{x}$ and $\bar{y}$ denote mean values. The 95% confidence limits for $pK_B$ are

$$pK_B = c \pm t_{(n-1)} \cdot SE(c) \qquad [9.16]$$

For example, $pK_B$ estimated by this method for the data shown in Fig. 9.3B is 6.57, with 95% confidence limits of 5.82 to 7.31.

Another method assumes a unit slope and calculates an individual value for $pK_B$ for each value of log(dr − 1) by the equation

$$pK_{B_i} = \log(dr_i - 1) - \log[B_i] \qquad [9.17]$$

and a mean $pK_B$ calculated from the resultant single estimates. For this method to be valid, it must be shown that the $pK_B$ values are essentially constant irrespective of log[B] and subject only to random error. Therefore, a regression of calculated $pK_B$ estimates from individual values of log(dr − 1) on log[B] should indicate no significant interdependence; Fig. 9.3C shows this regression for the data in Fig. 9.3B. No significant regression was obtained ($t = 0.6$, d.f. = 7, n.s.). Therefore, calculation of $pK_B$ with Eq. 9.15

is valid; the resulting estimate for $pK_B$ for the data calculated in this figure is $6.57 \pm 0.14$. The confidence limits of $pK_B$ then can be obtained by calculation of the mean $pK_B$ and an appropriate standard error from all of the estimates. Both of these methods also can use values of $(dr - 1)$ and $[B]$ (rather than logarithmic conversions).

Often experimental drugs are tested for which there is no prior knowledge of competitivity. In this setting, the slope is a critical parameter that is included in the calculations. Thus, even though an experimental slope is obtained that is not significantly different from unity, it can be included in the calculation of $pK_B$. Under these circumstances, $pK_B$ is obtained by a standard linear-regression analysis, with calculation of 95% confidence limits for the intercept as given in Chapter 6.

### Regressions with Slopes Different from Unity

Noncompliance of experimental Schild regressions with the Schild equation describing a straight line of slope equal to unity can signify one of four conditions: (i) the antagonism is not competitive, (ii) a drug-disposition mechanism or other nonequilibrium steady state obscures the competitive nature of the antagonism, (iii) the competitive antagonism of a heterogeneous receptor population subserving the same response is observed, or (iv) multiple drug properties are expressed in the concentrations used to make the measurements. The first alternative usually is considered only after elimination of the other three, because they can obscure true competitive antagonism to the point that it resembles true, not competitive, antagonism. The latter three conditions will be dealt with in some detail in later sections. It is important to detect nonequilibrium steady states, because these can obscure accurate measurement of all drug parameters. Often such steady states closely resemble true equilibria and are difficult to detect. This makes Schild analysis a valuable tool, because it furnishes a theoretical model to predict the behavior of agonists, antagonists, and receptors in true equilibria, thus giving a standard for comparison. If experimental data do not conform to the predictions of the Schild equation for a known competitive antagonist, then this will signify a veiled nonequilibrium steady state or a heterogeneous receptor population. Thus, in addition to providing a method to estimate $pK_B$, the second important function of the Schild regression is as a looking glass into agonist, antagonist, and receptor interactions to uncover veiled nonequilibrium steady states and/or receptor-population heterogeneity.

In experimental pharmacology, Schild regressions often are not linear or have slopes significantly different from unity. There are two ways to view such data; in one sense, this can be viewed as signifying a "failed" experiment in which conditions were not adequate to accurately measure the affinity of the antagonist. However, Schild regressions often are anomalous (nonlinear, or linear with slopes different from unity) because of inequilibrium between agonist, antagonist, and receptors. Therefore, in this light, the slope of the Schild regression can furnish valuable information about the reason why equilibrium was not achieved. This can be important, because nonequilibrium steady states can closely resemble true thermodynamic equilibrium, yet furnish totally spurious information about drugs and receptors. The presence of the antagonist perturbs such steady states, and the results can be compared to a model that assumes thermodynamic equilibrium (the Schild equation). If the experimental data do not conform to the model (linear regression with unit slope), then a nonequilibrium steady state may be unveiled. From this point of view, anomalous Schild regressions definitely will not be viewed as failed experiments, but rather as a valuable probe into the kinetics of drug-receptor interactions.

Given that the slope of the Schild regression can detect nonequilibrium steady states, the possibilities will be considered in cases in which the slope is less than, greater than, or equal to unity (but still yielding a spurious $pK_B$ value).

### Use of Antagonists to Detect Nonequilibrium Steady States

The Schild equation defines the relationship between the shift to the right in the agonist dose-response curve and the concentration of antagonist. As such, it can be a sensitive indicator of the secondary effects (in addition to receptor effects) of drugs (the agonist and/or the antagonist). For example, histamine produces relaxation of bethanechol-contracted rabbit trachea by activation of relaxant histamine H-2 receptors; this response is blocked competitively by the antagonist cimetidine. A Schild regression for cimetidine antagonism of histamine responses in this tissue is linear, with a slope of unity up to dose ratios of 160 (Fig. 9.4); at that point, nonlinearity is encountered. In this case, it has been determined that the concentrations of histamine (added as the hydrochloride salt) required to overcome cimetidine antagonism are sufficient to reduce the organ-bath pH, a chemical effect that produces non-H-2 receptor–mediated relaxation of the tissue; this accounts for the relative ineffectiveness of cimetidine. Thus, a chemical nonreceptor-mediated response to the agonist is detected by quantifying competitive antagonism with the Schild regression. Such nonspecific effects may augment or potentiate agonist responses and therefore cause underestimation of the dose ratio (slope < 1) or depress the tissue or otherwise block agonist responses nonspecifically and produce overestimation of the dose ratio (slope > 1). Whether or not the slope of the Schild regression deviates by being greater or less than unity clearly depends on the nature of the secondary effect. However, there are certain general nonequilibrium conditions that lead to predictable effects on the slopes of Schild regressions; these are worth considering separately.

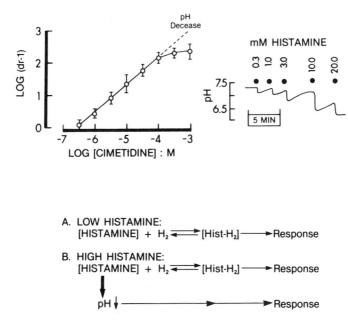

A. LOW HISTAMINE:
   [HISTAMINE] + $H_2$ ⇌ [Hist-$H_2$] → Response

B. HIGH HISTAMINE:
   [HISTAMINE] + $H_2$ ⇌ [Hist-$H_2$] → Response
   ↓
   pH ↓ ─────────────────────→ Response

**FIG. 9.4.** Schild regression for antagonism of histamine-induced relaxation of rabbit trachea by cimetidine. A linear regression with unit slope is obtained until concentrations of
histamine are attained that reduce the organ-bath pH; these concentrations correspond
to the nonlinear portion of the Schild regression (labeled pH decrease). The inability of
cimetidine to block the non-H-2 receptor–mediated relaxation produced by pH reductions
is shown in the schematic diagram. This cimetidine-resistant response is manifest in an
apparent loss of activity of cimetidine, resulting in underestimation in log(dr − 1) values
(Schild regression from ref. 23.)

Sometimes experimental Schild regressions have slopes less than unity;
agonist-removal mechanisms in tissues can be the causative factor. As discussed in Chapter 5, tissues often have mechanisms that remove agonist from
the receptor compartment and produce underestimation of agonist potency.
This occurs because only a portion of the agonist concentration added to the
organ bath is able to activate the receptors; the remaining fraction is removed
by the uptake mechanism. Detection and elimination of such uptake mechanisms are critical steps in receptor analysis; this often can be accomplished
pharmacologically by inclusion of uptake blockers in the medium bathing
the tissue (see Chapter 5). A practical aspect of this approach concerns the
detection of removal processes when no such inhibitor is available. If the
uptake process is saturable, one approach to this problem is with Schild
analysis; a slope less than unity for the Schild regression to a competitive
receptor antagonist can result when such agonist-uptake mechanisms are
saturated. In the absence of antagonist in a tissue with an agonist-removal
mechanism, the dose-response curve is produced by the residual agonist (the

amount that has escaped the uptake process) entering the receptor compartment. However, in the presence of a competitive antagonist, agonist concentrations must be elevated to produce responses, and if the elevated concentrations of agonist are sufficient to saturate the agonist-uptake process, underestimation of the antagonism will result. This is because, whereas only a portion of the agonist concentration could activate the receptors in the absence of antagonist, after saturation of the removal process almost all of the agonist added to the tissue activates receptors. In effect, the tissue is sensitized to the agonist by neutralization (by saturation) of the uptake process (Fig. 9.5). Under these circumstances, the antagonism is partially canceled by the tissue sensitization to the agonist, and the dose ratio is lower than would be predicted by the Schild equation. Figure 9.6A shows the effects of phentolamine as an antagonist of responses of rat anococcygeus muscle to norepinephrine. Figure 9.6B shows the resulting clearly anomalous Schild regressions (slope = 0.5, 0.2—0.7). This tissue is known to be highly innervated with a powerful neuronal uptake mechanism for norepinephrine. Blockade of this uptake process by desmethylimipramine (DMI) corrects the Schild regression to yield a slope of unity and the correct $pK_B$ (Fig. 9.6B). This strongly implicates saturation of the uptake mechanism as the factor that reduces the slope of the Schild regression for phentolamine in this tissue.

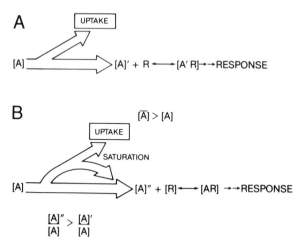

**FIG. 9.5.** Saturation of an agonist-uptake mechanism by competitive antagonism. **A:** In the absence of antagonist (control), a fraction of the agonist concentration does not reach the receptors and $[A]'/[A] < 1$. **B:** In the presence of antagonist, higher concentrations of agonist are required that saturate the uptake process. In this situation, most, if not all, of the organ-bath concentration enters the receptor compartment ($[A] \approx [A]''$). Therefore, the deficit in the control situation is removed; i.e., the effects of the agonist are effectively potentiated, and therefore antagonism is underestimated.

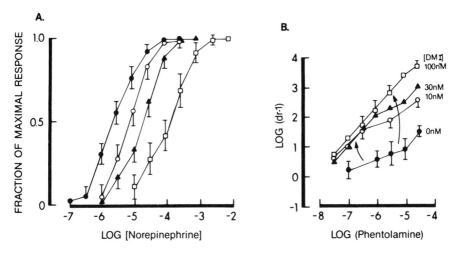

**FIG. 9.6.** Effects of uptake saturation and blockade on competitive antagonism. **A:** Antagonism of responses of rat anococcygeus muscle to norepinephrine by phentolamine. Ordinate: Contractions as fractions of the maximal response to norepinephrine. Abscissa: Logarithms of molar concentrations of norepinephrine. Responses in the absence (•, $N$ = 10) and presence of phentolamine at 0.1 (o, $N$ = 3), 1 (▵, $N$ = 4), and 10 μM (▢, $N$ = 3). **B:** Schild regression for blockade of norepinephrine responses in rat anococcygeus muscle by phentolamine. Regressions in the absence (•, $N$ = 18) and presence of DMI, a blocker of neuronal uptake of norepinephrine, at 10 (o, $N$ = 12), 30 (▵, $N$ = 10), and 100 nM (▢, $NL$ = 19). Bars represent SEM. (From ref. 22.)

These data illustrate two facets of Schild analysis. First, the parallel shifts to the right in dose-response curves for norepinephrine belie the nonequilibrium steady state in this tissue (only a fraction of the added norepinephrine reaches the receptors), and only by the Schild regression is this condition revealed. Second, totally erroneous estimates of the potencies of norepinephrine and phentolamine result from these nonequilibrium steady states. In addition, observation of the regression in the presence of various concentrations of DMI indicates at what concentration of DMI the nonequilibrium steady state is neutralized. In this case, phentolamine is known to be a competitive antagonist, with a $pK_B$ for α-adrenoceptors of 8.5. Therefore, observation of a linear Schild regression with a slope of unity and $pK_B$ of 8.5 in the presence of 100 nM DMI indicates that this concentration of uptake blocker is sufficient to eliminate the uptake process.

These effects can be modeled mathematically; Fig. 9.7A is a schematic representation of a tissue that removes the agonist $A$ from the receptor compartment by an uptake process [characterized by $J_{max}/(k_{in} \cdot K_m)$] and has receptors $R$ that are activated by the agonist to produce responses and are blocked competitively by antagonist $B$. The equation to predict the relative changes in the ratio of agonist concentrations in the organ bath ($[A_o]$) and

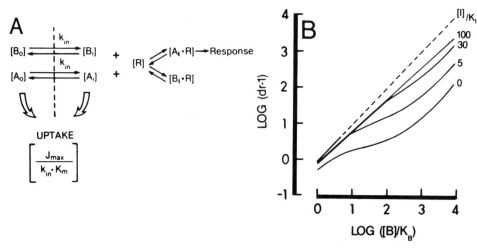

**FIG. 9.7.** Effects of uptake saturation on Schild regressions. **A:** Schematic diagram for a tissue possessing a saturable removal process for the agonist. Both agonist $[A_o]$ and antagonist $[B_o]$ diffuse into the receptor compartment with permeation constant $k_{in}$ and compete for receptor $[R]$. A saturable uptake process characterized by $J_{max}/(k_{in} \cdot K_m)$ removes agonist as it enters the receptor compartment. **B:** Theoretical Schild regressions according to Eq. 9.19. Regressions for a tissue with a removal mechanism for the agonist that produces a 30-fold deficit in agonist concentration at the receptor $[J_{max}/(k_{in} \cdot K_m) = 30]$ and after partial antagonism of this removal process by an uptake inhibitor $[I]$ ($[A_i]/K_m = 0.01$). (From ref. 22.)

receptor compartment ($[A_i]$) as functions of the antagonist concentration is

$$\frac{[A_o]}{[A_i]} = 1 + \frac{[B]}{K_B}\left[1 + \frac{\dfrac{J_{max}}{k_{in} \cdot K_m}}{1 + \dfrac{[A_i]}{K_m}\left(1 + \dfrac{[B]}{K_B}\right)}\right] \qquad [9.18]$$

where $K_B$ is the equilibrium dissociation constant for the antagonist-receptor complex. It can be seen from this equation that changes in $[B]$ can produce changes in the ratio $[A_o]/[A_i]$. The deficit of agonist caused by the uptake process at the receptor will tend to be greater in the absence of the antagonist, whereas at large values of $[B]/K_B$ the effects of the uptake process will be diminished (Fig. 9.5), these effects are shown in Fig. 9.7B. These particular regressions were calculated by a modification of Eq. 9.18 that includes a term $[I]/K_I$ that predicts the effects of prior inhibition of the removal process by an inhibitor $I$ before Schild analysis:

$$\frac{[A_o]}{[A_i]} = 1 + \frac{[B]}{K_B}\left[1 + \frac{\dfrac{J_{max}}{k_{in} \cdot K_m}}{1 + \dfrac{[A_i]}{K_m}\left(1 + \dfrac{[B]}{K_B}\right) + \dfrac{[I]}{K_I}}\right] \qquad [9.19]$$

where $K_I$ is the equilibrium dissociation constant for the inhibitor/site-of-removal complex. It can be seen from Eq. 9.19 and Fig. 9.7B that serial inhibition of the removal process cancels the effect of the process on the dose ratio and that complete inhibition leads to a theoretically correct Schild regression (linear, with slope of unity). The theory that models data obtained experimentally (Fig. 9.6B) predicts that Schild regressions distorted by an agonist-uptake process may be composed of linear portions with slope equal to unity and nonlinear portions with slope less than unity. It follows, therefore, that experimental observation of such Schild data would suggest the presence of an agonist-removal process in the tissue (Table 9.1A).

As seen in Figs. 9.6B and 9.7B, Schild regressions can be used to detect agonist-uptake mechanisms, and this may be important if a removal process is operative for which there is no selective inhibitor. However, even if there is a blocking drug for the uptake process, a second problem concerns the selectivity of the drug used to neutralize the uptake process; this will be dealt with in the next section.

There are nonequilibrium steady states that can produce Schild-regression slopes greater than unity. For example, if drug-receptor interaction, not diffusion, is rate-limiting in a pharmacologic experiment, then an inadequate period of time for equilibration of the receptors with the antagonist will produce Schild regressions with slopes greater than unity. This is because the rate of onset is concentration dependent. Therefore, lower concentrations require a

**TABLE 9.1.** *Use of Schild analysis to detect nonequilibrium steady states*

### A. Detection of agonist-uptake processes by Schild analysis

Schild analysis yields a regression with slope less than unity
Inhibitor of the agonist-uptake process increases the slope of the Schild regression
Concentration of uptake inhibitor that yields a linear Schild regression with the correct $pK_B$ for the antagonist is sufficient to eliminate the effects of the uptake process (i.e., achieve equilibrium conditions between agonist and receptors)

### B. Detection of heterogeneous receptor populations by Schild analysis

Different Schild regressions are obtained in a given tissue for the same antagonist when different agonists are used to produce responses
Nonlinearity and a slope less than unity may be obtained for the Schild regressions at dose ratios less than 10

### C. Detection of multiple drug properties by Schild analysis

Receptor blockade by uptake blockers produces linear Schild regressions with unit slope, but erroneously low $pK_B$ estimates
The potency of an antagonist that blocks an agonist-uptake process varies with the agonist used to produce the response and has a lower potency against agonists taken up by the uptake process (i.e., antagonist self-cancelation is observed)

greater time of onset to equilibrium than higher concentrations. Thus, whereas a dose of $2 \times K_B$ may require 1 hr to reach thermodynamic equilibrium with receptors, a dose of $100 \times K_B$ may require only 20 min. Therefore, if the Schild regression is determined after a 20-min equilibration, the effect of the low dose will be considerably underestimated, whereas that of the high dose will not; this type of error leads to a steepening of the Schild regression.

Calculations of dose ratios and corresponding Schild regressions at any time $t$ during the onset of the antagonist can be made with the following equation:

$$\log(dr_t - 1) = \log[B] - \log K_B$$
$$+ \log \left[ \frac{1 - \exp\{-k_2 ([B]/K_B + 1)t\}}{1 + ([B]/K_B) \cdot \exp\{-k_2 ([B]/K_B + 1)t\}} \right] \quad [9.20]$$

To illustrate this effect, Schild regressions for scopolamine antagonism of guinea pig ileal responses to carbachol were determined at various times of equilibration (Fig. 9.8A). The $k_2$ for scopolamine determined experimentally was $1.7 \times 10^{-4}$ sec$^{-1}$; Schild regressions calculated with Eq. 9.20 using this estimate of $k_2$ are shown in Fig. 9.8B.

Another situation in which the Schild-regression slope can be greater than unity is when there is a saturable removal mechanism in the tissue for the antagonist. This is shown schematically in Fig. 9.9A; the theoretical Schild

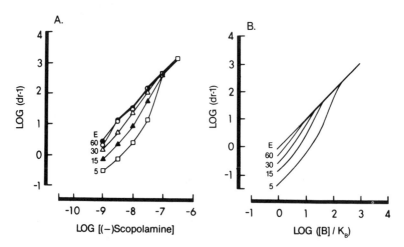

FIG. 9.8. Effects of temporal inequilibrium on Schild regressions. A: Schild regressions for antagonism of guinea pig ileal responses to carbachol by $(-)$-scopolamine. Regressions obtained after 5- (□), 15- (▲), 30- (△), 60- (○), and 90-min (●) equilibration periods. B: Calculation of theoretical regressions according to Eq. 9.23 using an experimentally obtained $k_2$ value for scopolamine of $1.7 \times 10^{-4}$ sec$^{-1}$. Numbers refer to time in minutes; E, equilibrium ($t > 240$ min). (From ref. 14.)

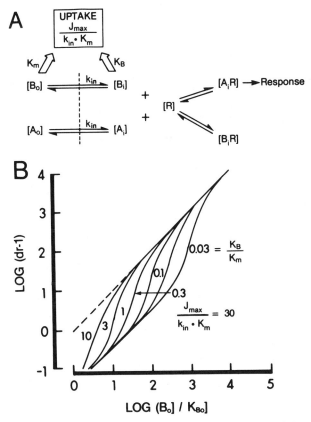

**FIG. 9.9.** Saturation of a removal mechanism for the antagonist. **A:** Schematic diagram for a tissue with a removal mechanism for the antagonist [B] characterized by $J_{max}/(k_{in}\cdot K_m)$. Antagonist is removed as it diffuses into the receptor compartment. **B:** Theoretical Schild regressions for a tissue that removes antagonist from the receptor compartment to produce an antagonist deficit of 30 [$J_{max}/(k_{in}\cdot K_m) = 30$]. Regressions (calculated with Eq. 9.21, shown for antagonists with varying affinities for receptors and for the site of removal; e.g., $K_B/K_m = 10$ characterizes an antagonist with a 10-fold greater affinity for the uptake site; $K_B/K_m = 0.1$ characterizes an antagonist with a 10-fold greater affinity for receptors. Nonlinear portions result from saturation of the removal mechanism. (From ref. 25.)

regression under these circumstances can be calculated by

$$\log(dr - 1) = \log\left\{\frac{K_m}{2}\left(\frac{[B_o]}{K_m} - \frac{J_{max}}{k_{in}\cdot K_m} - 1\right)\right.$$

$$\left. + \left[\left(1 + \frac{J_{max}}{k_{in}\cdot K_m} - \frac{[B_o]}{K_m}\right)^2 + \frac{4[B_o]}{K_m}\right]^{1/2}\right\} - \log K_B$$

[9.21]

where $J_{max}$ is the maximal rate of removal of the antagonist from the receptor compartment, $K_m$ is the Michaelis-Menten constant for antagonist removal, $k_{in}$ is the permeation constant for the antagonist into the receptor compartment, $K_B$ is the equilibrium dissociation constant for the antagonist-receptor complex, and $[B_o]$ is the concentration of antagonist in the organ bath. Calculations for theoretical Schild regressions for antagonists with various affinities for the receptor and uptake mechanism ($K_B/K_m$ = 10–0.03) are shown in Fig. 9.9B. The portions of regressions with slopes greater than unity indicate saturation of the removal process for the antagonist. Experimental evidence for such a mechanism was obtained in rabbit ileum for the antimuscarinic antagonist atropine, because this species is known to possess a unique esterase enzyme that degrades atropine. Figure 9.10A shows the nonlinear Schild regression for atropine in rabbit ileum, with resulting anomalous $pA_2$; the regression has a slope greater than unity. No such effect is observed in ileum from guinea pigs, a species known not to possess this metabolizing enzyme for atropine. In the presence of a great excess concentration for an alternative substrate, 4-methylbutyrate (to saturate the enzyme, thus preventing destruction of atropine), the regression is normalized (i.e., the slope of regression is reduced to unity) (Fig. 9.10B).

These analyses show how some nonequilibrium steady states in tissues can be detected by observation of anomalous Schild regressions. However, there are also situations in which nonequilibrium steady states can produce linear Schild regressions with slopes equal to unity. Therefore, it should be stressed that fulfillment of these criteria furnishes only presumptive evidence of competitivity, and there are nonequilibrium steady states that can still

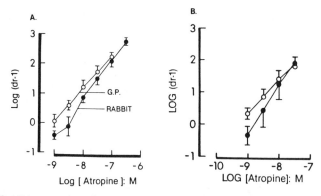

**FIG. 9.10.** Schild regressions for antagonism of responses of rabbit ileum to bethanechol by atropine. **A:** Schild regressions for atropine in rabbit (•, $N$ = 53) and guinea pig (o, $N$ = 14) ileum. The regression in rabbit ileum is nonlinear (test for linearity, $F$ = 28.1; d.f. = 1, 46; $p < 0.001$); the regression in guinea pig is linear, with a slope of 1.1 (0.95–1.2) and a $pK_B$ of 9.0 (8.9–9.2). **B:** Regressions in the absence (•, $N$ = 32) and presence (o, $N$ = 31) of 4-methylbutyrate (100 μM). The presence of the alternative substrate for atropinesterase changes the slope of the regression from 1.48 to 1.02. Bars represent SEM. (From ref. 25.)

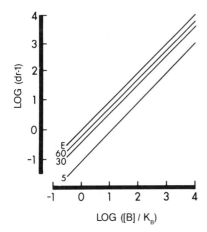

**FIG. 9.11.** Effects of temporal inequilibrium on a diffusion-limited system. Theoretical Schild regressions calculated with Eq. 9.22 for an antagonist with $k_{out} = 3 \times 10^{-4}$ sec$^{-1}$ in a tissue in which diffusion is rate limiting. Regressions calculated for times 5, 30, 60, and >240 min. (From ref. 13.)

much resemble thermodynamic equilibria and yield linear regressions with unit slopes, but spurious estimates of $pK_B$.

One such situation arises when the equilibration period for the antagonist is insufficient in a tissue in which diffusion, not drug-receptor interaction, is rate limiting. Under these circumstances, the Schild regression can be calculated by

$$\log(dr_t - 1) = \log[B] - \log K_B + \log(1 - e^{-k_{out}t}) \qquad [9.22]$$

where $k_{out}$ is a rate constant determining penetration of the antagonist out of the receptor compartment. The effects of equilibration time on a Schild regression for an antagonist-tissue system with $k_{out} = 3 \times 10^{-4}$ sec$^{-1}$ are shown in Fig. 9.11; the regressions are linear, with a slope of unity, but shifted to the right of the equilibrium regression for insufficient times of equilibration.

### Simulation of Biological Error for Single-Curve Schild Regressions

Usually, Schild analysis requires the determination of a control response, equilibration of the preparation with the antagonist, and the determination of another dose-response curve in the presence of the antagonist. From these data, a dose ratio of equiactive doses of agonist in the absence and presence of antagonist can be measured for use in Schild analysis. However, there are instances in which replication of dose-response curves is not practical; i.e., only one dose-response curve per tissue can be obtained. Under these circumstances the dose ratios must be obtained from the mean of the control dose-response curve and means of the various curves obtained in the presence of the antagonist. When this is done, however, there is no independent assessment of biological error for the dose ratios. Although there is an estimate of the error for the curve fit (see Chapter 6), no measure of the effects of pharmacologic differences in the estimate can be made. A method that statistically resamples the data can be used to, in essence, repeat the experiment many times and thus estimate biological error. With this technique, repeated samples (>1,000) are taken of control log $EC_{50}$ values and log $EC_{50}$ in the presence of antagonist and Schild regressions constructed. This yields a data set containing more than 1,000 estimates of the $pA_2$, slope of the Schild regression, and $pK_B$, if applicable. The distribution of these estimates then can be used as measures of error. Figure 9.12A shows the responses of guinea pig atria to the β-adrenoceptor agonist isoproterenol. Only one dose-response curve per tissue was obtained; therefore each curve represents an atrium from a different animal. The collective log $EC_{50}$ values were taken from these data and the bootstrap statistical resampling technique applied to produce the normal distribution of $pA_2$ values shown in Fig. 9.12B. The distribution of Schild regression slopes and $pK_B$ are shown in Fig. 9.12C and D, respectively. When these data are compared to dose ratios obtained from paired dose-response curves in the same atria, no significant difference was obtained. This demonstrates the potential value of this technique when, for technical reasons, only one dose-response curve per tissue can be obtained.

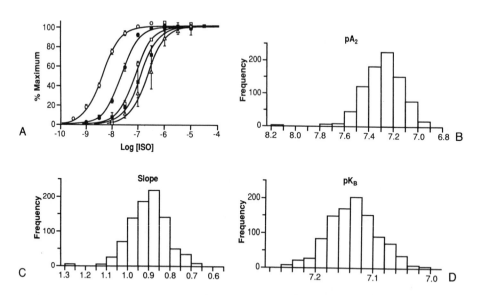

**FIG. 9.12.** Statistical resampling of data for the estimation of biological errors on Schild regressions. **A:** Dose-response curves for isoproterenol-induced positive inotropy in guinea pig left atria. Responses measured in the absence (o) and presence of atenolol 0.3 μM (•), 1 ≈ μM (□), 3 μM (■), and 10 μM (Δ). **B:** Distribution of $pA_2$ values obtained from resampling (>1,000) of dose ratios. Range 8.16–6.88; median 7.27. **C:** Distribution of Schild regression slopes. Range 1.29–0.52; median 0.9. **D:** Distribution of $pK_B$ estimates. Range 7.27–6.98; median 7.13. (From ref. 29.)

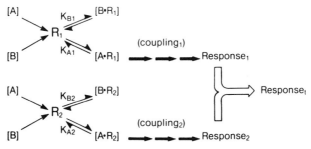

**FIG. 9.13.** Schematic diagram depicting competition of an agonist [A] and antagonist [B] for two receptors ($R_1$ and $R_2$) in the same tissue. It is assumed that both receptors subserve the same type of response; thus, the observed total stimulus is the sum of those produced by activation of $R_1$ and $R_2$.

## Antagonism of Heterogeneous Receptor Populations

Simple competitive antagonism assumes an agonist, antagonist, and homogeneous receptor population to be in equilibrium. If, however, the receptor population subserving the response is heterogeneous with respect to agonist binding or antagonist binding or both, then deviations from a simple, single $pK_B$–valued Schild equation may be observed. A hallmark of such a condition is that the Schild regression to a given antagonist varies with the agonist used to produce a response. For example, Fig. 9.13 is a schematic diagram of a tissue with two receptor types designated $R_1$ and $R_2$ that subserve the same type of response and an agonist that activates both receptor types with equal or varying affinities and/or intrinsic efficacies; the following theoretical calculation can be made.

There are theoretical and practical reasons why Schild analysis in functional tissues may be a more sensitive indicator of heterogeneous receptor systems than binding experiments. In the latter, the signals for each receptor type are of equal strength, namely, the disintegration of a radioisotope. Under these conditions, the relative density of the two receptor types and the relative selectivities of the radioligand and displacer dictate the observed kinetics and whether receptor heterogeneity will be detected. Also, radioligand studies detect receptor presence and not necessarily receptor function and/or importance. As shown in Chapter 2, relatively minor receptor populations in some tissues (e.g., rat adipose tissue) can control the bulk of the physiological response. Functional studies allow three further discriminators of receptor heterogeneity, namely, the intrinsic efficacy of the agonist, the relative efficiency of coupling of each receptor population, and the total sensitivity of the tissue to agonism in general (see Table 9.2). These added discriminators make functional Schild analysis a powerful tool to detect and study the physiological significance of heterogeneous receptor populations in tissues.

**TABLE 9.2.** *Discriminating factors for receptor subtypes in binding versus functional studies*

| Binding | Function |
|---|---|
| Radioactive ligand | Agonist |
| Selective affinity | Selective affinity |
| | Selective intrinsic efficacy[a] |
| Antagonist | Antagonist |
| Selective affinity | Selective affinity |
| Receptors | Receptors |
| Relative density | Relative density |
| | Coupling to transducers[a] |
| | Effector transduction |
| | Efficiency of transduction[a] |

[a] Additional discriminating factors for functional studies over binding studies.
From ref. 20.

The scheme depicted in Fig. 9.13 contains too many parameters to be a useful model for the quantitative study of heterogeneous receptor systems. However, an operational description of such systems has advantages in that general behavior patterns of heterogeneous receptor systems may be predicted. Figure 9.14A depicts a model whereby the effects of two receptor-mediated stimuli contribute to the overall organ response. No biochemical or pharmacologic significance is assigned to the differences in maximal strength and/or sensitivity of the two signals from the agonist since this would necessitate assumptions about unknown quantities such as relative receptor density and efficiency of receptor-coupling mechanisms. The relative strengths of the two stimuli are variable, as are their sensitivities to agonists and antagonists. The maximal strength of the secondary stimulus, relative to the maximal strength of the primary stimulus, is defined by a proportionality factor $\mu$, whereas the sensitivity of the organ to the secondary stimulus is variable. Thus, the concentrations of agonist that activate the receptor mechanisms to produce the secondary stimulus are related to those that produce the primary stimulus by a factor L. In the presence of a competitive antagonist for the two receptors, total stimulus to a tissue is given by:

$$S = \frac{[A]/K_A}{[A]/K_A + [B]/K_B + 1} + \frac{\mu \cdot [A]/(L \cdot K_A)}{[A]/(L \cdot K_A) + [B]/(\theta \cdot K_B) + 1} \quad [9.23]$$

where [B] denotes the molar concentration of the antagonist. All equilibrium dissociation constants for both the agonist and antagonist are for the primary receptor system. Under these conditions, the relative equilibrium dissociation constant for the antagonist-receptor complex of the primary receptor generating stimulus is denoted by $K_B$ and for the secondary receptor by $\theta \cdot K_B$. Therefore, the relative affinity of the antagonist for receptor 1 versus

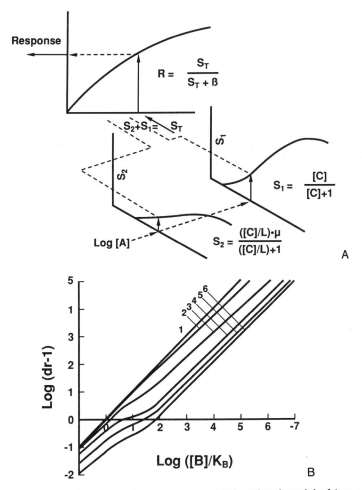

**FIG. 9.14. A:** Schematic representation of a general functional model of two receptor systems. A primary stimulus ($S_1$) is described by a standard Langmuir binding isotherm. A secondary stimulus ($S_2$) also is represented by a Langmuir isotherm but with a varying sensitivity to the agonist (factor $L$) and a varying maximal input to the total stimulus (factor $\mu$). Both stimuli are summed (to $S_t$) and processed by a general logistic function to tissue response. **B:** Theoretical Schild regressions for a two receptor system as measured in functional studies. Ordinates: Logarithms of equiactive dose ratios of agonist in the absence and presence of antagonist minus one. Abscissa: Logarithms of molar concentrations of antagonist expressed as a multiple of the equilibrium dissociation constant of the antagonist-receptor complex for one of the receptor types. Responses to agonist calculated from Eq. 9.23 and 9.24 with $L = 10$ and $\beta = 0.01$. Regressions shown for a single receptor population ($\mu = 0$, curve 1) and ones with increasing secondary input from another receptor system for which the antagonist has a 1/100-fold affinity. For these regressions, $\mu = 0.3$ (curve 2), 1.0 (3), 10 (4), 100 (5), and 1000 (6). (From ref. 20.)

receptor 2 is $\theta^{-1}$. It is further assumed that the relationship between the total receptor stimulus $S_t$ and tissue response is a rectangular hyperbolic function. Thus, the tissue response is given by a general logistic function:

$$R = \frac{S_t}{S_t + \beta} \qquad [9.24]$$

where $\beta$ is a fitting parameter with which the relative efficiency of tissue processing of the receptor stimulus by the tissue into response can be manipulated. With the use of Eq. 9.24, the overall tissue sensitivity can be manipulated without prior assignment of importance to the two receptor populations.

This model predicts the expected loss in antagonist potency that would be observed when the agonist in question activates a secondary receptor for which the antagonist has a lower affinity. This leads to a reduction in the expected dose ratio and a curvilinear Schild regression with portions of slope less than unity. Figure 9.14B shows theoretical Schild regressions for an antagonist with 100-fold selectivity for one of the receptor subtypes present in the tissue. It was assumed that the secondary receptor input was 10-fold less sensitive to the agonist ($L = 10$) and the final coupling constant for the total stimulus was $\beta = 0.01$. Regressions are shown for a single receptor system ($\mu = 0$, curve 1), and ones with increasing secondary receptor maximal input.

In multireceptor systems many factors could combine to produce differing relative stimulus input from an agonist that activates two receptors. Under these circumstances the locations and extents of nonlinear portions in Schild regressions for selective agonists would vary correspondingly. These factors are tissue, not only receptor, dependent; therefore the nonlinear portions in a set of Schild regressions from a number of tissues, when averaged, tend toward a general apparently *linear* Schild regression with a slope less than unity. A set of Schild regressions in two receptor systems in a number of tissues can be likened to traveling upon a surface of contours that vary with antagonist concentration ($\log([B]/K_B)$), extent of antagonism ($\log[dr - 1]$), and relative stimulus input from the two receptor systems (see Fig. 9.15; for this figure, this is modeled by changing $\mu$). The experimental determination of antagonist potency in two receptor systems with this technique can be likened to obtaining data points on a three-dimensional surface.

Schild analysis in functional systems may be a sensitive method of detecting heterogeneous receptor populations in tissues in that some generalities still may be independent of the nature of receptor coupling. Dose-response curves to agonists that activate two receptors in a tissue may still have Hill coefficients of unity since the relative stimulus input from the two receptor populations are processed by numerous cellular mechanisms to combine to a single signal. However, if a selective antagonist is used to shift the dose-response curve to the agonist into a different concentration range, then the relative input from the two receptor types may change when compared to

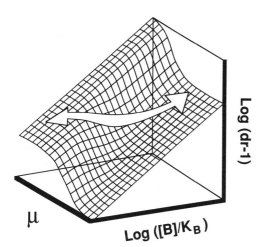

Log (dr-1)

μ

Log ([B]/K_B)

**FIG. 9.15.** Three-dimensional representation of a set of Schild regressions for two receptor systems. The maximal input of the secondary receptor system ($\mu$) is varied for an antagonist with 1,000-fold selectivity for one of the receptors over the other.

the control (no antagonist present) situation. Therefore the slope of agonist dose-response curves may change in two-receptor systems as a selective subtype antagonist changes the relative stimulus dynamics and shifts the dose-response curve. Another feature of mixed-receptor systems is the pattern of the errors in the experimental Schild regression. In single receptor systems, random errors in the experimentally introduced concentration of antagonist yield a corresponding random error in the observed dose ratio. The relative magnitude of these random errors is uniform along the concentration range of antagonist used to produce the Schild regression (Fig. 9.16A). However, in multireceptor systems the relative stimulus input from agonist activation of the various receptor populations varies with the concentration of agonist and selective antagonist. Therefore, as dose-response curves are shifted to the right by a selective antagonist, the relative input from the various receptor subtypes varies. This produces a dependence of the error, due to random differences in antagonist concentration, on the concentration of the antagonist; i.e., the errors on the ordinate values of Schild regressions will be heteroscedastic. This is shown in Fig. 9.16B, where the magnitudes of the errors vary with the antagonist concentration.

Dependence of agonist dose-response curve slope and Schild regression error are experimentally difficult to measure reliably. However, an experimentally accessible feature of Schild regressions in heterogeneous receptor systems is the dependence of selective receptor antagonist potency on the overall sensitivity of the tissue to receptor stimulation. A change in the overall sensitivity of a tissue to agonist stimulation may change the amplification characteristics of the two receptor inputs in a nonuniform manner that would, in turn, alter the *relative* contribution of the two receptor inputs. In two receptor systems, the two stimuli are processed and at some point summed in the biochemical stimulus-response machinery of the cell. The "power

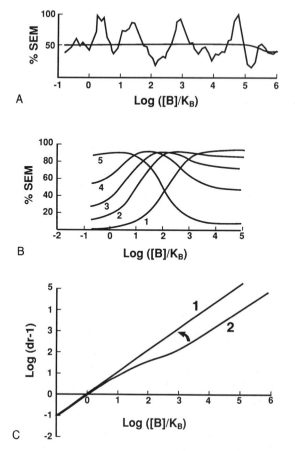

**FIG. 9.16.** Characteristics of single and dual receptor systems. **A:** Effects of 20% random error on antagonist concentration on ordinate values of a Schild regression in a single receptor system. Smoothed curve shows the homogeneity of the SEM with antagonist concentration. **B:** SEM for ordinate values of Schild regressions in a two receptor system with an antagonist with 1,000-fold selectivity for the primary receptor population and L = 1, $\beta$ = 0.01. Regressions shown for systems of varying maximal secondary receptor input: $\mu$ = 0.1 (curve 1), 1 (2), 3 (3), 30 (4), and 100 (5). Note how the magnitude of SEM varies with antagonist concentration. **C:** Effect of changing total tissue sensitivity to agonists on a Schild regression for a selective antagonist ($\theta^{-1}$ = 1,000, 5% secondary receptor input $\mu$ = 0.05, L = 0.5). Regression 2 for a highly coupled ($\beta$ = 0.03) tissue and regression 1 for the same system in which there has been a 10-fold loss of coupling efficiency for the *total* receptor population ($\beta$ = 0.3). (From ref. 20.)

amplifier'' (Chapter 2) of the tissue, which magnifies membrane signals into cellular response, grades the two receptor inputs to make a certain proportion of the total response mediated by each receptor population. If the strength of the power amplifier is altered, then the relative inputs from the two receptor systems also are subsequently altered but not necessarily in direct proportion to the initial input strength. In single receptor systems, the overall sensitivity of the tissue to agonists should not change the $pK_B$ of an antagonist. Therefore, if an alteration in the total sensitivity of a tissue to an agonist produces a change in the Schild regression for the antagonism of responses to that agonist by an antagonist, this would be indicative of agonist activation of a heterogeneous receptor population. In experimental terms, for example, this would predict that the treatment of a tissue system possessing two receptors with a drug that decreases tissue sensitivity also would alter the Schild regression to a selective antagonist. Figure 9.16C shows a Schild regression for a dual receptor system where the receptors are efficiently coupled to the stimulus-response mechanisms of the cells (regression 2; $\beta = 0.03$). The antagonism has a 1,000-fold greater affinity for one receptor system over the other, and it is assumed that the secondary receptor stimulus is 5% of the primary one with half the sensitivity to the agonist. The stimulus-response amplification factor has been chosen to enable the 5% receptor population to exert a significant agonist stimulus to the cell. Regression in Fig. 9.16C is the same tissue system in which the overall receptor-coupling sensitivity has been reduced by a factor of 10 ($\beta = 0.3$). Under these circumstances, the weak secondary receptor-stimulus input ($\mu = 5\%$) is effectively eliminated from the total stimulus to the agonist and the Schild regression essentially reflects blockade of the primary receptor population. This change in the Schild regression to an antagonist would not be observed in a tissue in which the response to the agonist was mediated by a single receptor population.

### Schild Regressions as Indicators of Multiple Drug Properties

As indicated in Chapter 1, drugs often are assumed to have one primary activity and thus to be selective. However, if a drug has two properties that are apparent in a common concentration range, interesting dissimilations can occur. It is important to differentiate the effects of multiple drug properties from multiple receptor effects, because the conclusions drawn from these two systems will differ considerably. Schild analysis is a useful tool for detecting multiple drug properties.

One problem to which this method can be applied is determination of the selectivities of drugs used to block agonist-uptake processes and thus achieve equilibrium in tissues. The selectivity of the uptake inhibitor can be judged by the ability or inability of such a drug to produce correction of the Schild regression. For example, although DMI is a fairly selective blocking agent for neuronal uptake of catecholamines, amitriptyline blocks neuronal uptake and $\alpha$-adrenoceptors with approximately equal affinities. This latter property produces shifts to the right in agonist dose-response curves that cancel tissue sensitization, and thus it prevents observation of the true potency of the agonist (i.e., $\phi < 10^4$ in Fig. 5.20).

This has practical ramifications for experiments in terms of detection of nonequilibrium steady states. For example, because of the affinity of amitriptyline for neuronal uptake and $\alpha$-adrenoceptors, this drug produces no effects on the sensitivity of rat anococcygeus muscle to norepinephrine (Fig. 9.17A). If observed experimentally, this profile would suggest the possibility that neuronal uptake in this tissue is not an important mechanism; a Schild regression can be used to differentiate this mechanism from one of concomitant uptake and receptor blockade. In this case, the fact that a second property of amitriptyline (receptor blockade) prevented this drug from unmasking the deficit in agonist concentration effect (i.e., by not producing significant

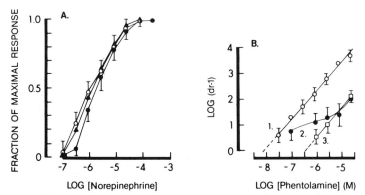

**FIG. 9.17.** Effects of agonist-uptake blockers with receptor-blocking properties. **A:** Effects of amitriptyline on dose-response curves for norepinephrine in rat anococcygeus muscle. Ordinate: Contractions as fractions of the maximal contraction to norepinephrine. Abscissa: Logarithms of molar concentrations of norepinephrine. Responses in the absence (•, $N = 9$) and presence of amitriptyline at 0.1 μM (○, $N = 3$) and 0.3 μM (▲, $N = 3$). **B:** Schild regressions for phentolamine antagonism of norepinephrine responses in rat anococcygeus muscle. Regression 1 is in the presence of complete uptake blockade (100 nM DMI); slope = 1.0 (0.9–1.2); $pK_B$ = 8.2 (7.6–8.7). Regression 2 is in the absence of uptake blockade; slope = 0.5 (0.2–0.7); $pK_B$ = 7.3 (5.3–9.8). Regression 3 is in the presence of amitriptyline at 1 μM, a concentration sufficient to effectively block uptake (as for DMI); slope = 1.0 (0.9–1.2); $pK_B$ = 6.5 (6.0–7.0). While the slope increases, $pK_B$ is grossly underestimated because of the receptor-blocking properties of amitriptyline. Bars represent SEM. (From ref. 21.)

potentiation of the agonist) was revealed by the fact that a linear Schild regression with unit slope that yielded the correct $pK_B$ was not obtained for phentolamine in the presence of amitriptyline (Fig. 9.17B). Instead, a significant underestimation of the potency of phentolamine was obtained in the presence of amitriptyline, indicating that a second property of the uptake blocker, not true thermodynamic equilibrium, was being observed (Table 9.1C).

Other examples of erroneous linear Schild regressions with slope of unity because of multiple drug properties can be found in antagonists that "self-cancel" by sensitizing the tissue to the agonist in the same concentration range needed for antagonism. One such drug is ambenonium, an antimuscarinic blocker ($pK_B$ = 6.1) that also is a competitive inhibitor of acetylcholinesterase ($pK_I$ = 6.4). This latter property sensitizes tissues to acetylcholine by blocking the degradation of this agonist. These two properties produce opposite effects on dose-response curves for acetylcholine (Fig. 9.18); thus, different degrees of self-cancellation of antagonism (by sensitization) will be obtained in various tissues, depending on the importance of acetylcholinesterase as a metabolizing enzyme. In a tissue with an avid cholinesterase activity, ambenonium will appear to be a weaker antimuscarinic blocker than in a tissue with low cholinesterase activity. Also, such differences will not be apparent for ambenonium antagonism of agonists not degraded by acetyl-

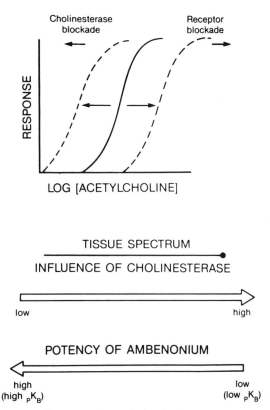

**FIG. 9.18.** Self-canceling effects of ambenonium on a dose-response curve for acetylcholine (schematic). Cholinesterase blockade produces potentiation, and receptor blockade produces antagonism of responses. In tissues with a powerful acetylcholinesterase mechanism, potentiation will be powerful, and the $pK_B$ for antagonism correspondingly underestimated.

cholinesterase (i.e., bethanechol); Table 9.3 shows the heterogeneity of $pK_B$ values for ambenonium as an antagonist of responses of various tissues to acetylcholine and the lack of tissue effects on antagonism of responses to bethanechol. In a tissue with a powerful cholinesterase-degrading mechanism for acetylcholine, such as guinea pig trachea, underestimation of the potency of ambenonium can be linked directly with the enzyme activity. This is shown in Fig. 9.19, where the potency of ambenonium as an antagonist of acetylcholine is increased by prior equilibration of trachea with the cholinesterase inhibitor neostigmine. A notable feature of these regressions is that they are linear and have slopes not significantly different from unity. Theoretical modeling of such systems indicates that Schild regressions for self-canceling drugs can be linear, with slopes of unity, over wide concentration ranges. The ratio of agonist concentrations in the organ bath and in the

**TABLE 9.3.** $pK_B$ *Values for ambenonium*

| Species | Tissue | $pK_B$ Acetylcholine[a] | Bethanechol[b] |
|---|---|---|---|
| Guinea pig | Ileum | 6.0 | 6.1 |
| | Trachea | 4.89 | 6.2 |
| | Tenia cecum | 5.2 | 6.0 |
| Rat | Anococcygeus muscle | 4.87 | 6.0 |

[a] Acetylcholine as the agonist.
[b] Bethanechol (not a substrate for acetylcholinesterase) as the agonist.

receptor compartment can be calculated by

$$\frac{[A_o]}{[A_i]} = \left(1 + \frac{[B_i]}{K_B}\right)\left[1 + \frac{\dfrac{J_{max}}{k_{in}\cdot K_m}}{1 + \dfrac{[A_i]}{K_m}\left(1 + \dfrac{[B_i]}{K_B}\right) + \dfrac{[B_i]}{K_B}\cdot\dfrac{K_B}{K_{BU}} + \dfrac{[I]}{K_I}}\right] \qquad [9.25]$$

where the ratio of equilibrium dissociation constants for the antagonist receptor and the site of agonist removal is given by $K_B/K_{BU}$, and $J_{max}/(k_{in}\cdot K_m)$ characterizes the removal mechanism for the agonist. Using Eq. 9.25, theoretical Schild regressions for self-canceling antagonists in a tissue that produces a 30-fold agonist deficit at the receptor $[J_{max}/(k_{in}\cdot K_m) = 30]$ have been calculated and are shown in Fig. 9.20; the regressions refer to antagonists with varying relative affinities for the uptake process and the receptors.

In general, it can be seen that a number of different types of nonequilibrium steady states and/or multiple drug properties can be made apparent by Schild analysis; a summary of these is given in Table 9.4. The use of Schild regres-

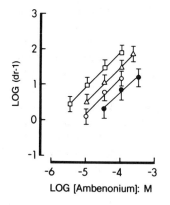

**FIG. 9.19.** Effects of serial blockade of acetylcholinesterase on Schild regressions for ambenonium. Schild regressions for antagonism of responses of guinea pig trachea to acetylcholine by ambenonium in the absence (●, $N = 24$) and presence of the acetylcholinesterase blocker neostigmine at 50 nM (○, $N = 8$), 0.3 μM (△, $N = 10$), and 3.0 μM (□, $N = 12$). Bars represent SEM. (From ref. 24.)

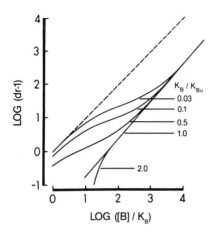

**FIG. 9.20.** Theoretical Schild regressions for antagonists that both sensitize the tissue to the agonist by blocking tissue degradation of agonist and block responses to the agonist by binding to receptors. Regressions calculated with Eq. 9.26, assuming a tissue that produces a 30-fold deficit of agonist at the receptor [$J_{max}/(K_{in} \cdot K_m)$ = 30]. Antagonists with varying affinities for the removal mechanism and receptors are shown; i.e., for $K_B/K_{BU}$ = 2.0, the antagonist has a twofold greater affinity for the site of removal; for $K_B/K_{BU}$ = 0.1, the antagonist has a 10-fold greater affinity for receptors.

**TABLE 9.4**

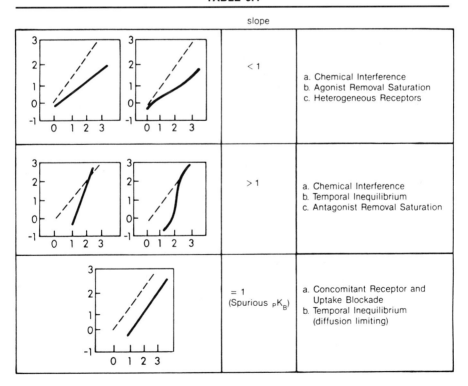

sions to detect such steady states and determine when they are corrected can be a valuable aspect of this method.

### Effects of Receptor Precoupling on Schild Regressions

As discussed in Chapter 8, there is evidence to suggest that some G protein–linked receptors couple spontaneously to G proteins, even in the absence of agonists. If the ligand used to block the effects of an agonist has differential affinity for the receptor $[R]$ and the receptor-transducer protein complex ($[R \cdot T]$, the precoupled receptor), then the observed antagonism will be a function of the extent of receptor precoupling, i.e., the relative proportions of $[R]$ and $[R \cdot T]$. Drugs with a selective affinity for $[R]$ over $[R \cdot T]$ can be thought to have "negative efficacy" (7) since they destabilize the agonist-stimulated ternary complexes (see Chapter 8). Spontaneous coupling produces a species ($[R \cdot T]$) for which the antagonist has a lower affinity; therefore a reduction in $[R \cdot T]$ and an increase in $[R]$ (destabilization of spontaneous coupling) yield a system more sensitive to antagonism by the negative antagonist. Therefore reduction in spontaneous coupling increases the apparent affinity of a drug with negative efficacy. For the opioid receptors in NG108-15 cells, receptors can be shown to be precoupled in isolated membranes but not in intact cell cultures, and there is experimental evidence to indicate that $Na^+$ destabilizes spontaneous coupling of opioid receptors with transducer proteins. Figure 9.21 shows the effect of $Na^+$ on the blockade of opioid receptors by the negative intrinsic efficacy drug ICI 174. As seen in Fig. 9.21, the $pA_2$ estimate for the negative antagonist ICI 174 in a receptor-precoupled system (absence of $Na^+$) is 6.78. The destabilization of precoupling by addition of $Na^+$ produces a $pA_2$ value for this antagonist of 7.43.

Receptor precoupling can depend on the tissue type and preparation of receptor system. In intact NG108-15 cells, the $pA_2$ for ICI 174 was found to be 7.5; the higher affinity of ICI 174 in cell culture indicates a lack of receptor precoupling in the intact system. It can be seen from these data that the

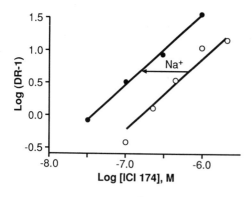

**FIG. 9.21.** Effects of receptor precoupling to transducer proteins on Schild regressions. Regressions obtained in membranes from NG108-15 cells for antagonism of the opioid agonist DADLE by the negative antagonist ICI 174. Regressions obtained in the presence of $Na^+$ (which destabilizes spontaneous association of opioid receptors for G proteins) and absence of $Na^+$ (replacement with $K^+$). (From ref. 7.)

estimation of $pK_B$ values by Schild analysis for this antagonist is dependent on the extent of receptor precoupling. As shown in reconstitution studies, this factor can depend on the relative levels of $[T]$ and $[R]$.

## THE CLARK PLOT: ANALYSIS BY THE METHOD OF STONE-ANGUS

Another method of estimating the affinity of a competitive antagonist for a receptor with advantages over Schild analysis has been described by Stone and Angus (37). The graphic representation of this method is termed the Clark plot. The Gaddum equation for competitive antagonism can be written in the form:

$$\rho = \frac{[A]/K_A}{[A]/K_A + [B]^n/K_B + 1} \tag{9.26}$$

where $\rho$ refers to the fractional receptor occupancy by the agonist $[A]$, and $[B]$ and $K_B$ refer to the antagonist. This equation can be written:

$$\frac{\rho}{1 - \rho} = \frac{K_B \cdot [A]/K_A}{K_B + [B]^n} \tag{9.27}$$

If response is a function of receptor occupancy, Eq. 9.27 implies that response is determined by a function of the ratio:

$$\text{Response metameter } R = f\left(\frac{[A]}{[B]^n + K_B}\right) \tag{9.28}$$

Stone and Angus (37) explored various functions for $f$, the simplest being the equation for a straight line:

$$y = a + b \cdot \ln\left(\frac{[A]}{[B]^n + K_B}\right) \tag{9.29}$$

Therefore, a fit of an appropriate linearization metameter for response (i.e., $\ln R$) to a line defined by Eq. 9.29 should yield fitted estimations of $K_B$ and $n$. Figure 9.22A shows dose-response data reported by Clark (5) in 1926 for atropine antagonism of acetylcholine in frog ventricular strips. The Clark plot for these data is shown in Fig. 9.22B.

There are advantages to the use of the Clark plot for the calculation of equilibrium dissociation constants for antagonists. A major one is the fact that Schild analysis puts undue emphasis on the control dose-response curve; i.e., every dose ratio is calculated repeatedly from the control. Therefore, errors in the location of the control dose-response curve are magnified throughout the analysis. Also, Schild analysis distills many data from both the control and shifted dose-response curves into a single estimate of the dose ratio. The Clark plot uses all data points from both curves, thereby

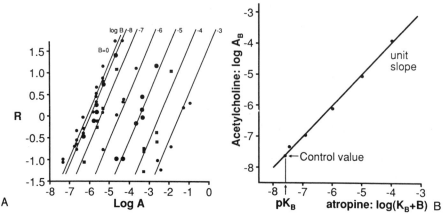

**FIG. 9.22.** Stone-Angus analysis of Clark's original data describing atropine antagonism of acetylcholine responses in frog heart. **A:** Dose-response curves for the effects of atropine on responses to acetylcholine. **B:** Clark plot for the data in A. (From ref. 36.)

increasing the accuracy of the fit. Also, a constant variance is assumed for $\log(dr - 1)$ values in Schild analysis, which, in turn, assumes that dose ratios nearer unity are determined more accurately than larger ones. An important practical advantage is the fact that single dose-response curves can be utilized for the Clark plot. This is useful for systems in which only one dose-response curve can be determined. Schild analysis usually is carried out in systems in which a control dose-response curve is obtained, a competitive antagonist added, and then a repeat dose-response curve in the presence of the antagonist is obtained to yield a dose ratio. Although the statistical method of bootstrapping the data can estimate biological error on single dose-response curve systems for Schild analysis (see previous section), this added step is not necessary for the Stone-Angus analysis.

A comprehensive approach to the study of competitive antagonism would be to use both the Clark plot and Schild analysis. The particular advantage of Schild analysis is the fact that it provides a convenient and graphically evident model of equilibrium kinetics between a single drug molecule and a single homogeneous receptor population, i.e., deviations from this model can be used to detect nonequilibrium steady states in systems, multiple activities of drugs, and heterogeneous receptor populations. If the undue emphasis of the control dose-response curve skews the estimate of the $K_B$, then this should be made evident in differences in the $K_B$ as measured with these two methods.

## PHARMACOLOGIC RESULTANT ANALYSIS

A technique, termed *resultant analysis*, has been introduced by Black and colleagues (4) that allows the measurement of the affinity of an antagonist for a receptor when that antagonist has other, and perhaps obscuring, actions. The principle on which this method is based is that if two competitive antagonists compete for the same binding site, then the mathematical models used to describe simple competitive antagonism can be used to calculate the expected dose ratio when both antagonists are present in the receptor compartment. This is similar in concept to the additive dose-ratio method presented by Paton and Rang (33) but differs in that the "test" antagonist is present during the measurement of the control dose-response curve. Therefore, any secondary actions of the test antagonist will not be a factor in the additive antagonism to that of the "reference" antagonist. For example, if a given test antagonist is present in the receptor compartment at a concentration of 10 times the $K_B$ for receptor antagonism, a 10-fold shift to the right of the control dose-response curve of the agonist should be observed. However, if this test antagonist has another property that sensitizes the tissue to the agonist (e.g., inhibition of agonist uptake) and if the given concentration of antagonist is sufficient to produce a fivefold shift to the left of the agonist dose-response curve, then only a *twofold* shift to the right would be observed, and the potency for receptor antagonism would be underestimated by a factor of 5. With resultant analysis, the test antagonist is included in the measurement of the control dose-response curve; thus the control is already shifted to the right by a factor of 10 and to the left by the fivefold increase in sensitization. Then, a second reference antagonist is added, for which the receptor $K_B$ would be known (and thus the expected dose ratio known as well), and the overall shift to the right is measured in the presence of both antagonists. Under these circumstances, both the control and shifted dose-response curves are under the influence of the sensitizing property of the test antagonist; therefore, under null conditions, this effect will cancel and only the additive receptor antagonism will be observed. Since the contribution of the reference antagonist ($[B_{ref}]/K_{Bref}$) and the concentration of the test antagonist ($[B_{test}]$) is known, the dose ratio is observed, the equilibrium dissociation constant of the test antagonist/receptor complex ($K_{Btest}$) can be calculated. Thus:

$$K_{Btest} = \frac{[B_{test}]}{(\text{dr} - 1 - [B_{ref}]/K_{Bref})} \qquad [9.30]$$

In practice this method can be more effective if a range of concentrations of reference and test antagonists is used. With this methodology, a test of the assumption of competitiveness also can be included in the analysis much like Schild analysis. Thus, in the presence of a reference antagonist ($[B']$) and a concentration $[C]$ of test antagonist, the resulting response is given by:

$$E' = f\left(\frac{[A']}{[A'] + K_A(1 + [B']/K_B + [C]/K_C)}\right) \qquad [9.31]$$

where $K_B$ and $K_C$ refer to the equilibrium dissociation constants of the antagonist-receptor complexes, $[A']$ is the molar concentration of the agonist, $K_A$ is the equilibrium dissociation constant of the agonist-receptor complex, and $f$ refers to the function associating receptor occupancy and tissue response. The response in the absence of the reference antagonist ($[B'] = 0$) is given by:

$$E = f\left(\frac{[A]}{[A] + K_A (1 + [C]/K_C)}\right) \tag{9.32}$$

Equal responses ($E' = E$) are assumed to result from equal receptor occupancies by $A$ and $A'$. Thus, Eqs. 9.31 and 9.32 can be equated and rearranged to:

$$\frac{[A']}{[A]} = r' = 1 + \frac{[B']}{K_B (1 + [C]/K_C)} \tag{9.33}$$

where $r'$ refers to equieffective concentrations of agonist ($[A]/[A']$) both in the presence of the test antagonist and in the absence ($[A]$) and presence ($[A']$) of the reference antagonist. The function $f$ cancels under the null conditions of equal responses; therefore the secondary effects of the test antagonist are expressed during the control and blocked (by the reference antagonist) dose-response curve and therefore do not affect the analysis.

In the absence of the test antagonist ($[C] = 0$), the dose ratios for equiactive agonist concentrations in the absence and presence of the reference antagonist are given by the Schild equation:

$$r = \frac{[B]}{K_B} + 1 \tag{9.34}$$

Relating equal dose ratios ($r' = r$) from Eqs. 9.33 and 9.34 and rearrangement yield:

$$\frac{[B']}{[B]} - 1 = y - 1 = \frac{[C]}{K_C} \tag{9.35}$$

the logarithmic metameter of which is:

$$\log(y - 1) = \log[C] - \log K_C \tag{9.36}$$

Therefore, an estimate of the equilibrium dissociation constant of the test antagonist-receptor complex can be obtained from a regression of $\log(y - 1)$ on $\log[C]$. In practice, Schild regressions are obtained for the reference antagonist in the absence and presence of various concentrations of test antagonist and the dextral displacement of the Schild regressions yields values for $y$. For example, isobutylmethylxanthine (IBMX) is known to be a competitive antagonist of purine receptors and also to inhibit phosphodiesterase. In cardiac tissue this latter factor produces positive inotropy. Since purines produce negative inotropy, changes in responses to purines caused by IBMX are difficult to interpret since it is not clear whether they are mediated by purine receptor antagonism or phosphodiesterase inhibition.

Therefore, the effects of IBMX, as a test antagonist, on the blockade of purine responses to the reference receptor antagonist 8-sulfophenyltheophylline (8-SPT) allow for determination of receptor effects. Since the IBMX is present from the control conditions, all phosphodiesterase effects are canceled. Under these conditions, the only difference between the control dose-response curve and the curve in the presence of the reference antagonist is receptor blockade by the reference antagonist. The potency of this antagonist is known, and thus the contribution to the observed dose ratio by the test antagonist can be determined from Eq. 9.30. Figure 9.23A shows the Schild regressions for 8-SPT in the absence and presence of three concentrations of IBMX. The resulting shifts of the Schild regressions (estimates of $y$) are shown as a function of the log IBMX concentrations in Fig. 9.23B. As can be seen from this figure, the regression is linear and has a slope not significantly different from unity. This indicates that the receptor blockade by IBMX is competitive and that the equilibrium dissociation constant of the IBMX-receptor complex ($K_C$) is 4 $\mu$M.

### Competitive Antagonism by Partial Agonists

Partial agonists are defined as drugs that produce submaximal tissue responses and competitively block the effects of agonists of higher intrinsic efficacies. It should be emphasized that agonism from partial agonists should be obtained at concentrations equal to those that produce blockade, because both agonism and antagonism result from interaction of a partial agonist with the receptor. An agonist response to a drug that occurs at concentrations greater than those that produce antagonism cannot be ascribed to interaction of the drug at a single receptor, according to present models of receptor theory, unless a significant threshold effect is operative (i.e., 50% receptor

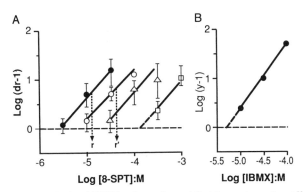

**FIG. 9.23.** Resultant analysis of IBMX antagonism of 2-chloroadenosine effects in guinea pig atria. **A:** Schild regressions for the reference antagonist 8-SPT in the absence (•) and presence of IBMX (10 [o], 30 [△], and 100 $\mu$mol/L [□]). **B:** Resultant plot for the regressions in A for IBMX. (From ref. 26.)

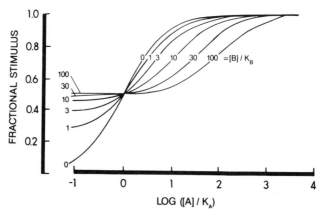

**FIG. 9.24.** Theoretical effects of a partial agonist on stimuli produced by a full agonist. The maximal response to the partial agonist is 0.5 that to the full agonist.

occupation by partial agonist before observable response). Figure 9.24 shows the effects of various concentrations of a partial agonist on dose-response curves for a full agonist. The dual effects of the partial agonist (i.e., producing a response and blocking the full agonist) can be seen in this figure; the shifts to the right in dose-response curves for the agonist can furnish dose ratios for Schild analysis. The question then arises, in which region of the dose-response curve for the agonist should these dose ratios be measured? Theoretical analyses suggest that measurement of the dose ratio that produces a half-maximal response to the full agonist provides the most unambiguous approach, although the intrinsic efficacy of the partial agonist still introduces an error factor into the estimate of $pK_B$. This error factor is proportional to the magnitude of the intrinsic efficacy of the partial agonist and also to the efficiency of coupling of the tissue stimulus-response mechanisms. In some cases the error due to the agonist effects of the partial agonist can be shown to be small. For example, dobutamine is a partial agonist for $\alpha$-adrenoceptors of rat anococcygeus muscle, producing 55% of the tissue maximal response. Figure 9.25A shows the effects of various concentrations of dobutamine on dose-response curves for norepinephrine in this tissue; the half-maximal concentrations of norepinephrine were used to furnish dose ratios for the Schild regression shown in Fig. 9.25C. In this same tissue, irreversible blockade of a fraction of the $\alpha$-adrenoceptor population eliminates responses to dobutamine; under these circumstances, this drug can be used as a competitive antagonist of norepinephrine responses (Fig. 9.25B). The dose ratios from this alkylated preparation were not affected by the dobutamine agonist response and yielded the Schild regression shown in Fig. 9.25C. The $pK_B$ estimates from both sets of data were not statistically significant, indicating that the partial-agonist activity of dobutamine in this instance did not introduce a significant error into the estimation of $K_B$ by Schild analysis.

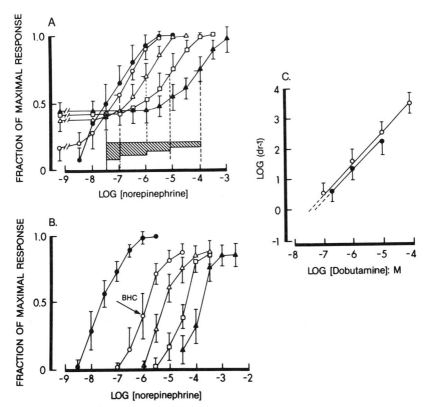

**FIG. 9.25.** Measurement of affinity of a partial agonist by Schild analysis. **A:** Antagonism of norepinephrine responses of rat anococcygeus muscle by the partial agonist dobutamine. Ordinate: Fractions of the maximal response to norepinephrine. Abscissa: Logarithms of molar concentrations of norepinephrine. Ordinate values immediately to the right of the ordinate axis represent agonist responses to dobutamine alone. Responses in the absence (●, $N = 8$) and presence of dobutamine at 0.1 (○, $N = 3$), 1 (△, $N = 2$), 10 (□, $N = 3$), and 100 μM (▲, $N = 3$). Histogram represents magnitudes of dose ratios as measured from half-maximal doses of norepinephrine. **B:** Antagonism of norepinephrine responses of rat anococcygeus muscle by dobutamine after pretreatment with the α-adrenoceptor alkylating agent $N,N'$-bis[6-(*O*-methoxybenzylamino)-*n*-hexyl]cystamine (BHC 10 μM for 20 min). Axes as for A. Responses in the absence of dobutamine before (●, $N = 9$) and after BHC treatment (○, $N = 8$) and in the presence of dobutamine at 0.2 (△, $N = 3$), 1 (□, $N = 2$), and 10 μM (▲, $N = 3$) after BHC treatment. *Arrow* represents level of measurement for dose ratios. **C:** Schild regression from data in A (●, $N = 11$) and B (○, $N = 8$). Bars represent SEM or range for $N < 3$. (From ref. 14.)

It is difficult to mathematically model estimates of the error in $K_B$ produced by agonist activity, because this varies with the nature and efficiency of stimulus-response coupling. For example, if the function relating stimulus and response is a rectangular hyperbola [$R = S/(S + 1)$], then it can be shown that the observed $K_B$ is related to the true $K_B$ by the equation

$$\text{observed } K_B = K_B(1 - \alpha_p)^{-1} \qquad [9.37]$$

where $\alpha_p$ relates to the intrinsic activity (maximal response to the partial agonist expressed as a fraction of the maximal response to the full agonist; see Chapter 8) of the partial agonist. It can be seen from this equation that the magnitude of the error factor depends on the magnitude of the maximal response to the partial agonist.

One experimental method to avoid this error is to partially depress the response capability of the tissue such that the partial agonist will not produce a response, but the full agonist will. Under these circumstances, the partial agonist can be used as a competitive antagonist, with $K_B$ estimated by Schild analysis. This can be achieved by partial alkylation of the receptor population or by physiological (functional) antagonism (see Chapter 10). Both of these approaches are useful, because a partial agonist has to activate more receptors to produce a response than does a full agonist. Therefore, serial depression of the response capability of a tissue will block responses to partial agonists before responses to full agonists. The effects of irreversible alkylation of increasing fractions of the receptor population are modeled in Fig. 9.26 for two agonists with a relative intrinsic efficacy ratio of 100:1. After 99% of the receptors have been activated, responses to the partial agonist are insignificant; at this point it can be used as a competitive antagonist of responses to the full agonist. This technique was used experimentally in Fig. 9.25B.

## ANTAGONISM OF INDIRECT AGONISTS

An indirect agonist produces a response by initiating release of an endogenous agonist (i.e., neurotransmitter) from within the tissue (Fig. 9.27A). A competitive antagonist may produce depression of the maximal response to such an agonist. For example, Fig. 9.27B shows the depression of the maximal response to the indirect agonist tyramine caused by propranolol. The

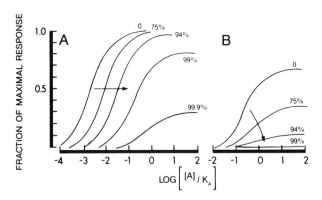

**FIG. 9.26.** Calculated effects of progressive receptor alkylation on responses to a full **(A)** and partial agonist **(B)**. Percentages refer to the portions of the receptor population alkylated. (From ref. 23.)

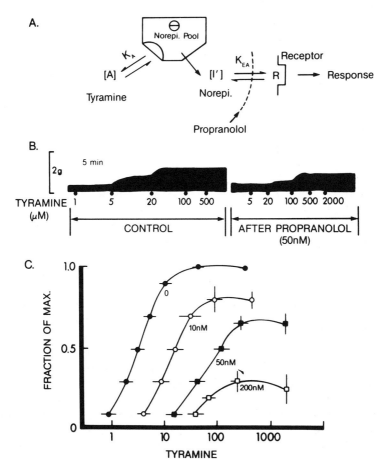

**FIG. 9.27.** Depression of maximal responses to tyramine by propranolol competitive antagonism. **A:** Schematic shows the sequence of response production by tyramine and site of intervention for propranolol. **B:** Sample dynograph tracing of electrically induced rat atrial contractions for tyramine in the absence and presence of propranolol. **C:** Mean dose-response curves for tyramine in rat left atria. Ordinate: Fractions of maximal control response to tyramine. Abscissa: Logarithms of molar concentrations of tyramine. Responses in the absence (●, $N = 17$) and presence of propranolol at 10 (○, $N = 5$), 50 (■, $N = 7$), and 200 nM (□, $N = 5$). Bars represent SEM. (From ref. 3.)

concentration-related shifts to the right and concomitant depressions of maxima of dose-response curves for tyramine are shown in Fig. 9.27C.

The receptor occupancy ($\rho$) produced by an indirect agonist $[A]$ that releases an endogenous agonist to occupy the receptors is

$$\rho = \left[ 1 + \frac{K_{EA}}{\Theta} \left( 1 + \frac{K_A}{[A]} \right) \right]^{-1} \qquad [9.38]$$

where $\Theta$ is the size of the available pool of endogenous agonist, $K_{EA}$ is the equilibrium dissociation constant for the endogenous agonist-receptor complex, and $K_A$ is the equilibrium constant for the complex between the indirect agonist and the site of release. It can be seen from this equation that if the pool of endogenous agonist is small or the endogenous agonist has a low affinity for the receptor (high $K_{EA}$), then maximal receptor occupancy by the indirect agonist may never be achieved. In the presence of a competitive antagonist [B], the receptor occupancy by an indirect agonist is given by

$$\rho' = \left[ 1 + \frac{K_{EA}}{\Theta} \left( 1 + \frac{K_A}{[A]} \right) \left( 1 + \frac{[B]}{K_B} \right) \right]^{-1} \qquad [9.39]$$

where $K_B$ refers to the equilibrium dissociation constant for the antagonist-receptor complex. It can be seen from this equation that the maximal receptor occupancy by the indirect agonist may further be depressed by a competitive antagonist. In practice, this means that competitive antagonists may produce depression of the maximal responses to indirect agonists concomitant with shifts to the right in dose-response curves. The magnitude of the maximal shift to the right in the dose-response curve before depression of maximal response is dependent on the efficiency of the mechanism of release of the indirect agonist, which itself is a function of the size of the pool of indirect agonist ($\Theta$) and the equilibrium dissociation constant for the indirect agonist-receptor complex ($K_{EA}$). Thus, if the pool is large with respect to $K_{EA}$ (high affinity), then $K_{EA}/\Theta$ will be small, and large shifts to the right in dose-response curves with no depression of maximal response will be observed. In contrast, if the pool of endogenous agonist is small or if the endogenous agonist has a low affinity for the receptors, a competitive antagonist may depress the maximal response at low concentrations (near $K_B$); these effects are shown in Fig. 9.28. Clearly, if there is efficient receptor coupling such

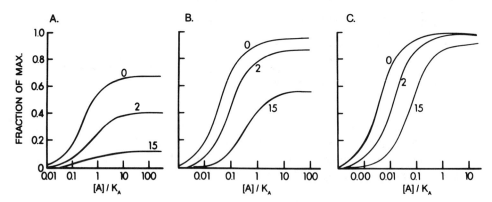

**FIG. 9.28.** Dependence of the fractional receptor occupancy by the endogenous agonist (ordinate scale) on the relative size of the pool of endogenous agonist ($K_{EA}/\Theta$). Abscissa: Logarithms of $[A]/K_A$. Numbers refer to values of $[B]/K_B$. (From ref. 3.)

that relatively small amounts of stimuli result in a maximal response, then this will tend to extend the maximal magnitude of parallel shift in dose-response curves before depression of maximal responses. In view of these variables, it is difficult to predict at which point a competitive antagonist will depress the maximal response to an indirect agonist. However, the alternative view, namely, that if a competitive antagonist does depress the maximal response to an agonist of unknown mechanism, then the release of an indirect agonist is implicated, can be useful in studies aimed at drug and receptor classification.

## REFERENCES

1. Ariëns, E. J., van Rossum, J. M., and Koopman, P. C. (1960): Receptor reserve and threshold phenomena. *Arch. Int. Pharmacodyn. Ther.*, 127:459–478.
2. Arunlakshana, O., and Schild, H. O. (1959): Some quantitative uses of drug antagonists. *Br. J. Pharmacol.*, 14:48–58.
3. Black, J. W., Jenkinson, D. H., and Kenakin, T. P. (1980): Antagonism of an indirectly acting agonist: Block by propranolol and sotalol of the action of tyramines on rat heart. *Eur. J. Pharmacol.*, 65:1–10.
4. Black, J. W., Gerskowitch, V. P., Leff, P., and Shankley, N. P. (1986): Analysis of competitive antagonism when this property occurs as part of a pharmacological resultant. *Br. J. Pharmacol.*, 89:547–555.
5. Clark, A. J. (1926): The antagonism of acetylcholine by atropine. *J. Physiol. (Lond.)*, 61: 547–556.
6. Clark, A. J. (1937): General Pharmacology. In; *Heffter's Handbook d-exp. Pharmacol., Erg., band 4.* Springer, Berlin.
7. Costa, T., Ogino, Y., Munson, P. J., Onaran, H. O., and Rodbard, D. (1992): Drug efficacy at guanine nucleotide-binding regulatory protein linked receptors: Thermodynamic interpretation of negative antagonism and of receptor activity in the absence of ligand. *Mol. Pharmacol.*, 41:549–560.
8. Furchgott, R. F. (1966): The use of beta-haloalkylamines in the differentiation of receptors and in the determination of dissociation constants of receptor-agonist complexes. In: *Advances in Drug Research*, edited by N. J. Harper and A. B. Simmonds, pp. 21–55. Academic Press, New York.
9. Furchgott, R. F. (1972): The classification of adrenoceptors (adrenergic receptors). An evaluation from the standpoint of receptor theory. In: *Handbook of Experimental Pharmacology, Catecholamines, Vol. 33*, edited by H. Blaschko and E. Muscholl, pp. 283–335. Springer-Verlag, Berlin.
10. Gaddum, J. H. (1937): The quantitative effects of antagonistic drugs. *J. Physiol. (Lond.)*, 89:7P–9P.
11. Gaddum, J. H. (1957): Theories of drug antagonism. *Pharmacol. Rev.*, 9:211–218.
12. Gaddum, J. H., Hameed, K. A., Hathway, D. E., and Stephens, F. F. (1955): Quantitative studies of antagonists for 5-hydroxytryptamine. *Q. J. Exp. Physiol.*, 40:49–74.
13. Kenakin, T. P. (1980): Effects of equilibration time on the attainment of equilibrium between antagonists and drug receptors. *Eur. J. Pharmacol.*, 66:295–306.
14. Kenakin, T. P. (1981): An in vitro quantitative analysis of the alpha adrenoceptor partial agonist activity of dobutamine and its relevance to inotropic selectivity. *J. Pharmacol. Exp. Ther.*, 216:210–219.
15. Kenakin, T. P. (1984): The relative contribution of affinity and efficacy to agonist activity: Organ selectivity of noradrenaline and oxymetazoline with reference to the classification of drug receptors. *Br. J. Pharmacol.*, 81:131–143.
16. Kenakin, T. P. (1984): The classification of drugs and drug receptors in isolated tissues. *Pharmacol. Rev.*, 36:165–221.

17. Kenakin, T. P. (1985): Schild regressions as indicators of nonequilibrium steady-states and heterogeneous receptor populations. *Trends Pharmacol. Sci.*, 6:68–71.
18. Kenakin, T. P. (1986): Tissue and receptor selectivity: Similarities and differences. In: *Advances in Drug Research, Vol. 15*, edited by B. Testa, pp. 71–109. Academic Press, New York.
19. Kenakin, T. P. (1987): What can we learn from models of complex drug antagonism in classifying hormone receptors? In: *Receptor Biochemistry and Methodology, Vol. 6, Perspectives on Receptor Classification*, edited by J. W. Black, D. H. Jenkinson, and V. P. Gerskowitch, pp. 169–184. Alan R. Liss, New York.
20. Kenakin, T. P. (1992): Tissue response as a functional discriminator of receptor heterogeneity: The effects of mixed receptor populations on Schild regressions. *Mol. Pharmacol.*, 41: 699–707.
21. Kenakin, T. P., and Beek, D. (1981): The measurement of antagonist potency and the importance of selective inhibition of agonist uptake processes. *J. Pharmacol. Exp. Ther.*, 219:112–120.
22. Kenakin, T. P., and Beek, D. (1982): A quantitative analysis of histamine $H_2$-receptor-mediated relaxation of rabbit trachea. *J. Pharmacol. Exp. Ther.*, 220:353–357.
23. Kenakin, T. P., and Beek, D. (1984): The measurement of the relative efficacy of agonists by selective potentiation of tissue responses: Studies with isoprenaline and prenalterol in cardiac tissue. *J. Auton. Pharmacol.*, 4:153–159.
24. Kenakin, T. P., and Beek, D. (1985): Self-cancellation of drug properties as a mode of organ selectivity: The antimuscarinic effects of ambenonium. *J. Pharmacol. Exp. Ther.*, 232: 732–740.
25. Kenakin, T. P., and Beek, D. (1987): The effects of Schild regressions of antagonist removal from the receptor compartment by a saturable process. *Naunyn Schmiedebergs Arch. Pharmacol.*, 385:103–108.
26. Kenakin, T. P., and Beek, D. (1987): Measurement of antagonist affinity for purine receptors of drugs producing concomitant phosphodiesterase blockade: The use of pharmacologic resultant analysis. *J. Pharmacol. Exp. Ther.*, 243:482–486.
27. Kenakin, T. P., and Black, J. W. (1978): The pharmacological classification of practolol and chloropractolol. *Mol. Pharmacol.*, 14:607–623.
28. Lemoine, H., and Kaumann, A. J. (1983): A model for the interaction of competitive antagonists with two receptor-subtypes characterized by a Schild-plot with apparent slope unity. *Naunyn Schmiedebergs Arch. Pharmacol.*, 322:111–120.
29. Lutz, M. W., Corsi, M., and Kenakin, T. P. (1992).
30. Mackay, D. (1978): How should values of $pA_2$ and affinity constants for pharmacological competitive antagonists be estimated? *J. Pharm. Pharmacol.*, 30:312–313.
31. Milnor, W. R. (1986): Limitations of Schild plots in a two receptor system: α-adrenoceptors of vascular smooth muscle. *J. Pharmacol. Exp. Ther.*, 238:237–241.
32. Munson, P. J., and Rodbard, D. (1980): Ligand: A versatile approach for the characterisation of ligand binding systems. *Anal. Biochem.*, 107:220–239.
33. Paton, W. D. M., and Rang, H. P. (1965): The uptake of atropine and related drugs by intestinal smooth muscle of the guinea pig in relation to acetylcholine receptors. *Proc. R. Soc. Lond. [Biol.]*, 163:1–44.
34. Rang, H. P. (1966): The kinetics of action of acetylcholine antagonists in smooth muscle. *Proc. R. Soc. Lond. [Biol.]*, 164:488–510.
35. Schild, H. O. (1949): $pA_x$ and competitive drug antagonism. *Br. J. Pharmacol.*, 4:277–280.
36. Stone, M. (1980): The Clark plot: A semi-historical study. *J. Pharm. Pharmacol.*, 32:81–86.
37. Stone, M., and Angus, J. A. (1978): Developments of computer-based estimation of $pA_2$ values and associated analysis. *J. Pharmacol. Exp. Ther.*, 207:705–718.
38. Suzuki, E., Tsujimoto, G., Tamura, K., and Hashimoto, K. (1990): Two pharmacologically distinct $\alpha_1$-adrenoceptor subtypes in the contraction of rabbit aorta: Each subtype couples with a different $Ca^{2+}$ signalling mechanism and plays a different physiological role. *Mol. Pharmacol.*, 38:725–736.

# 10

## Allotopic, Noncompetitive, and Irreversible Antagonism

*It is certain that all bodies whatsoever, though they have no sense, yet have perception; for when one body is applied to another, there is a kind of election to embrace that which is agreeable, and to exclude or expel that which is ingrate; and whether the body be alterant or altered, evermore a perception precedeth operation; for else all bodies would be like one another.*
                                                            —FRANCIS BACON, 1620

### ALLOTOPIC EFFECTS (ALLOSTERISM)

In 1909, Paul Ehrlich (8) wrote, "Substances can only be anchored at any particular part of the organism if they fit into the molecule of the recipient complex like a piece of mosaic finds its place in a pattern." A challenge to this lock-and-key view of drug-receptor interaction was offered as early as 1937 by Clark (4) who wrote, "It is necessary to postulate a complex receptor with which one drug can unite without displacing the other drug." The way in which two drugs could bind to and interact on a receptor surface without physical contact is by allosterism. This term was first used to describe the behavior of certain enzymes when the kinetics observed with those enzymes did not conform to the classical concepts of the time (19). It is defined as being the alteration of the activity of a protein (as an enzyme) by combination with another substance at a point other than the chemically active site. Substances that produce this effect are called allosteric effectors. From the point of view of industrial pharmacology, which seeks to design improved versions of endogenous molecules or the interference of the action of endogenous molecules, the differentiation of true active site competitiveness and allosteric effect can be important, because each mechanism presumably would involve different structure-activity relationships. In view of this, there are practical reasons for wanting to differentiate true competitiveness and allosterism. Before discussion of the various methods of differentiating these mechanisms, definition of terms is helpful.

*323*

In a classic paper on allosterism in enzyme systems, Monod et al. (19) outlined a differentiation of interactions between substrates and inhibitors. As shown in Fig. 10.1, the first scheme depicts true competitiveness, in which the substrate and inhibitor compete for the same amino acid residues for binding. In pharmacologic terms, these are the interactions described by the classic receptor theory equations derived by Gaddum and Schild (see Chapter 9). The second is a type of modified competitiveness in which the antagonist shares some but not all of the binding domain of the agonist and utilizes another domain as an anchor. This idea emanates from the observation that antagonists often are larger sterically than agonists. This situation was described by Monod et al. as direct interaction. The Charniere effect was an early description of this mechanism, whereby a region of the receptor was proposed to serve as an anchor for the antagonist, allowing the rest of the molecule to interfere with agonist binding by a hingelike competitive interaction (22). The thermodynamic rationale for this hypothesis was that van der Waals forces tightly bound the large aromatic regions of, in a specific

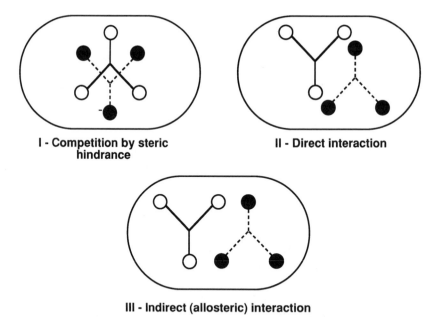

**I - Competition by steric hindrance**

**II - Direct interaction**

**III - Indirect (allosteric) interaction**

**FIG. 10.1.** Three theoretical types of interactions between molecules at the active catalytic site of an enzyme. **I:** True competitiveness in which the substrate (endogenous agonist for the receptor) and antagonist compete for binding to the same amino acid domain of the enzyme (receptor). **II:** Where the antagonist perhaps shares some but not all of the amino acid domain for binding to obscure the substrate binding to the catalytic site. **III:** Where the amino acid binding domains for the substrate (endogenous agonist) and the antagonist exist on separate parts of the enzyme (receptor) protein and the interaction between the two is allosteric. (From ref. 19.)

example, lachesine, to leave the polar side chain to compete for binding at the acetylcholine binding domain of cholinergic receptors. There are numerous examples of antagonists that structurally resemble the endogenous agonist but that also are more flexible molecules with large lipophilic groups. It might be supposed that these types of antagonist would block agonist response by scheme II. By this mechanism, some of the contact amino acids for the agonist and antagonist binding domains would differ. In terms of the definition of true allosterism, these antagonists would not be classified as allosteric effectors. The third possibility is what can be considered true allosterism (also referred to as allotopic interaction) in that the binding of the antagonist (allosteric effector) is at a site distinct and removed from the binding domain for the endogenous substrate (agonist) and that interference with agonist binding is achieved by a protein conformational change induced by the binding of the effector. It should be noted that the nature of the allotopic change can differ in this mechanism as well. The protein (receptor) may exist in different thermodynamically favorable conformations and the allosteric effector may discriminate between them (conformational selection; see Chapter 8). Another possibility would be that the allosteric effector may simply induce a degree of conformational modification to the protein, the intensity of which depends on the saturation of binding to the allosteric site (conformational induction).

There are two concepts involved in allosterism, namely, the exclusivity of binding sites for drugs and allosteric effectors on a receptor protein and cooperativity of binding. These ideas are complementary in that if binding to a receptor is cooperative, then it must also involve more than one site on the receptor. Therefore, the detection of allotopic effects can be achieved either by the detection and quantification of cooperative binding or the determination of separate binding sites on the receptor.

## ALLOSTERIC BINDING SITES

With the advent of cloning techniques and overexpression of proteins, adequate amounts of receptor can be isolated and sequenced and the tertiary structure assumed from hydropathicity data. The creation of point genetic mutations in receptors might allow the determination of critical amino acids in the function of drug receptors, and, from the relative location of these, the probability of competitive versus allotopic effects perhaps can be estimated. In an early discussion of allosteric effects in enzymes, Koshland (18) classified amino acids in an enzyme as being "contact amino acids," an intimate part of the active site for substrate binding; "contributing amino acids," those important for preservation of the tertiary structure of the active site but not playing a role in substrate binding; and "noncontributing amino acids," those not essential for enzyme catalysis but perhaps serving a structural role in the enzyme. This latter class Koshland also referred to as "junk" amino acids in terms of enzyme function in light of evidence that they could be enzymatically or chemically cleaved from the protein without a change in enzyme kinetics. Drug binding to these latter two categories of amino acids might constitute a mechanism of allosterism rather than pure endogenous agonist competition. Similarly, pharmacologic antagonists could bind to sites distinct from those utilized by the endogenous agonist (i.e., hormone, neurotransmitter) to alter binding and subsequent tissue response (Fig. 10.2). In terms of the current model of G protein–coupled receptors, drugs may bind to the cleft produced by the three extracellular loops, to the intramembrane spanning regions (e.g., muscarinic agonists, $\alpha_2$-adrenoceptor agonists $\beta_2$- adrenoceptor agonists) or theoretically to the cytoplasmic loops of the receptor. There also is evidence to suggest that some drugs approach the receptor in two-dimensional space by first dissolving into the lipid membrane (e.g., dihydropyridines, propranolol, amiodarone; see Chapter 4). If the intramembrane-spanning regions are indeed the binding domain for endogenous agonists, then the binding of antagonists to other regions of the receptor could constitute allosteric modulation. Point mutation studies, or those involving partial receptor purification, have produced different changes in the binding characteristics of agonists and antagonists. For example, a substitution in $\beta$- adrenoceptors of Asn at position 130 produces no effect on antagonist binding but a 10-fold increase in the affinity for agonists (9). In mutagenic studies with the hamster gene encoding $\beta$-adrenoceptors, replacements of aspartate-79 and asparagine-318 yielded mutants with wild-type affinities for antagonists but a 10-fold reduced affinity for agonists (24). These types of data suggest that many antagonists previously thought to compete for agonist binding at common domains may, in fact, be allosteric effectors. This conclusion would assume that the deletions affect separate regions of the receptor, some more relevant to the binding of one type of drug than another. It should also be stressed, however, that a deletion in one region of the receptor may produce a conformational change in another, therefore making it difficult to relate specific deletions to specific binding domains. A particularly striking

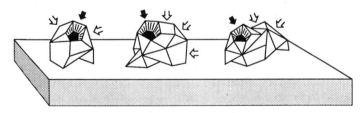

**FIG. 10.2.** Three hypothetical receptors possessing the same binding domain for the endogenous agonist but otherwise different sites for the binding of allosteric effectors. *Solid arrow*, endogenous agonist binding; *open arrow*, allosteric effector binding. (From ref. 17.)

**TABLE 10.1.** *Affinity of wild-type and mutant m1 receptors for [³H]NMS in the presence of gallamine*

| Gallamine (μM) | $K_i$ (pM) | |
|---|---|---|
| | Wild type | Asn 71 |
| 0 | 88 ± 4 | 82 ± 6 |
| 1 | 161 ± 14 | 97 ± 5 |
| 3 | 283 ± 2 | 133 ± 3 |
| 10 | 701 ± 27 | 274 ± 11 |
| 30 | 1793 ± 79 | 661 ± 40 |
| 100 | 3817 ± 57 | 1363 ± 25 |
| 300 | 3811 ± 156 | 1394 ± 156 |

From ref. 14.

illustration of the differences in amino acids required for competitive antagonist binding and allosteric effector binding can be seen in mutant muscarinic m1 receptors. Substitution of an aspartate residue at position 71, but not at positions 99 and 122, affects the affinity of the allotopic antagonist gallamine but not the affinity of the competitive antagonist radiolabeled [³H]-*N*-methyl-scopolamine ([³H]NMS) (see Table 10.1).

## PHARMACOLOGIC DETECTION OF ALLOTOPIC EFFECTS

Mass action kinetics predict the behavior of agonists and antagonists when they compete for common binding sites on receptors. When these predictions do not hold true (i.e., when apparently capricious changes in dose-response curves are observed), this either could be due to a nonequilibrium steady state in the receptor compartment, secondary effects of drugs, or allosteric modulation. It is worth considering the tools available to detect allosteric effects on receptors and the differentiation of these from other pharmacodynamics. The Langmuir binding isotherm for the binding of a single drug molecule to a single site (receptor) predicts a sigmoidal binding curve on a semilogarithmic axis with a slope coefficient of unity (see Chapter 1). Binding reactions that cannot be described by this model may then be the result of allotopic reactions in which the binding is positively cooperative (the binding of one drug molecule promotes the binding of subsequent drug molecules, with the slope coefficient of the binding curve greater than 1) or negatively cooperative (the binding of one drug molecule subsequently inhibits the binding of other drug molecules, with a slope coefficient less than 1). In radioligand binding experiments in which the amount of drug-receptor complex is measured directly, such slope coefficients may have relevance to molecular events at the drug-receptor level. The classic model of cooperative binding in biochemistry is the binding of oxygen to the hemoglobin tetramer. Figure

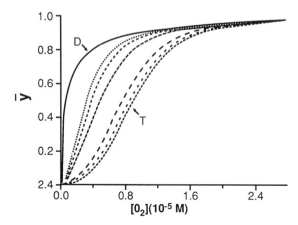

**FIG. 10.3.** The binding of oxygen to hemoglobin dimers (Hill coefficient for binding, $n =$ 1, curve D) and tetramers (Hill coefficient for binding, $N = 3.3$, curve T). Concentrations of hemoglobin range from 40 nM to 100 μM. (From ref. 1.)

10.3 shows the binding curves for oxygen to dimers and tetramers of hemoglobin. The changes in the shapes of the binding curves with changes in hemoglobin concentration indicate the increasing cooperativity with increased association of the protein chains. In functional studies, the slope of the dose-response curves may be determined entirely by receptor-effector coupling processes (see Chapter 11); therefore, these types of data cannot be relied on for information regarding possible allotopic effects.

Allotopic effects can be observed directly in binding studies. For example, Fig 10.4A shows the effect of the allosteric effector alcuronium on the binding of the muscarinic antagonist [³H]NMS. As can be seen from this figure, the binding of [³H]NMS is *stimulated* by alcuronium at lower doses and then inhibited to basal levels. This stimulation could occur either by an increase in the number of binding sites or an increase in the affinity of the receptor for [³H]NMS. Scatchard analysis of the binding of [³H]NMS in the absence and presence of alcuronium indicates that an increase in affinity of the receptor for [³H]NMS, probably by an allotopic mechanism, is produced by alcuronium (Fig. 10.4B).

A method that has been used to detect allosteric receptor effects is the quantitative and qualitative examination of the effects of antagonists on agonist dose-response curves. The classic technique for determination of antagonist competitiveness is by Schild analysis (see Chapter 9). By this method, if an antagonist produces parallel displacement of agonist dose-response curves with no alteration of the maximal response, then equiactive dose ratios can be calculated and used in the Schild equation. If a regression, according to a logarithmic metameter of the Schild equation, yields a straight line with a unit slope, then the behavior of the antagonist is consistent with

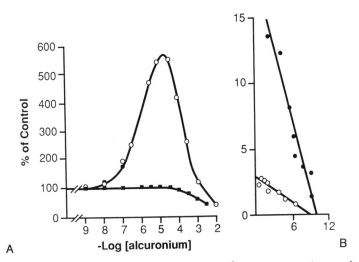

**FIG. 10.4.** Effect of alcuronium on specific binding of [$^3$H]NMS in membranes from rat atria (o) and submaxillary gland (■). **A:** Binding of 200 pM [$^3$H]NMS in the presence of a range of concentrations of alcuronium. **B:** Scatchard plot of the binding of [$^3$H]NMS in the absence (o) and presence (•) of alcuronium (10 μM). The change in slope with no change in abscissal intercept is indicative of a change in affinity of the receptor for [$^3$H]NMS and no increase in the number of binding sites. (From ref. 25.)

simple competitive antagonism. It is now well-known that kinetics showing that an antagonist produces a linear Schild regression with a unit slope are consistent with, but not proof of, competitiveness, since other mechanisms can produce similar effects. The strength of the Schild technique is that it provides a mathematically predictable paradigm of competitive behavior that true competitive antagonists must satisfy. The Schild equation predicts that a linear Schild regression with a unit slope should result over a very large concentration range of antagonist. Some tissue systems allow remarkable adherence to the theory. For example, in guinea pig ileum scopolamine produces a 10,000-fold shift to the right of cholinergic agonist dose-response curves with no depression of maximum. Deviations from competitive kinetics, as measured by the Schild technique, have been used as evidence of allosteric effects. Schild analysis can be used as a quantitative tool to detect allosterism under certain circumstances. For example, Clark and Mitchelson (5) showed that gallamine produced parallel displacement of carbachol and acetylcholine dose-response curves in guinea pig atria to yield a linear Schild regression of unit slope over a 30-fold concentration range. However, with higher concentrations of gallamine, this competitive behavior deviates dramatically and dose ratios of greater than 35 (for acetylcholine) could not be attained with this antagonist (Fig. 10.5). The apparent limiting antagonism of gallamine in the Schild regression indicates a saturation of binding to an allosteric site and the resulting maximal allotopic effect on agonist binding.

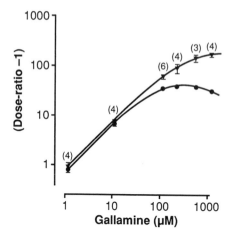

**FIG. 10.5.** Schild regressions for gallamine in guinea pig atria. Blockade of responses to acetylcholine (●) and carbachol (▼) by gallamine. (From ref. 5.)

Another approach to the detection of cooperativity is by the observation of the kinetics of binding. The rate of onset and offset of drugs from receptors can be determined experimentally and compared to first-order kinetic models (see Chapter 13). Thus, the receptor occupation by a drug should be temporally related in a linear fashion when plotted on a logarithmic scale (see Chapter 13). Similarly, the rate of offset of a drug from a receptor once bound should be related temporally by a distinctly defined relationship. However, if the binding of one drug molecule is affected by the previous binding of another, then these equivalences may not hold, and deviations from these predicted temporal relationships may be observed. Thus, if drugs bind in a positively cooperative manner, the rate of receptor occupancy should increase with time since the binding of drug will increasingly promote the binding of further drug molecules. Similarly, if binding is negatively cooperative, then the rate of offset of drug occupancy may differ with the experimental technique utilized to measure offset kinetics. Specifically, there are two practical radioligand binding methods to measure the rate of offset of a drug from a receptor. The first is to achieve a given equilibrium between a radioligand and a receptor and then to increase the volume of the reaction infinitely and measure the quantity of receptor-bound species with time. The second is to keep the volume of the reaction constant and add an essentially infinite concentration of nonradioactive ligand (which then will displace the radioactive counterpart ligand) and observe the kinetics of receptor occupancy. If the binding of one drug molecule affects the binding of another, then the rates of receptor offset by these two methods should differ because, in the first case, offset kinetics occur in the absence of ligand available for rebinding, whereas in the latter case, abundant ligand is available to elicit allotopic secondary binding behavior. For example, a large increase in the dissociation rate of receptor-bound insulin can be shown when the dissociation experiment is carried out in the presence of nonradioactive insulin (Fig.

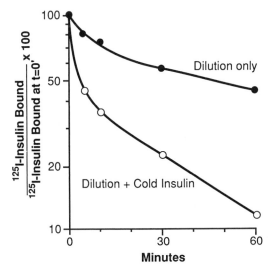

**FIG. 10.6.** Dissociation of [$^{125}$I]insulin receptor complex (50 pM) with time measured by "infinite" dilution and by dilution plus unlabeled insulin (0.17 μM) in IM-9 lymphocytes. Dissociation is considerably faster in the presence of excess insulin. (From ref. 6.)

10.6). These data have been interpreted as evidence for negative binding cooperativity by insulin for its receptor. In general, before dissociation kinetic data can be considered evidence for cooperative binding, the collisional limit of the system must be taken into account. The reader is referred to the section on collisional limits in Chapter 13 for further details.

## QUANTIFICATION OF ALLOSTERIC EFFECTS

A formal mathematical model of allotopic interactions between ligands on a receptor has been presented by Ehlert (7). Thus the binding of a ligand [A] and allosteric effector [B] to a receptor [R] can be thought of as:

$$[B] + [R] + [A] \overset{K_B}{\rightleftharpoons} [B{\cdot}R] + [A]$$

$$K_A \updownarrow \qquad \updownarrow \alpha K_A$$

$$[B] + [R{\cdot}A] \underset{\alpha K_B}{\rightleftharpoons} [B{\cdot}R{\cdot}A]$$

This defines a set of dissociation constants:

$$K_B = \frac{[B][R]}{[B{\cdot}R]} \qquad\qquad [10.1]$$

$$K_A = \frac{[R][A]}{[R{\cdot}A]} \qquad\qquad [10.2]$$

$$\alpha K_B = \frac{[B{\cdot}R][A]}{[B{\cdot}R{\cdot}A]} \qquad\qquad [10.3]$$

The total receptor occupancy by [A] is given by:

$$\rho_A = \frac{[A \cdot R] + [A \cdot R \cdot B]}{[R_t]} \qquad [10.4]$$

The conservation equation for $[R_t]$ is:

$$[R_t] = [R] + [B \cdot R] + [R \cdot A] + [B \cdot R \cdot A] \qquad [10.5]$$

where $[R_t]$ refers to the total concentration of receptors. Substitution and rearrangement yield the receptor occupancy for drug [A]:

$$\rho_A = \frac{[A] \cdot [R_t]}{[A] + K'_A} \qquad [10.6]$$

where $K'_A$ is a modified equilibrium dissociation constant for binding in the presence of the allosteric effector [B]. The extent of modification of $K_A$ by the effector is determined by the concentration of [B] and the equilibrium dissociation constant of the effector-receptor complex ($K_B$). Under these circumstances $K'_A$ is related to $K_A$ by:

$$K'_A = K_A \frac{K_B + [B]}{K_B + [B]/\alpha} \qquad [10.7]$$

where $\alpha$ is a cooperativity factor. As can be seen from Eq. 10.7, at maximal allosteric effector binding ($[B] \to \infty$), $K'_A/K_A \to \alpha$. If $\alpha > 1$, then the cooperativity is negative (i.e., the presence of the allosteric effector [B] increases the equilibrium dissociation constant for [A] and decreases affinity). Figure 10.7A shows binding curves for a ligand [A] in the absence and presence of an allosteric effector [B] with a cooperativity factor $\alpha = 10$. As can be seen from this figure, the allosteric effector produces dextral displacement of the curve similar to competitive antagonism, but, unlike the latter, a maximal shift is obtained (i.e., the value of $\alpha$, in this case a 10-fold shift).

If $\alpha < 1$, then the binding is positively cooperative (i.e., $K'_A < K_A$, the affinity of [A] is increased). Figure 10.7B shows the effect of a positively cooperative allosteric effect ($\alpha = 0.1$). As with Fig. 10.7A, the curves are parallel but shifted to the left up to a maximal shift ($\alpha = 0.1$ corresponds to a 10-fold shift to the left). The change in the binding constant $K_A$ can be visualized with a graphic representation of Eq. 10.7. In Fig. 10.7C, the changes in $K_A$ produced by both allosteric effectors ($\alpha = 10$ and 0.1) as a function [B] are shown.

It is considerably more straightforward to interpret allotopic phenomena in binding studies than it is with functional data because of the intervention of stimulus-response mechanisms and the assumptions necessary to nullify their effect. If it is known that the allosteric effector affects *only* agonist affinity and not efficacy, then the model described previously may be applied to functional data. However, if this is not known, then it cannot be assumed that the allosterically modified receptor interacts with the stimulus-response

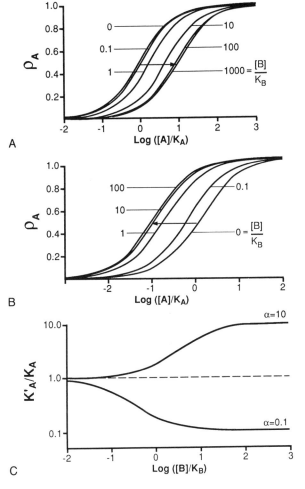

**FIG. 10.7.** The effects of allosteric effectors on the binding of a drug [A] to receptors. **A:** Negative cooperativity. Binding isotherms for [A] in the absence ($[B]/K_B = 0$) and presence of an allosteric effector with a cooperativity factor $\alpha = 10$. Note that the curves are parallel and the degree of dextral displacement of the isotherm has a limit. **B:** Positive cooperativity. Binding isotherms to [A] in the absence and presence of an allosteric effector with a cooperativity factor $\alpha = 0.1$. **C:** Dependence of the observed affinity of [A] (denoted $K'_A$ and shown as a ratio of the observed affinity and the affinity of [A] in the absence of allosteric effector) on the concentration of allosteric effector (both log scales). Ratios calculated from Eq. 10.7.

mechanisms of the cell in a fashion identical to the unmodified agonist-occupied receptor. If the efficacy of the agonist-receptor complex is modified, then the use of the above model requires that tissue stimulus *and* tissue responses be additive. This is rarely known for tissue systems, making interpretation of apparently allotopic interactions in functional tissues difficult.

## NONCOMPETITIVE ANTAGONISM

Another type of blockade of agonist response is interaction of an antagonist with a binding site intimately associated with the receptor, but distinct from the site for agonist binding. It is assumed that binding of the antagonist to this site precludes activation of the receptor by the agonist. Thus, the equilibrium between the agonist and remaining receptors is given by

$$[A] + \underset{(1-y-\rho_B)}{[R]} \underset{k_2}{\overset{k_1}{\rightleftharpoons}} \underset{y}{[A{\cdot}R]} \tag{10.8}$$

where $y$ and $\rho_B$ are the fractions of receptors bound by agonist and antagonist, respectively. The preclusion of agonist binding to receptors previously bound by antagonist is expressed by the fact that free agonist $[A]$ may bind to only a fraction $(1 - y - \rho_B)$ of the receptors. At equilibrium,

$$[A]{\cdot}(1 - y - \rho_B){\cdot}k_1 = k_2{\cdot}y \tag{10.9}$$

which rearranges to

$$y = \frac{[A{\cdot}R]}{[R_t]} = \frac{[A]}{[A] + K_A}(1 - \rho_B) \tag{10.10}$$

Calculating $\rho_B$ by the mass-action law, the equation for receptor occupancy by an agonist is

$$\frac{[A{\cdot}R]}{[R_t]} = \frac{[A]}{[A] + K_A} \cdot \frac{1}{1 + [B]/K_B} \tag{10.11}$$

As shown in Fig. 10.8A, removal of receptors for agonist activation by noncompetitive antagonism produces a progressive decline in agonist fractional receptor occupancy. Unlike competitive antagonism, in which excess concentrations of agonist allow maximal receptor occupancy by the agonist even in the presence of an antagonist, noncompetitive antagonism produces depression of maximal receptor occupancy by the agonist. However, the resulting effects on agonist responses may differ considerably because of the effects of stimulus-response coupling in tissues. For example, Fig. 10.8B shows the effects of noncompetitive antagonism of an agonist for which there is a large receptor reserve (stimulus-response curve shown in inset to Fig. 10.8B). In this tissue, 50% of the maximal response is produced by occupation of 1% of the receptors by the agonist, and 99% response by occupation of 1% of the receptors by the agonist, and 99% response by occupation of 10% of the receptors. Therefore, a noncompetitive antagonist at a concentration that will reduce agonist-receptor occupancy by 50% will not produce depression of the maximal response. Instead, a shift to the right in the agonist dose-response curve, much like what would be observed with a competitive antagonist, is observed. Because of the influence of tissue factors such as receptor number and efficiency of receptor coupling on the observed effects of noncompetitive antagonists, predictions from receptor theory concerning these agents are less useful. However, an equation for estimation of equilibrium dissociation constants for noncompetitive antagonist-receptor complexes can be derived in the same manner as equations describing irreversible antagonism for measurement of agonist $K_A$ (see Chapter 7). The fractional

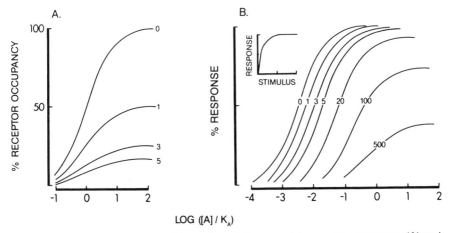

**FIG. 10.8.** Effects of a noncompetitive antagonist on agonist-receptor occupancy **(A)** and tissue response **(B)**, assuming a hyperbolic relationship between receptor stimuli and tissue responses (*inset*). Responses for B calculated for agonist with $\epsilon = 3.0$, $[R_t] = 1$, response = (stimulus)/(stimulus + 0.01). Numbers next to curves refer to values of $[B]/K_B$.

receptor occupancy by agonist $[A]$ in the presence of antagonist $[B]$ is given by Eq. 10.11. An equal receptor occupancy in the absence of antagonist ($\rho_B = 0$) is given by Eq. 9.7.

Assuming that equal fractional receptor occupancies lead to equal responses, equiactive concentrations of agonist can be related by equating Eqs. 9.7 and 10.11 to

$$\frac{[A]}{[A] + K_A} = \frac{[A']}{[A'] + K_A}(1 - \rho_B) \qquad [10.12]$$

where $[A']$ denotes the equiactive concentrations of agonist in the presence of antagonist. This rearranges to

$$\frac{1}{[A]} = \frac{1}{[A']} \cdot \frac{1}{1 - \rho_B} + \frac{\rho_B}{(1 - \rho_B) \cdot K_A} \qquad [10.13]$$

The equilibrium dissociation constant for the antagonist-receptor complex ($K_B$) can be derived from the mass-action law:

$$\rho_B = \frac{[B]}{[B] + K_B} \qquad [10.14]$$

A regression of $1/[A]$ versus $1/[A']$ yields a straight line of slope $(1 - \rho_B)^{-1}$ and intercept $\rho_B/(1 - \rho_B)K_A$. Therefore, relating $\rho_B$ to $K_B$ by Eq. 10.14, the $K_B$ for a noncompetitive antagonist can be derived as

$$K_B = \frac{[B]}{\text{slope} - 1} \qquad [10.15]$$

In practice, dose-response curves for the agonist are obtained in the absence and presence of noncompetitive antagonist, and the $K_B$ calculated with Eq. 10.15 is obtained from a regression of equiactive concentrations of agonist 1/[A] versus 1/[A'].

In accordance with the caveats raised regarding double-reciprocal regressions in Chapter 7, Eq. 10.13 can be rewritten

$$\frac{[A']}{[A]} = [A'] \cdot \frac{\rho_B}{(1 - \rho_B) \cdot K_A} + \frac{1}{1 - \rho_B} \qquad [10.16]$$

where

$$K_B = \frac{[B]}{\text{intercept} - 1} \qquad [10.17]$$

and also by

$$[A] = \frac{(1 - \rho_B)K_A}{\rho_B} - \frac{[A]}{[A']} \cdot \frac{K_A}{\rho_B} \qquad [10.18]$$

where

$$K_B = \frac{[B]}{(\text{slope/intercept}) - 1} \qquad [10.19]$$

In general, more accurate estimates of $K_B$ for noncompetitive antagonists are derived from experiments in which the maximal response to the agonist is depressed to less than 50% of the maximal response by the noncompetitive antagonist.

## IRREVERSIBLE ANTAGONISM

Antagonism that cannot be reversed by washing the tissue with a drug-free solution often is considered irreversible. Such an effect is seen with antagonists that form a chemical alkyl bond with the receptor; for example, β-haloalkylamines form a reactive species in solution (aziridinium ion) that alkylates protein readily. Irreversible antagonism is time-dependent; i.e., the longer the antagonist is in contact with the tissue, the greater the magnitude of the observed antagonism. Figure 10.9 shows the effects of successive 10-min exposures of guinea pig ileum to the alkylating drug dibenamine (1 nM) on histamine responses. Irreversible antagonists produce antagonism in much the same manner as noncompetitive antagonists, that is, preclusion of agonist activation of the receptor. However, an estimate of $K_B$ cannot be made with Eq. 10.13, because, unlike a reversible noncompetitive antagonist, an irreversible antagonist does not come to thermodynamic equilibrium during the course of a normal pharmacologic experiment.

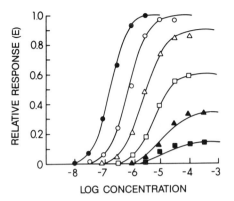

**FIG. 10.9.** Effects of equilibration time on magnitude of antagonism by an irreversible antagonist. Ordinate: Responses of guinea pig ileum to histamine as fractions of the maximal control response (absence of blockade) to histamine. Abscissa: Logarithms of molar concentrations of histamine. Responses before (•) and after five successive exposures of 10 min each to the histamine-receptor alkylating drug dibenamine (1 nM). Cumulative exposure times to antagonist are 10 (o), 20 (△), 30 (□), 40 (▲), and 50 min (■). (Data from ref. 1; graph redrawn from ref. 10.)

Because the rate constant for dissociation of an alkylating drug is insignificant compared with the rate constant for association, the degree of alkylation is time dependent. Therefore, all estimates of antagonist potencies must take account of the time of equilibration. It is difficult to quantify the potencies of irreversible antagonists because of this temporal dependence, which in turn is related to rate of diffusion into the tissue and the reactivity of the alkylating species. Estimates of potencies tend to be tissue, not receptor, dependent; for example, one quantitative scale uses the molar concentration of antagonist that reduces the maximal response to an agonist by 50% (denoted $pD_2'$). The limitations of this scale with respect to equilibration time and receptor reserve of the agonist are evident.

Irreversible alkylating agents such as β-haloalkylamines have been widely used as "chemical scalpels" to modify receptor density in tissues. Under strict conditions, β-haloalkylamines can be selective receptor inactivators, but care must be taken to scavenge the lipid-soluble, un-ionized parent drug with thiosulfate ion to remove residual leaching of drug from the tissue and subsequent further alkylation (2,20). For example, the long half-time of reversal from receptor alkylation by the β-haloalkylamine SY-14 (1,150 min$^{-1}$) is increased 5.75-fold by the presence of $10^{-4}$ M thiosulfate ion (200 min$^{-1}$, 16). In general, an intramolecule-assisted ester hydrolysis can account for the offset kinetics of alkylated β-haloalkylamine. However, if there is a pool of un-ionized β-haloalkylamine present in the tissue that functions as a depot for subsequent formation of aziridinium ion and further alkylation, then part of the receptor population will be competitively blocked by the aziridinium-ion complex, and a true condition of irreversible protein alteration will not exist. Instead, a complex condition will exist whereby part of the receptor population will be occupied by a reversible antagonist and part irreversibly alkylated. For example, Fig. 10.10 schematically shows an experimental system with two possible protocols. In both, a tissue has been exposed to a concentration of un-ionized phenoxybenzamine (POB) for a given time. This

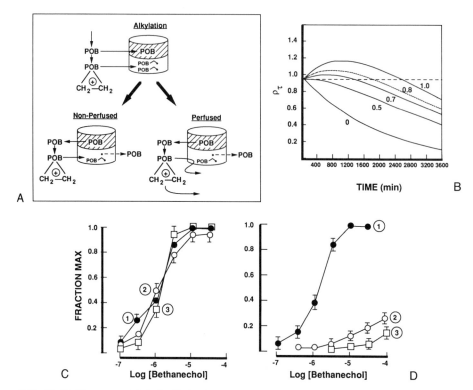

**FIG. 10.10.** The use of β-haloalkylamines as receptor alkylating agents. **A:** Schematic drawing of a tissue incubated with un-ionized POB. The drug diffuses into the tissue as the un-ionized species (*hatched area*) and also forms an aziridinium ion that binds reversibly to the receptor and subsequently forms an alkyl bond. In a closed system in which the medium is not constantly perfused or one in which there is not an excess of scavenging species (i.e., thiosulfate ion) for the aziridinium ion, the un-ionized POB may diffuse out of the tissue, form the aziridinium ion, and alkylate more receptors. This may occur concomitantly with an intramolecular hydrolysis of the alkylated species. In a perfused system (or one with an excess thiosulfate ion), the un-ionized POB is removed from the receptor compartment before it can alkylate the receptor. Under these circumstances, the intramolecular hydrolysis of the alkyl bond controls the rate of receptor regeneration. **B:** The receptor occupancy with time of a concentration of alkylating species that produces an initial receptor alkylation of 95%. Ordinate: Fractional receptor occupancy at time $t$. Abscissa: Time in minutes. Occupancies calculated with Eq. 10.20 assuming an offset rate constant of 0.0005 min$^{-1}$ and varying rates of diffusion from a tissue pool (numbers next to the curves in mmol/L$^{-1}$ min$^{-1}$). Receptor offset is considerably slower with a sizable diffusion from a tissue pool. **C:** Dose-response curves to bethanechol in guinea pig ileum longitudinal muscle strips (isotonic contraction). Ordinate: Shortening as a fraction of maximal shortening to bethanechol. Abscissa: Logarithms of molar concentrations of bethanechol. Repeat dose-response curves at time $t = 0$ (curve 1), 1 hr (curve 2), and a further 1 hr (curve 3). **D:** Dose-response curves as in C after receptor alkylation with POB. Curve 1 is the control, curve 2 after an exposure to POB (1 μmol/L for 5 min and 30-min washing with 100 μmol/L sodium thiosulfate and 30 min with drug-free solution) and curve 3 after a further 60-min washing with no thiosulfate ion present in the medium. After the 1-hr washing period without thiosulfate, there is an *increase* in the receptor blockade. (Data for C and D from Corsi and Kenakin, *unpublished*.)

leads to the irreversible alkylation of a portion of the receptor population and the formation of a pool of un-ionized POB in the preparation. In one tissue (Fig. 10.10A labeled perfused), constant removal of the un-ionized POB by perfusion or chemical scavenging of the newly formed aziridinium ion from this pool prevents this subsequent POB-receptor interaction from taking place. In the other scenario (Fig. 10.10A on the right), the tissue pool leaches out POB, which then reequilibrates with the medium in the receptor compartment and goes on to form active aziridinium ion. A simple model of the kinetics of receptor occupation, under these conditions, can be made where a zero-order receptor onset from the depot is concomitant with a first-order rate of receptor offset. The receptor occupancy is given by:

$$\rho_t = e^{-kt} \left( \frac{(\rho_0 (1 + D/K_B) + D/K_B)}{D/K_B(1 + e^{-kt}) + 1} \right) \qquad [10.20]$$

where $\rho_0$ denotes occupancy at time zero, $K_B$ equals the antagonist binding constant, $D$ represents the rate constant for release from the tissue depot, $k$ is the offset rate constant from the receptor and $\rho_t$ is the receptor occupancy at time $t$. Assuming specific rate constants, various temporal receptor occupancies can be calculated; some of those are shown in Fig. 10.10B. The numbers next to the calculated curves refer to the rate of diffusion of the un-ionized species from the tissue pool (magnitude of D in mmoles $L^{-1}$ $min^{-1}$). The receptor occupancy by the antagonist can actually *increase* over time if there is a sizable pool of un-ionized drug to leach out of the tissue (i.e., Fig. 10.10B for 0.001 mmoles $L^{-1}$ $min^{-1}$). This can be demonstrated experimentally in guinea pig ileum longitudinal muscle strips. Figure 10.10C shows that repeated dose-response curves to bethanechol can be obtained with minimal, if any, loss of responsiveness in this tissue. Partial alkylation of the receptor population with POB depresses the dose-response curve to bethanechol (Fig. 10.10D). After exposure to this alkylating agent, the unreacted aziridinium ion was scavenged by thiosulfate. However, after a further 1-hr washing without thiosulfate, the responses to bethanechol were *further* depressed, indicating a significant leaching out of POB from the tissue to produce further receptor alkylation. As a general precaution experiments with β-haloalkylamines require extraordinary care to ensure that a single population of alkylated receptor is left after treatment.

Another potential use for irreversible antagonists is for the detection and mapping of receptor types in tissues. To this end, antibodies to specific receptors have been raised in rabbits and subsequently used to displace radioligands. This technique has the advantage that exquisite specificity can be achieved. For example, fusion of the DNA fragment encoding a specific loop of the rat muscarinic m2 receptor to the gene for staphylococcal protein A yields a protein antigen capable of raising a polyclonal antibody to m2 receptors in rabbits. These antibodies can then be shown to displace [³H]quinuclidinyl benzilate (QNB) previously bound to a pure population of m2 receptors expressed in Chinese hamster ovary cells. Figure 10.11A shows the displacement with various lots of the antibody removed from rabbits at varying times. As can be seen from these data, immunoreactivity can be observed after the fifth bleed (bleeds taken every 2 weeks after a booster injection of antigen) and thereafter displaced QNB and by the seventh bleed, near 100% displacement was achieved. The antibody was shown to be extremely specific for the m2, as opposed to the four other gene products expressed muscarinic receptor subtypes (Fig. 10.11B). Treatment of rat heart and seven regions of rat brain with the receptor antibody revealed the relative density of m2 receptors shown in Fig. 10.11C. As can be seen from these data, rat heart contains nearly an exclusive population of m2 receptors, whereas the brain regions contain m2 receptors mixed with other subtypes

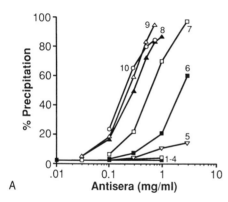

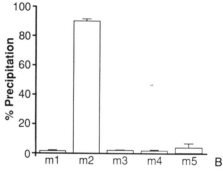

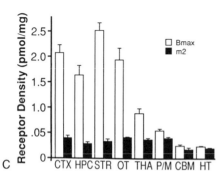

**FIG. 10.11.** Effects of an antibody for muscarinic m2 receptors. **A:** Titer curves of m2 antisera obtained from rabbits bled every 2 weeks after a booster injection. It can be seen that immunoprecipitation of muscarinic m2 receptors (expressed in CHO cells) is obtained by 10 weeks (fifth bleed) and maximal receptor immunoprecipitation occurs by the seventh bleed. **B:** Specificity of the m2 antisera. Immunoprecipitation is obtained only in membranes from CHO cells expressing m2 receptors and not in membranes containing m1, m3, m4, and m5 receptors. **C:** Distribution and density of m2 receptors in rat heart and brain. Relative density of m2 receptors and maximal binding of [3H]NMS (all muscarinic receptor subtypes) in cortex (CTX), hippocampus (HPC), striatum (STR), olfactory tubercle (OT), thalamus/hypothalamus (THA), pons/medulla (P/M), cerebellum (CBM), and heart (HT). Note how the muscarinic receptors in the heart are almost exclusively of the m2 subtype. (From ref. 15.)

(as measured by residual binding of QNB). This approach can be extremely useful in the study of receptor types and distributions.

There is a fine line between true irreversibility and essentially irreversible kinetics. Antagonists need not necessarily alkylate the receptor in order to bind tightly and dissociate slowly from the receptor. Within the time scale of agonist-receptor interaction, the antagonist binding could appear to be irreversible. Under these circumstances, the fractional receptor occupancy for the agonist could be important. An example of such pseudo irreversible antagonism is provided by scopolamine, a competitive but slowly reversible antagonist. In guinea pig ileum, scopolamine produces simple competitive antagonism of responses to the full agonist methylfurmethide. However, scopolamine produces a shift to the right and a depression of the maximal response to the partial agonist octyltrimethylammonium ($C_8$-TMA) (Fig. 10.12). This occurs because a "hemiequilibrium" state is attained between the receptors and $C_8$-TMA whereby this agonist, in the presence of scopolamine, can equilibrate with only a portion of the receptor population. The slow dissociation rate constant for scopolamine causes it to behave as an essentially irreversible antagonist of a fraction of the total receptor population. Because $C_8$-TMA is a partial agonist requiring 100% receptor activation to produce a maximal response, this hemiequilibrium state produces a depression of the maximal response. The equilibrium dissociation constant for the scopolamine-receptor complex still can be estimated by Eq. 10.13, 10.16, or 10.18; $K_B$ values for scopolamine were found to be 0.25 nM for antagonism of the full agonist (Schild analysis) and 0.24 nM and 0.21 nM for antagonism of $C_8$-TMA (Eq. 10.11).

The difference between pseudo irreversible blockade and true irreversible blockade is that the former can come to true equilibrium within the time constraints of a normal pharmacologic experiment, whereas the latter does not. Although the dissociation rate constant is low, the antagonist does disso-

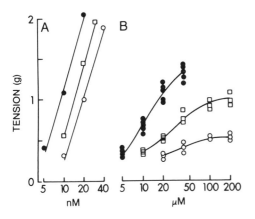

**FIG. 10.12.** Antagonism by scopolamine of guinea pig ileal responses to methylfurmethide **(A)** and $C_8$-TMA **(B)**. Ordinate: Grams of isometric tension. Abscissa: Nanomolar and micromolar concentrations of methylfurmethide and $C_8$-TMA, respectively (logarithmic scale). Responses in the absence (•) and presence of scopolamine at 0.16 nM (□) and 0.3 nM (○). Data points for methylfurmethide are means of six responses. (From ref. 21.)

ciate from the receptor, thereby allowing the drug to occupy a fraction of the receptor population according to the $K_B$. Because of this, Eq. 10.13 (and also 10.16 and 10.18) can be applied to pseudo irreversible blockade to estimate $K_B$ for such antagonists. Further discussion of hemiequilibrium states can be found in Chapter 13.

## REFERENCES

1. Ackers, G. K., Doyle, M. L., Myers, D., and Daugherty, M. A. (1992): Molecular code for cooperativity in hemoglobin. *Science*, 255:54–63.
2. Belleau, B. (1958): The mechanism of drug action at receptor surfaces. Part I. A general interpretation of the adrenergic blocking activity of β-haloalkylamines. *Can. J. Physiol. Pharmacol.*, 36:731–753.
3. Black, J. W., Jenkinson, D. H., and Kenakin, T. P. (1980): Antagonism of an indirectly acting agonist: Block by propranolol and sotalol of the action of tyramine on the heart. *Eur. J. Pharmacol.*, 65:1–10.
4. Clark, A. J. (1937): *General Pharmacology: Heffner's Handbook of Experimental Pharmacology, Erg-band 4.* Springer, Berlin.
5. Clark, A. L., and Mitchelson, F. (1976): The inhibitory effect of gallamine on muscarinic receptors. *Br. J. Pharmacol.*, 58:323–331.
6. De Meyts, P., Bianco, A. R., and Roth, J. (1976): Site-site interactions among insulin receptors. *J. Biol. Chem.*, 251:1877–1888.
7. Ehlert, F. J. (1988): Estimation of the affinities of allosteric ligands using radioligand binding and pharmacological null methods. *Mol. Pharmacol.*, 33:187–194.
8. Ehrlich, P. (1909): *Ber. Dtsch. Chem. Ges.*, 42:17–47.
9. Fraser, C. M., Chung, F-Z., Wand, C-D., and Venter, J. C. (1988): *Proc. Natl. Acad. Sci. U.S.A.*, 85:5478–5482.
10. Furchgott, R. F. (1966): The use of β-haloalkylamines in the differentiation of receptors and in the determination of dissociation constants of receptor-agonist complexes. In: *Advances in Drug Research*, edited by N. J. Harper and A. B. Simmonds, pp. 21–55. Academic Press, New York.
11. Furchgott, R. F. (1972): The classification of adrenoceptors (adrenergic receptors). An evaluation from the standpoint of receptor theory. In: *Handbook of Experimental Pharmacology, Catecholamines, Vol. 33*, edited by H. Blaschko and E. Muscholl, pp. 283–335, Springer-Verlag, Berlin.
12. Gaddum, J. H. (1957): Theories of drug antagonism. *Pharmacol. Rev.*, 9:211–218.
13. Gaddum, J. H., Hameed, K. A., Hathaway, D. E., and Stephens, F. F. (1955): Quantitative studies of antagonists of 5-hydroxytryptamine. *Q. J. Exp. Physiol.*, 40:49–74.
14. Lee, N. H., Hu, J., and El-Fakahany, E. E. (1992): Modulation by certain conserved aspartate residues of the allosteric interaction of gallamine and the m1 muscarinic receptor. *J. Pharmacol. Exp. Ther.*, 262:312–316.
15. Li, M., Yasuda, R. P., Wall, S. J., Wellstein, A., and Wolfe, B. B. (1991): Distribution of m2 muscarinic receptors in rat brain using antisera selective for m2 receptors. *Mol. Pharmacol.*, 40:28–35.
16. Kenakin, T. P., and Cook, D. A. (1976): Blockade of histamine-induced contractions of intestinal smooth muscle by irreversibly acting agents. *Can. J. Physiol. Pharmacol.*, 54:386–392.
17. Kenakin, T. P. (1990): Drugs and receptors: An overview of the current state of knowledge. *Drugs*, 40:666–687.
18. Koshland, D. E. (1960): The active site of enzyme action. *Adv. Enzymol.*, 22:45–97.
19. Monod, J., Wyman, J., and Changeux, J. P. (1965): On the nature of allosteric transitions. *J. Biol. Chem.*, 12:88–118.
20. Nickerson, M., and Gump, W. (1949): The chemical basis for adrenergic blocking activity in compounds related to dibenamine. *J. Pharmacol.*, 97:25–47.
21. Rang, H. P. (1966): The kinetics of action of acetylcholine antagonists in smooth muscle. *Proc. R. Soc. Lond. [Biol.]*, 164:488–510.

22. Rocha e Silva, M. (1969): A thermodynamic approach to problems of drug antagonism. I. Charniere theory. *Eur. J. Pharmacol.*, 6:294–302.
23. Stockton, J. M., Birdsall, N. J. M., Burgen, A. S. V., and Hulme, E. C. (1983): Modification of the binding properties of muscarinic receptors by gallamine. *Mol. Pharmacol.*, 23: 551–557.
24. Strader, C. D., Sigal, I. S., Register, R. B., Candelore, M. R., Rands, E., and Dixon, R. A. F. (1987): Identification of residues required for ligand binding to the β-adrenergic receptor. *Proc. Natl. Acad. Sci. U.S.A.*, 84:4384–4388.
25. Tucek, S., Musilkova, J., Nedoma, J., Proska, J., Shelkovnikov, S., and Vorlicek, J. (1990): Positive cooperativity in the binding of alcuronium and N-methylscopolamine to muscarinic acetylcholine receptors. *Mol. Pharmacol.*, 38:674–680.

# 11

# Methods of Drug and Receptor Classification

*"Mr. Holmes, how did you know it was there? Because I knew it was nowhere else."*—Sherlock Holmes, *The Adventure of the Second Stain*
— Sir Arthur Conan Doyle, 1886

*To consider that certain observations do not disprove a hypothesis does not amount to proof of a hypothesis; a statement that is readily apparent but frequently forgotten.*
—D. J. Finney, 1955

To a large extent, this chapter is concerned with differences between drugs and between drug receptors. Whereas Chapter 6 considers the statistical methods available to ascertain whether data sets are different, this chapter discusses the possible meaning of such differences in pharmacologic and physiological terms.

## POSSIBLE PHARMACOLOGIC SIGNIFICANCE OF DIFFERENCES

The primary tool in the process of drug and drug-receptor classification is the null hypothesis. This states that any observed difference arises strictly by chance; that is, there is no difference. Therefore, with no *a priori* reason to suppose that one hypothesis is more likely to be true than another, then, as the mathematician Laplace put it, an "equipartition of ignorance" should be made. Experimental data are then generated, in, it is hoped, an unbiased manner, and analyzed quantitatively to assess possible differences. From this, a probability ($p$) is generated that the observed difference, if any, would have been observed by chance. More correctly, $p$ is the probability that the observations would have been made if the null hypothesis were true. If, for example, there were no difference (when $p$ is small), then there are three possibilities: (i) an unlikely event has taken place, and the null hypothesis, although true, appears not to be true on the basis of the data (i.e., if $p <$ 0.01, then the experimenter happened upon that 1-in-100 instance that the observations belie a condition of no difference); (ii) the assumptions on which the test was based were faulty (i.e., biased sampling); or (iii) the null hypothesis is not true, and the true population means predicted by the two rival hypotheses being tested are different. For example, suppose the potency of the histamine H-1 receptor antagonist diphenhydramine is measured as a blocker of histamine responses in a given tissue to identify the receptors in that tissue. Previous data have classified diphenhydramine as a competitive antagonist of H-1 histamine receptors, with a $pK_B$ of 8.2 ($K_B = 6.3$ nM). This experiment then will test between two rival hypotheses: the histamine receptors are or are not of the H-1 type. These rival hypotheses generate two populations of data, the first being a set of $pK_B$ values of mean 8.2 (i.e., the experiment will sample from the same population), and the second being a set with a mean different from 8.2. The object of the experiment is to produce an adequate sampling to predict the true population mean and thus distinguish between the two hypotheses. The null hypothesis states that there is no difference between the means (the receptors in the tissue are of the H-1 type) and that the experimental data should yield a mean value of 8.2 (with confidence limits). Let us assume two alternative outcomes to this experiment: The first is that from a sampling of $N = 8$ the experimentally derived $pK_B$ is 7.4 ± 0.1 (mean ± SEM). The population value for true histamine H-1 receptors of 8.2 lies outside the 95% confidence limits of this sample mean (8.2–6.69). Therefore, according to the foregoing possibilities, the following could be true: (a) The random event (5-in-100 chance) occurred that the 7.4 estimate came from a population of mean 8.2 (i.e., the receptors in the tissue truly were H-1 receptors). In this case, a true null hypothesis (the receptors are H-1 receptors) was wrongly rejected; this is called an error of the first kind (type-1 error). (b) The sampling was improper and gave a biased value [i.e., 7.4 was an incorrect representation of the population mean, and indeed the tissue truly does have H-1 receptors, but our experiment was of insufficient quality to detect this (again a type-1 error). (c) The histamine receptors on the tissue are not of the H-1 type.

The alternative outcome could be that the sample mean for $pK_B$ is 7.9 ±0.2 ($N = 8$, confidence limits 8.3–7.43). Because 8.2 is within the 95% confidence limits of our sample mean, at the $p < 0.05$ level this would constitute no evidence to disprove the null hypothesis. If methodological or statistical factors have caused the sample mean of 7.9 to be an incorrect estimate of the population mean (either by chance or because of bad experimental design), then the null hypothesis would have been wrongly accepted; this is called an error of the second kind (type-2 error).

The outcome that no evidence has been generated to reject the null hypothesis raises a subtle point in pharmacologic and physiological research. In the

**TABLE 11.1.** $pK_B$ *Estimates for beta blockers*

| | Tissue | |
| --- | --- | --- |
| Drug | Guinea pig left atria ($\beta_1$) | Rat uterus ($\beta_2$) |
| Propranolol | 8.4 | 8.5 |
| Atenolol | 7.2 | 5.5 |
| | (7.4–6.8) | (5.0–6.0) |

example with histamine receptors, the erroneous assumption is that inability to disprove the null hypothesis means that the two receptors therefore are the same. With deference to the clear success of the fictional detective Sherlock Holmes, his reasoning in the quotation at the beginning of this chapter illustrates a flaw; i.e., "it" could have been somewhere where he did not look. As put by Finney (8), disproving the null hypothesis only furnishes evidence that our experiment was inadequate to detect a difference. The receptors may *not* be the same, but diphenhydramine is not capable of distinguishing them. For example, propranolol has a mean $pK_B$ for $\beta_1$-adrenoceptors and $\beta_2$-adrenoceptors of 8.4. This estimate would be obtained in a $\beta_1$-adrenoceptor-containing tissue such as guinea pig atrium and a $\beta_2$-adrenoceptor-containing tissue such as rat uterus (Table 11.1). Analysis of the $\beta$-adrenoceptors of these tissues therefore would imply only that propranolol could not distinguish the receptor types, not that the receptors were the same (which they are not). On the other hand, atenolol, which is $\beta_1$ selective, can distinguish these receptors (Table 11.1), illustrating the fallacy of interpreting the results with propranolol to mean that the receptors are the same.

## METHODS OF DRUG AND DRUG-RECEPTOR CLASSIFICATION

By classifying drugs and receptors, the properties of each can be quantified and ordered into a form suitable for prediction. Lack of classification can lead to chaos. For example, pilocarpine produces specific contractions of guinea pig ileum, and thus, strictly speaking, this tissue can be thought to have a "pilocarpine receptor." From similar data, the ileum can contain "acetylcholine receptors," "methacholine receptors," "carbachol receptors," and so on, for every foreign chemical that produces organ responses. These data are much less useful in this form than when they are organized, by methods of pharmacologic classification, into a more general order. In this case, the common $pK_B$ for atropine as an antagonist of all of these agonists allows a tentative grouping of the agonists as *cholinomimetics* stimulating *cholinergic receptors*. Of course, this does not mean that there are not subtypes of receptors within this classification, but until such time as evidence for subclassification can be generated, the group must be considered homogeneous. This process obviously is circular in that new receptor subtypes are classified with new drugs, and vice versa; there are two sets of unknown populations, those for drugs and those for the receptors with which they interact. Considering the rather limited number of chemicals with which cells have to deal routinely in the body, it can be assumed that the population of true receptors linked to stimulus-response mechanisms is much smaller than the number of possible chemical structures of drugs. The term "receptor" in this sense should be differentiated from "*acceptor*," which is a membrane protein that binds drug but is not linked to a response mechanism; i.e., a specific binding site is not necessarily a receptor. If pharmacologic data for a particular unknown chemical compound cannot be fit into existing classifications, the pharmacologist has a choice to reclassify the drug or the system with which it interacts (receptor). It would seem that a reasonable first approach would be one of strict *receptor parsimony*, in that a new receptor subtype should not be invoked until absolutely necessary. In fact, an element of wishful thinking (especially in the drug industry) often is introduced into pharmacologic literature, and new drugs tend to spawn new receptors somewhat prematurely. The attraction of this point of view is the convenient situation whereby the human body happens to possess specific response-linked binding sites for one's particular drug, thereby providing built-in specificity. The reasoning, in terms of drug development, behind this approach, and an approach oriented more toward examination of the properties of the drug, is quite different, as will be discussed in Chapter 13.

In general, the methods of classification to be discussed in this chapter relate to the classification of drugs as well as drug receptors, but with the emphasis that the presumably more variable component in a pharmacologic system is the drug. Thus, the bias in these procedures is to define the properties of drugs within the framework of existing receptor classifications until such time as this simply cannot be done without postulating a change in the physiological system. Although this can be a useful bias in the approach to classification, clearly it must not be inviolate; such a point of view would presuppose the untenable position that all of the existing receptors in cell membranes already have been discovered.

A theoretical differentiation may be made between receptor classifications by agonists and by antagonists. Natural physiological agonists such as hormones, neurotransmitters, and autacoids are strikingly uniform throughout mammalian species; thus, one would expect that their recognition sites (receptors) would correspondingly be uniform as well. But, depending on what one calls the receptor, this may apply only to the agonist recognition site, not necessarily the tertiary superstructure of the protein surrounding this site; i.e., the membrane-linked or surrounding protein structure near the agonist-binding site theoretically could vary with membrane composition,

**TABLE 11.2.** *Some autonomic-receptor classifications by antagonist*

| Receptor type | Natural agonist | Subclassification | Antagonist |
|---|---|---|---|
| Histamine | Histamine | H-1 | Diphenhydramine |
| | | | Mepyramine |
| | | H-2 | Cimetidine |
| | | | Ranitidine |
| $\alpha$-Adrenergic | Norepinephrine | $\alpha_1$ | Prazosin |
| | | $\alpha_2$ | Yohimbine |
| $\beta$-Adrenergic | Norepinephrine | $\beta_1$ | Atenolol |
| | | $\beta_2$ | ICI 118,555 |

cell type, organ type, or species. There is evidence that antagonists, which usually are larger and more hydrophobic molecules than agonists, may utilize binding sites surrounding the agonist recognition site either to bind and obscure agonist recognition sites or to alter them by allosteric modification of the tertiary protein conformation. If these surrounding sites are more variable with respect to origin, then greater heterogeneity with respect to antagonist binding may be encountered than for agonist binding. Support for this idea is found in the fact that the most definitive evidence for receptor subclassification has been obtained with antagonists (Table 11.2). In this light, use of the term "receptor" can be ambiguous, depending on whether the recognition sites for agonists or antagonists are being considered; agonist interactions may be relatively uniform within a given class of membrane proteins, whereas those of antagonists could be quite different.

Receptors can be classified in numerous ways, for example, by location (presynaptic or postsynaptic), mechanism (stimulatory or inhibitory for a particular enzyme), chemical messenger (cyclic AMP or cyclic GMP). This chapter focuses on classification by pharmacologic criteria, namely, classification on the basis of the quantitative properties that link drugs and receptors. Quantitative classification of drugs and drug receptors is carried out with null procedures, which, it is hoped, generate information specific to the drug-receptor interaction (i.e., the first transmission of the message between the drug and the cell). The basic approaches to this will be discussed separately.

### Agonist Potency Ratios

Historically, the relative potencies of agonists have provided a useful method for receptor classification. This method depends on the assumption that the relative equiactive concentrations of two or more agonists reflect only drug-receptor-related properties: the null method of employing equiactive doses allows cancellation of stimulus-response coupling processes. Therefore, for any one agonist recognition site, a series of agonists should always have the same relative potencies. The theoretical basis for this method lies in the dependence of agonist potency on the two drug-related parameters of affinity and intrinsic efficacy. If two agonists produce full tissue maximal responses in a tissue at concentrations well below the $K_A$ (i.e., there is a receptor reserve for the agonists), then $[A] \ll K_A$, and the equation for two such agonists reduces to

$$S_1 = \frac{\epsilon_1[A_1]}{K_{A1}} \quad \text{and} \quad S_2 = \frac{\epsilon_2[A_2]}{K_{A2}} \quad [11.1]$$

Assuming that equal responses result from equal stimuli, $S_1 = S_2$, and the potency ratio pr $= [A_2]/[A_1]$ becomes

$$R = \frac{[A_2]}{[A_1]} = \frac{\epsilon_1 \cdot K_{A1}}{\epsilon_2 \cdot K_{A1}} \quad [11.2]$$

Similarly, in terms of the operational model (Chapter 1), Eq. 11.2 becomes:

$$R = \frac{[A_2]}{[A_1]} = \frac{K_{A2} \cdot K_{E2}}{K_{A1} \cdot K_{E1}} \quad [11.3]$$

where $K_{E1}$ and $K_{E2}$ refer to the amount of agonist-receptor complex ($[A \cdot R]$) required for half-maximal response. This factor embodies the agonist-specific features of efficacy (intrinsic efficacy $\epsilon$) *and* the tissue-specific features of efficacy (efficiency of the stimulus-response mechanisms of the tissue). When analyses are carried out in the same tissue, then the tissue-specific aspects cancel and agonist-related efficacy determines the potency ratio.

The above relationships show that potency ratios are straightforward products of affinity and intrinsic efficacy for high-efficacy agonists in efficiently receptor-coupled systems (i.e., $[A] \ll K_A$). In cases in which this does not hold (receptor reserve cannot be assumed), potency ratios are more complex and may deviate from these simple equations. In terms of classic theory if $[A]/K_A$ cannot be ignored as an insignificant term, then Eq. 11.2 is:

$$\frac{[A_2]}{[A_1]} = \frac{[A_2](\epsilon_1 - \epsilon_2)}{\epsilon_2 \cdot K_{A2}} + \frac{K_{A2} \cdot \epsilon_1}{K_{A1} \cdot \epsilon_2} \quad [11.4]$$

This approaches the receptor reserve case when the two agonists are of comparable efficacy ($\epsilon_1 \rightarrow \epsilon_2$) or when $[A_2]$ is a highly potent, efficacious agonist and $[A_1]$ has a low affinity (i.e., potency of $A_2 \gg A_1$). Equation 11.4 in terms of the operational model is written:

$$\frac{[A_2]}{[A_1]} = \frac{K_{E2} \cdot K_2}{K_{E1} \cdot K_1} + \frac{[A_2](K_{E2} - K_{E1})}{K_1 \cdot K_{E1}} \quad [11.5]$$

Again in this case, the same generalities apply, namely, comparable efficacies or potency $A_2 \gg$ potency $A_1$ for the approximation to the receptor reserve case. For any given agonist-receptor pair, $\epsilon/K_A$ should be constant. Therefore, the $R$ for two agonists should be a drug-related constant unique for a given receptor. This is a valid assumption for full agonists, but not for comparisons between full and partial agonists, because the stimulus for the latter depends on the complete adsorption-isotherm/intrinsic-efficacy product (i.e., $[P] \nleqslant K_P$):

$$S = \frac{\epsilon_P \cdot [P]}{[P] + K_P} \qquad [11.6]$$

Figure 11.1 demonstrates the effects on receptor coupling of potency ratios for two agonists of different efficacies; when coupling is sufficient to allow full agonism, the potency ratios are constant, but as one agonist becomes incapable of producing the tissue maximal response, underestimation of the potency ratio results. This is because changes in receptor coupling produce

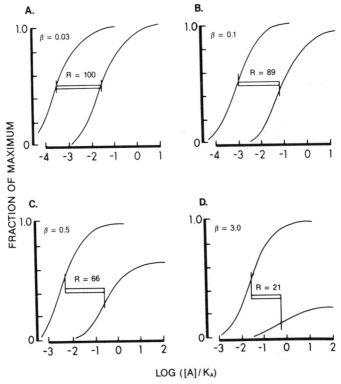

**FIG. 11.1.** Potency ratio for two agonists of relative efficacy 100 in tissues with different efficiencies of receptor coupling. Ordinates: Fractions of maximal tissue response. Abscissae: Logarithms of molar concentrations of agonist. Receptor coupling modeled by logistic function $R = S/(S + \beta)$, where $\beta$ is a fitting parameter, $S$ (stimulus) $= \epsilon/(1 + K_A/[A])$; relative efficacy of agonists is 100. **A:** $\beta = 0.03$. **B:** $\beta = 0.1$. **C:** $\beta = 0.5$. **D:** $\beta = 3$. Note how as the efficiency of receptor coupling decreases ($\beta$ increases); the potency ratio ($R$) for the two agonists decreases.

lateral displacements of dose-response curves along the concentration axis for full agonists, but only depression of the maximal response (with relatively little change in $EC_{50}$) for partial agonists. These considerations make calculation of potency ratios for receptor classification theoretically sound only for full agonists.

A much less rigorous form of this type of analysis sometimes is used to characterize receptors, namely, the use of rank order of potencies. Activation of a common receptor by a series of agonists will yield a unique set of potency ratios in a range of tissues possessing that receptor; the same rank order of potencies will always be found for these agonists. The converse, namely, that an identical order of potencies for a series of agonists in a range of tissues necessarily denotes a common receptor interaction, is not true. For example, angiotensin, norepinephrine, and 5-HT have the same rank order of potencies in rabbit aorta and rat portal vein (Fig. 11.2). However, these agonists are known to activate three separate receptor types in these

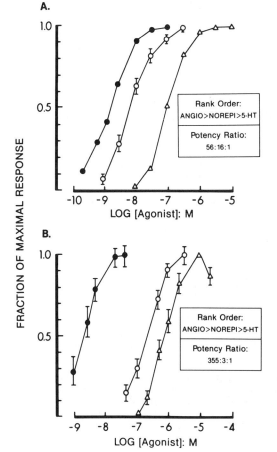

FIG. 11.2. Potency ratios and rank order of potencies for three agonists in rabbit aorta and rat portal vein. A: Rabbit aorta. (Data for angiotensin (●) from ref. 27; data for norepinephrine (○) from ref. 26; data for 5-HT (△) from ref. 23.) B: Rat portal vein. (Data for angiotensin (●) and norepinephrine (○) from ref. 4; data for 5-HT (△) from ref. 5.) Note that whereas the rank order of potencies is the same in both tissues, the potency ratios differ.

tissues, a fact made evident by their differing potency ratios. In general, rank orders of potencies yield crude and misleading data for drug and drug-receptor classification and should be avoided.

A specialized form of the use of agonist potency ratios for receptor classification uses optical isomers of drugs. It would be expected that the potency ratio for two optical isomers of agonists (or antagonists) would be constant for a given drug receptor; Fig. 11.3A demonstrates this for $(-)$ and $(+)$-norepinephrine in rabbit aorta and rat vas deferens (isomeric ratio is the same in both tissues). Figure 11.3B illustrates that once uptake and degradation

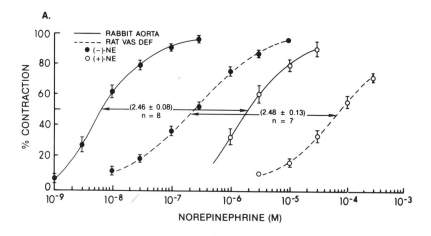

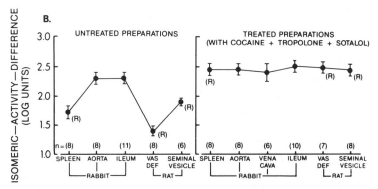

**FIG. 11.3.** Isomeric ratios for receptor classification. **A:** Dose-response curves for $(-)$- and $(+)$-norepinephrine (NE) from rabbit aorta and rat vas deferens. The potencies of the two isomers are nearly identical, indicating a common recognition site for norepinephrine in these tissues. **B:** Isomeric activity differences for $(-)$- and $(+)$-norepinephrine in various tissues. In the presence of norepinephrine uptake, degradation mechanisms, and β-adrenoceptors, the potency ratios vary among tissues, probably because of selective removal of $(-)$-norepinephrine by these processes ("untreated preparations"). When these are blocked by cocaine (10 μM), tropolone (30 μM), and sotalol (10–100 μM), the isomeric ratios are quite similar across species and tissues ("treated preparations"). (From ref. 26.)

mechanisms and other receptor types are eliminated as complicating factors, the isomeric ratios for $(-)$ and $(+)$-norepinephrine are quite consistent between species and tissue types.

In general, if agonist potency accurately reflects the $\epsilon/K_A$ ratio for a full agonist (i.e., if other factors such as agonist removal from the receptor compartment are neutralized), then quantitative estimates of agonist potency ratios can provide a most useful tool for classification. There are statistical procedures capable of enhancing the power of this method that warrant discussion.

### Quantitative Measurement of Agonist Potency Ratios

Measurement of the relative potencies of two agonists is straightforward and uses techniques of linear regression. However, certain special statistical procedures are required to estimate the error of the potency ratio. Parallel-line dose-ratio assays are designed to unambiguously measure relative locations along the log dose axis of the linear portion of a log dose-response curve. It is essential that such dose-response lines be parallel to make the potency ratio independent of the level of response; for this reason, the magnitudes of the responses should be matched as evenly as possible. Assuming that both agonists produce maximal tissue responses, then comparison of equable responses should maximize the likelihood of parallelism (Fig. 11.4A). Replicate values for responses at various dose levels allow statistical testing for deviations from parallelism. Whereas potency ratios can simply be determined graphically from two dose-response curves, balanced assays (such as $2 \times 2$ or $3 \times 3$ dose assays) have the advantage of statistically yielding the confidence limits for the estimate. The practical aspects of these procedures are best described by example.

The relative potencies of the $\alpha$-adrenoceptor agonists oxymetazoline and norepinephrine were measured in rat anococcygeus muscle with a $2 \times 2$ dose assay. The first step was to apply the doses to the tissues in an order determined by a Latin square to cancel the effects of the organ bath and the order of dosing. The doses were as follows: For oxymetazoline, $10^{-8}$ M $= X_{A1}$; $10^{-7}$ M $= X_{A2}$. For norepinephrine, $3 \times 10^{-8}$ M $= X_{B1}$; $3 \times 10^{-7}$ M $= X_{B2}$. Construction of the latin square and the results of the assay are shown in Table 11.3A and B; the response data are given in Table 11.3C. A two-way analysis of variance showed no significant effects of the order of dosing or the organ-bath location (Table 11.3D); thus, the results can be taken as relatively unbiased estimates of the responses.

The data then are reordered by dose (Table 11.3E), and the standard deviation of the error is calculated by a two-way analysis of variance carried out on the reordered data; this is shown in Table 11.3F. The quantities of interest are the means of squares and d.f. values for the residual errors. Next, a test

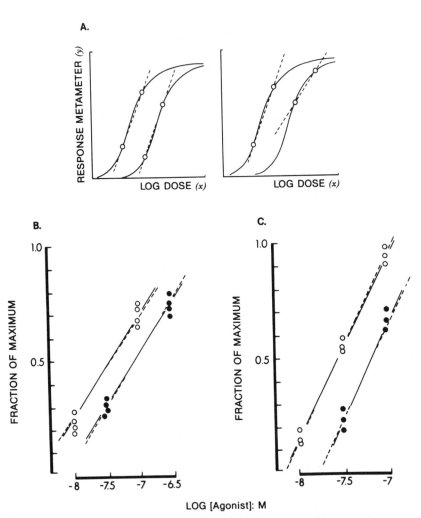

**FIG. 11.4.** Parallel-line assays for measurement of dose ratios. **A:** Illustration of how measurements at different levels of response may result in apparent deviations from parallelism; observations (o); straight-line fit to observations given by *solid lines*; true dose-response curves given by *broken lines*. (From ref. 6.) **B:** Results of a 2 × 2 dose assay on rat anococcygeus muscle to measure the relative potencies of oxymetazoline (o) and norepinephrine (●). Ordinate: Fractions of maximal tissue contraction. Abscissa: Logarithms of molar concentrations of agonist. Data analyzed in Tables 11.3 and 11.4. **C:** Results of a 2 × 3 dose assay in guinea pig ileum to measure the relative potencies of oxotremorine (o) and carbachol (●). Ordinate: Fractions of maximal isotonic shortening. Abscissa: Logarithms of molar concentrations of agonist. Data analyzed in Tables 11.5–11.7. For B and C, *broken lines* show individual regression lines for different sets of data points, and *solid lines* show the best-fit parallel straight lines.

**TABLE 11.3.** *2 × 2 Dose assay: oxymetazoline and norepinephrine in rat anococcygeus muscle*

A: Doses ordered and rotated by row

| Organ bath | Dose order | | | |
|---|---|---|---|---|
| | 1 | 2 | 3 | 4 |
| 1 | $X_{A1}$ | $X_{A2}$ | $X_{B1}$ | $X_{B2}$ |
| 2 | $X_{A2}$ | $X_{B1}$ | $X_{B2}$ | $X_{A1}$ |
| 3 | $X_{B1}$ | $X_{B2}$ | $X_{A1}$ | $X_{A2}$ |
| 4 | $X_{B2}$ | $X_{A1}$ | $X_{A2}$ | $X_{B1}$ |

B: Rows (3421) then columns (4132) randomized

| Organ bath | Dose order | | | |
|---|---|---|---|---|
| | 1 | 2 | 3 | 4 |
| 1 | $X_{A2}$ | $X_{B1}$ | $X_{A1}$ | $X_{B2}$ |
| 2 | $X_{B1}$ | $X_{B2}$ | $X_{A2}$ | $X_{A1}$ |
| 3 | $X_{A1}$ | $X_{A2}$ | $X_{B2}$ | $X_{B1}$ |
| 4 | $X_{B2}$ | $X_{A1}$ | $X_{B1}$ | $X_{A2}$ |

C: Doses applied to tissues and responses obtained (% max)

| Organ bath | Dose order | | | | Row totals |
|---|---|---|---|---|---|
| | 1 | 2 | 3 | 4 | |
| 1 | 74 | 33 | 29 | 71 | 207 |
| 2 | 25 | 74 | 69 | 25 | 193 |
| 3 | 21 | 64 | 79 | 36 | 200 |
| 4 | 69 | 23 | 28 | 66 | 186 |
| Column totals | 189 | 194 | 205 | 198 | 786 |

D: Two-way analysis of variance conducted to determine possible effects of organ-bath location or dosing order

| | SSq[a] | d.f. | MSq[b] | VR[c] |
|---|---|---|---|---|
| Between rows | 61.25 | 3 | 20.42 | $F_R = 0.024$ |
| Between columns | 34.25 | 3 | 11.42 | |
| Residual ($s^2$) | 7,730.25 | 9 | 858.91 | $F_C = 0.013$ |
| Total | 7,829.7 | | | |

**TABLE 11.3.** *Continued*

E: Data shown in Fig. 11.4B

| | Dose order | | | | Row totals |
|---|---|---|---|---|---|
| Organ bath | $y_{A1}$ | $y_{A2}$ | $y_{B1}$ | $y_{B2}$ | |
| 1 | 29 | 74 | 33 | 71 | 207 |
| 2 | 25 | 69 | 25 | 74 | 193 |
| 3 | 21 | 64 | 36 | 79 | 200 |
| 4 | 23 | 66 | 28 | 69 | 186 |
| Column totals | 98 | 273 | 122 | 293 | 786 |

F: Two-way analysis of variance on data ordered in part E

| | SSq | d.f. | MSq | VR |
|---|---|---|---|---|
| Between rows | 61.25 | 3 | 20.42 | $F_R = 1.15$ |
| Between columns | 7,604.25 | 3 | 2,534.7 | |
| Residual ($s^2$) | 160.25 | 9 | 17.8 | $F_C = 142$ |
| Total | 7,829.75 | 15 | 521.7 | |

[a] Sum of squares.
[b] Mean of squares.
[c] Variance ratio.

for parallelism (see Chapter 6) is run, and the common slope is calculated (Table 11.4).

The potency ratio is given by

$$R = \text{antilog}\left[(\bar{x}_A - \bar{x}_B) + \frac{\bar{y}_B - \bar{y}_A}{m_c}\right] \qquad [11.7]$$

where subscripts $A$ and $B$ refer to the two agonists, $\bar{x}$ is the mean dose, $\bar{y}$ is the mean response, and $m_c$ is the common slope for two straight regression lines between the two sets of data points. If the test for parallelism yields a significant value for $t$ (i.e., if the data points cannot be fitted to parallel lines), then this analysis cannot be done. For the example in Table 11.3C and Fig. 11.4B, that was not the case, and $R = 2.63$. The confidence limit for this estimate can be calculated for any confidence level; for example, at $p < 0.05$, $t = 2.26$ for 9 d.f. [this refers to the value of the residual mean square in Table 11.3D; d.f. = (rows − 1), (columns − 1)]. At this point, the confidence limits on this estimate can be calculated. A first statistic to determine is $g$:

$$g = \frac{t^2 \cdot s^2}{m_c^2(s_{XA}^2 + s_{XB}^2)} \qquad [11.8]$$

where $s$ refers to the means of squares of the residual error in the two-way analysis of variance for the ordered data (see Table 11.3D), and $s_x^2$ (for ago-

**TABLE 11.4.** *Test for parallelism in 2 × 2 dose assay shown in Table 11.3*

| [Oxotremorine] $x_A$ | Response $y_A$ | [Norepinephrine] $x_B$ | Response $y_B$ |
|---|---|---|---|
| −8 | 29 | −7.5 | 33 |
| −8 | 25 | −7.5 | 25 |
| −8 | 21 | −7.5 | 36 |
| −8 | 23 | −7.5 | 28 |
| −7 | 74 | −6.5 | 71 |
| −7 | 69 | −6.5 | 74 |
| −7 | 64 | −6.5 | 79 |
| −7 | 66 | −6.5 | 69 |

$\sum x_A = -60,$  $\sum y_A = 371,$  $\sum x_B = -56,$  $\sum y_B = 415$

$\sum x_A^2 = 452,$  $\sum y_A^2 = 21,125,$  $\sum x_B^2 = 394,$  $\sum y_B^2 = 25,313$

$n_A = 8,$  $\sum x_A y_A = -2,695,$  $n_B = 8,$  $\sum x_B y_B = -2,819.5$

$s_A = 15.29,$  $s_{XA}^2 = 2$  $s_B = 21.625,$  $s_{XB}^2 = 2$

$M_A = 43.75,$  $M_B = 42.75$

$s_P = 18.73,$  $t = 0.053$ (n.s.)

$W_A = 0.0171,$  $W_B = 0.0085$

$M_c = 43.42$  (common slope)

nists *A* and *B*) is given by

$$s_x^2 = \sum x^2 - \frac{\left(\sum x\right)^2}{n} \qquad [11.9]$$

For the example, $g = 0.012$. As in this case, when $g$ is small (i.e., when $1 - g$ approaches unity), the logarithms of the confidence limits (C.L.) for the potency ratio $R$ are given by

$$\log(C.L.) = \pm \frac{s \cdot t}{m_c}\left[\left(\frac{1}{n_A} + \frac{1}{n_B}\right) + \frac{(\bar{y}_B - \bar{y}_A)^2}{m_c^2(s_{XA}^2 + s_{XB}^2)}\right]^{1/2} \qquad [11.10]$$

which for the example is ±0.113. The confidence limits are obtained by adding and subtracting log(C.L.) from the logarithm of R; i.e., $R = 2.63$, log $R = 0.42$; 95% confidence limits = antilog(0.42 − 0.113) = 2.02, and antilog(0.42 + 0.113) = 3.41. If $1 - g$ does not approach unity, then a more rigorous form of Eq. 11.10 should be used for calculating the confidence limits. Under these circumstances,

$$\log(C.L.) = \pm \frac{s \cdot t}{m_c(1 - g)}\left[(1 - g)\left(\frac{1}{n_A} + \frac{1}{n_B}\right) + \frac{(\bar{y}_B - \bar{y}_A)^2}{m_c^2(s_{XA}^2 + s_{XB}^2)}\right]^{1/2}$$

$$[11.11]$$

**TABLE 11.5.** *2 × 3 Dose assay: oxotremorine and carbachol in guinea pig ileum*

| Organ bath | Oxotremorine (A) | | | Carbachol (B) | | Row totals |
|---|---|---|---|---|---|---|
| | $X_{A1}$ | $X_{A2}$ | $X_{A3}$ | $X_{B1}$ | $X_{B2}$ | |
| 1 | 12 | 55 | 94 | 23 | 70 | 254 |
| 2 | 19 | 59 | 90 | 19 | 65 | 252 |
| 3 | 15 | 53 | 98 | 28 | 61 | 255 |
| Column totals | 46 | 167 | 282 | 70 | 196 | 761 |
| $n$ | 3 | 3 | 3 | 3 | 3 | |
| $\sum x^2$ | 730 | 9,315 | 26,540 | 1,674 | 12,846 | |

Basically, the same procedure is used with a 3 × 3 dose assay, except that a test for linearity (see Chapter 6) can be included to determine if a parallel-line analysis can be allowed. Although a balanced assay (i.e., 2 × 2 or 3 × 3) is preferable, it may not always be possible; a 2 × 3 assay also can be used in basically the same manner as the previous example, except that a different analysis-of-variance table and calculation of $s$ are required. An example of a 2 × 3 assay is shown in Fig. 11.4C.

Two dose levels of carbachol (30 and 100 nM) and three dose levels of oxotremorine (10, 30, and 100 nM) were used to produce responses in guinea pig ileum. The doses were given randomly, and the response data collected and ordered as shown in Table 11.5. The calculation of $s$ is shown in Table 11.6 ($s = 15.66$). The test for parallelism (Table 11.7) indicates no significant difference between the best-linear-fit straight lines to the data points. The potency ratio for oxotremorine/carbachol, as calculated by Eq. 11.7, is 2.32; $g$ for a 95% confidence level = 0.112. The approximate confidence limits (Eq. 11.10) for the potency ratio (assuming $1 - g \approx 1.0$) are 4.08 to 1.32.

In general, accurate potency ratios can be calculated best when the following conditions are met: (a) The levels of response produced by the two agonists are comparable; this optimizes the condition of parallelism. Also, this

**TABLE 11.6.** *Analysis of variance for data in Table 11.5*

| | SSq | d.f. | MSq | VR |
|---|---|---|---|---|
| Between groups | 12,340.3 | 4 | 3,085.06 | |
| Within groups | 156.63 | 10 | 15.66 | $F = 197$ |
| Total | 12,496.93 | 14 | | |

**TABLE 11.7.** *Test for parallelism for data in Table 11.5*

| Oxotremorine | | Carbachol | |
|---|---|---|---|
| $x_A$ | $y_A$ | $x_B$ | $y_B$ |
| $-8$ | 12 | $-7.5$ | 23 |
| $-8$ | 19 | $-7.5$ | 19 |
| $-8$ | 15 | $-7.5$ | 28 |
| $-7.5$ | 55 | $-7$ | 70 |
| $-7.5$ | 59 | $-7$ | 65 |
| $-7.5$ | 53 | $-7$ | 61 |
| $-7$ | 94 | | |
| $-7$ | 90 | | |
| $-7$ | 98 | | |

| | | | |
|---|---|---|---|
| $\sum x_A = -67.5,$ | $\sum y_A = 495,$ | $\sum x_B = -43.5,$ | $\sum y_B = 275$ |
| $\sum x_A^2 = 507.75,$ | $\sum y_A^2 = 36{,}585,$ | $\sum x_B^2 = 315.75,$ | $\sum y_B^2 = 14{,}520$ |
| $n_A = 9,$ | $\sum xy_A = -3{,}594.5,$ | $n_B = 6,$ | $\sum xy_B = -1{,}897$ |
| $s_A = 3.32,$ | $s_{xA}^2 = 1.5,$ | $s_B = 4.51,$ | $s_{xB}^2 = 0.375$ |
| $M_A = 78.67,$ | | $M_B = 84$ | |
| $s_P = 3.80,$ | | $t = 0.77$ (n.s.) | |
| $W_A = 0.0185,$ | | $W_B = 0.00034$ | |
| $M_c = 78.77$ | (common slope) | | |

minimizes the $\bar{y}_A - \bar{y}_B$ term. It is assumed that both agonists produce the maximal response; this should be verified. (b) The term $g$ should be small; i.e., the slope of the line should be large relative to the standard deviation of the slope. (c) The term $s$, the error standard deviation, should be small; i.e., the responses should be as reproducible as possible. (d) The slope should be large to minimize the log(C.L.) term, as given by Eq. 11.10. (e) A symmetrical assay is optimum, because $(1/n_A + 1/n_B)$ is minimum when $n_A = n_B$. A large number of responses also will reduce this term. (f) The doses should be as far apart as possible to maximize $s_x^2$ (but still remain on the linear portions of the dose-response curves). If these conditions are met, unbiased potency ratios with appropriate confidence limits can be calculated.

## POTENCY RATIOS AND PROMISCUOUS RECEPTORS

The use of potency ratios tacitly assumes that the affinity and intrinsic efficacy of an agonist are solely drug receptor–related parameters that are not subject to the makeup of the measuring system. This assumption may not be valid in cases in which the receptor is able to activate two or more membrane-coupling proteins to produce responses. The physiological aspects of receptor pleiotropy with respect to coupling proteins are discussed in Chapter 8; this section will emphasize the ramifications for receptor classification with agonist potency ratios. The concept of a receptor specific–agonist potency ratio is valid in systems in which the coupling steps from receptor activation to tissue response are common to *all* agonists. Under these conditions, null procedures can be used to cancel their impact. However, this concept breaks down if part of the stimulus transduction chain involves cognitive aspects of the drug-receptor interaction (i.e., the recognition of *different* coupling proteins) with different agonists. For example, it has been speculated that the muscarinic receptor carbachol can produce agonist-receptor complexes capable of activating G proteins for potassium ion entry and increases in phosphoinositol turnover, whereas oxotremorine may be incapable of activating the latter G protein. Under these circumstances, the observed potency for each agonist will depend on the G protein present in the tissue being assayed, and this difference will not depend only on receptor type. Figure 11.5 shows a schematic representation of this effect for two agonists A1 and A2. The parameters for the calculations are such that A1 predisposes ternary complex formation with $G_1$ and A2 predisposes ternary complex formation more with $G_2$. Thus, in tissue I, which possesses $G_1$, the agonist A1 is more potent than A2, whereas in tissue II (which possesses $G_2$), the reverse is true. The equilibrium dissociation of the agonist-receptor complex for this simulation is constant, i.e., the receptor type in these two tissues is the same.

A more complex scenario is presented if the receptor can simultaneously activate more than one coupling protein in the membrane. If agonists predispose differing amounts of ternary complex with these mixtures, then the *relative quantities* of the different proteins in different membranes will determine agonist potency and therefore potency ratios. Figure 11.6 shows the simulated potency of two agonists that both predispose ternary complex formation for two G proteins but with differing potency. The relative amount of $G_1$ is reduced ($G_2$ constant) and the change in the potency of A1 (Fig. 11.6B) and A2 (Fig. 11.6C) shown. As can be seen from this figure, the location parameter of A1 is selectively more subject to the relative concentration of $G_1$, therefore if the relative quantities of these couplers were variable in different membranes, the relative potency of A1 and A2 would also vary. This could potentially lead to a situation in which agonists classify receptor-coupler pairs and not just receptor types (Fig. 11.7). Under these circumstances, one might expect differences between classification schemes with agonists and antagonists.

### Selective Agonism

An extreme example of agonist potency ratios, as used to classify receptors, is provided by selective production of responses by some agonists but

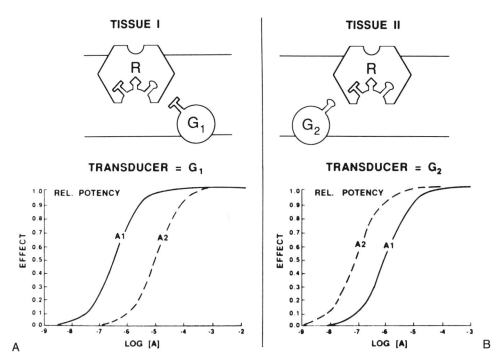

**FIG. 11.5.** Schematic diagram of the activation of a single receptor in different membranes containing two different coupling proteins $G_1$ (tissue I) and $G_2$ (tissue II) Both agonists promote ternary complex formation via a two-stage binding process (Chapter 7) in which $K_1$ denotes the equilibrium dissociation constant of the agonist-receptor complex ($[A{\cdot}R]$) and $K_2$ the equilibrium dissociation constant of the subsequently formed ternary complex. For agonist A1, $K_1 = 0.01$; $K_2 = 0.1$ for $G_1$ and $K_2 = 1$ for $G_2$. For agonist A2, $K_1 = 0.01$, $K_2 = 3$ for $G_1$ and $K_2 = 0.1$ for $G_2$. It can be seen from these parameters that A1 selectively promotes ternary complex formation with $G_1$ and conversely A2 promotes activation of $G_2$. **A:** Tissue I agonist A1 is 40-fold more potent than A2, whereas in tissue II **(B)**, this potency is reversed to 0.1. (From ref. 17.)

not others. The key factor in this type of analysis is the previous classification of the selective agonist. Thus, if agonist *A* is thought to be a selective agonist for receptor *A*, then it would be expected that the presence or absence of responses to agonist *A* would in turn reflect the corresponding presence or absence of receptor *A* in the tissue. There are two major assumptions in this reasoning that should be considered before the results of selective-agonist studies can yield useful information for classification. The first assumption is that the efficiency of receptor coupling in the tissue is sufficient to reveal a response to the selective agonist. This depends primarily on the intrinsic efficacy, not the affinity, of agonist *A* (see Chapter 8). For example, many pharmacologic data demonstrate that isoproterenol and prenalterol both are agonists of β-adrenoceptors, but that prenalterol has only 0.04 of the intrinsic efficacy of isoproterenol. In a well-coupled tissue such as rat isolated left atrium, both drugs produce agonist responses (Fig. 11.8A), but in canine

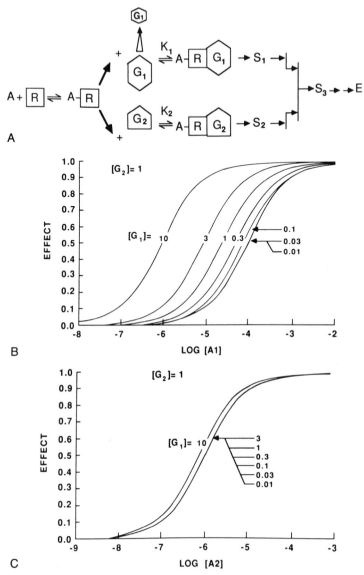

**FIG. 11.6.** The effects of reducing the relative concentration of $G_1$, with respect to $G_2$, in a membrane system containing both $G_1$ and $G_2$ that are both activated by a single receptor [R]. **A:** Schematic diagram of membrane components. **B:** Dose-response curves to agonist A1: $K_A$ for receptor binding = 0.01; $K_1$ for ternary complex formation with $G_1$ = 0.1; $K_2$ for ternary complex formation with $G_2$ = 1. [$G_1$] varied from 10 to 0.001, whereas [$G_2$] held constant. Agonist A1 is primarily $G_1$ dependent for response. **C:** Potency for [A2] in the same system. $K_A$ for receptor binding = 0.01; $K_1$ for ternary complex formation with [$G_1$] = 3; $K_2$ for [$G_2$] = 0.1. Agonist A2 is primarily $G_2$ dependent for response. (From ref. 18.)

**Analysis with Antagonists = 3 Receptor Types**

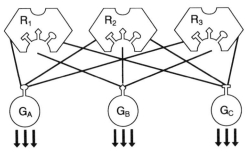

**Analysis with Agonists = 9 Receptor Types**

**FIG. 11.7.** Possible combinations of unique receptor-coupler pairs. Three receptor types are depicted that could interact with antagonists and thus be differentiated. If these three receptor types could variably interact with three different receptor-coupling proteins, then agonists theoretically could discern nine receptor-coupler pairs. Thus, the classification of these three receptors could take on an order of complexity not related solely to receptor type. (From ref. 17.)

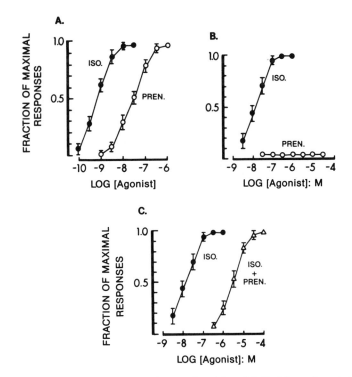

**FIG. 11.8.** Effects of isoproterenol and prenalterol in rat left atria and canine coronary artery. **A:** Rat left atria. Ordinate: Increased inotropy as fraction of maximal response to isoproterenol. Abscissa: Logarithms of molar concentrations of agonist. Responses to isoproterenol (•, $N = 6$) and prenalterol (○, $N = 6$). **B:** Canine coronary artery. Ordinate: Relaxation of maximal contraction to KCl as a fraction of induced tone. Abscissa: As for A. Responses to isoproterenol (•, $N = 4$) and prenalterol (○, $N = 4$). **C:** Blockade of responses of canine coronary artery to isoproterenol by prenalterol. Responses in the absence (•, $N = 4$) and presence (△, $N = 4$) of prenalterol (30 μM). Bars represent SEM (B and C from ref. 21.)

coronary artery, a tissue possessing the same type of β-adrenoceptor, only isoproterenol produces a response (Fig. 11.8A). Does this imply that the receptors for isoproterenol and prenalterol are different and that only those for isoproterenol are present in canine coronary artery? Actually, that is not the case; rather, the β-adrenoceptors in the canine coronary artery are not sufficiently coupled to generate a response to weak β-adrenoceptor stimuli. The clear interaction of prenalterol with the β-adrenoceptors can be demonstrated by blockade of isoproterenol responses by this drug (Fig. 11.8C). This can be a general method of verification (i.e., if a selective agonist does not produce a response in a tissue, it should be determined whether it produces blockade of a more powerful agonist in that same tissue).

The second assumption inherent in studies with selective agonists relates to the degree of selectivity assumed for the agonist. At the extreme, agonist $A$ can be assumed to be *specific* for receptor $A$, implying that it produces responses at no other receptor type. A much more common phenomenon is that agonist $A$ is *selective* for receptor $A$ in that it activates this receptor preferentially (i.e., the $\epsilon/K_A$ ratio is highest for receptor $A$), but at higher concentrations agonist $A$ may activate other receptor types. Therefore, the observed agonism must be verified to be due to activation of receptor $A$ by studies with antagonists. For example, the β-adrenoceptors of rat uterus have been shown to be of the $\beta_2$ subtype by a variety of techniques. Prenalterol, at one time thought to be a $\beta_1$ subtype–specific β-adrenoceptor agonist, produces powerful responses in rat uterus (Fig. 11.9A), leading to two possible interpretations: (a) the rat uterus contains previously undetected $\beta_1$-adrenoceptors, because a $\beta_1$-specific agonist produced a response (i.e., reclassify the system to tailor the drug). (b) Prenalterol is not a specific $\beta_1$ agonist, but rather also activates $\beta_2$-adrenoceptors (reclassify the drug to the system). In these cases, studies with antagonists are extremely helpful; Fig. 11.9B shows blockade of uterine responses to prenalterol by the $\beta_2$-selective agonist butoxamine, demonstrating that in this case prenalterol does possess intrinsic efficacy and affinity for $\beta_2$-adrenoceptors as well. The assumptions and verifications associated with the use of selective agonists for receptor classification are shown schematically in Fig. 11.10.

## Selective Receptor Desensitization

A technique related to selective agonism is the use of high doses of a given selective agonist to desensitize a tissue to that agonist (i.e., effectively remove receptor $A$). For example, if a test agonist $B$ produces a response in a tissue before, but not after, the tissue is desensitized to serotonin (by protracted exposure to a high dose of serotonin), the implication will be that agonist $B$ produces responses by activating serotonin receptors. Besides the obvious worry of cross-desensitization (i.e., do high doses of serotonin pro-

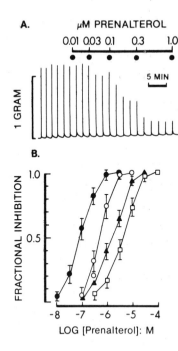

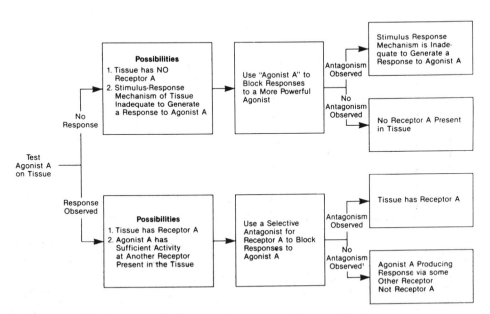

**FIG. 11.9.** Responses of rat uterus to prenalterol. **A:** Inhibition of electrically induced contractions of rat uterus by prenalterol. **B:** Blockade of prenalterol responses by the $\beta_2$-adrenoceptor-selective antagonist butoxamine. Ordinate: Inhibition of uterine contraction as a fraction of basal twitch height. Abscissa: Logarithms of molar concentrations of prenalterol. Responses in the absence (•, $N = 5$) and presence of butoxamine at 1 $\mu$M (○, $N = 3$), 3 $\mu$M (▲, $N = 3$), and 10 $\mu$M (□, $N = 3$). Bars represent SEM. (From ref. 13.)

'At least, none commensurate with the required $pK_B$ for antagonism of Receptor A

**FIG. 11.10.** Schematic diagram of possibilities when a selective agonist is used to classify an unknown receptor in a tissue.

duce desensitization of other receptors in the tissue?), this technique does not account for possible differences in intrinsic efficacies of the agonists involved. As pointed out in Chapter 8, and again earlier in this chapter, responses to the agonist of lower intrinsic efficacy are more subject to decreases in tissue response capability (i.e., reduction in receptor number or compromise of stimulus-response coupling). Figure 11.11 shows the effects of receptor loss (in this case, due to chemical alkylation, but analogous to receptor desensitization) on guinea pig ileal responses to the cholinomimetics oxotremorine and carbachol; oxotremorine has a lower efficacy (0.14 times), but higher affinity (24 times), for muscarinic receptors than does carbachol and thus is more potent. However, it can be seen that as receptor loss progresses, the responses to oxotremorine are preferentially depressed over those of carbachol. This experiment demonstrates a prediction from receptor theory that not all agonists will be equally affected by receptor desensitization. Therefore, in the experiment with agonist *B* and serotonin, if agonist *B* still had produced a response in a tissue refractory to serotonin, that would not necessarily have meant that agonist *B* did not activate serotonin receptors. Alternatively, agonist *B* could have an intrinsic efficacy for serotonin receptors greater than that of serotonin and thus still produce a serotonin receptor–mediated response. In general, differing intrinsic efficacies of agonists must be considered in classification studies by selective desensitization and/or receptor alkylation.

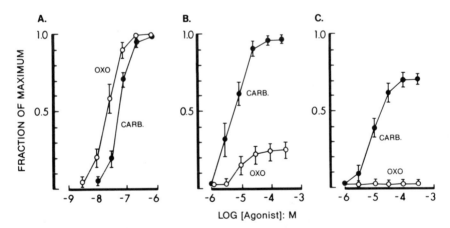

**FIG. 11.11.** Effects of diminution of receptor number on responses to drugs of different intrinsic efficacies. Ordinate: Isotonic contractions of guinea pig ileal longitudinal muscle strips as fractions of the maximal shortening to carbachol before receptor alkylation. Abscissa: Logarithms of molar concentrations of agonists. Oxotremorine (OXO) (o) has a greater affinity, but lesser intrinsic efficacy, as compared with carbachol (CARB.), for the muscarinic receptors. Responses before receptor alkylation (**A**, $N = 8$) and after progressive reduction of muscarinic receptor numbers by alkylation with POB at 10 μM for 12 min (**B**, $N = 4$) and 3 μM for 20 min (**C**, $N = 4$). Bars represent SEM.

## Differentiation of Affinity and Efficacy

Agonist potency ratios are useful for quantifying drug-receptor interactions because they reflect the ratio $\epsilon/K_A$. More rigorous analyses yield actual estimates of relative efficacies (Chapter 8) and agonist affinities (Chapter 7). Clearly, these constants can be used for drug and drug-receptor classification because they reflect the molecular interaction between the agonist and the receptor. For example, Table 11.8A shows the homogeneity of affinities measured for carbachol for muscarinic receptors in a range of isolated tissues. Table 11.8B shows different relative affinities and efficacies of catecholamines for subclasses of β-adrenoceptors. Measurement of actual affinities and relative efficacies of agonists requires more detailed analysis than that required for measurement of potency ratios, and in some cases the pharmacologic tools necessary for such measurements are not available. However, if these constants can be estimated, then additional valuable information regarding prediction of agonist effects across species and organ types can be gained (see Chapters 8 and 13). The fact that potency ratios truly reflect $\epsilon/K_A$ and are not dependent on the efficiency of receptor coupling only when the full tissue response can be attained (see Fig. 11.1) makes this approach somewhat more restrictive than measurement of relative $\epsilon$ and $K_A$.

**TABLE 11.8.** *Affinities and relative efficacies for agonists*

### A. Muscarinic receptors

| Agonist | Species | Tissue | $pK_A$[a] |
|---|---|---|---|
| Carbachol | Guinea pig | Ileum | 4.92[b] |
| | | Left atrium | 4.95[c] |
| | Rabbit | Aorta | 4.8[c] |
| | | Stomach fundus | 4.8[c] |

### B. β-Adrenoceptors[d]

| Agonist | Guinea pig atria (β₁) | | Rat uterus (β₂) | |
|---|---|---|---|---|
| | Rel. $K_D^b$ | Rel. ε | Rel. $K_D^2$ | Rel. ε |
| (−)-Isoproterenol | 1 | 1 | 1 | 1 |
| (−)-Epinephrine | 18.2 | 0.6 | 5.4 | 0.35 |
| (−)-Norepinephrine | 14.4 | 1.5 | 40.7 | 0.44 |

[a] $-\log K_A$
[b] From ref. 10.
[c] From ref. 9.
[d] From ref. 24.

## REACTION PRODUCT AS A RESPONSE

In most isolated tissue experiments, a steady-state response is observed as a tissue reaction to a constant production of stimulus. Under these conditions the rate of response production is not critical since the temporal relationship between agonist concentration and response can be visualized and the experimenter need only wait for a steady state to be obtained. Under these circumstances equiactive doses of compounds can be calculated. However, there are dose-response systems in which the *quantity* of product is used to measure drug activity. In these systems, if two agonists with different rates of response production are compared, then the kinetics of response may seriously affect the apparent equilibrium relative potency if true equilibrium is not achieved. For example, β-adrenoceptor agonists promote lipolysis in adipocytes. Lipolytic activity can be quantified *in vitro* by equilibrating fat cells in physiological medium with an agonist and then biochemically measuring the amount of glycerol released into the medium by the resulting lipolytic reaction. Under these circumstances, the total amount of glycerol produced is a measure of response, thus the time of incubation becomes a direct determinant of the magnitude of response. If two agonists with very different rates of onset are compared, the relative amounts of product made by each will differ. The rate of receptor occupation by the agonist is given by:

$$\rho_t = \rho_e(1 - e^{-(k([A]+K_A)t)}) \qquad [11.12]$$

where $\rho_t$ and $\rho_e$ is the receptor occupancy at time $t$ and at equilibrium, respectively, $t$ is time (in sec), $k$ is the rate of offset of the agonist from the receptor, $[A]$ is the molar concentration of the agonist and $K_A$ is the equilibrium dissociation constant of the agonist-receptor complex. Figure 11.12A shows the rate of receptor occupancy for two agonists $A_1$ (a fast onset agonist $k = 3 \times 10^{-3}$ sec$^{-1}$) and $A_2$ (a slower onset agonist $k = 3 \times 10^{-4}$ sec$^{-1}$) at concentrations sufficient to occupy 10% of the receptors in a given tissue. The magnitude of this quantity of product is given by the area under the curves shown in Fig. 11.12A and can be calculated with the integral of Eq. 11.12:

$$\rho_t = \rho_e \left( t + \frac{e^{-k([A]/K_A + 1)t}}{k([A]/K_A + 1)} - \frac{1}{k([A]/K_A + 1)} \right) \qquad [11.13]$$

Figure 11.12B shows the quantity of response produced by the two agonists $A_1$ and $A_2$. Note that the response to the slower agonist does not become a linear function of time until 8 min into the incubation time, 7 min longer than for the faster agonist. It can be seen from this figure that the agonist with the slower rate of onset (agonist $A_2$) requires approximately 10 min to attain the same rate of accumulation of stimulus as agonist $A_1$. It is this

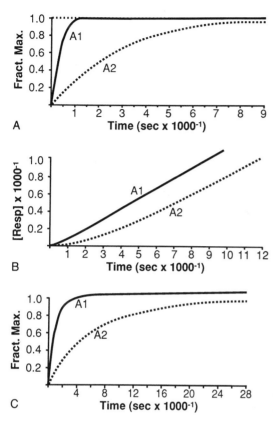

**FIG. 11.12.** Kinetics of response to two agonists of differing onset rates. **A:** Fractional receptor occupancy as a function of time to agonists A1 (*solid line*, fast) of offset $k = 3 \times 10^{-3}$ sec$^{-1}$ and A2 (*dotted line*, slow) $k = 3 \times 10^{-4}$ sec$^{-1}$. Concentrations chosen to produce 10% occupancy at equilibrium. **B:** Integral of receptor occupancy rate curves shown in A as calculated by Eq. 11.13. Response to A1 (*solid line*) and A2 (*dotted line*). **C:** Fractional response as a function of time produced by A1 (*solid line*) and A2 (*dotted line*).

difference in the quantity of response between these two agonists that will be translated to a difference in relative potency, and this disparity will diminish in importance as the time period for potency comparison is increased. From this it can be seen that once a steady-state rate of response is attained, the difference in the quantity of response produced at the initial stages of receptor occupancy will be less important to the relative magnitude of response as the total magnitude of the response (i.e., the time of equilibration) is increased. Thus, the initial differences in the magnitude of stimulus produced by drugs of differing kinetics of onset can be diminished by increasing the quantity of response (i.e., the equilibration time) on which the potency determination is made. This is illustrated by Fig. 11.12C where the effect of time on the quantity of response produced expressed as a fraction of the equilibrium response is shown. However, note that even after a 5-hr equilibration time, the response to the slower agonist does not reach the theoretical equilibrium response level. This is because of the "lost time" in terms of response production in the early stages of equilibration when receptor occupancy was submaximal. Therefore, the rate of onset can produce a permanent deficit of response to an agonist if the quantity of product is measured as an index of potency. The effects of this deficit can be reduced by increasing the equilibration time. Figure 11.13A and B shows the effect of equilibration time on the dose-response curves to both the fast ($A_1$) and to the slow ($A_2$) agonists. Note that as the time of equilibration is increased, the curve shifts to the left. Figure 11.13C shows the effect of equilibration time on the potency ratio of the fast and slow agonist. Therefore, if short equilibration times are used to construct the dose-response curves to these two agonists, it can be seen that the potency of the slower agonist will be selectively underestimated, thereby producing an artifactual overestimation of the potency ratio for the two agonists. This error in the potency ratio would, in turn, be potentially problematic for receptor classification.

## SHAPES OF DOSE-RESPONSE CURVES

Drug receptors are classified and compared with data that quantify the activity of agonists. Therefore, any feature of agonist activity that can serve to differentiate agonists can, in theory, be useful for differentiation of receptors. As noted in earlier chapters, the basic properties of affinity and intrinsic efficacy of agonists, when they can be measured reliably, can be useful for drug and drug-receptor classification. Other features of agonist activity such

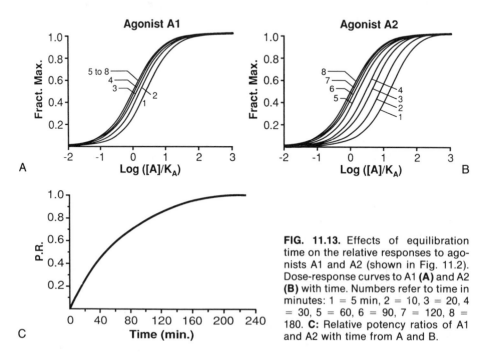

**FIG. 11.13.** Effects of equilibration time on the relative responses to agonists A1 and A2 (shown in Fig. 11.2). Dose-response curves to A1 **(A)** and A2 **(B)** with time. Numbers refer to time in minutes: 1 = 5 min, 2 = 10, 3 = 20, 4 = 30, 5 = 60, 6 = 90, 7 = 120, 8 = 180. **C:** Relative potency ratios of A1 and A2 with time from A and B.

as the shapes of the agonist dose-response curves, type of response, and sensitivity of response to physiological modification, also, under certain circumstances, may be used for receptor differentiation. However, the factors determining these properties of agonists depend on complex interactions of multiple physiological mechanisms; therefore the reliable use of these features of agonist activity for receptor classification is suspect and must be stringently tested.

Drug activity is quantified by dose-response curves, which, in turn, are characterized by the parameters of threshold, asymptotic maximum, location parameter ($EC_{50}$), and slope. This latter parameter also includes shape, as in whether a curve is a rectangular hyperbola or is best described by another function. In binding studies, there is some justification for the use of the slope and shape of the dose-response curve to infer molecular interactions at the drug receptor (see Chapter 12). In functional studies, this is not defensible in view of the fact that transducer functions, each with their own dose-response curves, intervene between the drug-receptor binding events and observed response. These transducer mechanisms can completely dictate the shape of dose-response curves making this feature of drug action unreliable for drug and drug-receptor classification. Intuitively, differences in the slopes for the dose-response curves in the same tissue (which share the *same* receptor-coupling mechanisms) might be used as evidence for differences at the receptor level, i.e., the two agonists activate a different population of receptors in the same tissue. However, before this can be considered seriously, interventions at the membrane level should be used to selectively alter the pattern of responses. The most common intervention is the addition of a receptor-selective competitive antagonist. For example, 2-chloroadenosine produces a biphasic dose-response curve in rat isolated kidney (Fig. 11.14A). One possible explanation for this pattern is the activation of adenosine A1 receptors to increase perfusion pressure and adenosine A2 receptors to reduce perfusion pressure by this agonist. This hypothesis is actually supported by the finding that dextral displacement of the dose-response curve by the adenosine receptor antagonist 8-SPT completely changes the relative effects of 2-chloroadenosine (see Fig. 11.14B). Unless the affinity for the two receptor subtypes mediating these two effects is identical, it would be expected that blockade of the receptor mixture would change the relative inputs from the two receptor populations and thus the shape of the dose-response curve. The change in the shape of the dose-response curves to 2-chloroadenosine in Fig. 11.14 suggests that this agonist activates two cell-surface receptors in this tissue.

This situation should be contrasted with complex dose-response curves resulting from the single-receptor activation of pleiotropic biochemical processes within cells. For example, it is well-known that intracellular second messengers such as cyclic AMP, $Ca^{2+}$, cyclic GMP, mediate many cellular responses. Usually, the pharmacologically observed response is the result of

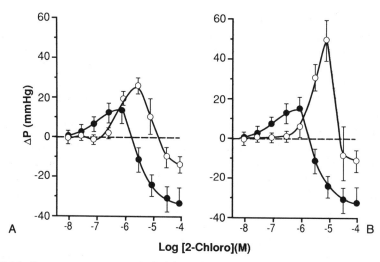

**FIG. 11.14.** Dose-response curves to 2-chloroadenosine (2-Chloro) in perfused rat kidney. Ordinates: Perfusion pressure. Abscissae: Logarithms of molar concentrations of 2-chloroadenosine in the perfusion medium. Response in the absence (●) and presence (○) of the adenosine receptor antagonist 8-SPT at a concentration of 3 **(A)** and 10 μM **(B)**. (From ref. 19.)

many second messenger–mediated biochemical processes within the cell. Some may be synergistic, as in the case of the release of intracellular calcium stores by the entry of "trigger" calcium through channels from the extracellular space. Some processes may be antagonistic, such as the activation of phosphodiesterase by calcium that has entered the cell through cyclic AMP–mediated phosphorylation of calcium channels. The activated phosphodiesterase degrades the cyclic AMP, thereby reducing the strength of the original signal (calcium entry). There are examples of when the strength of the receptor stimulus alters the *type* of cellular response, as would be the case when various second messenger–mediated processes have different thresholds and maximal outputs. For example, opioid receptors mediate the stimulation of GTPase *and* the inhibition of adenylate cyclase in NG108-15 cells. However, the GTPase response is more sensitive to diminution of opioid receptor number (i.e., a smaller effective receptor reserve) than the adenylate cyclase response (7). Presumably, this would suggest that a lower efficacy agonist could selectively stimulate only the most sensitive mechanism (i.e., inhibition of adenylate cyclase) and not both. Therefore, high- and low-efficacy agonists or the same receptor system would produce a different type of response in this cell type.

These complex response patterns can sometimes resemble receptor heterogeneity. For example, Fig. 11.15A illustrates a simple pleiotropic response model in which an initial stimulus modeled by a standard rectangular hyperbola feeds into a secondary saturable process with a different threshold and

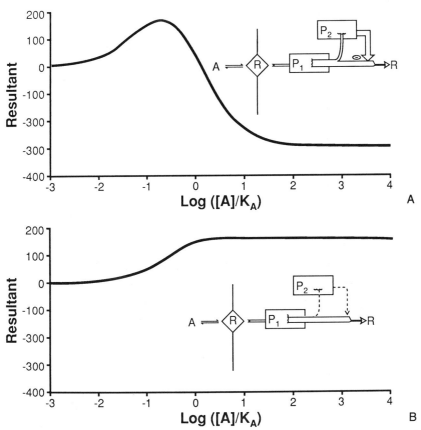

**FIG. 11.15.** Response output from a system in which the initial stimulus to the agonist ($P_1$) partially activates a secondary negative stimulus ($P_2$) to produce a response R. **A:** The strength of $P_1$ is sufficient to produce a significant negative stimulus. Response calculated from Eq. 11.14 with $M = 750$, $N = 500$, $K = 30$, and $L = 3$. **B:** The strength of the initial stimulus $P_1$ is reduced and insufficient to activate the negative stimulus. Parameters of Eq. 11.14 are the same as for A except that $M$ is reduced to 150.

maximal effect. This secondary process produces a negative stimulus and the cell responds with a summation of the stimuli. Thus, the receptor stimulus is the product of receptor occupancy ($\rho$) × the maximal stimulus output $M$. The factor $M$ includes the receptor density and the maximal output of the stimulus response apparatus for this process. The secondary stimulus responds to the first with $1/L$ sensitivity, a maximal output denoted by $N$, and a half-maximal value of $K$. Thus, the resultant response is given by:

$$\text{Response} = \frac{\rho \cdot M \cdot N}{\rho \cdot M + KL} - \rho L \qquad [11.14]$$

The output response from Eq. 11.14 can be made biphasic, as often is ob-

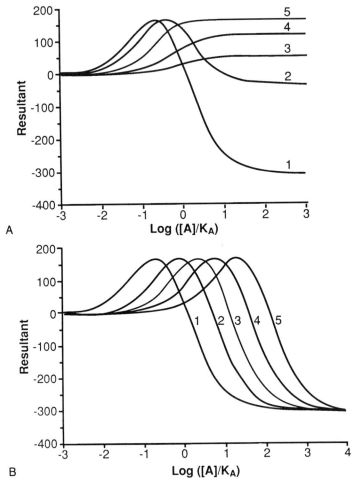

**FIG. 11.16.** Responses in a dual stimulus system (as shown in Fig. 11.15) calculated with Eq. 11.14. **A:** Effects of diminishing primary positive stimulus ($\rho_1$). Responses calculated with $N = 500$, $K = 30$, $L = 3$, and $M = 750$ (curve 1); 450 (curve 2); 150 (curve 3); 45 (curve 4); and 15 (curve 5). **B:** Effects of a competitive receptor antagonist on a biphasic response system. Response calculated with Eq. 11.14 with $M = 750$, $N = 500$, $K = 30$, $L = 30$ and in the absence (curve 1) and presence of competitive antagonist $[B]/K_B = 3$ (curve 2), 10 (curve 3), 30 (curve 4), and 100 (curve 5).

served experimentally. Figure 11.15A shows a biphasic dose-response curve to a pleiotropic response system with the constants defined in the figure legend. If an agonist has lower intrinsic efficacy and cannot generate a stimulus of sufficient strength to activate the secondary mechanism, then a single response pattern will be observed. Figure 11.15B shows the effect of a weaker agonist in which no biphasic curve is produced.

There are two characteristics of this type of dual stimulus-response model.

The first is the behavior of the dose-response curve to the alteration of the maximal initial stimulus, i.e., the efficacy of the agonist and the receptor density. Since the magnitude of the negative secondary stimulus is directly dependent on the magnitude of the initial receptor stimulus, reductions in driving power (i.e., agonist efficacy) or receptor number will also diminish the magnitude of the negative input. If, as is probable, the maximal output of the two systems ($M$ and $N$) and their sensitivity to the second messenger ($L$ and $K$) are not equal, then it would be unlikely that the two responses would diminish equally as efficacy and/or receptor number is reduced. Therefore, since the initial stimulus drives the secondary one, there should be an initial stimulus strength that produces only one of the responses. Figure 11.16A shows the effect of systematic decreases in the stimulus-producing power of the agonist on a pleiotropic system, as described by Eq. 11.14. Of note is the fact that the biphasic nature diminishes to a monophasic dose-response curve as the intrinsic efficacy of that agonist (reduction in $M$ in Eq. 11.14) decreases.

A second feature of biphasic systems controlled by a single receptor is the behavior of competitive antagonists. It would be predicted that blockade of the receptor for this effect would shift the dose-response curve to the right and preserve its biphasic nature (see Fig. 11.16B). This is because the biphasic response is a product of the initial stimulus and not the activation of a mixture of cell-surface receptors (see Fig. 11.14). For example, cholecystokinin (CCK) produces a biphasic response in guinea pig pancreatic acinar cells (Fig. 11.17A). Blockade of CCK receptors with the competitive antagonist proglumide analog 10 (CR 1409) produces parallel displacement of the dose-

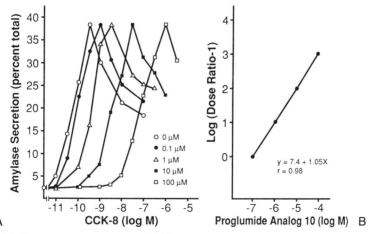

**FIG. 11.17.** Dose-response curves to CCK-8 in guinea pig acinar cells. **A:** Percentage of amylase secretion in the absence (0 µM) and presence of the CCK-8 receptor antagonist CR 1409 in the concentrations denoted in parentheses above each curve. **B:** Schild regression from the dose-response curves shown in A. (From ref. 28.)

response curves. Significantly, the biphasic nature of these dose-response curves is preserved in the same relative proportions throughout the concentration range of CCK. This suggests that the biphasic nature of the curve is related to the strength of the CCK stimulus and not a mixture of receptor subtypes. The simple competitive nature of the antagonism (Fig. 11.17B) further supports the involvement of a single receptor type mediating these two responses.

## CLASSIFICATIONS WITH ANTAGONISTS

As described in Chapter 9, measurement of the equilibrium dissociation constants for competitive antagonist-receptor complexes ($K_B$) theoretically is simpler than for agonists, because intrinsic efficacy is not a complication. Moreover, the Schild regression is a powerful tool with which to measure antagonist $K_B$ values. For these reasons, analyses with competitive antagonists have provided the framework on which most of the existing receptor classifications have been built. This section will discuss classification of drugs and receptors by the use of $K_B$ values, with the assumption that the Schild regressions are linear, with a slope of unity, i.e., that differences in antagonist potencies are not due to nonequilibrium steady states. These latter conditions were discussed in detail in Chapter 9.

There are basically two settings for analysis with competitive antagonists. The first relates to classification of receptors for agonists. For example, assume that two agonists, A and B, produce responses in a tissue, and the question is asked: Do these agonists activate a common receptor? In this case, the $pK_B$ for a competitive antagonist can be measured by Schild analysis with both agonists, and if the regressions are not different, then there is no evidence to suppose that agonists A and B do not activate the same receptor. The analysis of antagonism can be done conveniently by analysis of covariance of regression lines, because Schild analysis yields linearly related data. This is a distinct advantage over use of single $pK_B$ estimates, because much more information is used in the analysis. For example, a series of experiments was designed to study the efficiency of coupling of β-adrenoceptors in rat left atria. The agonists used were isoproterenol, prenalterol, pirbuterol, and terbutaline. Clearly, if receptor coupling was to be studied with these four agonists, it was essential to first determine that they produced responses in this tissue by activation of a common receptor. Therefore, Schild analysis with the selective $β_1$-adrenoceptor antagonist atenolol was conducted, and the question was asked: Does atenolol produce identical simple competitive antagonisms of responses to these four agonists in rat left atria? If the answer to this question was yes, then there was no reason to assume that the agonists activated anything other than $β_1$-adrenoceptors in these tissues to produce primary responses. Note this does not imply that no other receptors were present or that the agonists did not activate other

**TABLE 11.9.** *Analysis of covariance of multiple Schild regressions for atenolol*

| Log[atenolol] | $\log(dr - 1)$ | | | |
|---|---|---|---|---|
| | Isoproterenol (1) | Prenalterol (2) | Pirbuterol (3) | Terbutaline (4) |
| −6.5 | 1.12, 1.0, 1.0, 1.28, 0.9, 0.9 | 0.66 | 0.78, 0.84 | 0.95 |
| −6 | 1.64, 1.8, 1.3, 1.59, 1.0 | 1.38, 1.49 | 1.38, 1.38 | 1.28, 1.74 |
| −5.5 | 2.1, 1.89, 2.24 | 2.0, 2.1 | 2.0, 2.0 | 2.39, 1.84 |
| −5 | 2.84, 2.74, 2.54 | | | |
| $\sum y_i$ | 27.88 | 7.63 | 8.38 | 8.2 |
| $\sum y_i^2$ | 52.685 | 12.97 | 13.12 | 14.67 |
| $\sum xy_i$ | −159.15 | −44.06 | −49.09 | −47.56 |
| $n_i$ | 17 | 5 | 6 | 5 |
| $\sum x_i$ | −100.5 | −29.5 | −36 | −29.5 |
| $\sum x_i^2$ | 599.25 | 174.75 | 217 | 174.75 |
| $s_x^2$ | 5.18 | 0.7 | 1.0 | 0.7 |
| $s_{xy}$ | 5.67 | 0.96 | 1.19 | 0.82 |
| $s_y^2$ | 6.9618 | 1.33 | 1.42 | 1.22 |
| $m_i$ | 1.1 | 1.37 | 1.19 | 1.17 |
| $pA_{2i}$ | 7.39 | 7.0 | 7.17 | 7.3 |

receptors at doses greater than those required for the primary dose-response curve. Table 11.9 shows the data resulting from the analysis, and Fig. 11.18A shows the data points with corresponding separate Schild regressions. An analysis of covariance of multiple regression lines (according to Chapter 6) is shown in Table 11.10, and in this case no significant difference between the regressions was indicated. Thus, a common regression line (Fig. 11.18B) adequately describes the data, and no evidence is generated that the agonists activate anything other than $\beta_1$-adrenoceptors in this tissue.

The second major use of Schild analysis is for classification by antagonist potencies. Thus, an antagonist is found to have a unique $pK_B$ for a given receptor type and then is used to determine whether that receptor is present in other tissues. For example, propranolol has a $pK_B$ for $\beta$-adrenoceptors of 8.4. Therefore, if catecholamine responses in a tissue are antagonized by propranolol with a $pK_B$ of 8.4, then by implication the receptors mediating the catecholamine responses in that tissue will be $\beta$-adrenoceptors; i.e., there will be no evidence to suggest that they are not $\beta$-adrenoceptors. Thus, the $pK_B$ has a unique value for each receptor-antagonist pair. Differentiation

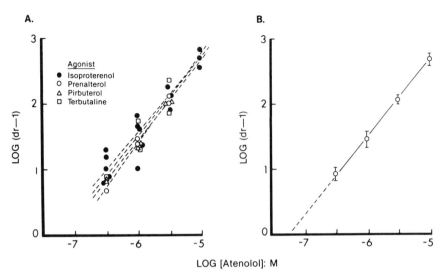

**FIG. 11.18.** Schild regressions for atenolol antagonism of rat left atrial responses to iso-proterenol, prenalterol, pirbuterol, and terbutaline. Ordinate: Logarithms of equiactive dose ratios for agonists in the presence and absence of atenolol − 1. Abscissae: Logarithms of molar concentrations of atenolol. **A:** *Broken lines* indicate individual best-fit linear regressions for the four agonists; data describing these regressions given in Table 11.9. **B:** All data points averaged for each concentration of atenolol, and the best-fit common Schild regression for all of the points is shown. Slope = 1.1; p$K_B$ = 7.25. (From T. P. Kenakin and M. S. McIntyre, *unpublished data.*)

**TABLE 11.10.** *Differences in slopes and elevations for data in Table 11.9*

| | SSq | d.f. | MSq |
|---|---|---|---|
| $F_{slope}$ = 0.4, d.f. = 3, 25 (n.s.) | | | |
| Differences in slope | | | |
| Due to common slope | 9.85 | 1 | |
| Differences between slopes | 0.05 | 3 | 0.0165 |
| Residual | 1.032 | 20 | 0.04128 |

| | $S_x^2$ | $S_{xy}$ | $S_y^2$ | SSq | d.f. | MSq |
|---|---|---|---|---|---|---|
| $F_{elev}$ = 1.26, d.f. = 3, 28 (n.s.) | | | | | | |
| Differences in elevation | | | | | | |
| Within groups | 7.52 | 8.64 | 10.93 | 1.003 | 28 | 0.036 |
| Total | 7.56 | 8.73 | 11.22 | 1.14 | | |
| Between groups | | | | 0.136 | 3 | 0.0453 |

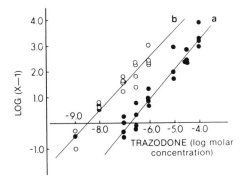

**FIG. 11.19.** Schild regressions for trazodone-induced antagonism of serotonin responses in rat uterus (o) and rat stomach strip (•). Ordinate and abscissa as for Fig. 11.18, with serotonin as the agonist. Slope for rat uterus = 0.99 (0.85–1.15); $pA_2$ = 8.49 (8.28–8.78). Slope for rat stomach strip = 1.19 (1.02–1.31); $pA_2$ = 6.74 (6.5–7.0). (From ref. 30.)

of receptors in tissues by means of antagonism also can utilize analysis of covariance of Schild regressions. Figure 11.19 shows Schild regressions for trazodone as an antagonist of serotonin responses in rat uterus and stomach strip. A relevant question would be: Are the receptors for serotonin the same in these two tissues? One approach to this question would be to analyze whether the potencies of trazodone as an antagonist of serotonin in these two tissues were the same; an analysis of covariance of the two Schild regressions can be used. The data are shown in Table 11.11, and the analysis of

**TABLE 11.11.** *Analysis of covariance for Schild regressions for trazodone antagonism of 5-HT responses (Fig. 11.18)[a]*

| log[trazodone] (M) | Rat [$\log(dr - 1)$] | | | | | | | |
|---|---|---|---|---|---|---|---|---|
| | Uterus [$\log(dr - 1)$] | | | | Stomach strip [$\log(dr - 1)$] | | | |
| −9.0 | −0.33, | −0.48, | −1.0 | | | | | |
| −8.0 | 0.53, | 0.65, | 0.7, | 0.8 | | | | |
| −7.0 | 1.25, | 1.55, | 1.67, | 1.8 | −0.55, | −0.36, | 0 | 0.24 |
| −6.5 | 2.3, | 2.1, | 1.84, | 1.4 | 0.8, | 0.36, | −0.1, | −0.24 |
| −6.0 | 3.0, | 2.44, | 2.3, | 2.26 | 1.36, | 0.95, | 0.85, | 0.8 |
| −5.0 | | | | | 3.0, | 2.0, | 2.0, | 1.73 |
| −4.5 | | | | | 2.86, | 2.38, | 2.38, | 2.38 |
| −4.0 | | | | | 3.93, | 3.33, | 3.2, | 3.0 |

| Uterus | | Stomach strip | |
|---|---|---|---|
| $x_1$ = log[trazodone] | | $x_2$ = log[trazodone] | |
| $y_1$ = log(dr − 1), uterus | | $y_2$ = log(dr − 1), stomach strip | |
| $\sum x_1 = -137$, | $\sum y_1 = 24.78$ | $\sum x_2 = -132$, | $\sum y_2 = 36.3$ |
| $\sum x_1^2 = 1{,}008$, | $\sum y_1^2 = 53.56$ | $\sum x_2^2 = 754$, | $\sum y_2^2 = 96.38$ |
| $n_1 = 19$, | $\sum xy_1 = -158.7$ | $n_2 = 24$, | $\sum xy_2 = -166.9$ |

[a] Data from ref. 30.

**TABLE 11.12.** *Calculation of analysis of covariance for trazodone Schild regressions*

|   |   | d.f. | $s_x^2$ | $s_{xy}$ | $s_y^2$ | d.f. | SSq | MSq |
|---|---|---|---|---|---|---|---|---|
| 1. | Within |  |  |  |  |  |  |  |
|   | Uterus | 18 | 20.16 | 19.98 | 21.24 | 17 | 1.44 |  |
|   | S. strip | 23 | 28 | 32.75 | 41.48 | 22 | 3.17 |  |
|   |  |  |  |  |  | 39 | 4.61 | 0.118 |
| 2. | Pooled | 41 | 48.16 | 52.73 | 62.72 | 40 | 4.99 | 0.125 |
|   |  |  |  |  |  | 1 | 0.38 | 0.38 |
| 3. | Overall | 42 | 79.19 | 56.5 | 63.18 | 41 | 22.86 |  |
|   |  |  |  |  |  | 1 | 17.87 | 17.87 |

Note: $F_{slope} = 0.38 \div 0.118 = 3.22$, d.f. $= 1, 39$; $F_{elevation} = 17.87 \div 0.125 = 142.96$, d.f. $= 1, 40$. .

covariance of regression lines is shown in Table 11.12. In this case, there is a highly significant difference between the potencies of trazodone in the two tissues, providing evidence to disprove the null hypothesis that the serotonin receptors in these two tissues are the same.

As pointed out in Chapter 9, observance of a linear Schild regression with unit slope constitutes evidence for simple competitive antagonism and also indicates that the calculated $K_B$ is a true representation of the equilibrium dissociation constant for the antagonist-receptor complex. However, there is a particular nonequilibrium steady state that warrants concern in such studies because it produces a linear Schild regression with unit slope, but an incorrect $pK_B$. This occurs when tissues are pretreated with drugs to induce agonist-receptor thermodynamic equilibria (i.e., uptake and degradation blockers) that themselves also block the receptors for the agonist. Discussed in Chapter 9, such drugs produce underestimations of antagonist potencies, because the control dose-response curve is already shifted to the right by a factor of $[B_U]/K_{BU} + 1$, where $[B_U]$ is the molar concentration of uptake blocker, and $K_{BU}$ is the equilibrium dissociation constant for the uptake-blocker-receptor complex (Fig. 11.20A). The observed dose ratios ($dr_{ob}$) for the antagonist $[B]$ in such a situation conforms to the following equation:

$$\log(dr_{ob} - 1) = \log[B] - \log K_B - \log\left(\frac{[B_U]}{K_{BU}} + 1\right) \quad [11.15]$$

The notable feature of this complication is that no alterations in slope occur, but rather the calculated $K_B$ is underestimated by a factor of $[B_U]/K_{BU} + 1$ (i.e., the Schild regression is shifted to the right along the $\log[B]$ axis). One example of this effect is shown in Fig. 11.20B, where the amitriptyline, a blocker of both the neuronal uptake of norepinephrine and $\alpha$-adrenoceptors, is used as a pretreatment for rat anococcygeus muscle in the Schild analysis of phentolamine. The resulting Schild regressions in the presence of amitrip-

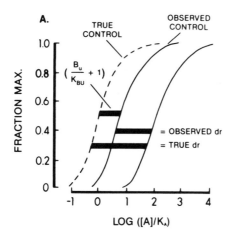

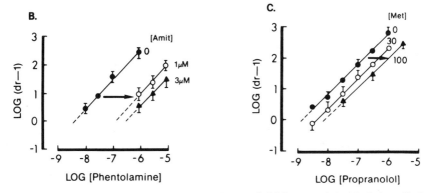

**FIG. 11.20.** Effects of prior receptor antagonism on Schild regressions. **A:** A drug $B_U$ that has appreciable receptor-blocking properties is equilibrated with the tissue as a pretreatment to attain equilibrium conditions; drug $B_U$ shifts the true dose-response curve (*broken line*) to the right by a factor of $[B_U]/K_{BU} + 1$. The tissue then is equilibrated with antagonist [B], and the dose ratio is measured from the *already shifted* control dose-response curve. The observed dose ratio ($dr_{ob}$) is an underestimation of the true dose ratio. **B:** Dextral displacement of the true Schild regression for the $\alpha$-adrenoceptor antagonist phentolamine in rat anococcygeus muscle by preequilibration of the tissue with amitriptyline (Amit), a drug with appreciable $\alpha$-adrenoceptor-blocking properties. Regressions in the absence ($\bullet$, $N = 13$) and presence of amitriptyline at 1 ($\circ$, $N = 9$) and 3 $\mu$M ($\blacktriangle$, $N = 9$). **C:** Dextral displacement of true Schild regression for the $\beta$-adrenoceptor antagonist propranolol in guinea pig trachea by the extraneuronal uptake blocker metanephrine (Met), a drug with appreciable $\beta$-blocking properties. Regressions in the absence ($\bullet$, $N = 15$) and presence of metanephrine at 30 ($\circ$, $N = 13$) and 100 $\mu$M ($\blacktriangle$, $N = 9$). (B and C from ref. 20.)

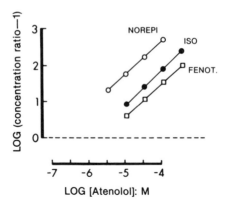

**FIG. 11.21.** Effects of heterogeneous receptor populations on Schild regressions. Schild regressions for atenolol in guinea pig ileum. Agonists used were norepinephrine (o, NOR-EPI), isoproterenol (•, ISO), and fenoterol (□, FENOT.). (From ref. 25.)

tyline are shifted to the right of the true regression for phentolamine. A similar effect is seen with metanephrine, a drug sometimes used to block extraneuronal uptake of catecholamines. This uptake blocker has $\beta$-adreno-ceptor-blocking properties that shift the Schild regression for propranolol in guinea pig trachea to the right of the true regression (Fig. 11.20C).

Complex effects can be observed with antagonists when agonists activate heterogeneous receptor populations to produce tissue responses; these really cannot be classed as nonequilibrium steady states, because the antagonist and agonist are in thermodynamic equilibrium with two receptors for which they have different activities. The effects on Schild regressions in heteroge-neous receptor systems are discussed in some detail in Chapter 9. However, it is worth reiterating that if a definitely nonlinear Schild regression is ob-served under equilibrium conditions, then agonist activation of a heterogene-ous receptor population is implicated. There are two features of such systems that warrant comment. The first relates to confirmation of receptor heteroge-neity. If two (or more) receptors are stimulated by the agonist, then the location of the Schild regression (i.e., apparent $pA_2$) should change when a different agonist is used to produce a response (unless the unlikely event occurs that both agonists have exactly the same relative affinities and efficac-ies for the two receptors). Figure 11.21 shows Schild regressions for the $\beta_1$-adrenoceptor-selective antagonist atenolol in guinea pig trachea, a tissue with a mixed $\beta_1/\beta_2$-adrenoceptor population. Considerable differences in the regressions are observed when different agonists (with different relative ac-tivities on $\beta_1$- and $\beta_2$-adrenoceptors) are used.

In general, classification of receptors and agonists by Schild analysis (and statistical methods to compare and analyze linear regressions) is a most use-ful and versatile process.

## REFERENCES

1. Ariëns, E. J., Beld, A. J., De Miranda, J. F. R., and Simmonis, A. M. (1979): The pharmacon-receptor-effector concept. A basis for understanding the transmission of information in biological systems. In: *The Receptors, A Comprehensive Treatise*, edited by R. D. O'Brien, pp. 33–91. Plenum Press, New York.
2. Black, J. W. (1981): Receptors in the future. *Postgrad. Med. J.*, 57:110–112.
3. Black, J. W. (1982): Receptor function and control. In: *Catecholamines in the Non-ischaemic and Ischaemic Myocardium*, edited by R. Riemersma and W. Oliver, pp. 3–12. Elsevier/North Holland, Amsterdam.
4. Cohen, M. L., and Wiley, K. S. (1977): Comparison of arteries with longitudinal and circular venous muscle from the rat. *Am. J. Physiol.*, 232:H131–H139.
5. Cohen, M. L., and Wiley, K. S. (1977): Specific enhancement of norepinephrine-induced contraction in rat veins after beta adrenergic antagonists. *J. Pharmacol. Exp. Ther.*, 201:406–416.
6. Colquhoun, D. (1971): *Lectures in Biostatistics*. Clarendon Press, Oxford.
7. Costa, T., Klinz, F-J., Vachon, L., and Herz, A. (1988): Opioid receptors are coupled tightly to G proteins but loosely to adenylate cyclase in NG108-15 cell membranes. *Mol. Pharmacol.*, 34:744–754.
8. Finney, D. J. (1955): *Experimental Design and Its Statistical Basis*. University of Chicago Press.
9. Furchgott, R. F. (1954): Dibenamine blockade in strips of rabbit aorta and its use in differentiating receptors. *J. Pharmacol. Exp. Ther.*, 111:265–284.
10. Furchgott, R. F. (1966): The use of β-haloaklylamines in the differentiation of receptors and in the determination of dissociation constants of receptor-agonist complexes. In: *Advances in Drug Research, Vol. 3*, edited by N. J. Harper and A. B. Simmonds, pp. 21–55. Academic Press, New York.
11. Furchgott, R. F. (1978): Pharmacological characterization of receptors. Its relation to radioligand-binding studies. *Fed. Proc.*, 37:115–120.
12. Kenakin, T. P. (1982): The Schild regression in the process of receptor classification. *Can. J. Physiol. Pharmacol.*, 60:249–265.
13. Kenakin, T. P. (1982): Theoretical and practical problems with the assessment of intrinsic efficacy of agonists: Efficacy of reputed beta-1 selective adrenoceptor agonists for beta-2 adrenoceptors. *J. Pharmacol. Exp. Ther.*, 223:416–423.
14. Kenakin, T. P. (1982): Organ selectivity of drugs. Alternatives to receptor selectivity. *Trends Pharmacol. Sci.*, 3:153–156.
15. Kenakin, T. P. (1984): The classification of drugs and drug receptors in isolated tissues. *Pharmacol. Rev.*, 36:165–221.
16. Kenakin, T. P. (1988): Are receptors promiscuous? Intrinsic efficacy as a transduction phenomenon. *Life Sci.*, 43:1095–1101.
17. Kenakin, T. P. (1989): Challenges for receptor theory as a tool for drug and drug receptor classification. *Trends Pharmacol. Sci.*, 10:18–22.
18. Kenakin, T. P., and Morgan, P. H. (1989): Theoretical aspects of single and multiple transducer receptor coupling proteins on estimates of relative potency of agonists. *Mol. Pharmacol.*, 35:214–222.
19. Kenakin, T. P., and Pike, N. B. (1987): An in vitro analysis of purine-mediated renal vasoconstriction in rat isolated kidney. *Br. J. Pharmacol.*, 90:373–381.
20. Kenakin, T. P., and Beek, D. (1981): The measurement of antagonist potency and the importance of selective inhibition of agonist uptake processes. *J. Pharmacol. Exp. Ther.*, 219:112–120.
21. Kenakin, T. P., and Beek, D. (1982): In vitro studies on the cardiac activity of prenalterol with reference to use in congestive heart failure. *J. Pharmacol. Exp. Ther.*, 220:77–85.
22. Lemoine, H., and Kaumann, A. J. (1983): A model for the interaction of competitive antagonists with two receptor subtypes characterized by a Schild plot with apparent slope unity. *Naunyn Schmeidebergs Arch. Pharmacol.*, 322:111–120.
23. Maayani, S., Wilkinson, C. W., and Stollak, J. S. (1984): 5-Hydroxytryptamine receptor in rabbit aorta: Characterization by butyrophenone analogs. *J. Pharmacol. Exp. Ther.*, 229:346–350.

24. McPherson, G. A., Molenaar, P., and Malta, E. (1985): The affinity and efficacy of naturally occurring catecholamines at β-adrenoceptor subtypes. *J. Pharm. Pharmacol.*, 37:499–501.
25. O'Donnell, S. R., and Wanstall, J. C. (1979): The importance of choice of agonist in studies designed to predict $\beta_2:\beta_1$ adrenoceptor selectivity of antagonists from $pA_2$ values on guinea-pig trachea and atria. *Naunyn Schmeidebergs Arch. Pharmacol.*, 308:183–190.
26. Patil, P. N., Patel, D. G., and Krell, R. D. (1971): Steric aspects of adrenergic drugs. XV. Use of isomeric activity ratio as a criterion to differentiate adrenergic receptors. *J. Pharmacol. Exp. Ther.*, 176:622–633.
27. Regoli, D., Park, W. K., and Rioux, F. (1974): Pharmacology of angiotensin. *Pharmacol. Rev.*, 26:69–123.
28. Vinayek, R., and Gardner, J. D. (1990): Receptor identification. In: *Biomembranes. Part V: Cellular and Subcellular Transport: Epithelial Cells. Methods in Enzymology, Vol. 191*, edited by S. Fleischer and B. Fleischer, pp. 609–639. Academic Press, New York.
29. Waud, D. R. (1968): Pharmacological receptors. *Pharmacol. Rev.*, 20:49–88.
30. Wrigglesworth, S. J. (1983): Heterogeneity of 5-hydroxytryptamine receptors in the rat uterus and stomach strip. *Br. J. Pharmacol.*, 80:691–697.

# 12

## Radioligand Binding Experiments

*Corpora non agunt nisi fixata [substances do not act unless bound].*
—PAUL EHRLICH, 1913

Until now, the indirect study of drug-receptor interaction has been emphasized. Data from functional studies with isolated tissues have unique advantages, as outlined in Chapter 3. However, there also are advantages to the direct study of ligand-receptor interactions, the major one being the ability to quantify the amount of drug-receptor complex ($[A \cdot R]$) without having to infer this quantity via null procedures in functional systems. However, it will be axiomatic that the biochemical procedures required to isolate and measure receptor binding *may* overlay an unphysiological aspect to the reactions; i.e., the biochemically characterized receptor may bear little resemblance to the receptor in the cell membrane of a functioning organ. This chapter discusses the measurement of reaction products at equilibrium. A further discussion of binding techniques for the determination of drug-receptor kinetics is given in the following chapter.

### DRUG-BINDING MODELS

It can be shown that the amount of drug bound ($[B]$) when a concentration $[A]$ of drug is brought into contact with $n$ binding sites is:

$$[B] = \frac{K_1 \cdot [A] + 2K_1 K_2 \cdot [A]^2 + 3K_1 K_2 K_3 \cdot [A]^3 \ldots + \ldots n \cdot K_1 \cdot K_2 \cdot K_3 \ldots \ldots K_n [A]^n}{1 + K_1 \cdot [A] + K_1 K_2 \cdot [A]^2 + K_1 K_2 K_3 \cdot [A]^3 \ldots + \ldots K_1 \cdot K_2 \cdot K_3 \ldots \ldots K_n [A]^n}$$

$$[12.1]$$

where $K_1$, $K_2$, $K_3$, . . . , $K_n$ are the stoichiometric equilibrium constants for binding of $[A]$ to each site. Equation 12.1 is valid if the affinity of $[A]$ is

different or the same for all sites, where there is positive or negative cooperativity, and when all of the sites are identical (i.e., binding of $[A]$ to a single
receptor population). In this latter instance $K_1 = K_2 = K_3 \ldots = K_n = K$
and Eq. 12.1 can be rewritten:

$$[B] = \frac{K \cdot [A] (1 + 2K \cdot [A] + 3K^2 \cdot [A]^2 + n \cdot K^{n-1} \cdot [A]^{n-1})}{1 + K \cdot [A] (1 + K \cdot [A] + K^2 \cdot [A]^2 + K^{n-1} \cdot [A]^{n-1})} \qquad [12.2]$$

Division of the numerator and denominator by $[A]^{n-1} K^{n-1}$ and assuming
that $1/[A]^{n-1} K^{n-1} \to 0$ yields:

$$[B] = \frac{[A] \cdot K \cdot n}{[A] \cdot K (1/[A] \cdot K + 1)} \qquad [12.3]$$

which simplifies to the well-known Langmuir adsorption isotherm for binding
to $n$ number of independent sites:

$$[B] = \frac{[A] \cdot K \cdot n}{1 + [A] \cdot K} \qquad [12.4]$$

where $K$ is the affinity constant defined as the rate of onset to the site divided
by the rate of offset from the site ($k_1/k_2$). Equation 12.4 is a mathematical
form for the description of a drug binding to $n$ identical sites with independent
and uniform affinity for each, i.e., the binding of a drug to one site does not
affect the binding of a drug to another site. A second model used frequently
in radioligand experiments is the binding of a drug to two independent and
noninteractive sites. Under these circumstances, binding is described by:

$$[B] = \frac{K_1 \cdot [A] \cdot n_1}{1 + K_1 \cdot [A]} + \frac{K_2 \cdot [A] \cdot n_2}{1 + K_2 \cdot [A]} \qquad [12.5]$$

where $n_1$ and $n_2$ refer to the two populations of binding sites and $K_1$ and $K_2$
the respective affinity constants for each site. It should be stressed that the
absence of cooperative effects and independence of binding between sites is
*assumed* with the use of this model. The fitting of binding data to an equation
of the form of Eq. 12.5 does not necessarily imply the presence of two independent binding sites $n_1$ and $n_2$. For example, it can be shown algebraically
that Eq. 12.1 of degree $n$ can be put into the form:

$$[B] = \frac{k_\alpha \cdot [A]}{1 + k_\alpha \cdot [A]} + \frac{k_\beta \cdot [A]}{1 + k_\beta \cdot [A]} + \frac{K_\sigma \cdot [A]}{1 + K_\sigma \cdot [A]} \qquad [12.6]$$

with a total of $n$ terms. When $n = 2$, Eq. 12.6 formally resembles Eq. 12.5
for two independent sites. However, the constants (e.g., $k_\alpha$, $k_\beta$) are *not* site-
binding constants but rather complex combinations of the actual binding
constants for the various sites (termed simulator binding constants). Therefore, good agreement of binding data to curves described by a two-term
adsorption isotherm such as Eq. 12.6 does not prove the existence of two

**TABLE 12.1.** *Constants for carbamyl phosphate binding to aspartate transcarbamylase*

| | |
|---|---|
| A. Stoichiometric binding constants (Eq. 12.1) | |
| $K_1 = 1.45 \times 10^6$ | $K_4 = 0.376 \times 10^5$ |
| $K_2 = 0.403 \times 10^6$ | $K_5 = 0.151 \times 10^5$ |
| $K_3 = 0.104 \times 10^6$ | $K_6 = 0.821 \times 10^4$ |
| B. Simulator binding constants (Eq. 12.6) | |
| $k_\alpha = 0.884 \times 10^6$ | $k_\epsilon = 0.259 \times 10^5$ |
| $k_\beta = 0.488 \times 10^6$ | $k_\phi = 0.218 \times 10^5$ |
| $k_\delta = 0.522 \times 10^5$ | $k_\gamma = 0.201 \times 10^5$ |

From ref. 12.

independent binding sites. For example, it is known that 6 M of carbamyl phosphate are bound per mole of aspartate transcarbamylase (i.e., there are six binding sites on the enzyme). Analysis of the binding with equation to the sixth power yields six binding constants (shown in Table 12.1A). The analysis can also be done with the alternative algebraic form of Eq. 12.1, namely, a six-term equivalent form of Eq. 12.6. This second analysis yields six simulator binding constants, shown in Table 12.1B. Considering experimental error, it would not be unreasonable to group simulator constants $k_\alpha$ and $k_\beta$ and constants $k_\delta$ to $k_\gamma$ into two groups and describe the binding with a two-term adsorption isotherm of the form of Eq. 12.6. In fact, a two-term equation fits the data very well. Therefore, although the statistical fitting of the data would be adequate with a two-term adsorption isotherm, the conclusion that there are two binding sites on aspartate transcarbamylase would be erroneous. In general, it is advisable to base binding models more on molecular mechanisms than on statistical fitting of the data. It will be assumed throughout this chapter that there is independent experimental evidence available to rationalize the use of single or multiple receptor-site models and that these are not utilized simply for reasons of statistical fit.

## DRUG BINDING

The major advantage of radioligand binding experiments is the ability to test the validity of the Langmuir binding isotherm model to the actual drug-receptor interactions observed experimentally. Thus, the production of the drug-receptor complex ($[A \cdot R]$) should be governed by the concentration of free ligand ($[A_f]$) and total unbound receptor ($[R_t]$) by the equations described in Chapters 1 and 7. It should be noted that the previous discussion on drug binding models uses affinity constants ($k_1/k_2$) for clarity of presentation, whereas the following discussion uses the more pharmacologically familiar equilibrium dissociation constants for depiction of binding activity ($k_2/k_1$, the reciprocal of the affinity constant):

$$[A \cdot R] = \frac{[A_f] \, [R_t]}{[A_f] + K_A} \qquad [12.7]$$

where $K_A$ is the equilibrium dissociation constant of the $[A \cdot R]$ complex. In general there are two types of radioligand binding experiments done to estimate the magnitude of $K_A$. The first is the saturation experiment, which requires a radioactive analogue of drug $[A]$ (denoted $[A^*]$) and measures the production of $[A^* \cdot R]$ directly. This is done by isolating this complex biochemically and measuring the difference between the amount of $[A^*]$ added and the amount of $[A^*]$ bound to the receptor. A second type of experiment is the displacement experiment in which a fixed quantity of radioactive drug is added to the receptor preparation (to produce an equilibrium quantity of $[A^* \cdot R]$ complex) and then another drug is added in fixed amounts to displace the radioactive ligand. Under these circumstances, assuming strict competitiveness, the affinity of the nonradioactive drug can be calculated by observing its potency as an antagonist of the radioactive ligand. For both of these approaches, the definition of "specific" binding of ligand to only the receptor sites is essential. Ideally, a nonradioactive compound known to bind to the same receptor population as the radioactive ligand but with a different chemical structure should be used to displace the radioactive ligand. This is because the radioactive ligand most likely will bind to the receptor sites as well as populations of other sites not related to the receptor (i.e., "nonspecific" binding). If the nonradioactive displacing drug is the same as the radioligand, then the receptors *and* the nonreceptor sites may tend to be defined as specific (receptor) binding. A different chemical structure for the nonradioactive displacing drug may reduce the common binding to the receptor population and thus reduce the measured nonspecific binding (see Fig. 12.1).

## Saturation Curves

A dose-response curve can be obtained with a radioactive ligand in a receptor system when the complex between the ligand and the receptor ($[A^* \cdot R]$) is isolated and quantified. The various methodological problems with the quantification of $[A \cdot R]$ complexes have been discussed at length elsewhere (1,3,4,13); thus it will be assumed that the practical obstacles to the measurement of radioligand binding have been considered. These are similar to those encountered in isolated tissue experiments, namely, the assumptions that a single site interaction of drug and receptor is being studied, that temporal equilibrium is achieved within the time span of the experiment, and that the concentration of either the receptor and/or the ligand is not altered during the experiment. In general, these obstacles may be less important than those

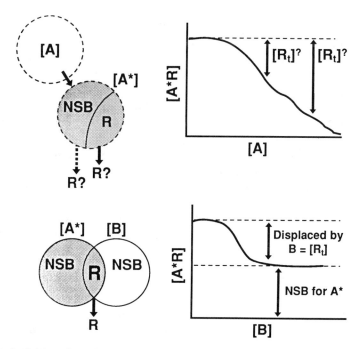

**FIG. 12.1.** Definition of specific binding of a radioactive ligand [A*] by excess nonradioactive [A] may define nonreceptor sites as receptors. Definition of specific binding by a chemically nonrelated receptor ligand may eliminate problems with [A*] binding to nonreceptor sites.

encountered in isolated tissue experiments because the experimental conditions of binding reactions can be more stringently controlled. The other side of this apparent advantage, however, is the fact that the manipulations required to achieve these conditions may make the resulting interactions less physiologically relevant.

Theoretically a saturation curve can be an experimental verification of the Langmuir adsorption isotherm of a substance binding to a surface (membrane-bound receptor). Thus, various concentrations of radioactive ligand [A*] are equilibrated with a given concentration of receptor and the resulting bound fraction (presumably [A*·R]) is measured by isolation of the protein bound ligand. As discussed above, it is well-known that many ligands bind to sites other than physiological receptors; thus parallel measurements in the presence of a specified concentration of nonradioactive ligand, assumed to bind to more than 99% of the receptors, are made. The difference is assumed to be specific binding of the radioactive ligand to the receptor population in the membrane preparation. The residual radioactivity not displaced by the excess nonradioactive ligand is assumed to represent nonspecific binding of the ligand to nonreceptor sites. It can be seen from this approach that the definition of specific binding is critical to these experiments since this defines the magnitude of the dependent variable, i.e., the response in functional experiments. Therefore, a fundamental difference in binding and functional experiments is the fact that the dependent variable in radioligand experiments is defined to a much greater extent than it is in functional ones in which essentially it is observed. The specific binding can be estimated by mathematical models that assume that specific binding is saturable (and thus defined by the Langmuir adsorption isotherm) and that nonspecific binding is nonsaturable and a linear function of ligand concentration. Under these circumstances, a curve representing total binding of ligand to a membrane preparation can be dissected into the receptor and nonspecific site binding portions. A more reliable estimate can be gained from the experimental estimation of nonspecific binding by the simultaneous measurement of ligand binding in the absence and presence of a nonradioactive ligand in sufficient quantity to occupy, for example, 99% of the receptors (i.e., $100 \times K_A$). Under these conditions, a simultaneous curve fitting of the total binding and the nonspecific binding can furnish a maximum number of measurements for the estimation of the quantity of $[A^* \cdot R]$ complex. A simultaneous curve-fitting procedure of the total binding (TB) and nonspecific binding (NSB) to the following equations will yield the parameters $a$ and $b$ of the saturable binding:

$$\text{TB} = \frac{a[A]}{b + [A]} + c[A] \qquad\qquad [12.8]$$

$$\text{NSB} = c[A] \qquad\qquad [12.9]$$

A detailed description of how the simultaneous fitting of Eqs. 12.8 and 12.9 to binding data allows the best determination of specific binding is given in Chapter 6 in the section on nonlinear curve fitting.

Saturation experiments allow the determination of the density of receptor sites (specific binding sites) under certain circumstances. Specifically, the maximum $[A^* \cdot R]$ measured equals the number of binding sites, but this value is impossible to obtain precisely (i.e., only when $[A^* \cdot R]$ equals infinity) and requires rigorous data even to estimate. The various forms of saturation curves are shown in Chapter 6, where it can be seen that what apparently is saturation on a linear abscissal scale may be far from saturation when viewed on a logarithmic scale (Fig. 6.14A versus B). In practical terms it may be difficult to obtain saturation since one usually is dealing with large numbers of radioactive counts and the difference between two large numbers, both subject to error, may be imprecise. The utilization of simultaneous fitting of total and nonspecific binding equations helps to reduce the impact of this problem.

A common transformation of saturation binding curves is the Scatchard plot (17). The adsorption isotherm is linearized by cross-multiplying the terms of Eq. 12.7 and dividing by $[A^*] \cdot K_A$. Thus, Eq. 12.7 becomes:

$$\frac{[A^* \cdot R]}{[A^*]} = \frac{[A^* \cdot R]}{K_A} + \frac{[R_t]}{K_A} \qquad [12.10]$$

A regression of specific binding (presumably $[A^* \cdot R]$), divided by the free concentration of radioactive ligand upon the bound specific binding, should yield a straight line with a slope of $K_A^{-1}$ and a y-intercept as an estimation of $[R_t]$. A major disadvantage in the Scatchard plot is the fact that it transforms data and thus distorts experimental error. This becomes especially a problem in Scatchard graphs since the y-axis combines dependent and independent variables. Moreover, Scatchard plots compress data at both ends of the regression with the result that estimates of $[R_t]$ by this method may be far short of true saturation. For example, Figure 12.2 shows saturation data in the form of a Scatchard plot and semilogarithmic saturation curve. It can be seen from this example that the abscissal intercept on the Scatchard graph is a poor representation of the true maximal number of binding sites. The Scatchard plot has been a useful indicator of complex binding phenomena, possible multiple binding sites, and methodological problems (e.g., deviations from equilibria). However, as is common with other transforms, the Scatchard plot is sensitive to bias in the data and often can be curvilinear simply because of statistical factors. For this reason, and with the advent of computer programs to fit nontransformed data to models, reliance on Scatchard plots now is less common.

## DISPLACEMENT CURVES

Another approach to the measurement of ligand affinity for receptors is with the displacement experiment. In these, a fixed quantity of radioactive ligand is equilibrated with the receptor preparation and then a range of concentrations of another ligand (which binds to the same receptor) is added to the medium. As the nonradioactive ligand displaces the radioactive one, the radioactivity associated with the receptor is reduced. Thus, the nonradioactive ligand $[B]$ competes with the radioactive ligand $[A^*]$ according to the standard equation for competitiveness (see Eq. 9.9):

$$[A^* \cdot R] = \frac{[A^*] \cdot [R_t]}{[A^*] + K_A (1 + [B]/K_B)} \qquad [12.11]$$

Figure 12.3 shows a saturation curve for the radioactive ligand and effects of a simple competitor on the saturation curve at various concentrations (dextral parallel displacement). This figure also shows the amount of radioactive complex ($[A^* \cdot R]$) produced by a concentration of radioactive ligand $[A^*]$ equal to the $K_A$ in absence and presence of various concentrations of nonradioactive competing ligand $[A]$. Such displacement-curve data can be fit to

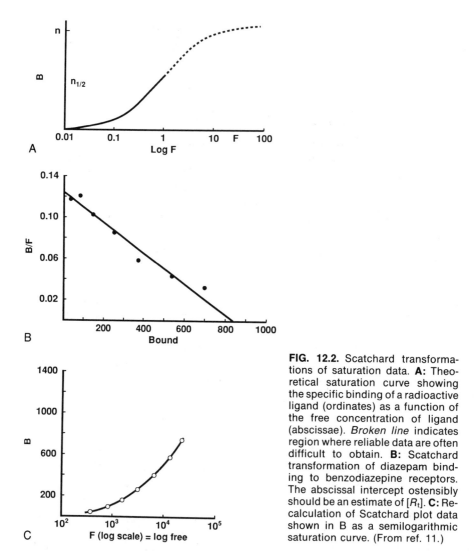

**FIG. 12.2.** Scatchard transformations of saturation data. **A:** Theoretical saturation curve showing the specific binding of a radioactive ligand (ordinates) as a function of the free concentration of ligand (abscissae). *Broken line* indicates region where reliable data are often difficult to obtain. **B:** Scatchard transformation of diazepam binding to benzodiazepine receptors. The abscissal intercept ostensibly should be an estimate of $[R_t]$. **C:** Recalculation of Scatchard plot data shown in B as a semilogarithmic saturation curve. (From ref. 11.)

Eq. 12.11 and, providing there is an accurate estimate of $K_A^*$, the $K_A$ for the nonradioactive ligand can be obtained.

## EFFECTS OF PROTEIN CONCENTRATION $[R_t]$

A common practical problem encountered experimentally is the effect of receptor concentration on the estimated parameters by both of these methods. In isolated tissue experiments conducted in large organ baths, the quan-

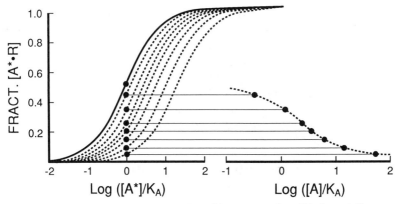

**FIG. 12.3.** Displacement of a radioactive ligand by a nonradioactive ligand. Curve on the left shows a saturation binding curve for a radioactive ligand. *Dotted lines* show this curve shifted by various concentrations of nonradioactive competitive antagonist. The points on the dotted curves show the radioactivity ([A*·R]) observed for one concentration of radioactive ligand in the presence of the competitive antagonist concentrations. These values for [A*·R], when plotted as a function of the concentration of competitive antagonist present in the medium, produce the displacement curve shown on the left.

tity of drug [A] bound to the receptor population usually is insignificant compared with the total pool of drug available in the bathing medium (see Chapter 5). Also, the presence of amplification mechanisms for receptor stimulus production into tissue response usually ensures that a small concentration of drug is required for the production of a measurable dependent variable (i.e., physiological response). In contrast, radioligand binding experiments elicit a constant signal (the disintegration of a radioactive ligand); therefore the strength of the signal is directly proportional to the density of the receptors. Also, the inevitable binding of the drug to other sites not physiologically relevant to the production of tissue response (i.e., nonspecific binding) makes the signal-to-noise ratio in binding experiments very important. One way to increase the strength of the signal in binding experiments is by increasing the density of receptors ($[R_t]$). However, indiscriminant increases in the concentration of receptor may invalidate Eq. 12.7 in terms of describing the binding reaction. Specifically, the concentration of drug [A] in Eq. 12.7 is assumed to be the *free* concentration available for stochastic interactions with free receptors at any instant. If the quantity of receptor is sufficiently large, such that binding of drug to the receptor *depletes* the available concentration of drug for binding to free receptors, then Eq. 12.7 becomes invalid. Specifically,

$$[A_f^*] = [A_t^*] - [A^* \cdot R] \qquad [12.12]$$

where $[A_t^*]$ refers to the total concentration of $[A^*]$ added to the medium. It can be seen from this equation that if the amount of drug binding to the receptor (the quantity of $[A^* \cdot R]$) is less than $[A_t^*]$, then $[A_t^*]$ approximates $[A_f^*]$. However, if $[A^* \cdot R]$ cannot be ignored, then Eq. 12.7 must be rewritten:

$$[A^* \cdot R] = \frac{([A_t^*] - [A^* \cdot R])\,[R_t]}{([A_t^*] - [A^* \cdot R]) + K_A} \qquad [12.13]$$

One solution for $[A^* \cdot R]$ in Eq. 12.13 is:

$$[A^* \cdot R] = \frac{1}{2}([A_t^*] + K_A + [R_t])$$

$$- \frac{1}{2}\sqrt{\{(-[A_t^*] - K_A - [R_t])^2 - 4[A_t^*]\,[R_t]\}}$$

$$[12.14]$$

From this equation it can be seen that the production of $[A^* \cdot R]$ complex from a fixed concentration of $[A_t^*]$ will be saturable as $[A^* \cdot R]$ depletes the available $[A^*]$ needed for binding. If $[A]$ were infinite (as is, for example, the effective case in large organ baths with an isolated tissue), then the specific binding of a radioactive ligand (the observed $[A^* \cdot R]$) will be a linear and unsaturable function of $[R_t]$. However, Eq. 12.14 predicts that as $[R_t]$ becomes large enough to bind a substantial quantity of $[A^*]$ so that $[A_f^*]$ is depleted, this linear relationship will collapse to a hyperbolic function. Therefore, a convenient test of the assumption that the quantity of receptor ($[R_t]$) does not appreciably affect the free concentration of ligand is a plot of specific binding $[A^* \cdot R]$ versus $[R_t]$, (usually expressed as the protein content of the membrane fragments). Figure 12.4 shows such a regression where the broken line indicates the theoretically predicted specific binding if the pool of $[A^*]$ were infinite and the solid line represents the experimental situation where $[R_t]$ becomes large enough to significantly affect $[A^*]$. The curved line was calculated as the binding of a concentration of radioligand equal to the $K_A$ ($[A^*] = K_A$) to a range of $[R_t]$ values expressed as multiples of $K_A$. It can be seen

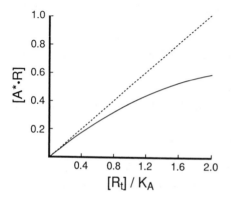

**FIG. 12.4.** The effects of $[R_t]$ on specific binding. Ordinate: Specific binding defined as $[A^* \cdot R]$. Abscissa: $[R_t]$ expressed as multiples of $K_A$. Data shown for binding of a ligand concentration equal to $K_A$. *Dotted line* shows the expected specific binding if the pool of ligand ($[A_t^*]$) was infinite. Hyperbolic function is true $[A^* \cdot R]$, as calculated by Eq. 12.14.

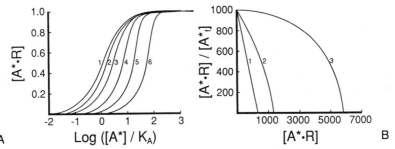

**FIG. 12.5.** Effects of [$R_t$] on saturation experiments. **A:** Saturation binding curves obtained at varying concentrations of [$R_t$] expressed as multiples of $K_A$. Curve 1 for [$R_t$] = 0.1 × $K_A$, 2 = $K_A$, 3 = 3 × $K_A$, 4 = 10 × $K_A$, 5 = 30 × $K_A$, and 6 = 100 × $K_A$. **B:** Scatchard plots shown for varying quantities of [$R_t$]. Curve 1 [$R_t$] = 0.1 × $K_A$, 2 = $K_A$, and 3 = 5 × $K_A$. Calculated with Eqs. 12.10 and 12.14.

from this figure that as [$R_t$] approaches the value of $K_A$, departure from linearity (i.e., [$A_f^*$] becomes less than [$A_t^*$]) occurs. Therefore to avoid the problems associated with deviating from simple Langmuir binding, radioligand binding experiments should be carried out in the linear region of Fig. 12.4 where it can be assumed that the concentration of radioactive ligand is not affected by binding to the receptor.

Figure 12.5A shows the effect of increasing concentrations of receptor on a saturation curve. As can be seen from this figure, the saturation curve shifts to the right in systems in which [$R_t$] approaches the value of $K_A$. For example, if [$R_t$] is 10 × $K_A$, a sixfold shift to the right of the true saturation curve occurs. It can be shown that the concentration of ligand required for half-maximal saturation of a receptor population (termed the [$A_{50}^*$]) is related to the true $K_A$ and the receptor concentration [$R_t$] by:

$$[A_{50}^*] = K_A + 0.5\,[R_t] \qquad [12.15]$$

Therefore, a plot of [$A_{50}^*$] values from a set of saturation curves from preparations with varying receptor concentrations [$R_t$] will yield a straight line. When this plot is extrapolated to zero protein ([$R_t$] = 0), the ordinate axis should yield the true $K_A$.

Scatchard analysis is particularly sensitive to [$R_t$] effects. As [$R_t$] approaches $K_A$, a convex nonlinearity is introduced into the plot. Since receptor heterogeneity produces curvilinearity in the opposite direction, this effect can mask mixed receptor populations when studied with this technique. Figure 12.5B shows the effects of increasing levels of [$R_t$] on Scatchard plots. Such sensitivity to technical concerns illustrates some of the shortcomings of data transformation.

Protein concentration also can affect displacement experiments. If the concentration of [$R_t$] is sufficiently high to abstract the radioactive ligand concentration during the binding experiment, then as a nonradioactive ligand displaces the labeled ligand, the free concentration of the radioactive ligand available for subsequent binding will increase. This will shift the displacement curve to another part of the saturation curve for the radioactive ligand and displacement will be underestimated. Under these circumstances, the concentration of the radioactive ligand-receptor complex $[A^* \cdot R]$ in the presence of the nonradioactive displacing ligand $[A]$ will be given by:

$$[A^* \cdot R] = \frac{([A_t^*] - [A^* \cdot R]) [R_t]}{[A_t^*] - [A^* \cdot R] + K_A + [B] \cdot K_A/K_B} \qquad [12.16]$$

Under these conditions, the concentration of radioactive ligand-receptor complex $[A^* \cdot R]$ is given by one solution of Eq. 12.16, which is:

$$[A^* \cdot R] = \frac{1}{2} \{[A^*] + [B] \cdot K_A/K_B + K_A(1 + \phi)\}$$

$$- \frac{1}{2} \sqrt{\{(-[A^*] - [B] \cdot K_A/K_B - K_A(1 + \phi)\}^2 - 4 K_A[A^*]}$$

$$[12.17]$$

where $\phi$ refers to $[R_t]$ as a multiple of $K_A$ ($\phi = [R_t]/K_A$). The net effect of large receptor concentrations in these experiments is a shift to the right of the displacement curve and a corresponding underestimation of the potency of the displacing ligand. Figure 12.6 shows the effects of $[R_t]$ on displacement curves.

In general, both saturation and displacement curves are a practical balance

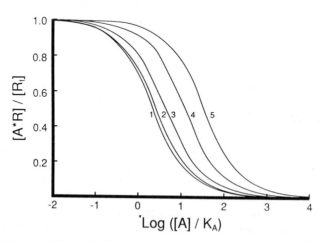

**FIG. 12.6.** Effects of $[R_t]$ on displacement curves. Ordinate: Fractional values of $[A^* \cdot R]$ in the absence ($[A^* \cdot R] = 1$) and presence of various concentrations of nonradioactive ligand $[A]$. Abscissa: Logarithmic scale of molar concentrations of $[A]$ as a fraction of $K_A$. Curve 1 for $[R_t] = 0.1 \times K_A$, $2 = K_A$, $3 = 3 \times K_A$, $4 = 10 \times K_A$ and $5 = 30 \times K_A$. Calculated from Eqs. 12.11 and 12.17.

between the smallest range of radioactivity that can confidently be ascribed to specific receptor binding and measured accurately and reproducibly and the smallest quantity of receptor to avoid the effects of excess $[R_t]$ on affinity estimations. One practical method of avoiding problems with excess $[R_t]$ is to increase the volume in which the binding reaction is carried out. Thus, the pool of available ligand $[A^*]$ approaches an infinite one much like the effect of placing a small isolated tissue in a large organ bath for functional studies.

## RADIOLIGAND BINDING FOR RECEPTOR CHARACTERIZATION

As with isolated tissues, the reliable measurement of the affinity of ligands can lead to the characterization of receptors and drugs. Once the technical difficulties of radioligand binding experiments have been overcome (see refs. 1, 3, 4, and 13 for further details), data interpretation can be less ambiguous than for functional studies. Presumably this is because the analysis is a more direct one in that the drug receptor interaction (i.e., measurement of the drug-receptor complex) need not be filtered through the response machinery of a functional system. However, the increased difficulties in data interpretation in physiological and pharmacologic terms (see Chapter 3) make the need for the correspondence of binding and functional data very important.

As with Schild analysis (Chapter 9), radioligand binding data are compared to the simplest model (i.e., binding to a single homogeneous population of receptors under equilibrium conditions) and interpreted from there. Specifically, if the data do not conform to this model, then more complex models are fit to the data in attempts to devise molecular mechanisms for the observations. For example, Fig. 12.7A shows some hypothetical binding data as a saturation curve. The dotted line is the best fit for a single receptor population model with noncooperative binding. As can be seen from this figure, the model of a single receptor population does not fit the data well, and this lack of correspondence leads to consideration of alternative models. The next most logical model is one for a heterogeneous population of independent binding sites. The mathematical interpretation of this model for saturation experiments is a summation of two hyperbolic functions:

$$\rho = \frac{[A]\cdot[R_{t1}]}{[A] + K_{A1}} + \frac{[A]\cdot[R_{t2}]}{[A] + K_{A2}} \qquad [12.18]$$

where $\rho$ represents the membrane-bound ligand, $[R_{t1}]$ and $[R_{t2}]$ represent the densities of the two binding-site populations, and $K_{A1}$ and $K_{A2}$ represent the equilibrium dissociation constants of the ligand-receptor complexes of the two receptors, respectively. A fit of the saturation data to Eq. 12.18 is more satisfactory in statistical terms (solid line Fig. 12.7A) and corresponds to the

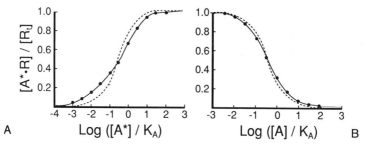

**FIG. 12.7.** Binding data fit with two receptor system models. **A:** Saturation binding data. *Broken line* indicates the best fit for ligand binding to a single receptor population. *Solid line* represents the fit for two independent receptor sites in a proportion of 29%:71% and respective $K_A$ values for each site of 0.11 and 0.97 according to Eq. 12.18. **B:** Displacement of a concentration of [A*], which produces 20% maximal [A*·R] by various concentrations of nonradioactive [A]: *Broken line* indicates the best fit of the data for binding to a single receptor population. *Solid line* indicates the best fit to a model of two independent receptor sites of relative proportion of 52%:48% and respective $K_A$ values of 0.11 and 1.1 as calculated with Eq. 12.19.

binding of the ligand to two independent sites of relative density of 29% ($K_{A1}$ = 0.011) and 71% ($K_{A2}$ = 0.97) in the membrane preparation.

These data also could be generated in displacement experiments. Figure 12.7B shows an experimental binding system studied with a low concentration of the radioligand and displaced by a range of concentrations of the same nonradioactive ligand. As can be seen from this figure, the data points do not correspond satisfactorily to a model of binding to a single receptor population (broken line Fig. 12.7B). These same data, however, could be fit to a model of two-receptor binding by a summation of hyperbolic functions similar to those in Eq. 12.18. Thus, the displacement of radioactive ligand [A*] from two receptor sites [$R_{t1}$] and [$R_{t2}$] by a nonradioactive ligand [B] is given by:

$$\rho = \frac{[A^*]\cdot[R_{t1}]}{[A^*] + K_{A1}(1 + [B]/K_{B1})} + \frac{[A^*]\cdot[R_{t2}]}{[A^*] + K_{A2}(1 + [B]/K_{B2})} \quad [12.19]$$

where the equilibrium dissociation constants of the ligand [A] and [B] for the two receptors [$R_{t1}$] and [$R_{t2}$] are $K_{A1}$ and $K_{A2}$, respectively. A fit of the data to Eq. 12.19 for this experimental system corresponds more closely and represents a better model for the experimental binding observed. As shown in Fig. 12.7B, the ligand appears to bind to two independent receptor sites (relative density of 52% and 48%) with respective equilibrium dissociation constants of 0.11 and 1.1. Such statistical improvement in fit of experimental data to a given model may constitute grounds to postulate that the ligand binds to two, rather than one, receptor in the membrane preparation. However, before this conclusion can seriously be considered, the possibility should be explored that different receptor *states* rather than different *recep-*

*tors* can account for the disparity of the data from the homogeneous receptor model.

## RADIOLIGAND STUDIES WITH COMPLEX LIGANDS: AGONISTS

As discussed in earlier chapters, a large family of receptors couples to membrane-bound transducer proteins to elicit cellular effect. If the interaction of a ligand with a receptor involves, either in a positive or negative fashion, the further interaction of the receptor with a membrane-bound transducer protein, then the kinetics of ligand binding may be complex and deviate from the Langmuir model. For discussion, these ligands will be termed complex ligands; the most commonly encountered complex ligands are agonists. In Chapter 7 (Agonist Affinity) it was shown how the two-stage coupling of an agonist-activated receptor to a transducer protein perturbs the equilibrium between the receptor and the agonist. The binding of the agonist then can be described by the following scheme:

$$[A] + [R_t] \stackrel{K_1}{\rightleftharpoons} [A \cdot R] + T \stackrel{K_2}{\rightleftharpoons} [A \cdot R \cdot T]$$

Thus, the production of a ternary complex ($[A \cdot R \cdot T]$) via a two-stage binding reaction consisting of agonist, receptor, and transducer protein effectively removes $[R_t]$ from the equilibrium reaction with $[A]$ and drives the reaction to the right. Under these conditions, more $[A \cdot R]$ is produced (due to the production of $[A \cdot R \cdot T]$) than normally would be allowed by $K_1$. If this occurs in a radioligand binding experiment, then the equilibrium dissociation constant of the apparent $[A \cdot R]$ complex will be underestimated (i.e., the ligand will appear to have a greater affinity for the receptor than $K_1$), and the experimentally observed affinity will depend on the magnitude of *both* $K_1$ and $K_2$. This can be observed as a shift to the left of a saturation binding curve or a displacement curve. The magnitude of these shifts is dependent on the equilibrium dissociation constant of the ternary complex ($K_2$) and the relative quantity of the coupling protein (i.e., $[R_t]/[T]$). For example, a striking 800-fold increase in the binding potency for the agonist oxotremorine is observed upon reconstitution of the receptor with the transducer protein $G_o$ (see Fig. 12.8).

There are two practical consequences of two-stage binding in radioligand experiments. One is that the heterogeneous receptor populations may appear to exist from mixtures of a single receptor in the complexed and uncomplexed form. A second is that the relative quantities of $[R_t]$ and $[T]$ will alter the observed affinity of the agonist ligand. Since this latter factor is a tissue-specific rather than receptor-specific phenomenon, such binding data may not be useful for receptor classification. It is worth discussing these two ideas separately. Depending on the relative values of $K_1$ and $K_2$ for a given ligand,

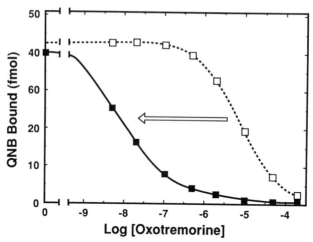

**FIG. 12.8.** Effects of coupling protein $G_o$ on the displacement of [$^3$H]L-quinuclidinyl benzi-late from muscarinic receptors in a reconstituted phospholipid vesicle. Purified muscarinic receptor (2 pmol) and $G_o$ (5.9 nmol of $\beta\gamma$ subunit and 3.4 nmol $\alpha_o$-IDP subunit) were reconstituted in 0.12 mg of phosphatidylcholine. Displacement curves shown for oxotre-morine in the presence (*solid line*) and absence (*broken line*) of $G_o$. *Arrow* indicates the shift to the left in the displacement curve produced by the presence of a coupling protein. (From ref. 8.)

mixtures of $[A \cdot R]$ and $[A \cdot R \cdot T]$ complexes may be produced in the membrane. If the ligand is radioactive, then these will be indistinguishable and would appear as two binding sites for the ligand in the preparation. The relative proportions of the two sites would depend on the relative magnitudes of $K_1$ and $K_2$ and the relative quantities of $[R_t]$ and $[T_t]$. Two-stage binding reactions can formally resemble two independent binding sites (i.e., receptors) as described by Eqs. 12.18 and 12.19. Figure 12.9 shows the same data previously fit in Fig. 12.7A by a summation of two hyperbolae (two indepen-dent receptors $[R_{t1}]$ and $[R_{t2}]$) and now alternatively fit to a single receptor binding to a transducer protein in the membrane with ligand $[A]$ having values of 1.0 and 0.01 for $K_1$ and $K_2$, respectively. These data were calculated for a system in which $[T] = 0.3 \times [R_t]$. It is important to distinguish these two alternatives since the latter is a consequence of the properties of the ligand, not necessarily the system, whereas the former is a property of the system. Under these circumstances, ligands that do not predispose ternary complex formation (such as pure antagonists) will not demonstrate binding specificity in a two-stage binding system, whereas they would in a heterogeneous recep-tor system (assuming that they did not have identical affinity for the two receptor types).

The idea that membrane components such as transducer proteins could control agonist binding potency stems from the availability of $[T]$ as a factor in the predisposition of the formation of $[A \cdot R \cdot T]$ and therefore the perturba-

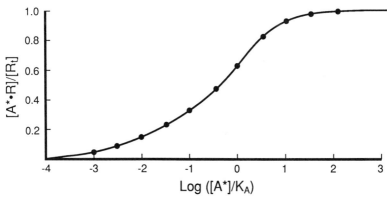

**FIG. 12.9.** Saturation data shown in Fig. 12.7A fit to an alternative model of a single receptor subsequently binding to a transducer protein $[T]$ in the cell membrane. The equilibrium dissociation constant for the $[A^* \cdot R]$ complex $(K_1) = 1.0$ and the equilibrium dissociation constant for the ternary complex $[A^* \cdot R \cdot T]$ $(K_2) = 0.01$. $[T]/[R_t] = 0.3$.

tion of the agonist-receptor binding. It is worth describing two hypothetical types of agonist at this point. The first resembles natural ligands (e.g., hormones, neurotransmitters) and can be called low affinity-high efficacy agonists. For these agonists, $K_2 < K_1$ such that they have a relatively low affinity for the bare receptor $([R_t])$ but once $[A \cdot R]$ is formed, this complex has a high affinity for $[T]$ and readily goes on to form $[A \cdot R \cdot T]$ if $[T]$ is present. The binding of these agonists is quite dependent on $[T]$ because of the low value of $K_2$. Figure 12.10A shows saturation curves for an agonist with $K_1/K_2$ of 100 $(K_1 = 1.0; K_2 = 0.01)$ in systems with varying quantities of $[T]$. As can be seen from this figure, differences in even relatively low ratios of $[T]$ to $[R_t]$ (i.e., a change of $[T]/[R_t] = 0.001$ to $0.01$) produces a significant shift to the left of the saturation curves. Also of note is the departure from monophasic curves as ternary complex formation becomes appreciable. Figure 12.10B shows the displacement of a concentration of $[A^*]$, which produces 20% total $[A^* \cdot R] + [A^* \cdot R \cdot T]$, by nonradioactive $[A]$ under conditions of varying ratios of $[T]/[R_t]$. As with saturation curves (Fig. 12.10A), the displacement curves are shifted to the left but, unlike saturation curves, the slopes of displacement curves are less subject to differences in $[R_t]/[T]$ ratios. In general, slope coefficients of displacement curves are less affected by heterogeneous receptor states than are saturation curves when the same ligand is used for the formation of $[A^* \cdot R]$ and for displacement.

A second type of agonist could be described as a high affinity-low efficacy one in which $K_2 \geq K_1$. Under these conditions, $[A]$ prefers to bind to the bare receptor $[R_t]$, although once the $[A \cdot R]$ complex is produced, there is a low but significant thermodynamic tendency to form $[A \cdot R \cdot T]$ (i.e., a favorable $K_2$). The affinity of these types of agonists would be less dependent on $[T]$; Fig. 12.10C shows a range of saturation curves for a high affinity-low

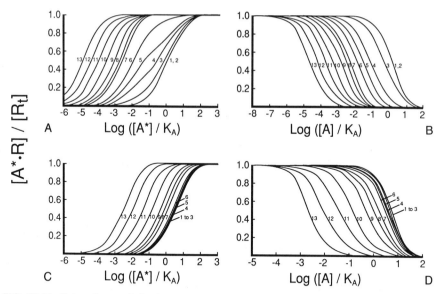

**FIG. 12.10.** Saturation and displacement curves in two-stage binding systems; effect of [T]. **A:** Saturation binding curves for a high-efficacy agonist ($K_1 = 1$; $K_2 = 0.01$) in systems of varying [T]. [$R_t$] = 1. Curve 1 [T] = 0.001, 2 = 0.01, 3 [T] = 0.1, 4 = 0.3, 5 = 0.5, 6 = 1.0, 7 = 3.0, 8 = 5.0, 9 = 10, 10 = 30, 11 = 100, 12 = 300, 13 = 1,000. **B:** Displacement curves for the systems shown in A. Effects of nonradioactive [A] on the binding of [$A^*$] chosen to produce 20% maximal [$A^* \cdot R$]. Numbers on curves as for A. **C:** Saturation binding curves for a low-efficacy agonist ($K_1 = K_2 = 1$) in systems of varying [$R_t$]/[T] ratios. Numbers on curves as for A. **D:** Displacement curves for agonist shown in C; numbers on curves as for A.

efficacy agonist ($K_1 = K_2 = 1$) under conditions of varying [T]/[$R_t$] ratios. Although shifts to the left of the saturation curves occur, they do so at higher ratios of [T]/[$R_t$]; i.e., it requires greater amounts of [T] to shift the saturation curves than for low affinity-high efficacy agonists. Figure 12.10D shows displacement curves of a concentration of [$A^*$] sufficient to produce 20% [$A^* \cdot R$] + [$A^* \cdot R \cdot T$] by nonradioactive [A] in systems of varying [T]. This differential sensitivity of binding affinity to levels of [T] for high- and low-efficacy agonists is illustrated in Fig. 12.11. Curve 1 is for a low affinity-high efficacy agonist ($K_1 = 1$; $K_2 = 0.01$). It can be seen from this curve that levels of [T]/[$R_t$] $\geq$ 0.05 produce greater than twofold increases in apparent affinity. Curve 2 on this figure shows the changes in potency of the low-efficacy agonist ($K_1 = K_2 = 1$) with varying quantities of [T]. For this agonist, differences in affinity are produced by [T] at levels considerably higher than those required for the high-efficacy agonist ([T]/[$R_t$] $\geq$ 1.5). From these calculations, it can be seen that, as the binding of these two types of agonist is studied in different membrane systems (with differing ratios of [T]/[$R_t$]),

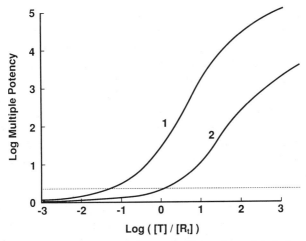

**FIG. 12.11.** Effects of $[T]/[R_t]$ ratios on observed affinity of agonists in two-stage binding systems. Ordinate: Negative logarithms of ligand concentrations that produce half-maximal binding expressed as a fraction of the value obtained in a single-stage binding system (i.e., $[T] \to 0$, binding according to $K_1$). Abscissa: Logarithms of varying $[T]/[R_t]$ ratios. Curves for a high-efficacy agonist (curve 1: $K_1 = 1$, $K_2 = 0.01$) and a low-efficacy agonist (curve 2: $K_1 = K_2 = 1$). *Dotted line* indicates a twofold changes in observed affinity.

there will be differential effects on the *relative* affinity of these agents. Therefore, these data would be unreliable for receptor characterization.

One hallmark of agonist binding is a complex binding curve resulting from the production of a mixture of $[A^* \cdot R]$ and $[A^* \cdot R \cdot T]$ species. This usually results in shallow binding curves of Hill coefficients less than 1. However, as seen from Figs. 12.10, if $[T]$ is very low, relative to $[R_t]$, then effectively very little $[A \cdot R \cdot T]$ will be produced and the Hill coefficient of the binding curve will be near unity. Similarly, if $[T]$ is greater than $[R_t]$, then effectively all of the species formed by the agonist will be $[A \cdot R \cdot T]$ and a Hill coefficient near unity will be observed for the binding curve. Therefore, a complex binding curve is *not necessarily* a condition for agonist binding. This becomes important in the detection of two-stage binding in experimental systems. These phenomena are straightforward for known agonists that produce measurable responses. However, it is theoretically possible that ligands could produce ternary complexes that may not produce visible responses either because the mechanisms required for the translation of the stimulus are not operative in the cell (or membrane) or the experimental techniques are insufficient to measure the response. Under these conditions, the binding of such silent agonists still would be complex, due to two-stage binding processes, but not obvious.

These phenomena are relevant to the classification of receptors by binding techniques. If agonist binding is used to characterize receptors, then ternary complex formation must be considered before distinct noninteractive receptor subtypes are postulated. If a complex binding curve for a ligand that does not produce a measurable response in a functional system is observed, then the possibility of "silent" agonism (i.e., the formation of nonresponse-producing ternary complexes) should be considered. This is because a potential problem comes when such agonists are used in systems of varying quantities of $[T]$. If $[T]$ is very low or very high, then the binding curves to these types of ligands would still have a Hill coefficient near unity yet demonstrate different $K_A$ values in systems of different $[T]$. Thus, the binding would be identical to that observed with an antagonist in preparations of different receptor subtypes.

Clearly, one method of avoiding the complications of two-stage binding reactions is to utilize pure antagonists for radiolabeling receptors and also to base receptor classifications solely on data with antagonists. As pointed out earlier, this may not be clear if the label or displacing agent does not produce an obvious response. Also, as will be seen in the next section, negative efficacy antagonists can still interfere with receptor-transducer protein pairs but not produce obvious responses in tissues. In practical terms, there may not be a pure antagonist radiolabel for the receptor. This is especially common with peptides in which the label usually is an iodinated derivative of the native ligand. However, there is an experimental procedure that in some cases may be used to detect two-stage binding reactions in radioligand experiments. When the ternary complexes involve G proteins, the destabilization of $[A \cdot R \cdot T]$ with excess GTP can be used to differentiate two-stage binding from discrete receptor subtype binding. As discussed in Chapters 7 (Agonist Affinity) and 8 (Agonist Efficacy), in the presence of excess GTP, effectively only the $[A \cdot R]$ complex will be observed under steady-state conditions in some systems. Therefore, if the binding curve to a ligand shifts to the right in the presence of GTP (or stable GTP analogue), then a two-stage binding should be considered. Figure 12.12A shows the effects of stable GTP analogue GMP-PNP on binding of β-adrenoceptor ligands. As can be seen from this figure GMP-PNP has no effect on the binding of the antagonist propranolol, a ligand that does not bind in a two-stage manner to form a ternary complex. However, the GTP analogue does shift the binding curve of the β-adrenoceptor agonist epinephrine in accordance with the cancellation of the second stage of binding to a ternary complex. The same type of effect is shown in Fig. 12.12B, where the displacement of [³H]dihydroalprenolol from β-adrenoceptors by the agonist isoproterenol is shown in the absence and presence of GTP. Whereas the binding curve in the absence of GTP is complex (i.e., best fit by two summed hyperbolic functions shown in Eq. 12.18) and appears to reflect binding to two sites (or two receptor states), the curve in the presence of GTP can be fit by a single hyperbola showing the agonist to have a lower affinity. This is consistent with the GTP effectively prevent-

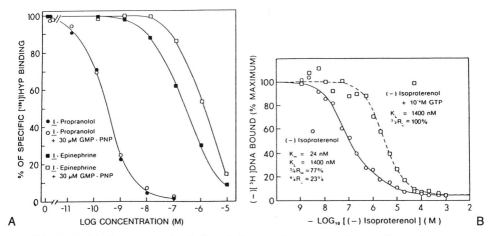

**FIG. 12.12.** Displacements of radioligands from β-adrenoceptors by agonists and antagonists. **A:** Displacement of [$^{125}$I]iodohydroxybenzylpindolol by the antagonist propranolol (•, ○), and the agonist *l*-epinephrine (■, □) in the absence (*closed symbols*) and presence (*open symbols*) of the guanine nucleotide GMP-PNP (guanylyl imidophosphate). (From ref. 14.) **B:** Displacement of [$^3$H]dihydroalprenolol (DNA) by the agonist (−)-isoproterenol in the absence (○) and presence (□) of GTP. In the absence of GTP, the Hill coefficient of the curve is less than unity. In the presence of GTP, the curve shifts to the right and has a Hill coefficient of unity. (From ref. 10.)

ing the accumulation and observation of the ternary complex and leaving only the production of [$A^*\cdot R$].

Two-stage binding can be misleading for receptor classification studies. For example, assume that saturation curves are obtained for two radioactive agonist ligands. Ligand A has low affinity ($K_1 = 1$) and high efficacy ($K_2 = 0.01$) and ligand B has high affinity ($K_1 = 0.1$) and low efficacy ($K_2 = 1$). Saturation curves done in membranes from a tissue with a low receptor to a G-protein ratio of 0.1 (i.e., [$R_t$] = 1; [$T$] = 0.1) show the affinity of ligand B to be 8.1 times greater than the affinity of ligand A (Fig. 12.13A). If displacement experiments were to be done in this same tissue for the displacement of the most potent ligand (i.e., ligand B at a concentration producing 20% [$A^*\cdot R$] + [$A^*\cdot R\cdot T$]) by both ligands A and B, virtually identical relative potencies would be observed (ligand B is 7.3 times more potent than ligand A; see Fig. 12.13B). However, these same experiments, done in membranes from another tissue with a different [$T$]/[$R_t$] ratio, could yield totally different results. Thus, in tissue II, which has a larger proportion of G protein ([$T$] = 30; [$R_t$] = 1), there is a *reversal* of relative potency for the two ligands. As shown in Fig. 12.13C saturation curves for the two ligands indicate that ligand B is 7.6 times *less* potent than ligand A in tissue II. As with tissue I, curves of both ligands displacing the most potent ligand (in this case, ligand A) show ligand B to be one-tenth as potent as ligand A, as with the saturation data.

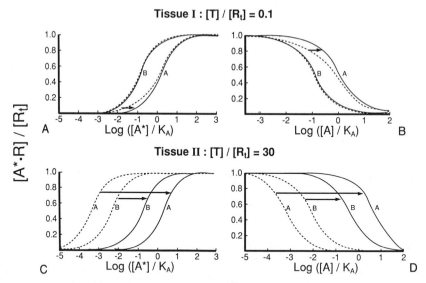

**FIG. 12.13.** Effect of GTP on binding curves for agonists in two-stage binding systems. **A:** *Broken lines* show saturation curves for a low affinity-high efficacy agonist ($K_1 = 1$; $K_2 = 0.01$: agonist A) and high affinity-low efficacy agonist ($K_2 = 0.1$; $K_2 = 1$: agonist B) in a tissue with a low $[T]/[R_t]$ ratio ($[T]/[R_t] = 0.1$, designated tissue I). *Solid lines* show the curves for the same agonists in the presence of a large excess of GTP (i.e., the second-stage binding reaction is canceled and binding depends only on $K_1$). *Arrows* indicate the effects of GTP on each agonist, respectively. **B:** Displacement curves for tissue I for the displacement of a concentration of the more potent radioactive agonist (agonist B), which produces 20% maximal $[A^* \cdot R] + [A^* \cdot R \cdot T]$. *Broken* and *solid lines* and *arrows* as for A. **C:** Saturation curves for agonists A and B in a different tissue with a large $[T]/[R_t]$ ratio ($[T]/[R_t] = 30$), designated tissue II. **D:** Displacement curves for displacement of a concentration of the more potent agonist (in this case, agonist A), which produces 20% maximal $[A^* \cdot R] + [A^* \cdot R \cdot T]$. Note for C and D the *reversal* in the relative potency of the two agonists in the presence of GTP.

Thus, the mixture of single receptor with two different densities of transducer [$T$] shows two agonist ligands to have completely different relative potency (and in fact different order of potency). Since the $[T]/[R_t]$ ratio is tissue, not receptor, dependent then these binding affinities do not constitute useful data for receptor classification.

As mentioned previously, if the coupling transducers are G proteins with catabolic GTPase activity, then carrying out these experiments in the presence of a large excess of GTP may cancel the second-stage binding, and the relative potency of the two ligands would reflect only $K_1$. Under these circumstances, a large excess of GTP would have little effect on tissue I since the effect of [$T$] is relatively small. Figure 12.13A and B (solid lines) shows the relative potencies of ligands A and B in the presence of a large quantity of GTP. As can be seen from these data, little difference in the relative potency of these ligands is observed. In contrast, the relative potency of the two ligands completely reverses in the presence of GTP in tissue II and more reflects that seen in tissue I. This is because the relative potency in this tissue is dominated by the transducer effect, and this is canceled in the presence of GTP. Figure 12.13C shows that, although ligand A is 7.6 times more potent than ligand B in the native membrane without GTP (dotted lines), the addition of GTP causes a *reversal* of relative potency such that ligand A is then 10 times less potent than ligand B (as observed in tissue I, solid lines). This same striking reversal of relative potency is observed in the displacement curves shown in Fig. 12.13D. These data illustrate the potential problems encountered when complex ligands such as agonists are used for binding.

It should also be noted that most of the Hill coefficients for the curves in the displacement experiments (Fig. 12.13B and D) are indistinguishable from unity; i.e., there is no obvious indication that the binding is a complex two-stage process. If ligands A and B were known to produce response in functional systems, then complex binding might be assumed. However, if these ligands did not produce a response in the systems tested but did promote ternary complex formation in some membranes, then the difference in relative affinity observed in tissues I and II could have been interpreted to mean that the receptors in the two tissues were different. Thus, a tissue difference ($[T] = 1$ versus $[T] = 30$) would have been interpreted as a receptor difference. These possibilities stress the importance of the classification of the pharmacologic tools used to classify receptors and the definitions of agonists and antagonists. They also illustrate the potential for GTP effects to distinguish one- and two-stage binding processes.

## RECEPTOR PRECOUPLING AND NEGATIVE INTRINSIC EFFICACY

Although some drugs can promote the formation of ternary complexes between receptors and coupling proteins (i.e., agonists), it is known that other drugs can *destabilize* the formation of such complexes. Under these circumstances, these still can be classified as complex ligands since the presence of transducer proteins affects receptor binding. As discussed in Chapter 8, these antagonists can be thought of as having negative intrinsic efficacy in that they have a higher affinity for the native receptor $[R]$ than for the receptor-transducer protein complex $[R \cdot T]$. This becomes important only when there is a substantial quantity of receptor spontaneously coupled to transducer protein (i.e., a measurable amount of $[R \cdot T]$ present in the membrane in the absence of ligand) or when the radioactive ligand is an agonist and is present in sufficient quantity to ensure that the negative antagonist must interact with the $[A \cdot R \cdot T]$ complex. Under these circumstances, the relative amounts of $[R]$ and $[T]$ and the magnitude of the spontaneous coupling constant between the receptor and the transduction protein can greatly affect the observed affinity of the negative efficacy antagonist. Figure 12.14A shows the effects of receptor-transducer coupling on the observed affinity of

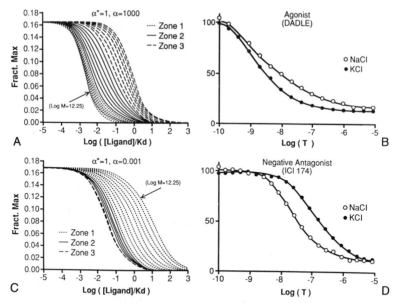

**FIG. 12.14.** Displacement curves for an agonist (**A** and **B**) and an antagonist with negative intrinsic efficacy (**C** and **D**) for the displacement of a radioactive pure antagonist. Ordinates: Additive values for $[A^*\cdot R\cdot T]$ and $[A^*\cdot R]$ where $[A^*]$ is the radioactive ligand. Abscissae: Logarithm of molar values for the nonradioactive displacing ligand divided by the equilibrium dissociation constant of the ligand-receptor complex. **A:** Theoretical calculations. Zones refer to regions where spontaneous coupling of receptor and transduction protein is favorable (Zone 1, $K_{eq}$ for $[R\cdot T] \leq [R]$), less favorable (Zone 2, $K_{eq} \geq [R]$), and nonsignificant (Zone 3, $K_{eq} \gg [R]$). **B:** Displacement of radioactive dinorphine bound to opioid receptors by the agonist DADLE ([D-Ala$^2$,D-Leu]enkephalin) in NG108-15 cell membranes. *Open circles*, experiments with NaCl (deactivation of spontaneous receptor coupling) and *filled circles*, experiments in which KCl was substituted for NaCl (promotion of spontaneous receptor coupling). **C:** Theoretical effects of the observed displacement affinity of an antagonist with negative intrinsic efficacy. **D:** Effects of the negative intrinsic efficacy antagonist ICI 174 ([$N,N'$-diallyl-Tyr,Aib$^{2,3}$]Leu-enkephalin) in a receptor-precoupled (KCl) and -nonprecoupled (NaCl) system from NG108-15 cell membranes. (From ref. 7.)

an agonist (i.e., a drug that promotes the formation of the ternary complex $[A\cdot R\cdot T]$). As can be seen from this figure, the spontaneous association of receptors with transducer protein (i.e., significant amount of $[R\cdot T]$) leads to an increase in the observed potency of the agonist as a displacing ligand. The relevant feature of these data for receptor-classification purposes is the fact that the extent of spontaneous receptor coupling (a tissue-specific and not necessarily receptor-specific phenomenon) determines the observed affinity of the agonist displacing ligand. The lower affinity of the agonist in the absence of spontaneous receptor coupling and higher affinity in the presence of significant amounts of $[R\cdot T]$ complex can be likened to the effects of excess guanine nucleotide (i.e., GTP shifts) on the cancellation of ternary complex formation. As discussed previously, excess GTP levels promote destabilization of ternary complex formation and the dominance of observed affinity on the equilibrium dissociation constant of the $[A \cdot R]$ complex. There is experimental evidence to show that opioid receptors can couple spontaneously to G proteins in some membranes and that $Na^+$ destabilizes the spontaneous $[R \cdot T]$ complexes. The effects of different levels of spontaneous receptor coupling can be seen in Fig. 12.14B where reduction in spontaneous formation of $[R \cdot T]$ (by replacement of $K^+$ with $Na^+$) produces a corresponding reduction in the observed affinity of the opioid agonist DADLE. Therefore, the observed affinity of DADLE in this system would depend on the extent of spontaneous receptor coupling, which, in turn, would depend on the relative quantities of $[R]$ and $[T]$ and the equilibrium dissociation constant of the spontaneous $[R \cdot T]$ complex.

A different effect is observed with antagonists with negative intrinsic efficacy. These drugs, which have a lower affinity for the $[R \cdot T]$ complex, have a lower observed affinity in spontaneously coupled receptor systems. Under these circumstances their observed affinity as displacers of radioactive ligand *decrease* with the extent of spontaneous receptor coupling or production of ternary complex by a radioactive agonist ligand. Figure 12.14C shows the effects of receptor precoupling on the observed affinity of an antagonist possessing negative intrinsic efficacy (the potential to destabilize ternary complex formation). Here it can be seen that the observed affinity of this type of ligand varies inversely with the propensity of the receptors to spontaneously form complexes with transduction proteins. Figure 12.14D shows the *increase* in observed potency of a negative antagonist (ICI 174) with the reduction of spontaneous receptor coupling with replacement of $K^+$ with $Na^+$. As with an agonist, the observed affinity of an antagonist with negative efficacy will depend on the measuring system and not only the receptor type.

## REFERENCES

1. Bennet, J. P., and Yamamura, H. I. (1985): Neurotransmitter, hormone, or drug receptor binding methods. In: *Neurotransmitter Receptor Binding*, edited by H. I. Yamamura, S. J. Enna, and M. J. Kuhar, pp. 61–89. Raven Press, New York.
2. Boeynaems, J. M., and Dumont, J. E. (1975): Quantitative analysis of the binding of ligands to their receptors. *J. Cyclic Nucl. Res.*, 1:123–142.
3. Burt, D. R. (1985): Criteria for receptor identification. In: *Neurotransmitter Receptor Binding*, edited by H. I. Yamamura, S. J. Enna, and M. J. Kuhar, pp. 41–60. Raven Press, New York.
4. Burt, D. R. (1986): Receptor binding methodology and analysis. In: *Receptor Binding in Drug Research*, edited by R. A. O'Brien, pp. 4–29. Marcel Dekker, New York.
5. Chang, K-J, Jacobs, S., and Cuatrecasas, P. (1975): Quantitative aspects of hormone-receptor interactions of high affinity. Effect of receptor concentration and measurement of dissociation constants of labelled and unlabelled hormones. *Biochim. Biophys. Acta*, 406: 294–303.
6. Costa, T., and Herz, A. (1989): Antagonists with negative intrinsic activity at σ opioid receptors coupled to GTP-binding proteins. *Proc. Natl. Acad. Sci. U.S.A.*, 86:7321–7325.

7. Costa, T., Ogino, Y., Munson, P. J., Onaran, H. O., and Rodbard, D. (1992): Drug efficacy at guanine nucleotide-binding regulatory protein-linked receptors: Thermodynamic interpretation of negative antagonism and of receptor activity in the absence of ligand. *Mol. Pharmacol.*, 41:549–560.
8. Florio, V. A., and Sternweis, P. C. (1989): Mechanism of muscarinic receptor action on $G_o$ in reconstituted phospholipid vesicles. *J. Biol. Chem.*, 264:3909–3915.
9. Hollenberg, M. D., and Cuatrecasas, P. (1979): Distinction of receptor from non-receptor interaction in binding studies. In: *The Receptors: A Comprehensive Treatise*, edited by R. D. O'Brien. Plenum Press, New York.
10. Kent, R. S., DeLean, A., and Lefkovitz, R. J. (1980): A quantitative analysis of β-adrenergic receptor interactions: Resolution of high and low affinity states of the receptor by computer modelling of ligand binding data. *Mol. Pharmacol.*, 17:14–23.
11. Klotz, I. M. (1982): Numbers of receptor sites from Scatchard graphs: Facts and fantasies. *Science*, 217:1247–1249.
12. Klotz, I. M., and Hunston, D. H. (1984): Mathematical models for ligand-receptor binding. *J. Biol. Chem.*, 259:10060–10062.
13. Limbird, L. E. (1985): *Cell Surface Receptors: A short Course on Theory and Methods.* Martinus Nihjoff, Boston.
14. Maguire, M. E., van Arsdale, P. M., and Gilman, A. G. (1976): Agonist-specific effect of guanine nucleotides on binding to the beta-adrenergic receptor. *Mol. Pharmacol.*, 12:335–339.
15. Molinoff, P. B., Wolfe, B. B., and Weiland, G. A. (1981): Quantitative analysis of drug-receptor interactions: II. Determination of the properties of receptor subtypes. *Life Sci.*, 29:427–443.
16. Munson, P. J., and Rodbard, D. (1983): Number of receptor sites from Scatchard and Klotz graphs: A constructive critique. *Science*, 220:979–981.
17. Scatchard, G. (1949): The attractions of proteins for small molecules and ions. *Ann. N. Y. Acad. Sci.*, 51:660–672.
18. Weiland, G. A., and Molinoff, P. B. (1981): Quantitative analysis of drug-receptor interactions. I. Determination of kinetic and equilibrium properties. *Life Sci.*, 29:313–330.

# 13

## Kinetics of Drug Action

*It is clearly unsatisfactory to attempt to relate structure to action if highly relevant information about kinetics is being ignored.*
—Sir W. D. M. Paton and H. P. Rang, 1966

The kinetics of drug actions observed *in vitro* can yield valuable information about drug-receptor interactions. Kinetics can be studied operationally, that is, simply to find out when a steady state is reached, or, under certain circumstances, the actual association and dissociation rate constants for drugs can be measured. This chapter outlines some of the techniques found useful in studying the kinetic parameters of drug actions.

### ATTAINMENT OF A STEADY STATE

As noted in Chapter 4, drugs diffuse more slowly in structured organs than in free solution, and the rates at which drug-induced steady states are attained in organs can vary considerably. However, useful information about drug constants is obtained only at thermodynamic equilibrium (or, at least, a steady state), such that the resulting values are not dependent on time. A practical problem then arises as to when these drug constants should be measured (i.e., When is equilibrium achieved?). A particularly relevant example concerns measurements of antagonist potencies (i.e., $pK_B$ or $pA_2$) where the resulting estimates have value only when they are independent of equilibration time (measurements made when equilibrium has been reached). Assuming first-order kinetics, a rate constant for the onset of antagonism can be calculated. For example, Fig. 13.1A shows the onset of $\alpha$-adrenoceptor blockade by phentolamine in rat vas deferens. The dose-response curve for the agonist (phenylephrine) is linearized by conversion to probits (see Chapter 6), and the best-fit straight line is calculated by linear regression. Responses to single doses of phenylephrine (100 $\mu$M) at various times after addition of phentolamine produce a series of decreasing responses as a func-

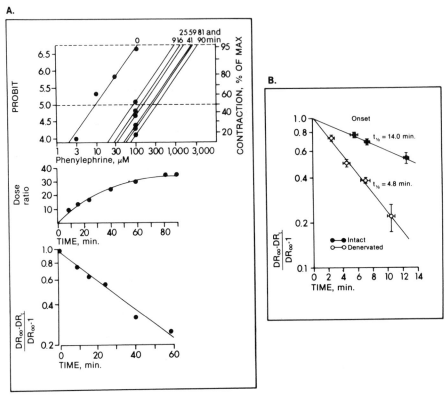

**FIG. 13.1.** Kinetics of onset of phentolamine blockade of α-adrenoceptors in rat vas deferens. **A:** Top panel shows dose-response curve for phenylephrine with ordinate values calculated as probits. The ordinate values in the absence of phentolamine (line closest to ordinate axis) defined the best-fit linear probit line. After addition of phentolamine, responses to 100 μM were obtained at various times thereafter. The declining responses to phenylephrine defined the positions of parallel probit lines representing the shifts in the dose-response curve obtained at those times. These parallel lines allowed calculation of the dose ratios shown in the middle panel. These dose ratios estimated at various times were used in Eq. 12.2 to estimate a first-order rate constant for antagonist diffusion into the receptor compartment (lower panel). **B:** Rate of onset of α-adrenoceptor antagonism by phentolamine in intact (•) and denervated (o) rat vasa deferentia. The faster rate of onset in denervated tissues indicates that the adventitia presents a substantial diffusion barrier for drugs. (From ref. 13.)

tion of time. Assuming that phentolamine is a competitive antagonist and thus produces parallel shifts to the right in phenylephrine dose-response curves, a series of parallel probit lines can be constructed from the equation for the control line and the depressed value for response; the displacement of these probit lines allows calculation of dose ratios for phenylephrine as functions of time. Figure 13.1A shows the probit lines and the relationship between dose ratio and equilibration time. Assuming a first-order rate of onset,

$$\frac{[B_e] - [B_t]}{[B_e]} = e^{-kt} \qquad [13.1]$$

where $[B_t]$ and $[B_e]$ are the concentrations of antagonist in the receptor compartment at time $t$ and at equilibrium, respectively, and $k$ is a first-order rate constant for the rate of onset. From Eq. 13.1, it can be shown that

$$\ln\left[\frac{dr_e - dr_t}{dr_e - 1}\right] = -kt \qquad [13.2]$$

where dr refers to dose ratio. Therefore, a plot of $\ln[(dr_e - dr_t) \div (dr_e - 1)]$ versus $t$ should yield a straight line of slope $-k$; this is shown in the bottom panel of Fig. 13.1A. One application of this type of measurement is in comparisons of diffusion rates into tissues. In Fig. 13.1B, the rates of onset for phentolamine, as quantified by this technique, are compared in intact and denervated (adventitia removed) rat vasa deferentia. The data clearly show a substantial diffusion barrier to be present in the adventitia in the form of a 2.9-fold increase in the rate constant for onset after denervation.

Empirical observation of the kinetics of drug antagonism can be useful also in terms of making evident multiple drug properties. Figure 13.2A shows the effects of 1 μM ambenonium on guinea pig tracheal response to acetylcholine; little change in steady-state responses to acetylcholine is observed. However, ambenonium is known to be a drug with dual self-canceling properties; i.e., it is a muscarinic-receptor antagonist (this will block acetylcholine responses) and an inhibitor of acetylcholinesterase, a degradative enzyme for acetylcholine (blockade of which will potentiate acetylcholine responses). The question then arises: Does the absence of an obvious effect on acetylcholine steady-state responses by ambenonium indicate a true lack of receptor interaction, or does it belie a cancellation of receptor blockade and agonist potentiation? The kinetics of onset of ambenonium can be useful in differentiating between these possibilities. Figure 13.2B shows steady-state guinea pig tracheal responses to a submaximal concentration of acetylcholine. In the top panel, the acetylcholinesterase blocker neostigmine is added, and a steady-state potentiation of responses is observed. The middle panel shows the effects of 1 μM ambenonium, and in this case, a biphasic response is obtained. Presumably, the initial potentiation indicates acetylcholinesterase blockade, and the latter decline in response is the receptor blockade; a similar pattern is shown in the lower panel for 10 μM ambenonium. In this case, additional information has been gained from observing the kinetics of ambenonium interaction; whereas steady-state responses depend on equilibrium dissociation constants (i.e., relative $K_B$ for receptors and $K_I$ for the degradative enzyme), the kinetics of response depend on the relative

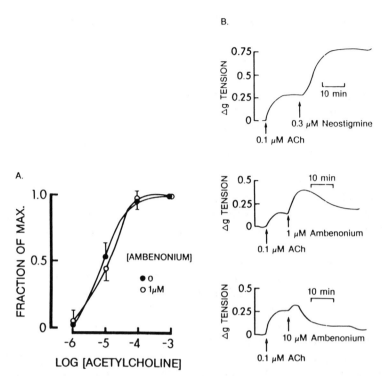

**FIG. 13.2.** Steady-state and temporal effects of ambenonium on guinea pig tracheal responses to acetylcholine. **A:** Dose-response curves from guinea pig trachea for acetylcholine in the absence (•, $N$ = 20) and presence (○, $N$ = 7) of ambenonium (3 μM). Bars represent SEM. **B:** Effects of cholinesterase inhibitors on steady-state contractions of guinea pig trachea to submaximal concentrations of acetylcholine. Ordinate: Tension in grams. Abscissa: Time in minutes. Effects of neostigmine (0.3 μM) and ambenonium (1 and 10 μM) on contraction to acetylcholine (0.1 μM). (From ref. 7.)

values for $k_{2B}$, $k_{1B}$, $k_{2I}$, and $k_{1I}$ (where $k_2$ and $k_1$ are rates of offset and onset, and $B$ and $I$ refer to receptors and enzyme, respectively); the addition of time as a variable dissects the process of attainment of a steady state and in this case allows a differentiation to be made.

Theoretical modeling of such processes allows certain general predictions; a model similar to the acetylcholine-ambenonium interaction described previously serves as an example. In this case, agonist [A] enters the receptor compartment and is taken up by a removal process of characteristic constants $J_m/k_{in} \cdot K_m$ ($J_m$ = maximal rate of removal, $k_{in}$ = permeation rate constant, and $K_m$ = Michaelis-Menten constant for removal), in addition to activating receptor $R$ to produce a response. Drug [B] has the dual properties of blocking the removal process (equilibrium dissociation constant $= K_{BI}$) and blocking receptors ($K_B$), with the ratio between the relative activities for these two processes given by $\phi = K_{BI}/K_B$. The relative rate of offset of $B$ from the uptake site ($k_{2I}$) and receptors ($k_{2B}$) is denoted $\xi = k_{2I}/k_{2B}$. Thus, if $\phi = 10$, $[B]$ has a 10-fold higher affinity for receptors than for the removal process; if $\xi > 1$, $[B]$ blocks the removal process more quickly than it blocks receptors. The effects of a concentration $[B]$ of such an antagonist on a steady-state preexisting submaximal stimulus by a constant concentration of agonist $[A]$ are given by

$$S_t = \exp\left\{1 + \frac{K_A}{[A]}\left[\frac{\left(1 + \frac{[B]}{\phi K_B} + \frac{J_m}{k \cdot K_m}\left\{1 + \frac{[B]}{\phi K_B}\exp\left[-k_2\left(\frac{[B]}{\phi K_B} + 1\right)t\right]\right\}\right)\left(1 + \frac{[B]}{K_B}\right)}{\left(1 + \frac{[B]}{\phi K_B}\right)\left(1 + \frac{[B]}{K_B}\left\{\exp\left[-\xi k_2\left(\frac{[B]}{K_B} + 1\right)t\right]\right\}\right)}\right]^{-1}\right\}$$

[13.3]

where $S_t$ is the stimulus at time $t$. Using Eq. 13.3, a variety of effects can be predicted for antagonists with differing relative potencies for receptors and removal mechanisms and various rates of blockade of these two processes. Figure 13.3 shows the effects of self-canceling antagonists; each panel is for a drug $[B]$, with a fixed ratio of affinities for the two sites ($\phi$), but differing rate constants for offset for the two processes ($\xi$ varies from 0.1 to 10). It can be seen that wide variations in relative parameters yield biphasic effects; these can become important from a practical point of view if the extreme peak responses differ considerably from steady-state levels and represent unwanted activities. For example, if a drug with dual properties is chosen as a candidate for therapy in humans on the basis of steady-state data alone, a possible danger with respect to the early phases of absorption of the drug (onset) might arise if an extreme peak response occurs that represents only one of the drug properties. Thus, the kinetics of onset and offset of the drug could render it therapeutically useless if $\xi$ were considerably greater than or less than unity.

Theoretical modeling of such systems indicates that biphasic responses will not be predicted if $\phi \times \xi \approx 1$ (i.e., if the product of the difference in rate constants for offset and the affinity ratio for the two processes approximates unity). This expression reduces to $k_{1B} \div k_{1I} \approx 1$ (i.e., the relative rate constants for onset for the two processes are approximately equal; no biphasic response will be observed whatever the relative potencies). The prediction of such biphasic effects for drugs with more than one property indicates a value for determining the kinetic constant $k_1$.

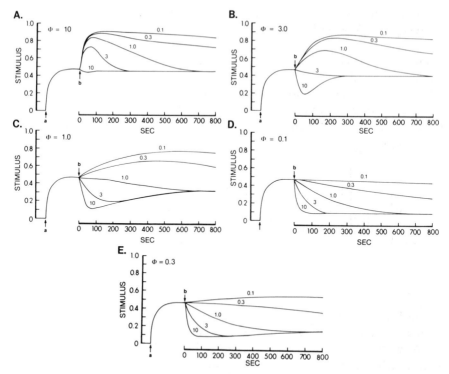

**FIG. 13.3.** Calculated effect of a self-canceling competitive antagonist on a steady-state stimulus to an agonist. Agonist added at point $a$ in a concentration of $[A]/K_A = 10$; antagonist added at point $b$ in a concentration of $[B]/K_B = 10$. It was assumed that $J_m/k_{in} \cdot K_m = 10$, and $k_2 = 6.0 \times 10^{-4}\ sec^{-1}$. Panels for five antagonists with varying relative potencies for the agonist-removal process and receptors: $\phi = 0.1$ **(A)**, 0.3 **(B)**, 1.0 **(C)**, 3.0 **(D)**, and 10 **(E)**. Numbers on the curves refer to the relative rate constants for dissociation of the antagonists from the receptors and uptake sites ($\xi = 10, 3, 1.0, 0.3,$ and 0.1). (From ref. 5.)

## KINETIC INDICATORS OF RESPONSE

There are a number of pharmacologic assays in which the activity of a drug is estimated from a kinetic experiment. For example, β-adrenoceptor agonists can be assayed for broncho-relaxant activity by precontracting an airway smooth muscle such as guinea pig trachea and then relaxing the precontraction with β-adrenoceptor agonist. It is tacitly assumed in these types of studies that the kinetics of response accurately mirror the kinetics of drug-receptor interaction. In many cases there is no reason to doubt that this assumption is valid especially if the results of a kinetic study are not significantly different from those of an equilibrium experiment. For example, Fig. 13.4A shows the dynagraph tracing of the spontaneous rate of beating of a guinea pig right atrium. Cumulative addition to the organ bath of the β-adrenoceptor agonist prenalterol produces tachycardia. As can be seen from

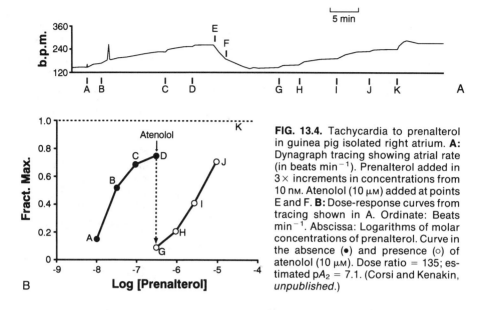

**FIG. 13.4.** Tachycardia to prenalterol in guinea pig isolated right atrium. **A:** Dynagraph tracing showing atrial rate (in beats min$^{-1}$). Prenalterol added in $3\times$ increments in concentrations from 10 nM. Atenolol (10 μM) added at points E and F. **B:** Dose-response curves from tracing shown in A. Ordinate: Beats min$^{-1}$. Abscissa: Logarithms of molar concentrations of prenalterol. Curve in the absence (•) and presence (○) of atenolol (10 μM). Dose ratio = 135; estimated $pA_2$ = 7.1. (Corsi and Kenakin, *unpublished.*)

this figure, addition of the β-adrenoceptor antagonist atenolol rapidly decreases atrial rate, presumably by blocking the β-adrenoceptors and displacing prenalterol. Readdition of more prenalterol in the presence of atenolol again produces tachycardia. Figure 13.4B shows the dose-response curves to prenalterol produced by the chart tracing in A. The important point is that the atenolol-induced shift in the dose-response curve yields an estimate for the $pK_B$ that is not significantly different from the estimate measured by Schild analysis under equilibrium conditions. Therefore, the kinetics of inhibition of prenalterol response by atenolol accurately tracked the kinetics of receptor occupancy by this antagonist.

There are cases, however, in which this assumption may not be valid. For example, β-adrenoceptor agonists produce sustained positive inotropy (Fig. 13.5A) and an increased rate of diastolic relaxation (Fig. 13.5B) in guinea pig left atria. Figure 13.5C shows the effects of the β-adrenoceptor antagonist atenolol on the positive inotropic response to isoproterenol. The rapid blockade of isoproterenol and resulting agreement of the response to what would be expected at equilibrium (Fig. 13.5C, inset) suggest that, like tachycardia in right atria, the kinetics of response inhibition agree with receptor occupation. In contrast, the relaxation response to isoproterenol does *not* mirror the kinetics of receptor occupancy. In this case, blockade of receptors by atenolol does not block the isoproterenol-induced relaxation (Fig. 13.5D) to produce the steady-state receptor obtained in equilibrium studies (Fig. 13.5D, inset). This suggests that there is a difference in the kinetics of decay of the receptor signal and the stimulus-response processing of that signal. In

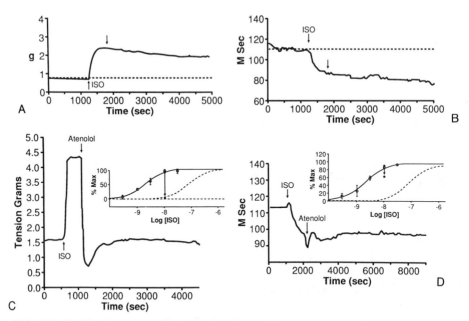

**FIG. 13.5.** Positive inotropy and lusitropy in guinea pig left atria to isoproterenol. **A:** Inotropic response to isoproterenol (10 nM) with time. A sustained increase in the peak force of contraction is obtained. **B:** Decreased time to 90% relaxation produced by the same dose of isoproterenol. A sustained lusitropic response is obtained. **C:** The effect of the β-adrenoceptor blocker atenolol (10 μM) on the steady-state response to isoproterenol. The single response data point is shown on the expected equilibrium shift of the dose-response curve to this dose of atenolol in the inset. **D:** The effect of atenolol (10 μM) on the steady-state lusitropic response to isoproterenol. The single data point is superimposed on the experimentally obtained shift of the lusitropic dose-response curve to isoproterenol produced by this dose of atenolol when the atria are preequilibrated with atenolol before exposure to isoproterenol. The response obtained in the kinetics study is different from that obtained in the equilibrium study.

the specific case of myocardial relaxation, it might be supposed that, although sustained positive inotropy requires a sustained receptor signal, relaxation may only require a burst of receptor activity to initiate the process. Thus, the elevation of cyclic AMP produced by β-adrenoceptor activation may serve to phosphorylate phospholamban, and once this occurs, the phosphorylated protein goes on to mediate sarcoplasmic reticulum ATPase (and myocardial relaxation). The kinetics of decay of relaxation may then rely on the rate of dephosphorylation of phospholamban and not on the termination of the initiating receptor signal.

## KINETIC MEASUREMENTS OF RATE CONSTANTS FOR ASSOCIATION AND DISSOCIATION

If drug-receptor interaction, not bulk diffusion, is rate limiting in an isolated-tissue preparation, then theoretically it is possible to measure the respective rate constants for antagonists for receptor onset and offset, and thus the $K_B$ ($k_2/k_1$). The interaction of a concentration of drug $[B]$ with a receptor $R$ can be depicted as

$$[B] + \underset{(1-\rho)}{R} \underset{k_2}{\overset{k_1}{\rightleftharpoons}} \underset{\rho}{[B{\cdot}R]} \qquad [13.4]$$

where $[B{\cdot}R]$ represents the "concentration" of drug-receptor complex, and $k_1$ and $k_2$ are the respective rate constants for onset and offset. The value $\rho$ represents the fraction of total receptors $R$ present in the form of the complex $B{\cdot}R$; the remaining fraction of receptor that is free for association with $[B]$ is $1 - \rho$. For the kinetics of onset (from Eq. 13.4),

$$\partial\rho/\partial t = k_1[B](1 - \rho) - k_2 \cdot \rho \qquad [13.5]$$

which on integration becomes

$$\rho_t = \rho_e(1 - \exp[-(k_1[B] + k_2)t]) \qquad [13.6]$$

where $\rho_t$ and $\rho_e$ are the fractional receptor occupancies at time $t$ and at equilibrium, respectively. Equation 13.6 rearranges to

$$\ln\left(\frac{(\rho_e - \rho_t)}{\rho_e}\right) = -(k_1[B] - k_2)t \qquad [13.7]$$

thus a regression of values of $\ln((\rho_e - \rho_t)/\rho_e)$ versus time should yield a straight line of slope $-(k_1[B] + k_2)$.

For the offset of antagonism (from Eq. 13.4),

$$\partial\rho/\partial t = -k_2 \cdot \rho \qquad [13.8]$$

which on integration becomes

$$\rho_t = \rho_e\, e^{-k_2 t} \qquad [13.9]$$

This equation rearranges to

$$\ln(\rho_t) = \ln(\rho_e) - k_2 \cdot t \qquad [13.10]$$

Thus, a regression of $\ln(\rho_t)$ on time yields a straight line of slope $-k_2$.

These equations suggest a practical method of measuring $k_1$ and $k_2$ directly: After a stable agonist dose-response curve is attained, several dose ratios during the onset and offset of antagonism by a constant concentration of $[B]$ are measured with time, and these furnish estimates of $\rho_t$ by the relation $\rho_t = (\mathrm{dr}_t - 1)/\mathrm{dr}_t$. Given temporal restraints in some tissues in terms of frequent measurements of responses, dr can be estimated by the matching of equiactive agonist doses (i.e., the agonist dose is increased as antagonism progresses to match the response to the agonist before antagonism). Figure 13.6 shows an experiment to measure the kinetics of onset and offset of methylatropinium as an antagonist of guinea pig ileal responses to acetylcholine. Table 13.1 shows the results of seven similar experiments, the resulting

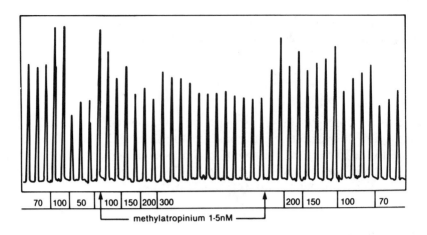

70 | 100 | 50 | 100 | 150 | 200 | 300                      | 200 | 150 | 100 | 70

methylatropinium 1-5nM

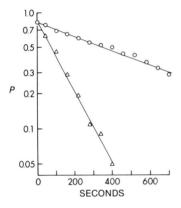

**FIG. 13.6.** Kinetics of onset and offset of methylatropinium blockade of acetylcholine responses in guinea pig ileal smooth muscle. **Top:** Contractions of guinea pig ileal smooth-muscle strips to acetylcholine; doses are picomoles added to a 10-mL bath. Methylatropinium (1.5 nM) added between *arrows* and dose of acetylcholine increased during onset and decreased over offset of blockade. **Bottom:** Kinetic analysis of data in upper panel. For onset (○), the ordinate is $(\rho_e - \rho_t)$ on a logarithmic scale. For offset, ordinate is $\rho_t$ on a logarithmic scale. (From ref. 11.)

**TABLE 13.1.** *Kinetic and equilibrium constants for acetylcholine antagonism by methylatropinium*

| Experiment | $k_1$ (sec$^{-1}$ mol$^{-1}$) | $k_2$ (sec$^{-1}$) | $k_2/k_1$ (= a) | Equilibrium[a] $K_B$ (= b) | b/a |
|---|---|---|---|---|---|
| 1 | $3.52 \times 10^6$ | $1.39 \times 10^{-3}$ | $0.4 \times 10^{-9}$ | $0.5 \times 10^{-9}$ | 1.25 |
| 2 | $3.4 \times 10^6$ | $1.72 \times 10^{-3}$ | $0.5 \times 10^{-9}$ | $0.46 \times 10^{-9}$ | 0.92 |
| 3 | $3.64 \times 10^6$ | $1.98 \times 10^{-3}$ | $0.54 \times 10^{-9}$ | $0.5 \times 10^{-9}$ | 0.93 |
| 4 | $4.49 \times 10^6$ | $1.65 \times 10^{-3}$ | $0.37 \times 10^{-9}$ | $0.47 \times 10^{-9}$ | 1.27 |
| 5 | $2.97 \times 10^6$ | $1.36 \times 10^{-3}$ | $0.46 \times 10^{-9}$ | $0.48 \times 10^{-9}$ | 1.04 |
| 6 | $3.2 \times 10^6$ | $1.85 \times 10^{-3}$ | $0.58 \times 10^{-9}$ | $0.47 \times 10^{-9}$ | 0.81 |
| 7 | $3.21 \times 10^6$ | $1.73 \times 10^{-3}$ | $0.54 \times 10^{-9}$ | $0.45 \times 10^{-9}$ | 0.84 |
| Mean | $3.5 \times 10^6$ | $1.67 \times 10^{-3}$ | | | 1.01 |
| SEM | $\pm 0.19 \times 10^6$ | $+0.09 \times 10^{-3}$ | | | $\pm 0.07$ |

[a] From $[B]/(dr_e - 1)$.
From ref. 11.

values of $k_1$ and $k_2$, and the calculated $K_B$ from the kinetic constants ($k_2/k_1$). These latter values compare favorably with the estimates of $K_B$ measured at equilibrium $\{[B]/(dr_e - 1)\}$, indicating that in these experiments, drug-receptor interaction, not diffusion, is rate limiting (see Table 13.1). Figure 13.7 gives an example of a similar measurement of onset, except that partial dose-response curves are used to measure $dr_t$.

Clearly, if bulk diffusion, as opposed to drug-receptor interaction, is rate limiting, such measurements will not yield correct estimates of $k_1$ and $k_2$, but the internal confirmation that $k_2/k_1$ should equal the $K_B$ derived under equilibrium conditions (correct only if drug-receptor kinetics are rate limiting) allows the distinction to be made. A practical question arises at this point: Why make the more complicated measurements of $k_1$ and $k_2$ when it is much simpler to measure $K_B$ under equilibrium conditions? Part of the answer to this question is given in the quotation from Paton and Rang at the beginning of this chapter, namely, that changes in chemical structure affect the molecular properties of drug-receptor binding, and a finer differentiation of these can be made on the basis of studies of kinetics. Paton and Rang (11)

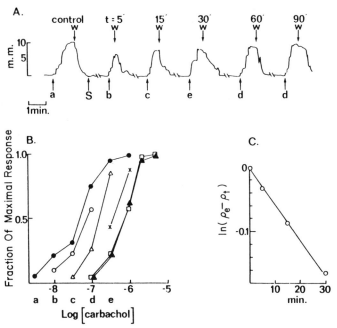

**FIG. 13.7.** Onset of (−)-scopolamine antagonism of guinea pig ileal smooth-muscle responses to carbachol. **A:** Isotonic contractions to carbachol at concentrations a to d shown on abscissa scale of B. w, wash, S, (−)-scopolamine (3 nM) readded after every wash. Responses tested at 5, 15, 30, 60, and 90 min. **B:** Dose-response curves from A; a progressive shift to the right in the presence of scopolamine with time was observed. The resulting dose ratios furnished calculated values for $\rho_t$ and $\rho_e$. **C:** Kinetic analysis of data in B. (From ref. 4.)

**TABLE 13.2.** *Heats of activation and reaction for lachesine-receptor interaction*

|  | 30.5°C | 37.5°C | Ratio | Enthalpy change (kcal mol$^{-1}$) |
|---|---|---|---|---|
| $K_B$ (M) | $0.95 \times 10^{-9}$ | $1.25 \times 10^{-9}$ | 1.3 | 7 |
| $k_2$ (sec$^{-1}$) | $0.96 \times 10^{-3}$ | $1.93 \times 10^{-3}$ | 2.0 | 17 |
| $k_1$ (sec$^{-1}$ mol$^{-1}$) | $1.01 \times 10^6$ | $1.54 \times 10^6$ | 1.5 | 10 |

From ref. 11.

commented further: "Using rate constants, one could begin to relate to the association rate those structural features likely to be important for access from a distance, such as charge and charge distribution, orientation and configuration, or hydration; and to the dissociation rate, those features important at short range, particularly van der Waals forces." For example, quaternization of the nitrogen of atropine to methylatropinium has no effect on the dissociation rate constant (for atropine, $k_2 = 1.8 \times 10^{-3}$ sec$^{-1}$ and for methylatropinium, $k_2 = 1.7 \times 10^{-3}$ sec$^{-1}$), but it produces a twofold increase in the rate of association (for atropine, $k_1 = 1.8 \times 10^6$ sec$^{-1}$ mol$^{-1}$, and for methylatropinium, $k_1 = 3.5 \times 10^6$ sec$^{-1}$ mol$^{-1}$). In a series of alkyltrimethylammonium compounds with similar cationic heads differing only in the length of the alkyl chain, the association rate constant $k_1$ does not vary appreciably; this is to be expected, because the long-range effects of the cationic charge should be most important for the association between drug and receptor. However, the differences in the alkyl chains will be expected to affect the van der Waals forces at close range and hence the disso-

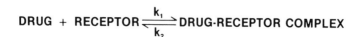

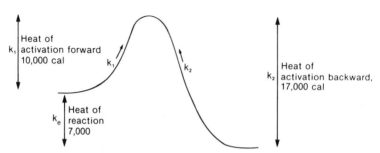

**FIG. 13.8.** Energy diagram for lachesine-receptor interaction in guinea pig ileum. Kinetic measurements made at 30.5°C and 37.5°C furnished heats of activation and reaction (Table 13.2). (From ref. 11.)

ciation rate constant. In agreement with this prediction, kinetic experiments show that $k_2$ diminishes by a factor of 2.65 per methylene group added to the molecule. Such insights into the molecular effects of structural changes may assist organ chemists in the design of drug molecules.

Another application of kinetic measurements concerns the possibility of deriving information about the thermodynamics of drug-receptor events. This can be done by varying the temperature at which experiments are done and thereby calculating activation energies for association and dissociation; Table 13.2 shows the results of such experiments for the antimuscarinic drug lachesine, and Fig. 13.8 shows the estimated heats of activation and reaction. However, the maximal acceptable temperature ranges for most isolated tissues are limited and thus restrict this approach in physiological experiments.

## KINETICS OF ADJUSTMENT OF RECEPTOR OCCUPANCIES BY TWO DRUGS

A given concentration $[B]$ of antagonist occupies a fraction of the existing receptor population $(\rho_B)$ according to the mass-action law:

$$\rho_B = \frac{[B]}{[B] + K_B} = \frac{[B]/K_B}{[B]/K_B + 1} \qquad [13.11]$$

In the presence of a concentration of agonist $[A]$, a readjustment of receptor occupancy occurs, and the receptor occupancy by the antagonist at equilibrium is given by

$$\rho_{B+A} = \frac{[B]/K_B}{[A]/K_A + [B]/K_B + 1} \qquad [13.12]$$

The important aspect of these equations is the time required for the condition described by Eq. 13.12 to occur (i.e., how quickly the relative receptor occupancies of the agonist and antagonist can readjust for true competitivity to be observed). This presents a theoretical problem with practical consequences. The problem arises when attempts are made to describe drug-receptor events with calculated kinetic constants. For example, the competitive antagonism of responses to the muscarinic agonist methylfurmethide in guinea pig ileum by atropine assumes that in the interval between when methylfurmethide enters the organ bath and when a steady-state response is achieved, the relative receptor occupancies for methylfurmethide and atropine adjust to conform to Eq. 13.12. However, the half-time for dissociation of atropine is 7 min, which is considerably longer than the time span required for production of the methylfurmethide response in this tissue (4–5 sec). To accommodate this finding, it must be assumed that the receptor occupancy by methylfurmethide needed to produce the response is negligible with respect to the existing receptor pool (i.e., large receptor reserve). However, atropine is capable of producing a 100,000-fold shift to the right in the methyl-furmethide dose-response curve in this tissue, leading to the unlikely supposi-tion that the receptor reserve for this agonist is 99.99999%. This presents a paradox: How can such a large shift ($10^4$-fold) to the right (with no depression of maximal response) in the methylfurmethide dose-response curve be pro-duced by atropine if this agonist requires a fractional receptor occupancy greater than $\rho_A = 0.00001$ and if the $k_2$ for atropine is insufficient to allow receptor-occupancy readjustment in the time scale for production of peak response (5 sec)? The critical factors in the analysis are the relative dissocia-tion rate constants ($k_2$) for the agonist and antagonist and the receptor occu-pancy required for the agonist to generate a response. If it is assumed that the agonist $k_2$ is greater than that for the antagonist ([A] is a fast-acting drug with respect to [B], a relatively slow-acting drug), then on addition to the organ bath, [A] will equilibrate quickly with the free-receptor pool (i.e., the fraction not occupied by [B]) according to its own kinetic constants. The remaining equilibration of [A] with the rest of the receptor pool depends on the dissociation rate constant for the antagonist $B$. The kinetics of readjust-ment of receptor occupancy by a slow drug ($B$, antagonist) in the presence of a fast drug ($A$, agonist) are described by

$$\rho_{B(t)} = \rho_{B+A} - (\rho_{B+A} - \rho_B) \exp\left[-k_2\left(\frac{[B]/K_B + [A]/K_A + 1}{[A]/K_A + 1}\right)t\right] \quad [13.13]$$

where $\rho_{B(t)}$ is the receptor occupancy by the antagonist at time $t$, $\rho_{B+A}$ is the antagonist occupancy in the presence of [A] at equilibrium (Eq. 13.12), $\rho_B$ is the initial antagonist occupancy at equilibrium in the absence of $A$ (Eq. 13.11), and $k_2$ is the dissociation rate constant for the antagonist [B]. It can be seen from Eq. 13.13 that the occupancy by the antagonist declines from $\rho_B$ to $\rho_{B+A}$ exponentially, with a rate constant not equal to $k_2$ (i.e., for atropine, a value reflected by the $t_{1/2}$ of 7 min), but rather with a rate constant that may be very much greater than $k_2$:

$$\text{readjustment rate constant} = k_R = -k_2 \frac{[B]/K_B + [A]/K_A + 1}{[A]/K_A + 1} \quad [13.14]$$

As seen from this equation, the rate of reequilibration of receptor occupan-cies among the agonist, the antagonist, and the receptor pool depends on two factors: the fractional receptor occupancy required by the agonist to achieve a response and the magnitude of $k_2$, the dissociation rate constant for the antagonist. This first factor is made evident if Eq. 13.14 is rewritten as

$$k_R = k_2 \cdot \left(\frac{[B]}{K_B}(1 - \rho_A) + 1\right) \quad [13.15]$$

where $\rho_A$ is the receptor occupancy by the agonist. It can be seen from this equation that $k_R$ will exceed $k_2$ by decreasing amounts as $\rho_A$ approaches unity. This has the consequence of producing flattened dose-response curves for agonists that require large receptor occupancies in the presence of slow antagonists. Figure 13.9 shows the theoretical time course for agonist-receptor occupancy in the presence of an antagonist with $k_2 = 1.8 \times 10^{-3}$ sec$^{-1}$ (i.e., atropine) for three different agonist occupancies. The top panel of this figure shows the time course for an agonist occupancy of 0.001 in the presence of increasing multiples (1 to $10^4$) of a concentration of antagonist equal to the $K_B$. Because the receptor occupancy required by the agonist is so low (0.001), virtually immediate receptor occupancy is achieved in the presence of an antagonist concentration producing even a $10^4$-fold shift to the right in the dose-response curve. The middle panel of Fig. 13.9 shows the time course for receptor occupancy if the agonist occupancy is somewhat higher (0.1). It can be seen that after the initial occupation of the free receptors by the agonist, the time course for readjustment of occupancy is much slower (on the order of 10–15 sec). The bottom panel ($\rho_A = 0.1$) shows an even slower time course for adjustment of receptor-agonist occupancy. Clearly, in the cases of $\rho_A = 0.01$ and 0.1, agonist occupancy is far from equilibrium at 5 sec (the time scale for response), and the disparity becomes more pronounced as the antagonist concentration is increased. If the response characteristics of the tissue are such that increasing occupancies over periods of up to 60 to 80 sec are reflected accurately, then the response to the agonist will be observed to become slower as the antagonist shifts the dose-response curve to the right. However, for many tissues, rapid desensitization or other factors will preclude observation of the equilibrium response that reflects the true

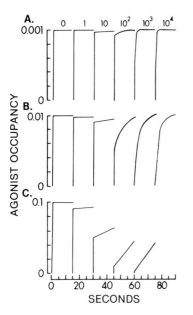

FIG. 13.9. Calculated time course for receptor occupancies by a fast-acting agonist in the presence of increasing concentrations (1 to $10^4$ as multiples of $K_B$) of atropine ($k_2 = 1.8 \times 10^{-3}$ sec$^{-1}$). A: Agonist occupancy at equilibrium ($f_A = 0.001$); occupancy reaches 95% of equilibrium value within 5 sec at all antagonist concentrations. B: Agonist occupancy at equilibrium = 0.01. C: Agonist occupancy at equilibrium = 0.1. The initial steep rise in occupancy reflects the occupancy of free receptors not occupied by atropine, and the secondary phase reflects the readjustment of occupancy between agonist and antagonist. Note that for $\rho_A = 0.01$ and 0.1, the agonist occupancy is far from the equilibrium value at 5 sec. (From ref. 12.)

equilibrium agonist occupancy; therefore, the dose-response curve to the agonist can be depressed by a slow competitive antagonist. This effect will be more pronounced with partial agonists than with highly efficacious full agonists, because the former drugs require greater receptor occupancies to produce responses (high $\rho_A$). Thus, a hemiequilibrium state results wherein the agonist equilibrates with only a portion of the available receptor pool; an example of this is given in Chapter 10 (Fig. 10.12).

The other factor that determines the rate of readjustment of receptor occupancies (and hence the likelihood of a hemiequilibrium state and subsequent depression of the dose-response curve) is the magnitude of $k_2$. As indicated by Eq. 13.14, the rate of adjustment of receptor occupancy is directly proportional to $k_2$; thus, depression of agonist dose-response curves should be more pronounced with slower acting than with faster acting antagonists. This is illustrated in Fig. 13.10 by the effects of equiactive (in terms of equilibrium receptor occupancy) concentrations of the muscarinic-receptor antagonists of $C_{11}$-trimethylammonium ($C_{11}$-TMA) and atropine on dose-response curves

|           | pK$_B$ | k$_2$ (s$^{-1}$) | k$_2$-Ratio |
|-----------|--------|------------------|-------------|
| Atropine  | 8.9    | $1.79 \times 10^{-3}$ | 1   |
| C$_{11}$TMA | 5.6  | $9.5 \times 10^{-3}$  | 5.3 |

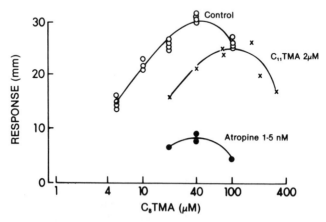

FIG. 13.10. Blockade of muscarinic responses in guinea pig ileal smooth muscle to $C_8$-TMA by slow- and fast-acting antagonist. Ordinate: Isotonic shortening in millimeters. Abscissa: Logarithms of molar concentrations of $C_8$-TMA. Responses in the absence (○, control) and presence of equiactive concentrations of the fast-acting antagonist $C_{11}$-TMA (×, 2 μM) and slow-acting antagonist atropine (●, 1.5 nM). Table gives the relative dissociation rates for these antagonists. (From ref. 11.)

to the agonist $C_8$-TMA. Far less depression of the maximal response to $C_8$-TMA is produced by $C_{11}$-TMA (as compared with atropine), in accordance with the 5.3-fold greater dissociation rate constant for $C_{11}$-TMA as compared with atropine (Fig. 13.10). Hemiequilibrium conditions should especially be considered in receptor-classification studies in which a given antagonist produces competitive blockade of one agonist and seemingly noncompetitive blockade of another. Similarly, competitive blockade versus apparent noncompetitive blockade of a given agonist by a given antagonist in different tissues may not reflect differences in receptors as much as differences in receptor numbers or coupling efficiencies (i.e., different $\rho_A$ values).

## KINETICS OF ONSET AND OFFSET IN BINDING EXPERIMENTS

Radioligand binding experiments hold advantages over functional experiments in the study of drug-receptor interactions because the quantity of drug-receptor complex can be quantified directly. However, care still must be taken to ensure that the assumptions in the use of mass action kinetics are not violated. An experimentally accessible approach to the measurement of ligand-receptor onset is by the pseudo first-order method of onset kinetic measurement. This technique utilizes an excess of radioligand such that the concentration of binding ligand does not change appreciably during the course of binding ($[A] \gg [R]$). This makes the second-order bimolecular reaction between ligand and receptor essentially first order. This approach also takes the dissociation of bound ligand into consideration, thereby utilizing the whole time course of association. Under these circumstances, the rate of onset is given by:

$$\frac{d[A \cdot R]}{dt} = k_1 [A][R] - k_2[A][R] \qquad [13.16]$$

According to Eq. 13.7, the integral of the differential Eq. 13.7 is:

$$\frac{[A \cdot R]_e}{[A \cdot R]_e - [A \cdot R]_t} = e^{(k_1[A] + k_2)t} \qquad [13.17]$$

where $[A \cdot R]_t$ and $[A \cdot R]_e$ refer to the quantities of ligand-receptor complex at time $t$ and equilibrium, respectively. Thus, association can be graphed with time, as shown in Fig. 13.11A. Often the relationship is linearized with the logarithmic metameter of Eq. 13.17:

$$\ln \left[ \frac{[A \cdot R]_e}{[A \cdot R]_e - [A \cdot R]_t} \right] = (k_1[A] + k_2)t \qquad [13.18]$$

According to Eq. 13.18, onset would be a straight line with time (Fig. 13.11B). The right-hand portion of Eq. 13.18 can be rewritten as $k_{obs} \cdot t$, where $k_{obs}$ refers to an observed rate constant comprised of $k' + k_2$ and ($k' = k_1[A]$).

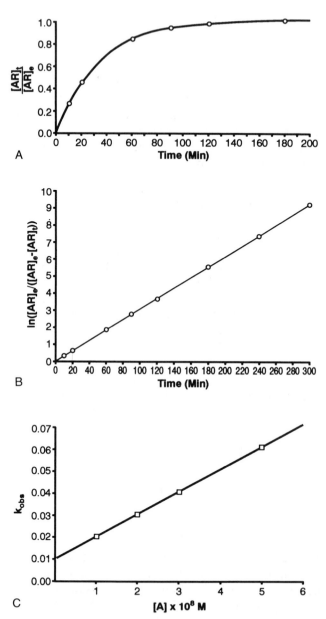

**FIG. 13.11.** The measurement of the rate of onset of a ligand in a radioligand binding study. **A:** A plot of the formation of $[A \cdot R]$ complex with time for a ligand with $k_1 = 10^6$ $sec^{-1}$ $mol^{-1}$ and $k_2$ of 0.01 $sec^{-1}$ at a concentration of 20 nM. **B:** A plot of the linear metameter (Eq. 13.18) of the plot shown in A. **C:** Determination of true $k_1$ by redetermination of $k'$ values for onset of a range of concentrations of ligand. The true $k_1$ is the ordinate intercept of this plot.

Thus, $k_1$ could be calculated from an onset experiment by nonlinear fitting to Eq. 13.17 or a linear fit to Eq. 13.18 and substitution of $k_2$ found by independent means. Alternatively, a series of onset experiments could be carried out at various concentrations of ligand and the observed rate constant ($k_{obs}$) plotted as a function of $[A]$. Under these circumstances, the resulting straight line (assuming simple kinetics of a single onset process) would have a slope of $k_1$ and an ordinate intercept of $k_2$ (Fig. 13.11C).

If it cannot be assumed that the concentration of free ligand is equal to the concentration added, i.e., binding depletes $[A]$, then the second-order equation for onset must be utilized:

$$\ln\left(\frac{[A \cdot R]_e \, ([A]_t - [A \cdot R]_t \, [A \cdot R]_e/[A]_t)}{[A]_t([A \cdot R]_e - [A \cdot R]_t)}\right) = k_1\left(\frac{[A]_t \, [R]_t - [A \cdot R]_e t}{[A \cdot R]_e}\right) \quad [13.19]$$

Experimentally, the rate of offset of ligand from the receptor is more readily measurable. In practice, a binding reaction is carried to equilibrium (equilibrium amount of $[A \cdot R]$ formed) and then the medium either (effectively) infinitely diluted or a large excess of competing nonradioactive ligand added (or both) and the amount of $[A \cdot R]$ followed with time. The rate of decay of $[A \cdot R]$ is given by:

$$\frac{d[A \cdot R]}{dt} = -k_2[A \cdot R] \quad [13.20]$$

The integrated form of which is:

$$\ln\frac{[A \cdot R]_t}{[A \cdot R]_e} = -k_2 t \quad [13.21]$$

Thus a plot of fractional $[A \cdot R]$ complex with time should yield a straight line with a slope of $k_2$. Deviations from linearity may indicate that some of assumptions made are invalid. Specifically, curvature of a plot according to Eq. 13.21 could result if there is incomplete reversibility, two or more phases of reversible dissociation, heterogeneous binding sites, or binding cooperativity. This latter possibility is often tested for by comparing the dilution and excess ligand methods of offset to see if differences are observed in the offset rate constant. If there are, this may indicate cooperative binding since the presence of ligand versus absence of ligand (infinite dilution) should not affect a simple single site offset (see Chapter 10). However, differences between these methods also could be due to reactions approaching the collisional limit (see following section).

## BINDING AT THE COLLISIONAL LIMIT

The biological reactivity of biological systems may be adjusted by the orientation and proximity of reactive sites (receptors) on membranes. As shown in scheme 13.22 (see also scheme 7.1), the binding of a ligand [A] to a receptor can be described as a two-step process:

$$A + R \underset{k_{D2}}{\overset{k_{D1}}{\rightleftharpoons}} A{\cdot}R^* \underset{k_-}{\overset{k_+}{\rightleftharpoons}} A{\cdot}R \qquad [13.22]$$

where the initial step is the diffusion of the ligand to the receptor (controlled by $k_{D1}$ and $k_{D2}$) and the second step is the binding of [A] to the receptor characterized by the first-order rate constants $k_+$ and $k_-$.

The collisional limit is reached when the surface is uniformly reactive, and every collision between the ligand and receptor results in a binding event. This occurs because a ligand will collide with a surface and then diffuse in the vicinity of the surface and recollide several times before escaping into the bulk solution. When the density of receptor sites is high, the probability of binding during this diffusion process approaches 1 (see Fig. 13.12). Considering the binding of a ligand to receptors on a membrane particle, the probability of escaping the surface without a binding event is given by:

$$P_{\mathrm{esc}} = \frac{\pi a}{(n_s + \pi a)} \qquad [13.23]$$

where $r$ is the radius of a single site, $a$ is the radius of the entire membrane particle, and $n$ is the number of vacant sites per particle. The probability of binding becomes $1 - P_{\mathrm{esc}}$ or:

$$P_{\mathrm{bnd}} = \frac{n_s}{n_s + \pi a} \qquad [13.24]$$

The rate constant for the collision between two spherical bodies is given by Smoluchowski's equation (see Chapter 7, Eq. 7.2), therefore the rate constant for a fruitful collision on a membrane particle is this rate constant multiplied by the probability of binding (Eq. 13.24):

$$k_f = \frac{4\pi N D a}{1,000}(P_{\mathrm{bnd}}) \qquad [13.25]$$

where $N$ is Avogadro's number and $D$ is the sum of the particle diffusion coefficients. The velocity of the forward binding reaction then is given by the second-order reaction $k_f[A][C]$ where [C] is the concentration of membrane particles.

Substituting Eq. 13.24 into Eq. 13.25, $k_f$ becomes:

$$k_f = \frac{4ND}{1,000}\left(\frac{n\pi r a}{na + \pi a}\right) \qquad [13.26]$$

When $n$ is small (few vacant sites per particle, low receptor density), then $nr \ll \pi a$ and the forward rate constant follows normal bimolecular kinetics:

$$k_f = \frac{4ND}{1,000}r \qquad [13.27]$$

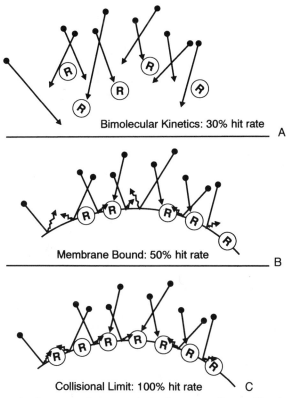

**FIG. 13.12.** Schematic diagrams of systems behaving according to bimolecular kinetics **(A)**, and approaching **(B)** and at **(C)** the collisional limit where every collision with the surface results in binding to a receptor. The relative locations and trajectories of the particles are the same for A–C. The collision rate for A is 30%; for B (same number of receptors but oriented on a membrane), 50%; C (more receptors and all oriented on a membrane), 100%.

However, if the receptor density is very high or the target size on the receptors is large, then $nr \gg \pi$ and the collisional limit for the rate of association
is reached. Under these circumstances, $k_f$ is given by:

$$k_f = \frac{4ND}{1,000}\, \pi a \qquad\qquad [13.28]$$

In practice, $k_f$ varies between these two extremes.

Shown in Fig. 13.13A are different time courses for the onset of the binding
of a ligand to receptors on a particle the size of a platelet. The different
curves refer to binding to a particle of the same size with different receptor
densities. Whereas the low receptor density systems would best be described
with bimolecular kinetics (Eq. 13.27), the high receptor density systems
would more resemble the collisional limit (Eq. 13.28). Figure 13.13B shows
the initial binding velocities for receptors on a cell the size of a platelet under

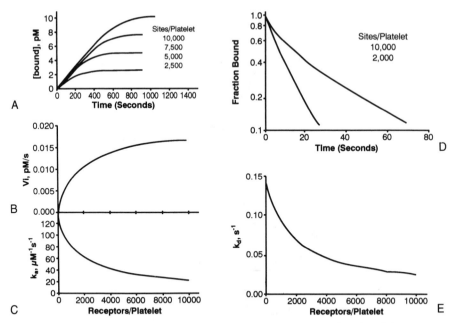

**FIG. 13.13.** The collisional limit for membrane-bound receptors. **A:** Simulated time course for pseudo first-order onset for 100 pM ligand with 0.001 pM cells. Receptor concentrations varied from 10,000 to 2,500 receptors per cell. **B:** Initial reaction velocities for the system shown in A. **C:** Apparent bimolecular rate constants for the system in A with changing receptor densities. **D:** Dissociation rates for reactions at the collisional limit. Time course for dissociation of ligand from receptors on cells. All receptors occupied at time zero. **E:** Limiting dissociation rates (for dissociation from the last 10% of the occupied receptors) for systems with different receptor densities. This formally resembles what would be observed with negative binding cooperativity. (From ref. 1.)

conditions of varying receptor density. With few receptors, the binding rate increases linearly with receptor number as predicted by bimolecular kinetics. However, at high receptor densities (high values of $n$), the reaction velocity approaches the collisional limit; i.e., by about 3,000 to 4,000 receptors per cell, the initial velocity approaches a limit that is independent of receptor concentration. The dependence of the measured association rate constants on receptor density for the system in Fig. 13.13B is shown in Fig. 13.13C. As can be seen from this figure, the variable rate constants for association with receptor density are clearly deviant from what would be predicted by a bimolecular rate expression. These data indicate that for systems with more than 5,000 binding sites per particle, what is measured experimentally may not be the true association rate constant but rather the rate constant for the collisional limit.

The dissociation of ligand from the receptor varies with particle radius and number of vacant receptors and is the product of the equilibrium dissociation constant ($K_A = k_-/k_+$) and the probability of the ligand escaping the receptor ($P_{esc}$):

$$k_r = K_A P_{esc} (3D/r^2) \qquad [13.29]$$

As with association, at the collisional limit $Nr \gg \pi a$ and the rate constant for offset becomes:

$$k_r = (1/n)(3\pi aD/r^3)K_A \qquad [13.30]$$

From this equation it can be seen that as $n \to \infty$, the probability of a ligand diffusing away from a receptor and rebinding to another vacant receptor becomes so high that $k_r \to 0$. If $\pi a \gg nr$, then normal bimolecular kinetics apply and

$$k_r = (3d/r^2)K_A \qquad [13.31]$$

In general, collisional limits predict that cell-bound receptors will produce dissociation kinetics that are much slower than those observed for soluble receptors. Furthermore, the relationship between receptor occupancy and time will be curvilinear. This is because at the early stages of offset when more of the receptors are occupied by ligand, little reassociation of ligand with free receptors will occur. However, as offset progresses, the probability of a dissociated ligand finding a free receptor increases and offset is slowed. Figure 13.13D shows the offset kinetics for a cell the size of a platelet containing 10,000 and 2,000 receptors. The collisional limit is approached in the 10,000 receptor density cell. The dependence of offset rate constant on receptor number (for a given target cell size) is shown in Fig. 13.13E.

It should be noted that, whereas the relative particle size and receptor density can greatly affect the kinetics of receptor binding, they do not affect parameters describing equilibrium binding. Table 13.3 shows that the terms sensitive to collisional limits, namely, the probability of binding and escape, cancel to the same term ($\pi a/nr$), thus the $K_I$ would be the same in either a normal bimolecular kinetic system or one demonstrating collisional-limit kinetics.

The collisional limit should be considered in kinetic experiments designed to detect binding cooperativity. As discussed in Chapter 10, a difference in

**TABLE 13.3.** *Probability of binding for bimolecular association and the collisional limit*

| Probability | Collisional limit | Bimolecular reaction |
|---|---|---|
| $P_{bind}$ | $nr/(nr + \pi a)$ | As $nr \ll \pi a$ |
|  | $nr \gg \pi a$ | $P_{bind} \to nr/\pi a$ |
|  | $P_{bind} \to 1$ |  |
| $P_{esc}$ | $\pi a/(nr + \pi a)$ | $nr \ll \pi a$ |
|  | $P_{esc} \to \pi a/nr$ | $P_{esc} \to 1$ |
| $P_{esc}/P_{bind}$[a] | $\pi a/nr$ | $\pi a/nr$ |

[a] Condition at equilibrium.

the offset kinetics when measured in a system in which the equilibrium bound ligand-receptor complex is allowed to dissociate into an infinitely diluted medium versus one in which an excess of nonradioactive ligand is added to promote dissociation could herald binding cooperativity. However, these two conditions also greatly affect binding of dissociated ligand to free receptors and thus a difference can be shown between bimolecular kinetics systems and those at the collisional limit. Specifically, although there is no difference in offset kinetics measured by competition ($V_{competition}$) and dilution ($V_{dilution}$) in a bimolecular kinetic situation ($\pi a \gg nr$), at the collisional limit, where $nr \gg \pi a$, $V_{competition}/V_{dilution} = nr/(\pi a + 1)$. Thus, a difference would be observed by these two methods that would depend on receptor density and not cooperative binding. In general, the collisional limit should be considered for all membrane-bound receptor systems.

## BINDING KINETICS OF TWO COMPETITIVE LIGANDS

In radioligand studies, the reaction between the drugs and receptors often is most easily initiated by the addition of membrane preparation to a milieu of buffer, radioligand, and competitor. Unlike experiments in which the response can be continually monitored and a steady state can be observed, binding reactions are terminated at some time point that assumes equilibrium. With single ligand experiments, the rate of onset and offset of a ligand can be measured readily. In two ligand experiments, the relative rates of onset and offset are potentially more complex and can be important in terms of affecting approach to equilibrium and the observation of pseudoequilibria. The effect of time on two-ligand steady states can be important if these steady states are not true equilibria since the relative potency of the radioligand and the displacing drug then will be erroneous. The two concomitant binding reactions for a radioligand ([$A^*$]) and nonradioactive displacing drug ([$B$]) can be written:

$$A^* + R \underset{k_2}{\overset{k_1}{\rightleftharpoons}} A^* \cdot R$$

$$B + R \underset{k_4}{\overset{k_3}{\rightleftharpoons}} B \cdot R$$

where $k_1$ and $k_3$ are the forward association constants for the radioligand and displacer, respectively, and $k_2$ and $k_4$ the respective off-rate constants. For simplicity, these calculations will be for concentrations of ligands that are not substantially depleted by membrane binding ($<10\%$). The above binding reactions lead to the following equations:

$$\frac{d[A^* \cdot R]}{dt} = k_1[A^*][R] - k_2[A^* \cdot R] \qquad [13.32]$$

$$\frac{d[B{\cdot}R]}{dt} = k_3[B][R] - k_4[B{\cdot}R] \tag{13.33}$$

$$[R] = [R_t] - [A^*{\cdot}R] - [B{\cdot}R] \tag{13.34}$$

where $[R]$ is the concentration of free receptors and $[R_t]$ the total concentration of receptors. Solving the differential equations leads to the expression that describes the amount of radioligand receptor complex $[A^*{\cdot}R]$ with time:

$$[A^*{\cdot}R]_t = \frac{k_1[R_t][A^*]}{K_F - K_S}\frac{k_4(K_F - K_S)}{K_F\,K_S} + \frac{(k_4 - K_F)e^{-K_Ft}}{K_F} - \frac{(k_4 - K_S)e^{-K_St}}{K_S} \tag{13.35}$$

where:

$$K_A = k_1[A^*] + k_2$$

$$K_B = k_3[B] + k_4$$

$$K_F = 0.5\{(K_A + K_B) + \sqrt{(K_A - K_B)^2 + 4k_1k_3[A^*][B]}\}$$

$$K_S = 0.5\{(K_A + K_B) - \sqrt{(K_A - K_B)^2 + 4k_1k_3[A^*][B]}\}$$

It can be seen that Eq. 13.35 reduces to the Gaddum equation for competitive antagonism (Eq. 9.6) as equilibrium is reached (i.e., as $t \to \infty$).

It can take considerably longer to reach equilibrium in the presence of a displacing drug than with radioligand alone, suggesting caution in reliance solely on kinetics studies with the radioligand. In general, two extremes can be considered: $k_4 \ll k_2$ (displacer dissociates from the receptors more slowly than the radioligand) and $k_4 \gg k_3$ (radioligand dissociates more slowly than the displacer). In the case in which the displacer is slower than the radioligand, the kinetics of the radioligand do not matter, and the equilibration time depends solely on $k_4$ (equilibrium reached at $1.75/k_4$) (Fig. 13.14A). However, in the latter case ($k_4 \gg k_3$), the time required to reach equilibrium depends on the concentration of the radioligand. This is also the case in the absence of displacer (Fig. 13.14A, curve marked radioligand alone) but, as can be seen from this figure, the equilibration can be markedly slower in the presence of a displacer and the disparity in equilibration times increases with increasing radioligand concentration (curves $k_2 \ll k_4$ versus radioligand alone, Fig. 13.14A).

The relative kinetics of the radioligand and displacer can profoundly affect the location of displacement curves and therefore the estimation of the potency of displacing drugs. Figure 13.14B shows the calculated log ($IC_{50}$) values for a displacing drug of set $K_i$ but varying rates of onset and offset. As can be seen from this figure, if the displacer is faster in onset and offset than the radioligand, then it will overshoot its equilibrium receptor occupancy and appear more potent than it really is (see bottom curves Fig. 13.14B for rapid $k_3,k_4$). If the displacer is slower than the radioligand, then the

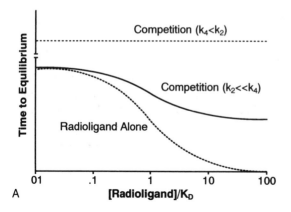

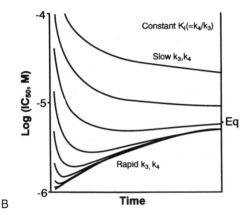

**FIG. 13.14.** The kinetics of concomitant radioligand and displacer in binding experiments. **A:** Time required for equilibrium to be reached (ordinate) as a function of the radioligand concentration for a displacer with slower offset kinetics (*broken line,* $k_4 < k_2$) and faster offset kinetics ($k_2 \ll k_4$) than the radioligand. **B:** Effect of onset and offset kinetics on the potency of a displacing drug (as the log ($IC_{50}$) with time. (From ref. 9.)

equilibrium $IC_{50}$ will be approached monotonically. In view of the potential differences in the kinetics of radioligand/displacing drug mixtures, it can be seen that the kinetics of displacement experiments may not always mirror saturation kinetics of the radiolabel.

## DRUG-RECEPTOR INTERACTIONS *IN VIVO*

If information about drug-receptor interaction is required from an *in vivo* system, then the kinetics of drug-receptor interaction as well as the kinetics of drug delivery and removal from the receptor compartment necessarily must be considered. Clearly the concentration of drug in the receptor compartment is more subject to the effects of restricted diffusion and various degradation, uptake, and removal mechanisms of the organism. In effect, estimations of drug potency are "snapshots" of an ever-changing profile of biological activity in response to the drug. In view of this, assumptions must be made as to the correspondence between the concentrations entering the access system to the relevant organ and the concentrations presented to the receptor after distribution and degradation. These necessary assumptions are a mandatory caveat to the application of *in vivo* data to molecular mechanisms at the receptor level.

As discussed in Chapter 9, the estimate of the potency of competitive antagonists is made solely from two parameters: the molar concentration of antagonist in the receptor compartment and the magnitude of the dextral displacement of the agonist dose-response curve produced by the antagonist. In general, the sensitivity of the system to agonist is measured, the antagonist is absorbed and dispersed throughout the *in vivo* system (given, e.g., intravenously or orally) and then the sensitivity to agonist measured again. The multiple increases in the doses of agonist required for equiactive responses (dr) then can be used to estimate antagonist potency as it is done in isolated tissue systems (via Schild analysis; see Chapter 9). A special problem to *in vivo* systems is the fact that the measurements are made from a heterogeneous collection of systems (i.e., different organs) and the antagonist must diffuse into a number of different receptor compartments to reach the receptors.

The concentration of a drug perfusing into a receptor compartment of volume $V$ with a flow rate (i.e., circulation) $Q$ is given by:

$$[C_t] = [C_o] \cdot (1 - e^{-(Q/V) \cdot t}) \qquad [13.36]$$

where $[C_o]$ is the antagonist concentration at the point of entry (i.e., in the circulation) and $t$ refers to time. The time courses of drugs perfusing into receptor compartments of different effective volumes are shown in Fig. 13.15A. Here it can be seen that at high values of $Q/V$ (e.g., $Q/V = 0.3$), the concentration of antagonist may effectively be equal to that of the central compartment at one time point (e.g., 20 min) and be only 20% of that concentration in another compartment (i.e., $Q/V = 0.01$ at 20 min). If the selectivity of the antagonist is being determined, the pharmacokinetics and not the receptor profiles can be dominant. For example, if a cardioselective β-adrenoceptor blocker is being tested for antagonism of catecholamine responses in the heart and the airways (determination of possible bronchospasm), then it must be clear that the central compartment of antagonist has completely equilibrated with both receptor compartments (i.e., the heart and the airway smooth muscle).

Differences in receptor compartment concentrations due to diffusion kinetics can be overcome by long equilibration times, but only if the antagonist is not concomitantly removed from the receptor compartment. In most systems the antagonist diffuses into the receptor compartments from the central compartment and is also eliminated from the body. A simple approximation of this process can be made by assuming a first-order elimination of the antago-

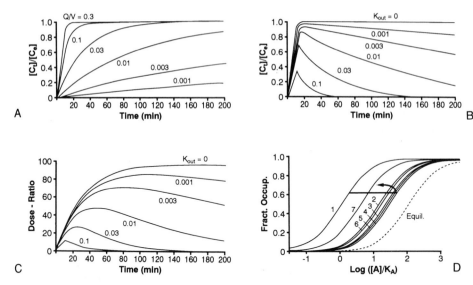

**FIG. 13.15.** Effects of diffusion and diffusion plus a first-order removal mechanism on receptor-compartment concentrations of antagonists. **A:** Effects of varying flow rate to volume ratios ($Q/V$ = 0.3–0.001 as denoted by the numbers on the curves) on the receptor-compartment concentration of drug. **B:** Effects of a first-order rate of removal ($k_{out}$ = 0–0.1 as denoted on curves) from the receptor compartment in a system with $Q/V$ = 0.3. Ordinates for A and B: Receptor compartment concentrations as fractions of the concentration at the site of entry. Abscissae: Time in minutes. **C:** Effects of diffusion plus a first-order removal process on antagonism produced by a competitive antagonist *in vivo*. Ordinate: Equiactive dose ratios for agonists produced by the antagonist. Abscissa: Time in minutes. Calculations for a concentration of antagonist 100 times the equilibrium dissociation constant of the antagonist-receptor complex in a system of $Q/V$ = 0.03. Antagonist removal rates vary ($k_{out}$ = 0–0.1 as denoted on curves). **D:** Effects of an antagonist on agonist dose-response curves in the presence of a first-order removal mechanism for the antagonist ($k_{out}$ = 0.03; $Q/V$ = 0.03). Ordinate refers to fractional agonist response; abscissa to logarithms of molar concentrations of agonist expressed as fractions of the equilibrium dissociation constant for the agonist-receptor complex. Dose of antagonist = 100 times $K_B$ (i.e., equilibrium dose ratio = 101). Curves calculated for various time points from injection of antagonist (1 = control, 2 = 5, 3 = 10, 4 = 20, 5 = 40, 6 = 60, 7 = 120 min as denoted on the curves). *Broken line* indicates dose-response at 120 min in the absence of antagonist removal (true equilibrium dose ratio). (From ref. 6.)

nist with a rate constant designated $k_{out}$:

$$[C_t] = [C_o] \cdot (e^{-k_{out}t}) \cdot (1 - e^{-(Q/V) \cdot t}) \qquad [13.37]$$

Under these circumstances, unless $k_{out}$ is considerably less than $Q/V$, then an appreciable steady-state concentration of antagonist may never be obtained in the receptor compartment. As shown in Fig. 13.15B, different rates of removal of antagonist from the receptor compartment can lead to conditions in which the central compartment concentration is *not* obtained.

Assuming a rapid first-order onset of the antagonist to the receptor, the concentrations calculated with Eq. 13.37 can be converted to dose ratios for antagonism. For a system in which $Q/V = 0.3$ and receptor compartments of varying rates of antagonist removal, it can be seen that the true equilibrium dose ratio may not be observed for removal rates of $k_{out} > 0.001$; see Fig. 13.15C). Under these circumstances, the true potency of an antagonist may be underestimated. For example, Fig. 13.15D shows dose-response curves in the absence and presence of an antagonist infused into a system at concentration of 100 times the $K_B$ (thus producing an equilibrium dose ratio of 100). It was assumed that the $k_{out}$ was 0.01. It can be seen from this simulation that the true potency is not observed and also that an *apparent* steady state (see curves 2 to 6 over 55 min) is obtained, which falls short of the true equilibrium.

The kinetics of onset of an antagonist *in vivo* are clinically relevant. The first-order rate of onset of a drug for a receptor is given by:

$$\rho_t = \rho_e (1 - e^{-(k_{on}[C] + k_{off}) \cdot t}) \qquad [13.38]$$

where [C] refers to the molar concentration of antagonist, $k_{on}$ and $k_{off}$ refer to the rates of onset and offset, respectively, from the receptor, and $\rho_t$ and $\rho_e$ refer to the fractional receptor occupancy at time $t$ and equilibrium, respectively. Curve 1 of Fig. 13.16 shows the time course of the fractional receptor occupancy for a drug with $k_{on}$ $10^5$ min$^{-1}$ mol$^{-1}$ and $k_{off} = 0.001$ min$^{-1}$. In the case in which diffusion is faster than the rate of receptor onset, these constants would represent the onset rate in all *in vivo* systems, thus yielding a predictive clinical parameter. However, in the case in which diffusion is rate limiting, then the first-order rate of receptor occupancy is modified by

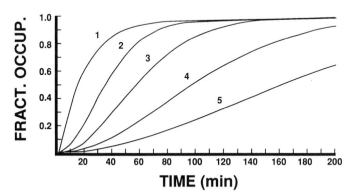

**FIG. 13.16.** Effects of diffusion on the observed kinetics of antagonism. Ordinate: Fractional receptor occupancy for 100 times the $K_B$ concentration of antagonist (99% receptor occupancy). Abscissa: Time in minutes. Rate constants for the antagonist: $k_{on} = 1 \times 10^5$ min$^{-1}$ mol$^{-1}$; $k_{off} = 0.001$ min$^{-1}$. Curve 1 calculated for free diffusion (the rate constant for diffusion exceeds the first-order rate constant for onset to receptors). The kinetics of antagonism under these circumstances are dependent on receptor interaction. Curves 2 to 5 represent increasing $Q/V$ ratios (restricted access into the receptor compartment). Curve 2, $Q/V = 0.03$; 3 = 0.01; 4 = 0.003; 5 = 0.001. (From ref. 6.)

the kinetics of diffusion. The rate of receptor occupancy in a compartment of volume $V$ fed by flow rate $Q$ is:

$$\rho_t = \rho_e \left(1 - e^{-(k_{on}[[C]\cdot\{1 + \exp[(Q/V)\cdot t]\}]k_{off})\cdot t}\right) \qquad [13.39]$$

Curves 2 to 5 of Fig. 13.16 demonstrate the effect of restricted diffusion on the time course of receptor occupancy. The relative ease of diffusion into various receptor compartments can prolong the rate of receptor onset even from an antagonist diffusing from a common central compartment. Therefore, a steady state for one organ response (i.e., one receptor compartment) may not necessarily imply the presence of a steady state in another. This makes the use of data from kinetically dependent systems suspect for drug-selectivity assessment.

## REFERENCES

1. Abbott, A. J., and Nelsestuen, G. L. (1988): The collisional limit: An important consideration for membrane-associated enzymes and receptors. *FASEB J.*, 2:2858–2866.
2. Bennet, J. P., and Yamamura, H. I. (1985): Neurotransmitter, hormone, or drug receptor binding methods. In: *Neurotransmitter Receptor Binding*, edited by H. I. Yamamura, S. J. Enna, and M. J. Kuhar, pp. 61–89. Raven Press, New York.
3. Burt, D. R. (1986): Receptor binding methodology and analysis. In: *Receptor Binding in Drug Research*, edited by R. A. O'Brien, pp. 4–29. Marcel Dekker, New York.
4. Kenakin, T. P. (1980): Effects of equilibration time on the attainment of equilibrium between antagonists and drug receptors. *Eur. J. Pharmacol.*, 66:295–306.
5. Kenakin, T. P. (1986): Tissue and receptor selectivity: Similarities and differences. In: *Advances in Drug Research, Vol. 15*, edited by B. Testa, pp. 71–109. Academic Press, New York.
6. Kenakin, T. P. (1992): The study of drug-receptor interaction in in vivo systems. In: *The In Vivo Study of Drug Action*, edited by C. J. Boxtel, N. H. G. Holford, and M. Danhof, pp. 1–15. Elsevier, Amsterdam.
7. Kenakin, T. P., and Beek, D. (1985): Self-cancellation of drug properties as a mode of organ selectivity: The antimuscarinic effects of ambenonium. *J. Pharmacol. Exp. Ther.*, 232: 732–740.
8. Limbird, L. E. (1985): *Cell Surface Receptors: A Short Course on Theory and Methods.* Martinus Nijhoff, Boston.
9. Motulsky, H. J., and Mahan, L. C. (1984): The kinetics of competitive radioligand binding predicted by the law of mass action. *Mol. Pharmacol.*, 25:1–9.
10. Paton, W. D. M. (1961): A theory of drug action based on the rate of drug-receptor combination. *Proc. R. Soc. Lond. [Biol.]*, 154:21–69.
11. Paton, W. D. M., and Rang, H. P. (1966): The kinetic approach to drug antagonism. In: *Advances in Drug Research, Vol. 3*, edited by N. J. Harper and A. B. Simmonds, pp. 57–80. Academic Press, New York.
12. Rang, H. P. (1966): The kinetics of action of acetylcholine antagonists in smooth muscle. *Proc. R. Soc. Lond. [Biol.]*, 164:488–510.
13. Ruffolo, R. R., Jr., and Patil, P. N. (1979): Kinetics of alpha-adrenoceptor blockade by phentolamine in the normal and denervated rabbit aorta and rat vas deferens. *Blood Vessels*, 16:113–168.
14. Van Ginneken, C. A. M. (1977): Kinetics of drug receptor interaction. In: *Kinetics of Drug Action*, edited by J. M. Van Rossum, pp. 357–411. Springer-Verlag, Berlin.

# 14

## Drug Design and Discovery

Drug-receptor interactions offer a fascinatingly complex subject for study; the discovery of useful entities for treatment of diseases in humans must be considered an important objective in this endeavor. The term *drug discovery* may be somewhat of a misnomer in pharmacology, because it conveys a sense of searching for something that is already there, but not yet found. That viewpoint would unfortunately put pharmacologists in a passive mode in which they would need only to hone their discriminative assays, and eventually the drugs would come to them (i.e., random screening). That approach does not use to advantage a vast array of information, both theoretical and practical, regarding drug-organ interactions that can be applied to the drug discovery process. A strong element of creativity in drug design that utilizes principles of drug-receptor theory can only be beneficial; in this sense, random searching (screening) should be deemphasized wherever rational concepts of drug selectivity can be exploited. This chapter discusses some principles that may be useful in the initial design and subsequent improvement of drugs.

### DEFINITION OF THE OBJECTIVE

The initial step is definition of the objective (i.e., the importance of asking the right questions in order to obtain the desired answers is intuitively obvious). The impetus for a drug design and discovery program may come from a therapeutic need (i.e., we need a cardiotonic drug for treatment of congestive heart failure with a greater therapeutic ratio than digitalis, because this disease is responsible for hundreds of thousands of deaths annually). Another approach may initiate a program based on the properties of a defined chemical structure. For example, catecholamines possess a myriad activities stemming from stimulation of both α- and β-adrenoceptors; some of these activities may be beneficial (i.e., bronchodilation, cardiac inotropy, lipolysis) and some detrimental (hypertension, tachycardia, muscular tremor), so the

*441*

problem becomes one of eliminating the unwanted while retaining the useful properties of these molecules. A number of possibilities, based on the two fundamental properties of drugs, affinity and efficacy, can be defined; in the case of sympathomimetics, these activities produce α- and β-adrenoceptor agonism and antagonism. Figure 14.1 shows some of the possible uses for such drugs. The attractive feature of this approach is the increased number of therapeutic endpoints from a single chemical structural type; presumably this will increase the possible success-to-effort ratio for the organic chemist, because a single structural type may have therapeutic utility in a greater number of disease states.

Alternatively, the impetus for a drug discovery program may stem from a defined but unsolved pharmacologic problem. This approach led to the discovery of one of the most important classes of therapeutic entities of this century, the beta blockers. Prior to 1960, the subclassification of adrenergic receptors into α and β subtypes was based on the classic studies with agonists and the hypothesis of Ahlquist. The synthesis of ICI 38,174 (pronethalol) in 1960, the first pure beta blocker (in the sense of possessing no intrinsic efficacy for β-adrenoceptors), led to the final definition of β-adrenoceptors as a functional adrenergic receptor subtype. This obviously significant event was brought about by a research group led by James Black at the Pharmaceuticals Division of ICI, which was formed to investigate a pharmacologically unanswered question, as stated by Black in 1959: "the search for compounds which will block cardiac sympathetic responses constitutes a clear-cut pharmacological problem." To be sure, the motivation to solve this problem had both theoretical and practical bases, namely, the idea that the oxygen deficit in the heart in angina pectoris could be canceled by decreasing the oxygen demand of the myocardium (by β-adrenoceptor blockade), as opposed to the alternative approach at that time, namely, to increase oxygen delivery to the heart by vasodilatation. However, the ubiquitous presence of beta blockers in the physician's armamentarium today could not have been foreseen at the time of initiation of the search for beta blockers, and in this sense, the discovery of the unique pharmacologic entity preceded realization of the therapeutic potential (i.e., the discovery of a unique drug precedes its application to disease states). From this point of view, the discovery of unique pharmacologic entities can be justified before the actual association of the discovery program with a defined therapeutic need, as put by Black and Stephenson (6) in the first paper on pronethalol: "We are hoping that this compound will be sufficiently active to examine some pharmacological and clinical problems."

## APPROACHES TO DRUG DESIGN

It is clear that one approach to drug discovery is random testing of chemicals in batteries of physiological tests. The effort-versus-success ratio in

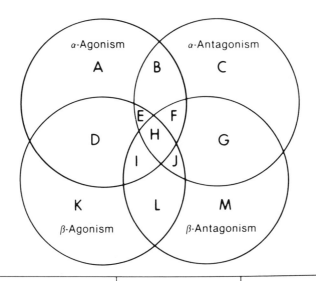

| Alpha-Adrenoceptors | Beta-Adrenoceptors | Possible Indication |
|---|---|---|
| A   full agonist | | |
| B   partial agonist | | shock, trauma |
| C   antagonist | | hypertension |
| D   full agonist | full agonist | |
| E   partial agonist | full agonist | acute cardiac decompensation |
| F   partial agonist | antagonist | nasal decongestion, glaucoma, shock, CPR[1] |
| G   antagonist | antagonist | hypertension |
| H   partial agonist | partial agonist | lipolysis |
| I   full agonist | partial agonist | |
| J   antagonist | partial agonist | asthma, hypertension, CHF[2] |
| K | full agonist | asthma |
| L | partial agonist | asthma |
| M | antagonist | hypertension, angina, glaucoma |

1.  Cardiopulmonary Resuscitation
2.  Congestive Heart Failure

FIG. 14.1.  Possible combinations of activities for adrenergic receptors and some theoretical therapeutic applications.

these procedures usually lies far to the inefficient. The most negative aspect of random screening is the lack of useful data from most of the experiments. A successful pharmacologic experiment advances knowledge irrespective of whether the hypothesis being tested is supported or negated. Thus, these can be termed two-way experiments, in that useful information is obtained that determines the design of the next experiment no matter what the result. Random screening can be considered a succession of one-way experiments in that success is attained only if the substance is active; an inactive substance does not indicate what the next experiment should be, only that the structure is inactive. The following approaches to rational drug design often do allow for two-way experiments, in that hypotheses regarding structural changes in substances already known to be active or postulated to encompass multiple activities can be tested.

There are several approaches to the design of new drugs. One originates from isolation and study of natural products from plant or animal substances previously known to be of therapeutic benefit. Perhaps one of the earliest such substances is described in the Ebers papyrus (circa 1550 B.C.): "another for night blindness in the eyes: liver of ox, roasted and crushed out, is given against it. Really excellent." It is now known that night blindness often results from lack of vitamin A, for which liver is a prime source. The active constituents of medicinal plants can be isolated and characterized and then improved to optimize useful therapeutic effects and diminish unwanted activity. One example of where this approach has been fruitful is the development of the useful local anesthetic procaine from the addicting and toxic natural product cocaine found in erythroxylon coca (Fig. 14.2A). Another is the development of ampicillin from the natural substance penicillin G, which is unstable to gastric acid and is degraded by the enzyme penicillinase (Fig. 14.2B). The bioavailability of the useful cardiac glycoside digoxin is greatly improved by the addition of an acetyl or methyl group on the trisaccharide side chain (Fig. 14.2C).

In some cases, the side effects of drugs can suggest new structural entities for treatment of other diseases. For example, the antibacterial drug carbutamide was found to have an antidiabetic side effect leading to the development of tolbutamide (Fig. 14.3A). The antibacterial sulfanilamide has an antiedemal effect in patients with congestive heart failure; in this case, the drug also is an antagonist of the enzyme carbonic anhydrase. This activity was developed and resulted in the synthesis of the diuretic furosemide (Fig. 14.3B).

Another approach is to improve (with respect to a desired activity profile) a naturally occurring substance in the body (i.e., hormone). For example, the β-adrenoceptor-stimulating properties of the naturally occurring neurotransmitter norepinephrine are greatly amplified in the catecholamine isoproterenol; this profile is enhanced further in the metabolically stable drug salbutamol, which is useful for treatment of asthma (Fig. 14.4A). Another example

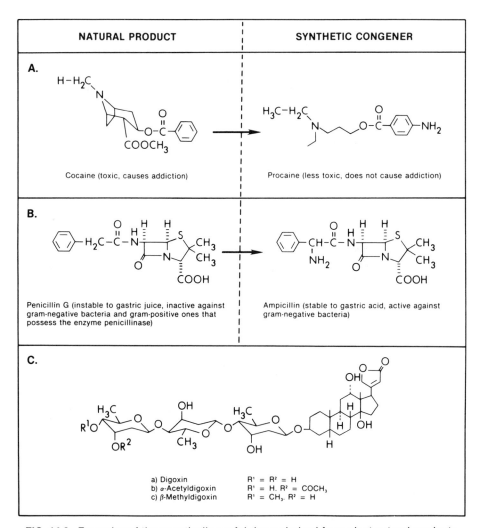

| NATURAL PRODUCT | SYNTHETIC CONGENER |
|---|---|
| **A.** Cocaine (toxic, causes addiction) | Procaine (less toxic, does not cause addiction) |
| **B.** Penicillin G (instable to gastric juice, inactive against gram-negative bacteria and gram-positive ones that possess the enzyme penicillinase) | Ampicillin (stable to gastric acid, active against gram-negative bacteria) |
| **C.** a) Digoxin — R¹ = R² = H<br>b) α-Acetyldigoxin — R¹ = H. R² = COCH₃<br>c) β-Methyldigoxin — R¹ = CH₃. R² = H | |

**FIG. 14.2.** Examples of therapeutically useful drugs derived from plant natural products.

of a natural hormone providing the lead for a useful synthetic drug is the synthesis of (+)-norgestrel after progesterone (Fig. 14.4B).

Physiological processes unique to organs or pathological conditions can be used to develop selective drugs; for example, the inability of bacteria (as opposed to host cells) to utilize presynthesized folic acid offers a method of producing antibacterials. Because bacteria must synthesize folic acid from $p$-aminobenzoic acid, inhibition of this synthetic pathway (by sulfonamides, for example) produces selective destruction of bacteria, with no consequences to the host (the antimetabolite theory). Hitchings and associates

| PROTOTYPE | PRODUCT OF SIDE EFFECT |
|---|---|
| **A.** | |
| $H_2N$—⟨⟩—$SO_2$-NH-$\overset{\overset{O}{\|\|}}{C}$-NH-$C_4H_9$ | $H_3C$—⟨⟩—$SO_2^-$NH-$\overset{\overset{O}{\|\|}}{C}$-NH-$C_4H_9$ |
| Carbutamide (antibacterial activity, antidiabetic side effect) | Tolbutamide (antidiabetic activity, no antibacterial effect) |
| **B.** | |
| $H_2N$—⟨⟩—$SO_2NH_2$ | ⟨O⟩—$CH_2$-$\overset{H}{N}$—⟨Cl, HOOC⟩—$SO_2NH_2$ |
| Sulfanilamide (antibacterial, diurectic side effect) | Furosemide |

**FIG. 14.3.** Examples of therapeutically useful drugs that originated from side effects of drugs designed for other applications.

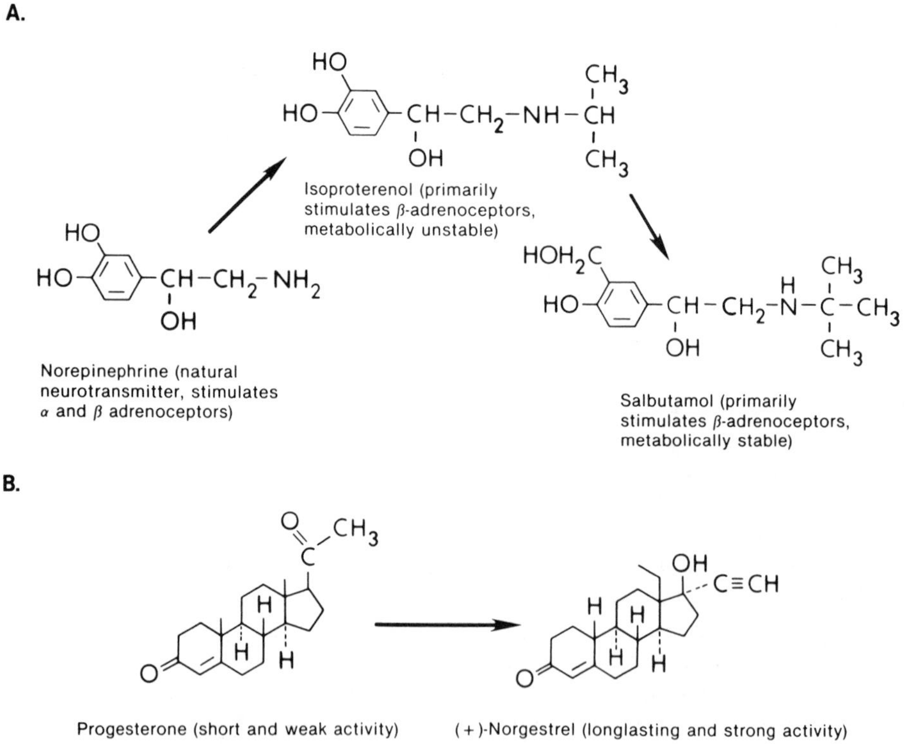

**A.**

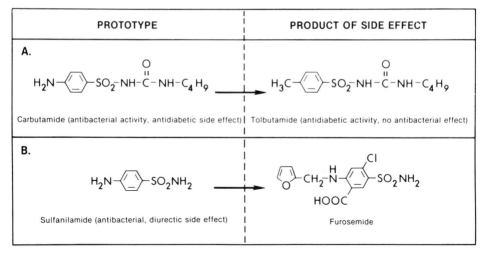

Isoproterenol (primarily stimulates β-adrenoceptors, metabolically unstable)

Norepinephrine (natural neurotransmitter, stimulates α and β adrenoceptors)

Salbutamol (primarily stimulates β-adrenoceptors, metabolically stable)

**B.**

Progesterone (short and weak activity)   (+)-Norgestrel (longlasting and strong activity)

**FIG. 14.4.** Examples of chemical modification of naturally occurring hormones to produce therapeutically useful drugs.

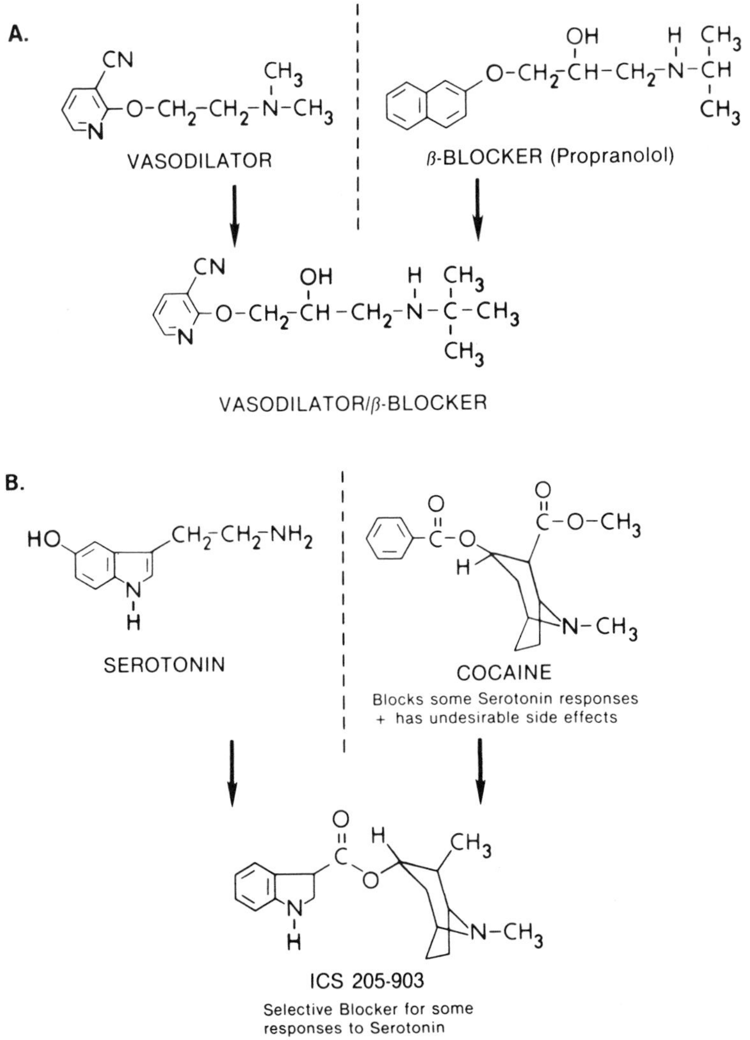

**FIG. 14.5.** Examples of drug symbiosis: combination of two structural types to produce a unique chemical entity. **A:** Compound with vasodilating and beta-blocking properties, as described by Baldwin et al. (2). **B:** Design of ICS 205-903, as described by Richardson et al. (18).

used this theory to great advantage to produce drugs that interfere with nucleic acid metabolism. The result was incorporation of fraudulent nucleic acids into genetic material that in turn prevented cell replication. This mechanism was successful against quickly dividing cells, such as those found in acute lymphoblastic leukemia and chronic granulocytic leukemia, and was extended to produce drugs useful for malaria, gout, and organ transplantation.

**TABLE 14.1.** *Some important chemical structures en route from the natural agonist for H-2 receptors, histamine, to cimetidine, the clinicallly useful antagonist of H-2 receptors*

| Compound | Structure | Antagonist *in vitro* $K_B{}^a$ $10^{-6}$ M | Activity *in vivo* $ID_{50}{}^b$ μg mol/kg |
|---|---|---|---|
| Histamine | $CH_2-CH_2-NH_2$ on imidazole (H-N...N) | — | — |
| Nᵉ-Guanylhistamine: the "lead"; a weakly active partial agonist | $CH_2CH_2NHCNH_2$, $\overset{\parallel}{+NH_2}$ on imidazole (HN...N) | 130 | 800 |
| SK&F 91486: lengthening the side chain increases activity | $CH_2CH_2CH_2NHCNH_2$, $\overset{\parallel}{+NH_2}$ on imidazole (HN...N) | 22 | 100 |
| SK&F 91581: thiourea analogue is much less active as an antagonist, but is not an agonist | $CH_2CH_2CH_2NHCNHMe$, $\overset{\parallel}{S}$ on imidazole (HN...N) | 115 | c |
| Burimamide: lengthening the side chain again dramatically increases antagonist activity | $CH_2CH_2CH_2CH_2NHCNHMe$, $\overset{\parallel}{S}$ on imidazole (HN...N) | 7.8 | 6.1 |
| Metiamide: introducing —S— in the side chain and CH₃ in the ring alters imidazole tautomerism and increases activity | $CH_3$, $CH_2SCH_2CH_2NHCNHMe$, $\overset{\parallel}{S}$ on imidazole (HN...N) | 0.92 | 1.6 |
| Guanidine isostere: replacing C = S by C = CH gives a basic side chain and reduces activity | $CH_3$, $CH_2SCH_2CH_2NHCNHMe$, $\overset{\parallel}{+NH_2}$ on imidazole (HN...N) | 16 | 12 |
| Cimetidine: introducing a CN substituent reduces basicity and increases activity | $CH_3$, $CH_2SCH_2CH_2NHCNHMe$, $\overset{\parallel}{N-CN}$ on imidazole (HN...N) | 0.79 | 1.4 |

[a] Dissociation constant $K_B$ determined *in vitro* on guinea pig right atrium against histamine stimulation.

[b] Activity *in vivo* as an antagonist of near-maximal histamine-stimulated gastric acid secretion in anesthetized rats using a lumen-perfused preparation. The $ID_{50}$ is the intravenous dose required to produce 50% inhibition.

[c] No antagonism seen in an intravenous dose as high as 256 μM/kg.

From ref. 8.

Incorporation of two activities into one molecule theoretically can produce useful drugs. Given the appropriate balance of properties, such a drug will be absorbed, metabolized, and excreted at one rate; this has advantages over multiple-drug therapy, in which various rates are involved. One example in which this method produced a useful entity was the design of a vasodilator/ beta blocker combination for therapy for hypertension (Fig. 14.5A). Another example of successful application of this technique was the design of ICS 205-903, a potent antagonist of some neural effects of serotonin that may have application in treatment of migraine. Previously it was known that cocaine antagonized some neural responses to serotonin, but the central effects of cocaine prevented therapeutic application of this activity. By designing a structure that incorporated the structural elements of cocaine with those of serotonin (Fig. 14.5B), a highly selective serotonin antagonist was obtained that lacked the disadvantages of cocaine.

Two precedents for the design of drug-receptor antagonists were set by Black and colleagues in their discoveries of beta blockers and histamine H-2 receptor antagonists. In both cases, the initial premise was that the receptor recognized the agonist; therefore, the object was to begin with the agonist structure and then retain affinity and eliminate intrinsic efficacy. The agonist structure was systematically altered until a blocker with no intrinsic efficacy was obtained. A sequence of the key compounds leading to the clinically useful histamine H-2 receptor antagonist cimetidine is shown in Table 14.1.

There is much evidence available to demonstrate that even at the present state of the art, rational drug design is feasible and has been successful. As stated earlier, it is preferable to employ two-way experiments as opposed to a program of random screening, in order to achieve a rational approach to drug discovery.

## SELECTIVITY BY CONCENTRATION BIAS AND VOLUME OF DRUG DISTRIBUTION

One method of obtaining organ selectivity with drugs is to produce a concentration bias with respect to the amount of drug in the desired organ and the rest of the organism. Sometimes this can be achieved by the choice of route of drug entry to such susceptible organs as the skin (topical application), lungs (aerosal delivery), nasal passages (inhalation), eyes (eyedrops), or gastrointestinal tract (oral administration). For example, β-adrenoceptor agonists produce bronchodilation for the treatment of asthma but also disturbing tachycardia and digital tremor. A concentration bias produced by aerosal delivery greatly reduces the risks of these side effects. A similar favorable bias is produced for the reduction of intraocular pressure with the β-adrenoceptor blocking drug timolol. In this case, cardiovascular system depression is greatly reduced by ocular application. However, unless concentration bias by route administration is linked to selective degradation or excretion, eventually the bias will be lost as the drug is absorbed and distributes throughout the body.

By limiting the volume of distribution of a drug, selectivity sometimes can be achieved. For example, the triprolidine is a potent antihistamine ($pK_B$ = 10.2) and, like all antihistamines, produces sedation and impairment of mental acuity at some doses. However, by chemical addition of an acrylic acid moiety to produce acrivastine, a molecule that does not cross the blood-brain barrier into the brain was created. Thus, oral administration limits acrivastine distribution to the periphery with no concomitant sedation.

The lipid solubility of a drug can greatly modify its distribution and duration of action. The equilibration of the long-acting β-adrenoceptor agonist salmeterol is one example of the striking effects of dissolution into cell membranes (see Chapter 5). Another is the antimuscarinic selectivity of atropine due to selective distribution. It is known that atropine is 14 times less potent in producing inhibition of gastric secretion by virtue of a concentration gradient loss into the gastric juice. Thus, lower plasma levels of the less lipid-soluble antimuscarinic pirenzepine produce equal inhibition of gastric secretion because pirenzepine, unlike atropine, is not lost through the oxyntic cell.

## PRODUCTION OF ACTIVE DRUGS (PRODRUGS)

Another method of controlling drug distribution is by the use of prodrugs (i.e., chemicals that are substrates for biological enzymes). Thus, active drug molecules can be produced by selective enzymatic degradation in particular organs; i.e., the organ itself becomes an effective factory for the production of an active drug. For example, epinephrine produces a reduction of intraocular pressure for the treatment of glaucoma, but this catecholamine does not penetrate the cornea readily, making it unstable and short acting. However, the congener dipivalylepinephrine is well absorbed through the cornea, and enzymatic hydrolysis produces the active species at the site of action (Fig. 14.6A). This makes dipivalylepinephrine 17 times more potent in reducing ocular pressure than the parent drug epinephrine. The degradation of the naturally unstable enzymatically produced epinephrine in the eye reduces leakage into the general circulation and thus the production of side effects.

The passage of drugs through the blood-brain barrier can be enhanced by methods such as latentiation, i.e., the conversion of hydrophilic drugs into lipid-soluble drugs usually by masking hydroxyl, carboxyl, and primary amino groups. A concentrating effect then can be achieved if the hydrophilic parent is released by enzymatic hydrolysis in the brain and the drug cannot cross back into the periphery. For example, heroin, a lipid-soluble diacetyl derivative of morphine, crosses the blood-brain barrier at a rate 100 times

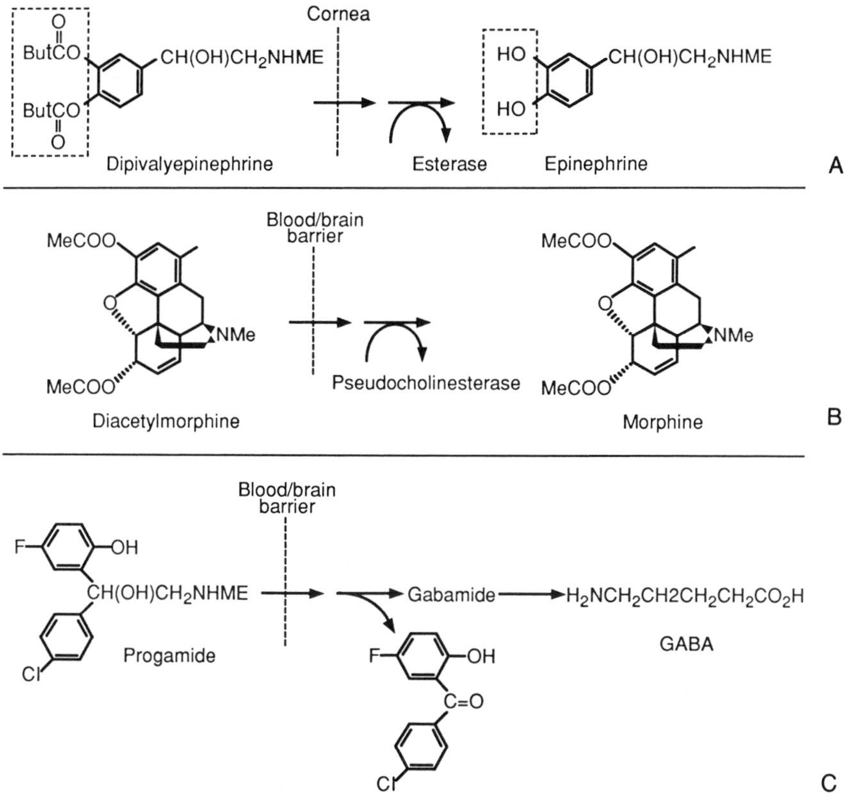

**FIG. 14.6.** Prodrugs for bioselectivity. **A:** Dipivalylepinephrine readily passes through the cornea of the eye and then becomes hydrolyzed to the active drug for the treatment of glaucoma. **B:** Heroin (diacetyl derivative of morphine) passes through the blood-brain barrier at a rate 100 times faster than morphine. Once in the brain, it is hydrolyzed, and subsequently trapped, to morphine. **C:** The Schiff-base progamide enters the CNS and releases GABA in the brain. (From ref. 13.)

faster than its polar parent. Once heroin enters the brain, precapillary pseudo cholinesterase produces deacetylation back to morphine (Fig. 14.6B). Latentiation also can be used to selectively deliver gamma-aminobutyric acid (GABA), a drug not easily deliverable to the CNS, across the blood-brain barrier. However, the Schiff-base progamide crosses into the CNS to release active GABA for the treatment of diseases such as depression, anxiety, Alzheimer's disease, parkinsonism, and schizophrenia.

If a particular enzyme-conversion mechanism is associated with a specific organ, then organ selectivity may be achieved by targeting a particular enzyme. For example, the kidney has a high level of γ-glutamyl transpeptidase and aromatic L-amino acid decarboxylase activity. Therefore, delivery of γ-glutamyldopa to the kidney releases high levels of the vasodilator dopa to the kidney, thus producing levels five times higher than those in the periphery and a selective renal vasodilation.

## METHODS TO ENHANCE ORGAN SELECTIVITY

Often it is desirable to produce a drug action that is directed toward a particular organ, tissue, or pathological tissue state. Application of pharmacokinetics to selectively distribute drugs can be quite useful. At the cellular level, certain aspects of drug-receptor theory and drug disposition can be exploited to achieve organ selectivity. The production of a drug response can be separated into three basic processes, as shown in Fig. 14.7. The first is the delivery of drug into the receptor compartment; referring to Fig. 14.7, this depends on whether there are removal processes (i.e., uptake or metabolic degradation processes) for the drug (A) and the relative ease of permeation into the receptor compartment (B). The second is the drug-receptor interaction; a complicating factor is whether or not the drug interacts with other receptors to functionally modify the primary response (C). The third (for agonists only) is translation of the receptor stimulus into a tissue response, a process determined by the cellular factors of receptor density and the efficiency of stimulus-response coupling (D). Interference with one or more of these processes could result in synergy or self-cancellation of properties that could in turn result in organ selectivity.

Degradative metabolic processes can affect drug actions by altering the concentration of drug in the receptor compartment. For example, neuronal uptake of norepinephrine can greatly attenuate the receptor-compartment concentration of this agonist in the rat anococcygeus muscle. If neuronal

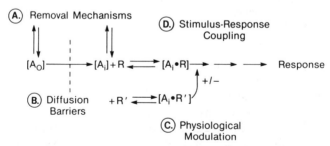

**FIG. 14.7.** Schematic diagram of production of organ responses by drug A. The concentration of agonist A in the extracellular space $[A_o]$ diffuses into the receptor compartment (process B); en route, an active or passive mechanism may remove the drug from the compartment (process A), allowing a residual concentration $[A_i]$ in the receptor compartment. This concentration activates the primary receptor $R$, but also could activate receptor $R'$; the result of this latter process (C) could modulate or potentiate the primary response resulting from activation of receptor $R$. Last, the primary stimulus from activation of $R$ by $[A_i]$ is processed by the tissue into a measurable response (process D). (From ref. 11.)

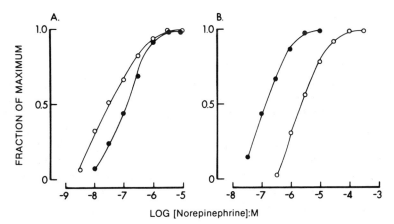

**FIG. 14.8.** Responses of rabbit aorta and rat anococcygeus muscle to norepinephrine. Ordinate: Contraction as a fraction of the maximal contraction to norepinephrine. Abscissa: Logarithms of molar concentrations of norepinephrine. **A:** Relative potencies of norepinephrine in rat anococcygeus muscle (o) and rabbit aorta (•); neuronal uptake processes are blocked with desmethylimipramine (0.3 μM). These curves represent the true relative sensitivities of these tissues to norepinephrine. **B:** Relative potencies in rabbit aorta (•) and rat anococcygeus muscle (o) when neuronal uptake of norepinephrine is not blocked. A striking reversal of relative sensitivities of these tissues to norepinephrine is produced by the more avid neuronal uptake of norepinephrine in rat anococcygeus muscle. (From ref. 11.)

uptake is blocked, norepinephrine is more potent in the rat anococcygeus muscle than in rabbit aorta (Fig. 14.8A). However, when uptake is not blocked, it can be seen from Fig. 14.8B that the selective neuronal uptake of norepinephrine in rat anococcygeus muscle makes norepinephrine considerably less potent as an agonist in this tissue. This type of selective potency translates *in vivo* for drugs that are substrates for degradative processes. Mechanisms related to neurotransmission usually have associated with them the disposal processes for the neurotransmitter (i.e., neuronal uptake of catecholamine or acetylcholinesterase). Therefore, substrates for these processes would be expected to be degraded to a greater extent in the vicinity of highly innervated receptors. For example, the cardiac sinoatrial node (for the control of cardiac rate) is more densely innervated than the bulk of the myocardium. Under these circumstances, it would be expected that a substrate for the neuronal uptake process would be somewhat less potent for production of rate changes as opposed to inotropy (myocardial muscle-cell activation), because the nerves at the sinoatrial node would tend to remove the substrate agonist out of the receptor compartment before it activated receptors. This can be shown for norepinephrine, a substrate for sympathetic neuronal uptake; neuronal uptake is implicated as the factor causing the selectivity, because selectivity is abolished by cocaine, a blocker of the uptake process. In general, it can be supposed that incorporating a metabolically active ligand into a drug that produces an inactive metabolite on metabolism could yield organ selectivity. For example, the short-acting β-adrenoceptor-blocking agent Esmilol is degraded by plasma cholinesterase. This might have utility in the control of intraocular pressure if applied topically, because beta blockade would be achieved in the eye, where it is needed, but not in the periphery. This selectivity would result from degradation of Esmilol in the plasma once the drug diffused out of the ocular space.

A drug that interacts with two tissue processes may produce organ selectivity by virtue of the fact that the two processes may not have the same dominance ratio in any two organs. For example, as pointed out in Chapter 9, ambenonium blocks enzymatic degradation of the neurotransmitter acetylcholine (by blockade of acetylcholinesterase, process A in Fig. 14.7) and also blocks muscarinic receptors. The former activity potentiates the acetylcholine response, whereas the latter inhibits it; therefore, there is the potential for self-cancellation. The extent of the self-cancellation (i.e., potentiation versus blockade) depends on the relative importance of acetylcholinesterase-mediated destruction of acetylcholine and muscarinic-receptor activation; because these effects differ for various tissues, there is the potential for organ selectivity. In the case of ambenonium, organ selectivity from self-cancellation of drug properties is observed. Figure 14.9A–C shows the antagonism responses of acetylcholine in three isolated tissues produced by a given concentration of ambenonium (100 μM); a 16-fold range of dose ratios is produced by this single concentration. The diversity can be linked to the relative importance of acetylcholinesterase as a degradative mechanism for acetylcholine in each tissue. This is made evident by the inverse relationship between the potency of ambenonium as a muscarinic-receptor blocker and the magnitude of the deficit of acetylcholine in the receptor compartment produced by acetylcholinesterase in various tissues (Fig. 14.9D). It would be difficult to predict the resulting organ selectivity *in vivo*, as the cancellation of antagonism would be dependent on both the avidity of acetylcholine removal and the rate of permeation of acetylcholine to the receptor. This latter factor depends, among other things, on the route of drug entry, making it difficult to compare *in vitro* and *in vivo* results. However, by the incorporation of the two drug activities in ambenonium, a profile of selectivity has been achieved. This is illustrated by the Venn diagrams shown in Fig. 14.10. The large set is the total number of organs under autonomic control and the smaller subset (shaded area) is for the organs exercising this control through muscarinic $M_1$ receptors. This subset is further subdivided by the anticholinesterase properties of ambenonium to the intersection of the subset under $M_1$ receptor control and those organs having a high acetylcholinesterase activity.

Another type of self-cancellation of drug properties may stem from functional interactions. For example, dobutamine is an agonist for both vascular α-adrenoceptors mediating contraction and β-adrenoceptors mediating relaxation. In isolated canine saphenous veins, dobutamine produces no obvious

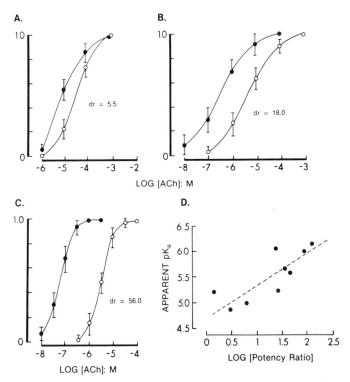

**FIG. 14.9.** Heterogeneous muscarinic-receptor blockade by ambenonium in various tissues. Ordinates for **A** to **C**: Response as a fraction of the maximal response to acetylcholine. Abscissae for **A** to **C**: Logarithms of molar concentrations of acetylcholine. Effects of 100 µM ambenonium on dose-response curves to acetylcholine in rat anococcygeus muscle (dose ratio = 5.5) (A), guinea pig tenia cecum (dose ratio = 18) (B), and guinea pig ileum (dose ratio = 56) (C). **D:** Inverse correlation between the potency of ambenonium as a muscarinic antagonist ($pA_2$, ordinate) and the importance of acetylcholinesterase as a metabolizing enzyme in various tissues. A measure of this latter activity was made by comparison of the sensitivities of the tissues to acetylcholine and bethanechol, a muscarinic agonist not degraded by acetylcholinesterase. When acetylcholinesterase was not a factor in the control of receptor-compartment concentrations of acetylcholine, then acetylcholine was 150 times more potent than bethanechol (log potency ratio = 2.18). In tissues in which acetylcholinesterase selectivity decreased the potency of acetylcholine, the potency ratio decreased. Abscissa values reflect the relative importance of acetylcholinesterase in the control of sensitivity of a tissue to acetylcholine; linear-regression analysis indicates a significant relationship; $t = 3.2$, d.f. = 7, $p < 0.025$. (From ref. 14.)

change in vascular tone; this apparent lack of receptor activity can be delineated into concomitant contraction and relaxation by addition of appropriate blocking agents (Fig. 14.11), indicating self-cancellation by receptor activation. In general, by judicious choice of which processes are unique to or especially important to various organs, dual properties may be designed into drugs to take advantage of synergy or self-cancellation.

As seen in Chapter 8, agonist responses to low-efficacy agonists are more

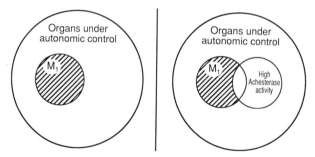

**FIG. 14.10.** Subsets of the organs affected by a standard muscarinic $M_1$ receptor antagonist (*shaded area*) and organs with high cholinesterase activity. The intersection between the two subsets defines a new subset in which antagonists with properties of interaction with $M_1$ receptors and cholinesterase. (From ref. 13.)

dependent on the efficiency of tissue stimulus-response mechanisms than are those to high-efficacy agonists. If intrinsic efficacy could be equated to a weight placed on one end of a lever, and the resulting displacement of the lever equated to the tissue response, a high-efficacy agonist could be thought to exceed the tissue maximal response and thus function as a full agonist in most tissues. The points along the lever at which displacements are observed could be viewed as tissues of different stimulus-response coupling efficiencies (i.e., the closer to the fulcrum, the lower the coupling efficiency). Figure 14.12A schematically shows the expected dose-response curves for a high-efficacy agonist in these tissues. The efficiency of receptor coupling determines where along the concentration axis the dose-response curves are located, and the tissue maximal response is obtained in all tissues. Figure 14.12B shows the same situation for a low-efficacy agonist (from Fig. 1.4);

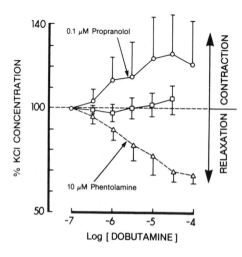

**FIG. 14.11.** Effects of dobutamine in canine isolated saphenous vein. Ordinate: Change in vascular muscle tone. Abscissa: Logarithms of molar concentrations of dobutamine. There is little detectable response to dobutamine in untreated tissues ($\square$, $N = 3$). However, when relaxant $\beta$-adrenoceptor effects are blocked by propranolol, a concentration-dependent contraction is observed ($\circ$, $N = 4$). Similarly, when contractile $\alpha$-adrenoceptor effects are blocked by phentolamine, a concentration-dependent relaxation results ($\triangle$, $N = 4$). Thus, the absence of visible response results from self-cancellation of receptor effects. (From ref. 9.)

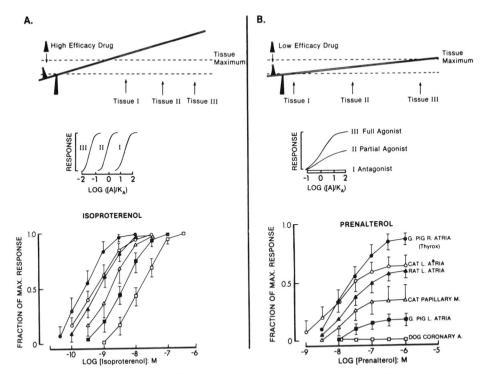

**FIG. 14.12.** Effects of high- and low-efficacy agonists in different tissues. Displacement of the lever balance to the left of the fulcrum represents the stimulus, and that to the right represents the amplified response. Where along the lever the amplified displacement is viewed represents the amplification factor (i.e., increasing efficiency of coupling as displacement is viewed farther to the right of the fulcrum). The displacement of the lever is in proportion to the weight; this represents the intrinsic efficacy of the drug. **A:** High-efficacy agonist (large weight) produces more than sufficient stimulus to produce maximal responses in all tissues; in consequence, only the locations of the dose-response curves vary with different receptor coupling efficiencies. An example of this is the range of dose-response curves to isoproterenol in various tissues (symbol code for tissues shown in B for prenalterol). **B:** Low-efficacy agonist (low weight). In this case, the lever displacement is within the range in which the vantage point is more important (i.e., depending on the efficiency of receptor coupling, drugs may be full or partial agonists or antagonists). An example of this is the range of responses of various isolated tissues to prenalterol (0.04 the intrinsic efficacy of isoproterenol). (Dose-response curves from ref. 10.)

in this case, the receptor-coupling efficiency can have a more profound effect on the observed agonist activity. Depending on the stimulus-response coupling, a low-efficacy drug may be an antagonist, partial agonist, or full agonist. Figure 14.12 also shows data from a series of isolated tissues for the high-efficacy β-adrenoceptor agonist isoproterenol and the low-efficacy (0.04 that of isoproterenol) agonist prenalterol. Whereas isoproterenol is a full agonist in all of the tissues, the maximal responses to prenalterol range from zero to 85% of maximum. In general terms, this means that greater organ selectivity

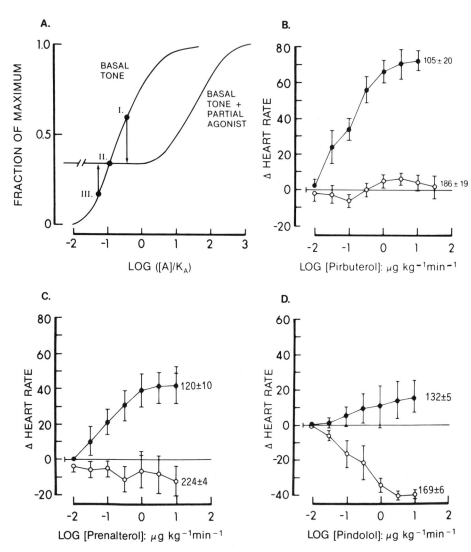

**FIG. 14.13.** *In vivo* effects of partial agonists. **A:** Theoretical dose-response curves *in vivo* for an endogenous full agonist in the presence and absence of a partial agonist. Dose-response curves to the endogenous agonist (labeled "basal tone") represents the population of basal responses *in vivo* to a population of basal levels of endogenous agonist. In the presence of a partial agonist, this relationship changes to the curve designated "basal tone + partial agonist." In preparations of high basal tone, the partial agonist produces a decreased response (I). In preparations in which the basal tone equals the response to the partial agonist, no change will be seen (II), and in preparations of low basal tone, an agonist response will be observed (III). **B** to **D:** Ordinates: Changes in basal heart rates in anesthetized cats. Abscissae: Logarithms of intravenous infusion concentrations of partial agonists. Data shown for cats with high basal heart rates (o; anesthetic = urethane/pentobarbital) and low basal heart rates (•; anesthetic = chloralose/pentobarbital). Numbers next to curves represent the mean basal heart rates for the preparations (±SEM). Changes in heart rates to pirbuterol (B), prenalterol (C), and pindolol (D). The propensity to produce tachycardia is in direct proportion to the relative efficacies of these partial agonists (pirbuterol > prenalterol > pindolol), and bradycardia is inversely related to this parameter. (From ref. 11.)

can be expected of low-efficacy agonists as opposed to high-efficacy agonists.

This approach could be useful for selectively attaining agonism in different tissues; low-efficacy agonists would tend to produce agonist responses only in efficiently receptor-coupled tissues. However, a complicating aspect of this approach would be the antagonism of endogenous agonists produced in less efficiently coupled organs. Whereas agonism for a low-efficacy drug may not be observed in organs with inefficient receptor coupling, receptor antagonism will be produced if concentrations greater than the $K_A$ are present in the receptor compartment. Thus, the effects of a partial agonist can be quite complex *in vivo*, where organs are under physiological hormonal and neural tone. Figure 14.13A shows the theoretical effects of a low-efficacy agonist in organs under basal physiological tone. The curve labeled "basal tone" represents the observed responses for the population; i.e., if the cat heart rate is the relevant parameter, then some cats will be under low catecholaminergic tone (low heart rates) and some under high tone (high heart rates). The responses of the population in the presence of a given concentration of partial agonist are shown in the same figure (basal tone + partial agonist). In terms of the observed responses, in high-tone cats a drop in heart rate (point I) will occur, in low-tone cats an increased rate (point III) will be seen, and if the response to the partial agonist happens to equal the basal tone, no change in rate will occur (point II). The changes in heart rates in cats to three β-adrenoceptor partial agonists of differing relative efficacies (pirbuterol > prenalterol > pindolol) are shown in Figs. 14.13B–D. The choice of anesthetic produces high-tone preparations (high sympathetic tone due to catecholamine release with urethane/pentobarbital anesthesia) and low-tone preparations (low cardiac rate, chloralose/pentobarbital anesthesia). The diversity of responses (from tachycardia to bradycardia) to the various partial agonists demonstrates the importance of the interrelationship between intrinsic efficacy and basal physiological tone. In general, partial agonists can be modulators of physiological responses, increasing low basal tone and decreasing high basal tone to a common level.

## PRINCIPLES OF RECEPTOR THEORY IN DRUG TESTING

Ultimately, a chemical compound is tested in an appropriate physiological system for activity, and a value judgment is made concerning the result. If a selective response is observed, it will be possible that the compound possesses truly novel activity (i.e., is a "key" to the understanding of a biological process), but there are distinct advantages to knowing how a valuable compound achieves selectivity. Knowledge of the mechanism of action may greatly assist the organic chemist in the search for structural changes to enhance activity. For example, metanephrine is a beta blocker of guinea pig

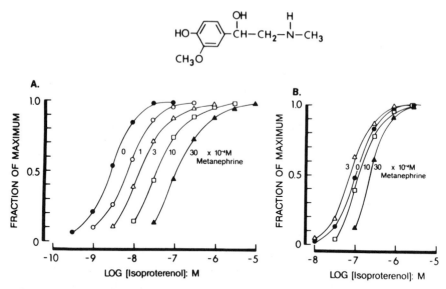

**FIG. 14.14.** β-blocking properties of metanephrine in cardiac and tracheal smooth muscle. Ordinates: Responses as fractions of the maximal response to isoproterenol. Abscissae: Logarithms of molar concentrations of isoproterenol. Effects of metanephrine in guinea pig atria (**A**) and guinea pig trachea (**B**). Responses in the absence (•) and presence of metanephrine at 100 μM (o), 300 μM (Δ), 1 mM (□), and 3 mM (▲).

atrial responses to isoproterenol (Fig. 14.14A), but demonstrates considerably weaker activity in guinea pig trachea (Fig. 14.14B); from these data, it appears that metanephrine is a cardioselective beta blocker. If this is the desired target, then the chemist has the structure of metanephrine (and those leading up to that structure) as a data base for future modification to enhance activity. However, in this case, the cardioselectivity of metanephrine stems not from receptor selectivity but rather from a self-cancellation of responses in trachea as opposed to atria. Metanephrine, in addition to being a beta-blocking drug, potentiates isoproterenol responses by blocking extraneuronal uptake of catecholamines; this latter activity cancels beta blockade. Because extraneuronal uptake of isoproterenol affects receptor-compartment concentrations of isoproterenol in trachea much more than in atria, a proportionately greater self-cancellation of beta blockade is observed in trachea. The value of knowing this mechanism of action is that an expanded data base is provided from which the chemist may draw to enhance this profile; now all blockers of β-adrenoceptors and extraneuronal uptake of catecholamines become relevant to the design process (Fig. 14.15).

Another example in which delineation of the mechanism of action was beneficial came from studies of the relationship of the selective inotropy of dobutamine, a catecholamine derivative, to agonist activity at α-adrenoceptors. Catecholamines such as isoproterenol produce concomitant cardiac ino-

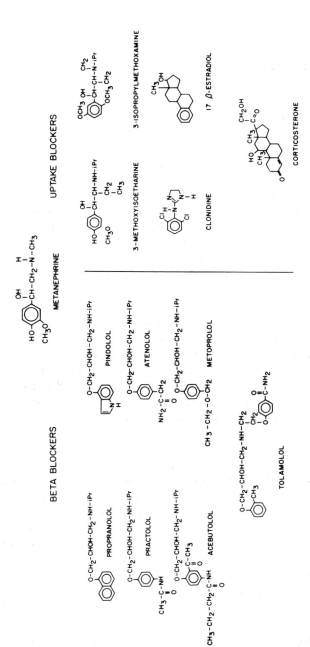

**FIG. 14.15.** Chemical structure of metanephrine, a competitive antagonist of β-adrenoceptors and of extraneuronal uptake of catecholamines. Chemical structures of other β-adrenoceptor blockers and inhibitors of extraneuronal uptake shown may assist the organic chemist in efforts to enhance the dual activities of the metanephrine molecule.

tropy and tachycardia; this latter property limits the use of such drugs as cardiotonics. Figure 14.16A shows the increases in heart rate obtained for measured positive inotropic responses to isoproterenol in anesthetized cats. The data for dobutamine (Fig. 14.16A) demonstrate less tachycardia for common increases in inotropy, showing this agonist to be a selectively inotropic catecholamine; this raises the question of the mechanism of the selectivity. If dobutamine activates a β-adrenoceptor subtype unique to inotropy, then it would be presumed that further structural modification of the molecule would enhance this activity and produce an even more selective cardiotonic. However, in the case of dobutamine, prior treatment of anesthetized cats with the α-adrenoceptor-blocking drug phentolamine greatly reduces the selective inotropy (Fig. 14.16B), indicating mild α-adrenoceptor activation, and resulting modulation of reflex tachycardia, to be the mechanism of the selective inotropy. The value in knowing this lies in the fact that this mechanism is self-limiting; i.e., further α-adrenoceptor activation would produce further modulation of tachycardia, but also a damaging pressor response, which would make the drug of no use therapeutically. Therefore, further structural modification of dobutamine to achieve inotropic selectivity in this case would not appear to be worthwhile.

An important consideration in the testing of agonists in isolated tissues is the relative dependence of potency on affinity and efficacy. For example, consider two agonists, A and B, with A having five times the intrinsic efficacy but one-fifth the affinity of B. In an efficiently coupled tissue (high receptor density and/or efficient stimulus-response mechanisms), these agonists would be equipotent (Fig. 14.17, left). However, in an inefficiently coupled tissue, the responses to B, the drug of lower intrinsic efficacy, would be selectively attenuated (Fig. 14.17, right), giving a totally different impression of the relative activities of these two drugs. Therefore, if compound B were being tested for activity in the efficiently coupled tissue (assuming A was a standard), then it would be assumed that the compound had activity comparable to that of the standard. However, if the inefficiently coupled tissue were used as the test system, the compound might be discarded as being weakly active compared with the standard. A more relevant question is which of these tissues would more likely resemble the effects in humans. These factors would suggest that testing in tissues of varying coupling efficiencies would be useful to determine how much of an agonist's potency depends on efficacy and how much on affinity.

As discussed in Chapter 2, the relative power of various tissues can be useful to detect intrinsic efficacy of drugs. Thus, low-efficacy agonists may not produce responses in poorly receptor-coupled tissues, but may demonstrate "surprising" agonism in other, more efficiently coupled systems. Also, there are instances in which drugs have more than one action, and this duality (or in some cases multiplicity) masks or modifies the observed effects. This is

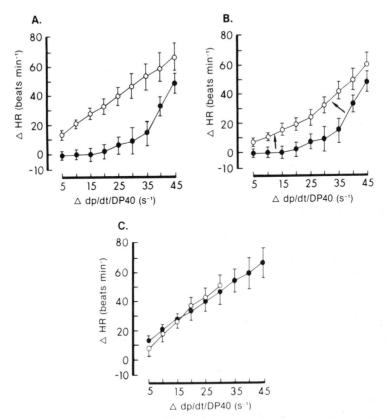

**FIG. 14.16.** Tachycardia for catecholamine-induced increases in cardiac inotropy in anesthetized cats. Ordinates: Increases in basal heart rate in beats min$^{-1}$. Abscissae: Increases in basal inotropic state as the first derivative of an isovolumic left ventricular pressure increase of 40 mm Hg. **A:** Tachycardia for increased inotropy to isoproterenol (o, $N = 6$) and dobutamine (•, $N = 5$); dobutamine demonstrates inotropic selectivity (i.e., less tachycardia for increased inotropic state) over isoproterenol in this preparation. **B:** Effects of phentolamine ($\alpha$-adrenoceptor-blocking agent) on tachycardia to dobutamine; responses in the absence (•, $N = 5$) and presence (o, $N = 4$) of phentolamine. *Arrows* show the shift in the curve; when $\alpha$-adrenoceptors are blocked, dobutamine produces more tachycardia for given increases in inotropy after phentolamine. **C:** Effects of phentolamine on tachycardia to isoproterenol. Responses in the absence (•, $N = 6$) and presence of phentolamine (o, $N = 4$); in this case, $\alpha$-adrenoceptor blockade produces no change in the tachycardia produced by isoproterenol for given increases in inotropy. (From ref. 15.)

important to delineate since the combination of properties in another receptor system of differing relative emphasis may be completely divergent from that of the test system. Therefore, there are practical advantages to manipulating systems in order to maximize the ability to detect these drug actions. There are pharmacologic approaches to the amplification and simplification of drug action in tissue systems.

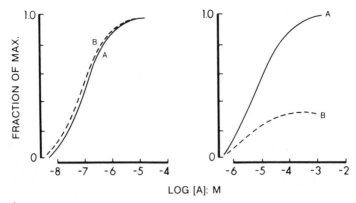

**FIG. 14.17.** Effects of efficiency of receptor coupling and/or receptor density on responses to a high-efficacy low-affinity agonist (**left**) and a low-efficacy high-affinity agonist (**right**). Receptor stimulus given by $S = \epsilon \cdot [R_t]/(1 + K_A/[A])$; for A, $\epsilon = 3$, $K_A = 10^{-5}$ M; for B, $\epsilon = 0.6$, $K_A' = 2 \times 10^{-6}$ M. Response modeled by $S/(S + 0.1)$. In the high receptor–density preparation on the left ($[R_t] = 1.0$), both agonists are equiactive. In the low receptor–density preparation on the right ($[R_t] = 0.03$), agonist B (lower efficacy) is considerably less active.

One example is in the testing of type IV phosphodiesterase inhibitors to elevate intracellular levels of cyclic AMP *in vivo* and thereby produce positive cardiac inotropy for therapy of congestive heart failure. One potential problem in the testing of such compounds is the difference between the therapeutic situation and the controlled testing systems used to screen drugs. Specifically, in humans with congestive heart failure, there are circulating levels of catecholamines stimulating β-adrenoceptors to produce elevation of cyclic AMP. Under these circumstances, inhibition of the catabolic enzyme (for cyclic AMP) phosphodiesterase would produce a net increase in the availability of this second messenger with the therapeutic result of increased cardiac inotropy. However, in the common test system for inotropic compounds, namely, an isolated cardiac preparation, the basal β-adrenoceptor stimulation is not present, thus the potential beneficial effects of phosphodiesterase inhibition may not be evident. One potential approach to this problem would be to introduce a low level of β-adrenoceptor stimulation into the system to simulate the *in vivo* situation. The effects of a powerful β-adrenoceptor agonist such as isoproterenol would be difficult to control (across tissue systems) because of variation in receptor density, the efficiency of receptor coupling in various tissues, and the high intrinsic efficacy of isoproterenol. However, the use of a *low* intrinsic efficacy agonist (such as prenalterol) could be useful. Specifically, a concentration of a low-efficacy agonist could be chosen to maximize receptor occupancy, thereby confining the resulting agonism to the intrinsic efficacy of the stimulating agonist. This would give a more uniform low-level stimulation since the factor of varying receptor occupancy would not be relevant (i.e., occupancy could be set at

>99%). Figure 14.18A shows the effect of the type IV phosphodiesterase inhibitor fenoximone on electrically stimulated isometric contractions of guinea pig left atria. As can be seen from this figure, little positive inotropy to fenoximone is observed. However, the same test in the presence of the low-efficacy β-adrenoceptor agonist prenalterol unmasks a powerful inotropy. It should be noted that prenalterol itself does *not* produce substantial positive inotropy in this tissue. Presumably the small elevation of intracellular cyclic AMP is insufficient to produce positive inotropy (see Fig. 14.18A) when the catabolic phosphodiesterase enzymes present in the cytosol are not blocked. However, blockade of this degradatory mechanism by fenoximone increases the cytosolic cyclic AMP to the point where positive inotropy results. Thus, the pretreatment with prenalterol sensitizes the atria to the positive inotropic effects of fenoximone. This activity correlates with the observed positive inotropy seen with this drug *in vivo* (see Fig. 14.18B).

*In vivo* the effects of drugs can be modified by basal hormone- or neurotransmitter-mediated tone. As with fenoximone (above), preconditioning of the test system sometimes may amplify the desired response. This approach can be extremely useful for the prediction of drug effect *in vivo*. For example, it is known that adenosine is involved in renal ischemia and acute renal failure. The probable mechanism of action is a decreased renal blood flow due to vasoconstriction. *In vitro* experiments in isolated perfused kidney show no vasoconstriction to adenosine-receptor agonists, only a vasodilation at high doses. Therefore, the *in vitro* preparation is an unsuitable model for the pathology observed *in vivo*. Adenosine agonists are known to activate at least two types of receptor, one mediating vasoconstriction (by inhibition of adenylate cyclase, A1 receptors) and another vasorelaxation (by activation of adenylate cyclase, A2 receptors). Therefore, pretreatment of the perfused kidney with the α-adrenoceptor agonist methoxamine and then partial relaxation of the vasculature of the same preparation with the adenylate cyclase activator forskolin produce a tissue with vasoactive tone controlled by adenylate cyclase (Fig. 14.18C). Under these circumstances adenosine receptor activation of A1 receptors inhibits adenylate cyclase and allows the methoxamine contractile stimulus to override cyclic AMP tone, and a vasoconstriction is observed. Similarly, A2-receptor stimulation produces an additive excitation of adenylate cyclase and further override of methoxamine contraction (further vasorelaxation). Therefore, the pretreated kidney more resembles the *in vivo* state in which it is under neuronal and hormonal control of vascular tone. As shown in Fig. 14.18D, the adenosine-receptor agonist 2-chloroadenosine produces vasoconstriction at low doses and vasorelaxation at high doses, consistent with A1-and A2-receptor activation. This is in contrast to the nonpretreated kidney, in which no vasoconstriction to this agonist is observed (Fig. 14.18D).

As discussed in Chapter 3, the advent of binding techniques in cell culture and the ability to clone and express human receptors in surrogate cell lines

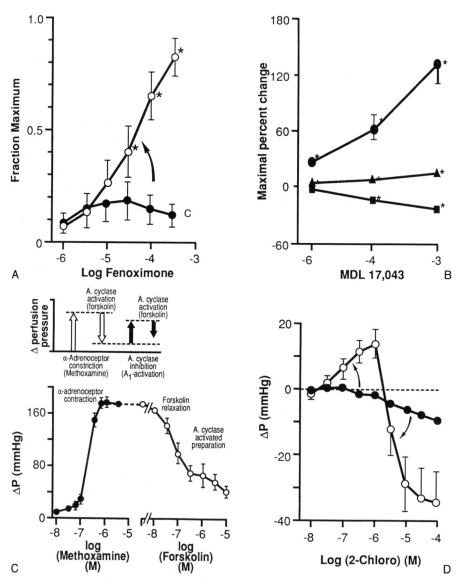

**FIG. 14.18.** Modification of test systems to detect drug activity. **A:** Effects of the phosphodiesterase inhibitor fenoximone on cardiac inotropy in guinea pig isolated left atria *in vitro*. Positive inotropy in the absence (•) and presence (○) of the weak β-adrenoceptor agonist prenalterol. Prenalterol has no significant inotropic effect in this preparation. (From ref. 17.) **B:** The effects of fenoximone on cardiac contractile force (•), heart rate (▲) and mean blood pressure (■) anesthetized dogs. (From ref. 7.) **C:** Enhancement of vascular reactivity of kidney vasculature with pretreatment with methoxamine (to produce vasoconstriction) and forskolin (to produce vasodilatation). With these treatments, the blood vessels in the kidney are under adenylate cyclase control and respond to agonists that block adenylate cyclase. **D:** Effects of 2-chloroadenosine on perfusion pressure in rat kidneys under basal conditions (•) and after pretreatment with methoxamine and forskolin (○). The dual activity of 2-chloroadenosine, namely, the activation of adenylate cyclase by A2 receptors and inhibition of adenylate cyclase by A1 receptors, becomes evident in the pretreated preparation. (C and D from ref. 16.)

allow for the screening of chemical compounds in customized test systems. There may be practical advantages to choosing some of these systems over others. For example, it has been shown that some antagonists possess negative efficacy in that they destabilize ternary complex formation. There are therapeutic scenarios in which such drug activity may be an advantage. For example, as shown in mutation studies on the $\alpha_{1B}$-adrenoceptor, substitution of any amino acid at position 293 produces a basally active receptor that produces inositol-phosphate turnover in the absence of hormone. It might be supposed that such mutations occur physiologically and may be involved in pathological states (e.g., some cancers). Therefore, an antagonist with negative efficacy would have the advantage of decreasing the basal activity of such mutants as well as blocking the hormonally induced activity. Also, if receptor precoupling to transducer proteins occurs to varying extents in different organs, then an antagonist with negative efficacy will demonstrate greater organ selectivity than a neutral antagonist. This differentiation may be therapeutically advantageous under certain circumstances. With the new technology of recombinant receptor systems, it may be possible to *create* drug-testing systems for the detection of negative antagonism. As shown in Fig. 3.11, the reconstitution of receptors and G proteins can produce systems in which spontaneous coupling of receptors and transducers occurs naturally. Such systems could be valuable for the detection of negative efficacy for antagonists.

## REFERENCES

1. Austel, V., and Kulter, E. (1980): Practical procedures in drug design. In: *Drug Design, Vol. 10*, edited by E. J. Ariens, pp. 1–69. Academic Press, New York.
2. Baldwin, J. J., Lumma, W. C., Jr., Lundell, G. F., Ponticello, G. S., Raab, A. W., Engelhardt, E. L., Hirschmann, E. L., Sweet, C. S., and Scriabine, A. (1979): Symbiotic approach to drug design: Antihypertensive β-adrenergic blocking agents. *J. Med. Chem.*, 22: 1284–1290.
3. Black, J. W. (1981): Receptors in the future. *Postgrad. Med. J.*, 57:110–112.
4. Black, J. W. (1982): Receptor function and control. In: *Catecholamines in the Nonischaemic and Ischaemic Myocardium*, edited by R. Riemersma and W. Oliver, pp. 3–12. Elsevier/North Holland, Amsterdam.
5. Black, J. W., Duncan, W. A. M., Durant, C. J., Ganellin, C. R., and Parsons, E. M. (1972): Definition and antagonism of histamine $H_2$-receptors. *Nature (Lond.)*, 236:385–390.
6. Black, J. W., and Stephenson, J. G. (1962): Pharmacology of a new adrenergic beta-receptor-blocking compound (nethalide). *Lancet*, 2:311–314.
7. Dage, R. C., Roebel, L. E., Hsieh, C. P., Weiner, D. L., and Woodward, J. K. (1982): The effects of MDL 17,043 on cardiac inotropy in the anesthetized dog. *J. Cardiovasc. Pharmacol.*, 4:500–512.
8. Ganellin, C. R., and Durant, G. J. (1981): Histamine $H_2$-receptor agonists and antagonists. In: *Burgers Medicinal Chemistry, Vol. III*, edited by M. E. Wolf, pp. 487–552. Wiley, New York.
9. Kenakin, T. P. (1982): Organ selectivity of drugs. Alternatives to receptor selectivity. *Trends Pharmacol. Sci.*, 3:153–156.
10. Kenakin, T. P. (1984): The classification of drugs and drug receptors in isolated tissues. *Pharmacol. Rev.*, 36:165–222.

11. Kenakin, T. P. (1985): Drug and organ selectivity: Similarities and differences. In: *Advances in Drug Research, Vol. 15*, edited by B. Testa, pp. 71–109. Academic Press, New York.
12. Kenakin, T. P. (1989): Macromolecular targets for drug action. In: *Comprehensive Medicinal Chemistry, Vol. 1, Targets for Biologically Active Molecules*, edited by C. Hansch, pp. 195–208. Pergamon, Oxford.
13. Kenakin, T. P. (1989): The concept of bioselectivity. In: *Comprehensive Medicinal Chemistry, Vol. 1, Targets for Biologically Active Molecules*, edited by C. Hansch, pp. 209–222. Pergamon, Oxford.
14. Kenakin, T. P., and Beek, D. (1985): Self-cancellation of drug properties as a mode of organ selectivity: The antimuscarinic effects of ambenonium. *J. Pharmacol. Exp. Ther.*, 232: 732–740.
15. Kenakin, T. P., and Johnson, S. F. (1984): The importance of the α-adrenoceptor agonist activity of dobutamine to inotropic selectivity in the anaesthetized cat. *Eur. J. Pharmacol.*, 111:347–354.
16. Kenakin, T. P., and Pike, N. B. (1987): An in vitro analysis of purine-mediated renal vasoconstriction in rat isolated kidney. *Br. J. Pharmacol.*, 90:373–381.
17. Kenakin, T. P., and Scott, D. L. (1987): A method to assess concomitant cardiac phosphodiesterase inhibition and positive inotropy. *J. Cardiovasc. Pharmacol.*, 10:658–666.
18. Richardson, B. P., Engel, G., Donatsch, P., and Stadler, P. A. (1985): Identification of serotonin M-receptor subtypes and their specific blockade by a new class of drugs. *Nature*, 316:126–131.
19. Shelley, J. H. (1983): Creativity in drug research. II. *Trends Pharmacol. Sci.*, 4:323–325.
20. Shelley, J. H. (1983): Creativity in drug research. III. *Trends Pharmacol. Sci.*, 4:361–362.
21. Shelley, J. H. (1983): Creativity in drug research. I. *Trends Pharmacol. Sci.*, 4:283–284.

# Subject Index

Aqueous approach, of drugs to receptors,
129–134,169
lipid concentration and, 170–171
Arecoline, biphasic inotropic response,
263,264
Ariëns theory, 16–17,255–258
Arithmetic means, 188
Arteries
contraction measurement, 109,110–112
perfusion pressure measurement,
110–112
Aspartate transcarbamylase, 387
Association rate constant
collisional limit and, 432
for diffusion, 222
kinetic measurement, 418–423
in rate theory, 25
Atenolol
β-adrenergic receptor interaction, 346
competitive antagonism, 376–377,378
Atropine, 7
acetylcholine antagonism, 311,312
antimuscarinic selectivity, 450
nonlinear Schild regression, 296

**B**
Bacteria, folic acid synthesis, 445
Basal heart rate, variance analysis,
184–186
Bessel function, 152–153
Beta-adrenergic receptors. *See* β-
Adrenergic receptors
Beta blockers, discovery, 442
Bias, in experimental design, 176,177
Binding. *See also* Coupling; Drug-receptor
theories; Radioligand binding
experiments
biochemical, 9
kinetics, 427–436
membrane versus aqueous approach,
129–134
models, 237,385–387
single-site receptor model, 237
stages, 221–222
by surface adsorption, 166–169
two-stage, 229–238
Bioassay, 70–72,89–91
Biological error simulation, 297–298
Bladder, adrenergic-receptor density
variability, 103–104
Blood-brain barrier, enhanced drug
passage, 450–451
Blood vessels
bioassay studies, 89,91
rapidity of drug response, 134
Boltzmann's equation, 128,223,224,225
Bolus injection, in drug diffusion, 120
Bond energy, 223,224

Boundary-layer effects, 121
BRL 37344, lipolytic responses, 57,58
Buchheim, Rudolf, 2
Bupranolol, equilibrium dissociation
constants, 11–12
Burimamide, structure, 448

**C**
Calcitonin gene-related peptide, membrane
binding, 216–218
Calcium
cholinergic agonist sensitivity and, 65
as second messenger, 372
stimulus-response mechanisms and, 55
Calcium channels, cardiac, 50,51
Calcium uptake, carbachol effects, 50,52,
53
Calibration curve, 196–197
Carbachol
atrial biphasic dose-response, 263,265
calcium uptake effects, 50,52,53
contractile response effects, 52
desensitization-related binding decrease,
73,74
as G-protein activator, 360
ileal sensitivity, 65
intrinsic efficacy, 366
muscarinic receptor affinity, 367
potency ratio, 358,359
receptor occupancy effects, 52
receptor reserves, 47
relative efficacy, 367
scopolamine antagonism, 294,421
Carbamyl phosphate, binding constants,
387
Carbonic anhydrase, antagonist, 444
Carbutamide, as tolbutamide prototype,
444,446
Cardiotonics, side effects, 460,462
Catecholamines
stability in solutions, 120,121
as tachycardia cause, 460,462,463
Catechol-O-methyltransferase, 155,156
Cell cultures, 70–87
passage number, 74–75
Central tendency measures, 181–188
Charniere effect, 324
Chemical antagonism, 279
Chemical compound screening, 465,467
Chemical structure
drug-response binding and, 421
potency and, 7,8
Chimeric receptors, 72
2-Chloroadenosine, biphasic dose-response
curve, 371,372
Cholecystokinin, octapeptide, biphasic
dose-response curve, 375–376
Cholinergic receptors, 346
density during ontogeny, 42,43

Cholinesterase, as esmilol degrader, 454
Cholinomimetics, 346
Cimetidine
  histamine antagonism, 288,289
  structure, 448,449
Clark plot, 311–312
Classification
  of drugs. *See* Drug classification
  of receptors. *See* Receptor classification
Cloned adrenergic receptors, 71–72
Cloned cell systems, receptor/G-protein
    ratios, 78–81
Clonidine, concentration range, 3,4
Closed ion channels, 32–35
Cocaine
  multiple properties, 1
  norepinephrine interaction, 154,156,159,
    160,161
  serotonin interaction, 447,449
  synthetic congener, 444,445
Cofactors, 22,55,65
Collisional limit
  binding at, 429–434
  in cooperative binding, 331
Collision-coupling model, 251
Common slope, 202–203
Competitive antagonism, 278–322,415–416
  Clark plot analysis, 311–312
  definition, 278–279
  by indirect agonists, 318–321
  mechanisms, 324
  by partial agonists, 315–318
  potency
    *in vivo*, 437
    measurement, 283–287,437
  in radioligand displacement, 391,393
  receptor classification and, 376–382
  receptor occupancy adjustment in,
    423–427
  receptor-selectivity, 371
  resultant analysis, 312–318
  reversible
    definition, 280–281
    measurement, 281–311
  uptake mechanisms and, 289–293
Concentration bias, 449–450
Concentration gradients
  agonist potency and, 147–149
  in bulk diffusion, 118
  chemical effects on, 120–121
  drug entry route and, 42–43
  saturability and, 145
  in tissues, 123–124,145–146
  uptake inhibition effect, 150–165
Concentration range, 1
  specificity relationship, 3,4
Concentration-response curves. *See also*
    Drug concentration
  drug removal and, 157–158
  general logistic function, 61–64

occupation theory, 17
  sigmoidal, 32,33
Confidence limits, 181–182
  of regression line, 194–196
Conformational induction, 229,249,250
Conformational selection, 229,249–252,325
Congestive heart failure
  animal models, 93–95
  cardiac inotropy, 464
  isoproterenol receptor occupancy, 48–49
Contraction, measurement, 106,107,108,
    109
Control experiments, 101–102
Control response, 178
Cooperativity, 37
  two-state model, 32–35
Correlation coefficient, 211
Coulombic interactions, 223
Coupling
  agonist efficacy and, 456–459,462–465
  agonist potency ratio and, 350–351
  cell-to-cell, 134–135,150
  intracellular compartmentalization and,
    57–61
  partial agonist affinity and, 241,242
  in pathological conditions, 48–49
  receptor density measurement and,
    41–43,44
  spontaneous, 310
  stimulus-response. *See* Stimulus-
    response mechanisms
Covariance analysis, 205–211
Cross-desensitization, 364,366
Crossover design, 179–180
Cumulative frequency analysis, 190–191,
    205,207
Cyclic AMP. *See* Adenosine-3'5'-cyclic
    monophosphate
Cylinder tissue shape
  concentration gradients, 146
  drug diffusion into, 124


**D**

Debye's function, 222–223
Degrees of freedom, 181,182
Dependent variables, 188–189,211
  straight-line analysis, 191–199
Desensitization
  efficacy and, 366
  receptor density measurement and, 42
  saturation consequence, 154,156
  selective, 364,366
  in whole-cell systems, 73,74
Diacetylmorphine, blood-brain barrier
    passage, 450–451
Diazepam
  as adenosine-uptake blocker, 163,164,
    200–201,202
  benzodiazepine receptor binding, 392